Neuroscience for Rehabilitation

Neuroscience for Rehabilitation

2
EDITION

Edited by

Helen Cohen, EdD, OTR, FAOTA

Assistant Professor
Bobby R. Alford Department of Otorhinolaryngology
    and Communicative Sciences
Baylor College of Medicine
Houston, Texas

with 29 contributors

Illustrations by

Jamie Huffman, BS, AMI

Akron City Hospital
Akron, Ohio

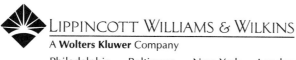

LIPPINCOTT WILLIAMS & WILKINS
A **Wolters Kluwer** Company

Philadelphia · Baltimore · New York · London
Buenos Aires · Hong Kong · Sydney · Tokyo

Acquisitions Editor: Margaret M. Biblis
Assistant Editor: Amy Amico
Project Editor: Gretchen Metzger
Production Manager: Helen Ewan
Production Coordinator: Patricia McCloskey
Design Coordinator: Nicholas Rook
Indexer: Nancy Newman
Illustrators: Jerry Cable, Jennifer Smith

Edition 2

Library of Congress Cataloging in Publications Data

Neuroscience for rehabilitation / edited by Helen Cohen ; with 29
     contributors, –– 2nd ed.
          p.   cm.
     Includes bibliographical references and index.
     ISBN 0-397-55465-6 (alk. paper)
     1. Neurosciences.   2. Rehabilitation.   I. Cohen, Helen Sue.
     [DNLM: 1. Nervous System Physiology.   2. Nervous System Diseases –
     – rehabilitation.   3. Nervous Systgem––physiopathology.
     4. Rehabilitation.   5. Behavior––physiology.   WL 102 N5059 1999]
     RC341.N437   1999
     616.8′043––dc21
     DNLM/DLC
     for Library of Congress   98-24809
                                                                    CIP

Care has been taken to confirm the accuracy of the information presented and to describe generally accepted practices. However, the authors, editors, and publisher are not responsible for errors or omissions or for any consequences from application of the information in this book and make no warranty, express or implied, with respect to the contents of the publication.

     The authors, editors, and publisher have exerted every effort to ensure that drug selection and dosage set forth in this text are in accordance with current recommendations and practice at the time of publication. However, in view of ongoing research, changes in government regulations, and the constant flow of information relating to drug therapy and drug reactions, the reader is urged to check the package insert for each drug for any change in indications and dosage and for added warnings and precautions. This is particularly important when the recommended agent is a new or infrequently employed drug.

     Some drugs and medical devices presented in this publication have Food and Drug Administration (FDA) clearance for limited use in restricted research settings. It is the responsibility of the health care provider to ascertain the FDA status of each drug or device planned for use in their clinical practice.

To all the people who have encouraged me to think,
to question, and to wonder

Contributors

Robert N. Alder, MS, OTR
Assistant Professor
Department of Occupational Therapy
College Misericordia
Dallas, Pennsylvania

Douglas A. Baxter, PhD
Assistant Professor
Department of Neurobiology & Anatomy
University of Texas Medical School
Houston, Texas

Mary Frances Baxter, MA, OTR
Assistant Professor
School of Occupational Therapy
Texas Woman's University
Houston, Texas

Kirk W. Barron, PhD
Assistant Professor
Department of Physiology & Biophysics
University of Oklahoma Health Sciences Center
Oklahoma City, Oklahoma

Robert W. Blair, PhD
Associate Professor
Department of Physiology & Biophysics
University of Oklahoma Health Sciences Center
Oklahoma City, Oklahoma

Thérèse Cabana, PhD
Professor, Chairman
Sciences Biologiques
Universite de Montreal
Montreal, QC, Canada

Joseph W. Cheu, DO, PhD
Instructor of Physical Medicine & Rehabilitation
Departments of Physical Medicine &
    Rehabilitation and Neurosciences
University of Medicine and Dentistry of
    New Jersey
Newark, New Jersey

F. Richard Clemente, PhD, PT
Associate Professor
Department of Physical Therapy
John G. Rangos School of Health Sciences
Duquesne University
Pittsburgh, Pennsylvania

Helen Cohen, EdD, OTR, FAOTA
Assistant Professor
Bobby R. Alford Department of Otorhino-
    laryngology & Communicative Sciences
Baylor College of Medicine
Houston, Texas

Cecilia M. Fox, PhD
Assistant Professor
Department of Biology
Wingate University
Wingate, North Carolina

Charles R. Fox, OD, PhD, FAAO
Assistant Professor
Director of Optometry Services
Department of Ophthalmology
University of Maryland, Baltimore
School of Medicine
Baltimore, Maryland

Marion E. Frank, PhD
Professor, Biostructure & Function
Program Director, Connecticut Chemosensory
    Clinical Research Center
School of Dental Medicine
University of Connecticut Health Center
Farmington, Connecticut

Janneane F. Gent, PhD
Research Associate
Taste & Smell Center
Department of Biostructure & Function
School of Dental Medicine
University of Connecticut Health Center
Farmington, Connecticut

Jean M. Held, EdD, PT
Associate Professor and Chair
Department of Physical Therapy
University of Vermont
Burlington, Vermont

Meenakshi B. Iyer, PhD, OTR/L
Clinical Assistant Professor
Department of Occupational Therapy
Division of Rehabilitation Sciences
State University of New York at Stony Brook
Stony Brook, New York

S. Essie Jacobs, PhD, OTR
Assistant Professor
Department of Kinesiology
Occupational Therapy Program
University of Wisconsin-Madison
Madison, Wiscoz nsin

Lynette A. Jones, PhD
Principal Research Scientist
Department of Mechanical Engineering
Massachusetts Institute of Technology
Cambridge, Massachusetts

Sharon L. Juliano, OTR, PhD
Professor
Department of Anatomy & Cell Biology
Uniformed Services University of the Health
 Sciences
Bethesda, Maryland

Christiana M. Leonard, PhD
Professor of Neuroscience
University of Florida Brain Institute
Gainesville, Florida

Deborah L. Lowe, PhD
Formerly, Research Associate
Department of Anesthesiology

University of Wisconsin Hospitals & Clinics
Madison, Wisconsin

Debra F. McLaughlin, PhD
Research Fellow
Department of Anatomy & Cell Biology
Uniformed Services University of the Health
 Sciences
Bethesda, Maryland

Andrew R. Mitz, PhD
Neurophysiologist/Biomedical Engineer
Laboratory of Neurophysiology
National Institute of Mental Health
Poolesville, Maryland

Sheila A. Mun-Bryce, PhD, OTR/L
Research Associate
Department of Neurology and Occupational
 Therapy Program
School of Medicine
University of New Mexico
Albuquerque, New Mexico

Tim Pay, PT
Staff Therapist
Department of Physical Therapy
Fletcher Allen Health Care
Burlington, Vermont

Linda L. Porter, PT, PhD
Associate Professor
Departments of Anatomy & Cell Biology
 and Neuroscience
Uniformed Services University of the Health
 Sciences
Bethesda, Maryland

William F. Sewell, PhD
Associate Professor
Program in Neuroscience and Department of
 Otology and Laryngology
Harvard Medical School
Boston, Massachusetts

Susan E. Shore, PhD
Research Assistant Professor
Department of Otolaryngology
Medical College of Ohio
Toledo, Ohio

and
Adjunct Assistant Research Scientist
Kresge Hearing Research Institute
University of Michigan
Ann Arbor, Michigan

Allan Siegel, PhD
Professor of Neurosciences and Psychiatry
Departments of Neuroscience and Psychiatry
University of Medicine and Dentistry of
    New Jersey
Newark, New Jersey

David L. Somers, PhD, PT
Assistant Professor
Department of Physical Therapy
John G. Rangos School of Health Sciences
Duquesne University
Pittsburgh, Pennsylvania

Carolee Winstein, PT, PhD
Assistant Professor
Department of Physical Therapy
University of Southern California
Los Angeles, California

Foreword

Effective rehabilitation must take into account the current understanding of how the nervous system participates in normal and abnormal behavior. Much of what is understood about neuroscience has been learned in the past few decades. Unfortunately, there is usually a long delay between new discoveries in basic neuroscience and application of these discoveries in the clinic. It is not easy to bridge the gap between basic neuroscience and clinical rehabilitation, since it demands that instructors are well-grounded in both worlds. Too often, students of rehabilitation have a good understanding of basic neuroscience concepts, but have difficulty applying these concepts to their clinical course work and practice.

This text will help relieve the frustration of students of rehabilitation who are attempting to apply the basic principles of neuroscience directly to their study and practice of clinical therapeutic exercise. The goal of physical and occupational therapists is to enhance human movement and function by assessing, preventing, and treating disorders of motor behavior. Therapists reach this goal by using clinical problem solving, which depends on their own understanding of basic sciences such as neurophysiology and neuroanatomy. Therapists use neural adaptation and learning to optimize existing motor potential, unmask residual function, and facilitate recovery due to neuroplasticity. The better therapists understand the relationship between basic neurosciences and human motor function or dysfunction, the better prepared they will be to reach their therapeutic goals.

This is an exciting period for the rehabilitation professional, since it is now possible as never before to apply neuroscience theories and experimental results directly to the rehabilitation process. This text helps bridge the gap between our current understanding of neuroscience and how this understanding is important for practical rehabilitation. A better understanding of neuroscience is necessary if the disciplines of physical and occupational therapy are to continue to progress from technologies of skilled hands to professions of problem solvers.

Fay B. Horak, PhD, PT
Senior Scientist
Neurological Sciences Institute
Professor of Physiology and Neurology
Oregon Health Sciences University

Preface

-
-
-
-
-
-
-
-

This book was written for the benefit of allied health professionals, especially for therapists—the usually unheralded professionals who strive daily to improve the quality of life for other people. To be the colleague of such insightful, giving people is both a great pleasure and a great frustration. Although we have much to offer we also have much more to learn; hence the original impetus for this book.

Margaret Rood, OTR, RPT, a great therapist and pioneer in neurorehabilitation, once exhorted therapists to consider the complex neural mechanisms underlying any successful response to treatment and not merely to be technicians.[1] This book is based on that idea—to develop better treatment paradigms to provide better care for our patients, we can and should start by understanding the nervous system and how it controls behavior. The success of the first edition of this text suggests that rehabilitation professionals agree.

This book introduces the anatomy and physiology of the nervous system. Discussion focuses on physiology, because many excellent atlases are available to supplement the anatomical figures given here. To help the reader retain the information, each chapter includes some discussion of why the material is relevant to the clinician. This book is not intended to serve as the main text for courses on neurorehabilitation, although it may be useful as a bridge between the science and practice in some cases. The astute reader will notice some omissions: some deliberate, to keep the text at a reasonable size and level for students; others reflect the current state of our knowledge. Neuroscience is still in its infancy, and many questions remain to be asked and answered. In this text we present some of what we know, what we suppose, and what remains to be learned.

Based on the feedback from instructors using the first edition, the second edition has been updated and modified. This edition has an expanded introductory section, with more material on gross anatomy, updated material on the neuron, and additional chapters on neurotransmitters and the support structures and processes of the system. The section on the sensory systems, especially the somatic senses, has been expanded. The chapters on the special senses and on motor control have been updated and expanded as well. The number of chapters in the section on higher cognitive functions has been reduced, but the current chapters have been updated and expanded, and give an introduction to the diversity of work in this field. Finally, the section on the life span has been expanded, and the chapters on development and recovery of function have been updated. The detailed glossary has been retained and the reference lists for each chapter have been expanded.

The importance of neuroscience and the ability to understand the brain was highlighted by the United States Congress, which declared the 1990s to be the Decade of the Brain.[2] As we draw near the close of the decade, we can appreciate how far we have come in this century, and how far we have yet to go. The contributors to this book have made significant contributions to that effort. Perhaps some readers of this book will eventually contribute to neuroscience, too.

The contributors to this book are neuroscientists. Some of them are also clinicians; two are former clinicians; some of the others teach allied health students. All of the contributors have written about topics in which they have special expertise, and all of them bring to their work a fascination with the science and a willingness to share it with nonscientists who will incorporate their work into their approaches to clinical practice. Writing a chapter can be an arduous task but the contributors to this text have done so enthusiastically; they have produced a book that should help rehabilitation professionals begin the new millennium with a greater understanding of neuroscience than we had just a few years before. As their editor I am grateful for the work of such gifted people and I hope their endeavors will help rehabilitation professionals move into the 21st century.

Helen Cohen, EdD, OTR, FAOTA
Houston, Texas

References

1. Rood MS. The use of sensory receptors to activate, facilitate, and inhibit motor response, autonomic and somatic in developmental sequence. In: Sattely C, ed. *Study Course VI, Third International Congress, World Federation of Occupational Therapists.* Dubuque, IA: William C. Brown Company, 1962:26–37.
2. Public Law 101–58. July 25, 1989. *Congressional Record.* Vol. 135. 1989.

Acknowledgments

The successful production of a textbook requires the assistance of many people. As the editor I am particularly grateful for the assistance of two wonderful librarians, Aletta Moore, MLIS, and Kathlyn L. Reed, MLIS, PhD, OTR, FAOTA, both of whom have shared their love of books and understanding of information sources with me. Margo B. Holm, PhD, OTR, FAOTA, and the ever-helpful health science administrators at the National Institute on Deafness and Other Communication Disorders/ NIH—Daniel A. Sklare, PhD, Beth Ansel, PhD, and Judith A. Cooper, PhD—provided invaluable assistance in finding some contributors for the second edition. Margaret Waltner and the excellent staff at Lippincott Williams & Wilkins provided invaluable assistance. Andrew Allen, PhD, worked hard at convincing me to do a second edition. My work was partly supported by the Clayton Foundation for Research.

Contents

-
-
-
-
-
-
-
-

section two
SENSORY SYSTEMS

KIRK W. BARRON, PhD, and ROBERT W. BLAIR, PhD

section four
HIGHER COGNITIVE FUNCTIONS

ALLAN SIEGEL, PhD, and JOSEPH W. CHEU, DO, PhD

section five
THE LIFE SPAN

Neuroscience for Rehabilitation

BASIC PROCESSES

Introduction: Getting the Brain in Mind

HELEN COHEN, EdD, OTR, FAOTA

**A Brief History of Neuroscience
and Rehabilitation**

Prehistory

Brief Sketch of Neuroscience History

Organizational Principles

Structural and Functional Relationships

Functional Principles

Structural Principles

Clinical Correlations

• • •

If you are a professional in one of the rehabilitation specialties, or if you are studying to become one, then you need to understand how the nervous system controls behavior. If, in your career, you will help someone who has a problem that affects her capacity to use her nervous system—a person with brain damage, an elderly person with age-related problems, a person with mental retardation, a person with a psychiatric disorder, a person with hear-

ing loss, a person with visual impairment, a person with a language disorder, a person with diabetes or some other systemic disorder, a person with burns, or a person with orthopedic problems that might affect sensation or muscle strength—then you should understand how the nervous system helps a person to function. In other words, if you plan to work with anyone who is not superhuman, you need to understand the nervous system, because every potential client or patient may have a nervous system that might have been compromised.

Most complex tasks are easy to perform when you break them down into their component parts and then tackle the parts one at a time. Rehabilitation professionals are skilled at breaking down tasks into their component parts so their patients can learn them easily. This skill is known as "activity analysis." If you can do activity analysis, if you can figure out how to break down an activity into small parts that can be addressed one at a time, then you can learn neuroscience. Initially, many people are intimidated when they consider learning this material. Do not be intimidated. Use your activity analysis skills and study the information here in small increments, one chapter at a time.

This book is an introduction to the nervous system. It is primarily a physiology book, because it primarily addresses function. It also discusses anatomy, because to understand function you must also understand structure. All of the facts discussed in this book have been discovered through painstaking research by individual neuroscientists, driven by their own curiosity about this remarkable system. In the long time frame of written history, we have learned a tremendous amount in a short period, but we still have much more to learn. The next section puts the current level of knowledge in context for you, by introducing the history of neuroscience and its relationship to rehabilitation.

A Brief History of Neuroscience and Rehabilitation

The history of neuroscience fills volumes in any medical library, covering a diverse range of topics and virtually the entire history of civilization. This material is worthy of study because understanding the development of ideas and the context in which insights have been won helps to clarify our current level of knowledge and to find the way to future work. A noted investigator has provided an elegant example of the valuable insights from history in his introduction to a text on vestibular disorders.[1] Cohen outlined an important conceptual argument that contributed to the discovery of the vestibular system and to virtually all of the current research questions in basic and clinical vestibular science. For students, clinicians, and investigators in any field, having such an understanding is essential for knowing how to weave the thread of current research findings into the fabric of the science, an expression paraphrased from a professor who, no doubt, paraphrased it from someone else. This brief section in this chapter merely introduces the complex history of neuroscience. For more complete overviews of this field, see some of the texts listed at the end of this chapter.[2-5]

Prehistory

Ancient Egyptians noticed the space-occupying structure that we call the brain, and noticed that le-

sions of the brain impair behavior, but they developed no theories about these relationships, so a thousand years passed before more progress was made. A millennium after the Egyptians, Greek physicians realized the relationship of motor and sensory nerves to the brain, but they did not develop a method to study it. Many centuries after them, Leonardo da Vinci developed a methodology for studying the structure of the brain and, like the Greeks, he related the spirit to the brain, but he did not communicate his insights.

From the work and the oversights of these early observers, we can learn some important lessons that are still relevant today both to neuroscience and to rehabilitation. Without a theoretic framework within which to organize their observations, the ancient Egyptian physicians could make little progress in understanding the brain. Of course, perhaps in their culture they had little need to understand it; we may never know. We do know, however, that their observations—no matter how astute—did not advance the state of knowledge. The lesson: observation without the organizational context of good theory does not further understanding. The failure of the ancient Greeks to develop a methodology for studying the nervous system teaches us another lesson: theory alone, without organized methods for testing theory, does not facilitate further understanding. In failing to communicate the results of his research, da Vinci—arguably one of the greatest geniuses ever known and a man many centuries ahead of his time—erred too, or perhaps made a deliberate omission. The lesson: failure to communicate insights or findings does not advance knowledge. Because he kept his findings to himself, da Vinci's work had no impact on our understanding of the brain and behavior, so his work in this field remains a historical curiosity rather than a significant contribution to neuroscience.

Brief Sketch of Neuroscience History

Two hundred years after da Vinci, and without knowing of da Vinci's work, Descartes introduced the concept that the brain could be dissected and studied; among his ideas he gave an early example of a flexor withdrawal reflex. After Descartes, Willis—for whom the Circle of Willis is named (see Chapters 2 and 5)—made the first observations that some functions can be localized to some parts of the brain. In the 18th century, a time of great scientific as well as political revolutions, Pourfour du Petit showed that nerves control motion, and Whytt demonstrated that a small spinal cord section can control a reflex. In the 19th century Broca, Jackson, and others confirmed and extended Willis' observations on localization of function.

Until late into the 19th century, investigators thought that the brain was made of a reticular network, or an indivisible brain substance, and hence the name for part of the brainstem: the reticular formation. We know now that the brain is made of individual cells and structures, but that idea, the so-called cell theory of the brain, is relatively recent and did not become accepted without considerable controversy. Proof of this theory depended on technologic progress. It required the development of light microscopes so that the great early neuroanatomists, such as Schwann, Purkinje, and Ramon y Cajal, could image the cells that make up the brain and describe their individual characteristics. Today we take the cell theory of neuroanatomy for granted, but the concept took 70 years, much argument, and many improvements in technology to become accepted.

Meanwhile, in the late 19th century and early 20th century, other investigators were doing groundbreaking work that established the bases for areas of study that are still important today. For example, many later studies of sensation and movement were based on Sherrington's studies of sensory and motor physiology. Other investigators, such as Head, Franz, and Lashley, did the first work underlying neuropsychology and neurologic rehabilitation. Many treatment paradigms in use for rehabilitation today are based on the findings from these early studies.

In the latter two thirds of the 20th century, several social, political, and technical issues coalesced. Improved medical care leading to increased survival of brain-injured soldiers after World War II and increased survival of civilian patients after brain damage led to increased public concern over the effects of brain damage on function; at the same time, the development of improved technology facilitated more sophisticated experimental paradigms. Also, more stable political and economic systems in the industrialized nations of the world have allowed more resources to be available for research. These factors resulted in increased interest in neuroscience and increased availability of research funds, eventually producing an extraordinary increase in our understanding of the nervous system and our ability to use this information for treatment of people with nervous system disorders. Although clinical practice in-variably lags behind the basic science by several years, the science is the basis for improved medical care and treatment paradigms for neurological rehabilitation.[6]

Organizational Principles

You have already learned some fundamental concepts about the nervous system, all of which were considered outlandish at one time or another. You know that the nervous system controls behavior, that it can be studied objectively and systematically, that the nervous system is made of individual cells, and that some control functions of the nervous system are partially localized in some areas of the brain. As you read this book, try to think of how scientists have learned about each part of the nervous system. Remember that each chapter is necessarily an overview of the most important concepts, but each chapter represents many years of study by many investigators. The rest of this section reviews some other general concepts that you should keep in mind as you read this book.

Structural and Functional Relationships

Structure and function, anatomy and physiology, are inextricably linked. For teaching purposes, anatomy and physiology are often separated, and many texts discuss only one or the other. For example, the many atlases of gross anatomy describe only structure. Many physiology texts discuss function almost exclusively. You should try to remember that the structure/function duality is merely a didactic convenience. In reality, structure allows function and function gives meaning to structure. You will notice many examples of this idea in this text, such as the description of different cell types that have different responses in the cochlear nucleus in the chapter on the auditory system (Chapter 9).

Functional Principles

Purposiveness
The Nobel prize-winning neurophysiologist, Ragnar Granit, wrote that the overriding organizational concept of the nervous system is "purposiveness."[7]

Purpose relates the behavior or function—of individual cells, groups of cells, entire organs, or whole human beings—to the surrounding environment and gives meaning to behavior. This concept is familiar to rehabilitation professionals, who concern themselves with the purposiveness of their clients' behavior. Function or purposiveness is a hallmark of normal motor behavior. Normal movement is characterized by goal-directedness.[8,9] The aimless movements of athetoid fingers and toes and the meaningless, self-stimulating arm-waving of autistic children are obviously pathologic because they are not goal directed.

Granit has explained that purposiveness is a point of view, or frame of reference. We can consider the problem of learning, including motor learning, as a form of adaptation, which has meaning within the context of purposiveness. Motor learning and the underlying cellular processes that mediate adaptation occur because they allow the individual to adapt to changing conditions in the environment. As you read this book, try to think about the "purpose" for each part of the system and the reason it works the way it does. If you consider those reasons as a frame of reference, you will be able to organize and remember the material.

Systems Organization
The entire nervous system, including the brain, spinal cord, and peripheral nerves, is one large mechanism for the purpose of generating and controlling behavior. Purposiveness in structure and in function is evident in this system in many different ways, because the nervous system has many different levels, anatomically and functionally. Many years ago, Norbert Wiener, a brilliant engineer, described how systems, in general, can be understood.[10] The concepts from his work have provided new ways to understand the structure and function of the nervous system. This engineering approach to neuroscience has spawned a subspecialty, computational neuroscience, in which engineers and mathematicians try to determine generic rules for the function of different aspects of the nervous system. These rules take the form of mathematical models, which suggest experimental paradigms to test them empirically; the data from those experiments can then be used to refine the mathematical models.

Functional Mechanisms. The brain is the government of the body. In the United States the federal government has three branches, each performing a different function. The administrative branch has different departments that are really convenient administrative subdivisions to perform different tasks. For example, the National Institutes of Health (NIH) is a mechanism for supporting research to improve the health of the population; the Internal Revenue Service is a mechanism for collecting the funds needed by the government to operate, including the research funds disbursed by the NIH. Within each administrative division, smaller mechanisms may operate for more specific purposes. For example, the NIH has 18 independent institutes, each dedicated to research on a different set of problems. Each administrative mechanism in government is really a collection of individual people, with many different occupational roles. For example, the National Aeronautics and Space Administration employs astronauts, cafeteria workers, engineers, physiologists, scuba divers, and secretaries. All of those people work toward the goal of gleaning new knowledge from the exploration of outer space, but people in different job categories have different roles to play in that effort.

In the same way, the nervous system has many mechanisms, each made of collections of individual neural and nonneural cells that perform different functions, connected so that together the entire unit performs a specific function. As you read this book, you will learn about many functional mechanisms and different kinds of cells that mediate those functions.

Systems Theory
Levels of Analysis. Wiener's work on systems theory and the subsequent research by other investigators has taught us that any system can be studied and considered at various levels of analysis. Thus, the nervous system can be studied from the tiniest level of structure, the molecule, which is important to understanding the mechanism of the cell membrane, to the largest level of structure, the whole person in the environment. In between are many other levels, including the level of the specific motor behavior (e.g., the vestibuloocular reflex), the level of the functional system (e.g., one sensory system such as the vestibular system), the level of the group of nerve cells (e.g., the superior vestibular nucleus), the level of the individual cell (e.g., the single hair cell in the vestibular labyrinth), and the level of part of a cell (e.g., the mitochondrion). Like a Russian matryoshka doll, another level of analysis is always inside. To understand the behavior of the whole person in the environment, we must understand

the behavior of the nervous system at all of these levels.

This task is not trivial. For each different level of analysis different research techniques are used, and the work at one level of the system may not elucidate the next level of the system. This concept has direct application to rehabilitation professionals, who are concerned with disease and disability. The NIH has recognized that an understanding of the pathophysiology of disease does not explain the handicap that can result because these issues are at different levels of the person system.[11] In neuroscience, with the development of improved laboratory technology to look at successively lower levels of the system, the tendency in some research areas has been toward work at the lower levels while ignoring work at the higher levels. Unfortunately, as Granit has pointed out, this increase in knowledge at lower levels does not translate to increased understanding at higher levels, and may even be accompanied by relative losses at higher levels. Some therapists have made the opposite mistake: thinking that work only at the highest levels of analyses is worth considering.

The work at every level of analysis is important. When different levels of analysis can be related, as in some of the current work on aggression and rage, then we finally approach an understanding of how the nervous system controls behavior. As you read this text, try to determine at what level of analysis the material should be considered and how that level relates to the rest of the system.

Emergent Properties. In the nervous system, the isolated actions of individual nerve cells, or even nuclei, may be of little significance. New kinds of behavior, however, emerge from the unified actions of many cells in many centers. For example, cognition, the act of thinking, emerges from the unified actions of various parts of the brain. Granit has explained that the properties of consciousness cannot be explained simply by the physiology of the nervous system. Thus, consciousness is an **emergent property.** It is an example of the concept that the structure and function of lower levels of the system cannot explain the structure and function of higher levels.

Distributed Control. At any one time, the nervous system coordinates many different activities. The system must control voluntary motor activities, such as walking or reaching, cognition and movement to produce speech and interactive language, as well as

homeostatic regulation. All of this activity can happen simultaneously. Consider, for example, what you might be doing while chatting with a colleague over a cup of coffee. While you generate language to converse, you reach for your coffee cup, drink the coffee, and digest it. At the same time as you attend to the conversation and drink the coffee, you sense some discomfort from sitting in one position for too long, so you shift your weight to relieve the pressure. At various moments different centers may be in more control, as one or another specific task dominates your attention. Therefore, the nervous system must have multiple centers of control, and must be able to switch among them as needed.

Control within subsystems is also distributed. For example, as you will learn in the motor control chapters, several centers at different levels of the system control different aspects of so-called voluntary movement. Disrupting any of those centers leads to movement disorders. At any point in a movement, one or more centers may control the action. Some centers are essential for planning movement; some centers are required for initiating movement; some centers are essential for fine-tuning the movement parameters, such as timing or smooth coordination of muscle groups. The control center changes as the action sequence unfolds.

Redundant Representations. Information may be represented in the nervous system in several forms at the same time. Data about the same thing come into the system along several different routes, and may be processed along parallel pathways. For instance, we know that an orange is an orange because it looks, feels, smells, and tastes like an orange. Any one of these facts identifies the orange as that particular variety of fruit. To identify it, only one of those bits of information is really necessary, yet all are available. At different times, one or another bit of information about the orange may be the most useful. Thus, the orange has some built-in duplication of information and the nervous system has many ways to obtain information about the orange. This redundancy is not only useful under normal circumstances, it can be useful to the disabled person, and to the astute therapist caring for that person.

Parallel and Serial Processing. Some information travels linearly up or down through the levels of the system. This way of handling information is known as **serial processing.** For example, one rainy day I stepped in a puddle. The message went from my foot, where I experienced the water, up a nerve in my leg to my spinal cord, up the spinal cord to the very top of my brain, where I interpreted the information and decided to move my foot out of the puddle. Then a message went down to my spinal cord, to another set of nerves to my leg, and I moved my foot out of the puddle. This simplified description illustrates serial processing. A different way of handling information is **parallel processing,** which may be illustrated by considering the definition of the orange discussed earlier. If an orange is defined as an edible object with a particular shape, texture, range of tastes, and range of colors, then you know you are holding or eating an orange when you experience two or more of those attributes simultaneously. Each attribute is different, processed by different sensory systems, but messages about them may be received by the brain simultaneously, along different, parallel, pathways—hence the term, parallel processing.

Feedback. The nervous system keeps itself informed through the use of feedback mechanisms. When the brain gives a command, a copy of that command, a corollary discharge,[12] is sent to other parts of the brain to keep the entire system informed about what should happen. Then, when the event occurs, feedback is sent to the command center informing it that the event did occur. The command center can then compare the original command with the results and decide what further action to take. On a simpler level, various pathways connect one nerve cell to the next cells but also to previous nerve cells, giving a cell the opportunity to affect the activity of an earlier cell in the pathway.

Integration. The nervous system does not merely take in information and generate automatic responses. Instead, information is processed and reprocessed repeatedly. Based on feedback, the ability of the nervous system to take in information can be fine-tuned. A signal that is reported veridically at one level of the system may be interpreted and changed at another level, based on other input. For example, at centers deep in the brain that receive information about vision, other information about touch or sound may affect how those nerve cells respond and signal to other cells.[13] Thus, although many rehabilitation treatment techniques are based on the old notion that sensory input and motor output are directly and

linearly related,[14] we know now that the situation is far more complex.

Adaptation. A hallmark of the nervous system is its remarkable ability to learn or to change behavior, at most levels of the system. Humans and lower animals are able to adapt their responses to environmental demands as those demands change and as their own physical capabilities change. Animal species who are unable to adapt become extinct, such as dinosaurs. People who are unable to adapt are handicapped. Rehabilitation professionals are employed to help people learn to adapt when they are unable to do so by themselves.

The ability to learn new information—to modify something in the nervous system so that new information is retained or to perform old tasks in new ways—is what allows you to read this text with the reasonable expectation that by the time you have finished it you will understand something about how the nervous system works. The ability to adapt to changes in our physical morphology allows us to remain independent across most of the life span, despite alterations in size, shape, strength, and visual acuity. These changes occur at the level of the cell membrane, at the level of individual cells, in reflexes, and in observable motor behavior.

Structural Principles

Localization of Function

The purpose of your nervous system, as a whole, is to generate and control your behavior. Different parts of the nervous system, such as the occipital lobe of the cerebral cortex—the part of the brain at the back of your head—have different functions that are supported by differences in structure. For example, the occipital lobe performs sophisticated interpretation of visual information that allows you to read and interpret this page. Visual information is initially detected by the retina of the eye, processed by several other centers, and then sent to the visual cortex in the occipital lobe for further interpretation. Under a light microscope, this visual cortex, unlike other areas of cortex, appears to be striated, or striped, and hence it is called "striate cortex." This striped effect occurs because the structure of the cortex in this area is somewhat different than in other areas, owing to the presence of a particularly large number of cells in one layer. The visual cortex also receives a unique set of information, or input. You will learn more about the details of the visual cortex later in this book. What you should remember from this section is that a defined area of the brain has unique functions, and unique structural properties in that area underlie its unique functions.

Topographic Organization. Information to and from various places maintains some spatial distinctiveness. This concept is most apparent in the senses related to touch because the centers that receive information about things touching the skin have representations of the body surface, so that different areas can be distinguished from each other. This specific representation of the body surface is most apparent in the uppermost layers of the brain, but is true at other levels, too.

Hemispheric Specialization. The phylogenetically newer sections of the brain have some spatial division of labor. In most people, the areas concerned with language are larger on one side of the brain and the areas concerned with spatial perception are larger on the other side of the brain. Although the popular press has made much of this issue, the application of this concept has limits. Except for some patients who have had surgery to section large areas of the brain, usually to treat uncontrollable seizure disorders, no one is truly "left-brained" or "right-brained."

Layers and Columns

Phylogenetic Layers. Because humans developed from more primitive animals that are lower on the phylogenetic scale, our nervous systems have retained many of the features of those other nervous systems. Consequently, the human nervous system has many features that are phylogenetically quite old. For this reason, most research on the nervous system may be done with lower animals and the results applied to humans.

Some structures in the human brain have probably been added to the basic design. In general, newer structures have been added on top of older structures, so that older structures are deeper inside the brain, and lower down. The structures that are, literally, on the top of the brain have developed more recently on the scale of evolution. Of course, we rely on different kinds of information than some other animals, so some other structures have probably also been lost. For example, rats depend heavily on smell for orientation and relatively little on vision, so relatively large parts of their brains process olfactory information. We rely much less on smell and much more on vision. Not surprisingly, our brains have relatively larger centers for vision than for olfaction. The original structures seem to have remained, although those structures seem to have become adapted for other purposes, and newer structures have been added to them. Therefore, the study of neuroscience is complicated by the fact that although we have many features in common with lower animals, we are not simply more complicated models of the same thing. Instead, the essential design features may remain, but the structure has been altered significantly.

Anatomic Layers. Some structures in the brain are made of layers of cells, within which different kinds of processes take place, each of which affects the information that is transmitted. These layers form some of the anatomic bases for some of the functional principles discussed previously. For example, a large group of cells known as the superior colliculus is deep inside the brain. When the cells are stained so that they can be viewed easily, layers of cells, like the layers of an onion, are obvious. Different processes take place in the deep and superficial layers.

Columnar Organization. Many parts of the nervous system are organized in vertical columns, particularly the older areas. For example, the groups of cells involved in taste form a long column in the base of the brain. Also in the base of the brain, the groups of cells that control eye movements are located one above the other, in a broken column. These groups of eye movement cells are connected by a large network of pathways, the medial longitudinal fasciculus.

Structural Specialization

The body has different organs that have specialized anatomic features for different purposes, and within cells, different organelles have specialized structures that perform different functions. So, too, in the nervous system specialized structures mediate different functions. For example, parts of nerve cells have specific functions, nerve cells in cell groups have different shapes that reflect different functions, and the structures of entire regions of the brain display specialization that supports specific functions of those areas.

Convergence and Divergence

In the event of a natural disaster, such as a hurricane, information from many individual sources is sent in to the Federal Emergency Management Agency. There, the agency director integrates the information, sends the integrated information up to the President, and also sends information and decisions to other parts of the government. In other words, information converges on the agency, where it is processed, and then diverges to other parts of the government, either for further processing and decision making or to levels where decisions will be carried out. In the same way, information enters the nervous system from thousands of individual neurons and converges on centers, where it may be processed for control of low-level motor behavior, it may be transmitted to other centers, or it may be combined with other information and then sent on to a variety of other centers.

Clinical Correlations

Most chapters in this book have sections that introduce you to the clinical relevance of the science in the chapter. For some topics, making those connections may be easy; for other chapters, understanding the relationships between the chapter topic and clinical problems may be more difficult. All of this material is relevant to the clinician because to be a whole person requires a complete nervous system. The Clinical Correlations sections are here to aid you in understanding why you need to understand the material.

An individual person is a system, with many layers of organization. This book introduces some of the many layers and mechanisms of one system within the larger system. Because the nervous system controls behavior, damage to any layer, structure, or mechanism in the system produces disordered behavior. To understand how to rehabilitate a person, to help someone learn to modify his or her behavior, you must understand how the nervous system contributes to normal behavior. With that knowledge comes the foundation for rational approaches to rehabilitation.

REFERENCES

1. Cohen B. Foreword. In: Baloh RW, Halmagyi GM, eds. *Disorders of the vestibular system*. New York: Oxford University Press, 1996:v–vii.
2. Sherrington CS. *The integrative action of the nervous system*. Cambridge: Cambridge University Press, 1947.
3. McHenry LC. *Garrison's history of neurology*. Springfield, IL: Charles C Thomas, 1969.
4. Corsi P, ed. *The enchanted loom: chapters in the history of neuroscience*. New York: Oxford University Press, 1991.
5. Finger S. *Origins of neuroscience: a history of exploration into brain function*. New York: Oxford University Press, 1994.
6. Cohen H, Reed KL. Looking back: the development of neuroscience and rehabilitation. *Am J Occup Ther* 1996;50:561–568.
7. Granit R. *The purposive brain*. Cambridge, MA: MIT Press, 1977.
8. Bernstein N. *The co-ordination and regulation of movements*. Oxford: Pergamon Press, 1967.
9. Whiting HTA, ed. *Human motor actions: Bernstein reassessed*. Amsterdam: Elsevier, 1984.
10. Wiener N. *Cybernetics or control and communication in the animal and the machine*. Cambridge, MA: MIT Press, 1961.
11. National Institute of Child Health and Human Development. *Research plan for the National Center for Medical Rehabilitation Research*. NIH Publication No. 93–3509. Bethesda, MD: U.S. Department of Health and Human Services, Public Health Service, National Institutes of Health, National Institute of Child Health and Human Development, 1993.
12. Sperry RW. Neural basis of the spontaneous optokinetic response produced by visual inversion. *Journal of Comparative and Physiological Psychology* 1950;43: 482–489.
13. Stein BE, Meredith MA. *The merging of the senses*. Cambridge, MA: MIT Press, 1993.
14. Rood MS. The use of sensory receptors to activate, facilitate, and inhibit motor response, autonomic and somatic in developmental sequence. In: Sattely C, ed. *Study course VI, Third International Congress, World Federation of Occupational Therapists*. Dubuque, IA: William C. Brown Company, 1962:26–37.

GENERAL REFERENCES

When beginning a new field of study, knowing where to obtain information is essential. This section lists some of the many excellent books and periodicals available.

Journals/Periodicals

Reviews of Current Topics

Annual Review of Neuroscience. Published annually, this periodical includes serious reviews of a few topics each year.

The Behavioral and Brain Sciences. This journal publishes in-depth reviews, with commentaries by other investigators in the field. This format is helpful for learning about controversies and unresolved issues in the field.

Progress in Brain Research. This journal publishes in-depth reviews on current topics in the neurosciences.

Trends in Neuroscience. This journal publishes brief, cogent reviews by established scientists about current issues and topics in the neurosciences. This publication keeps neuroscientists abreast of developments outside of their own research specialties. Therefore, it is relatively accessible to nonspecialists.

Periodicals: Research Papers

The vast number of periodicals publishing research papers related to neuroscience precludes a complete listing, but a few that you should know about are listed here.

Neuroscience. The official journal of the Society for Neuroscience.

Experimental Brain Research. One of the major journals publishing neuroscience research.

Journal of Comparative Neurology. A major journal that publishes research on neuroanatomy.

Journal of Neurophysiology. One of the major journals publishing neuroscience research.

Science. The official journal of the American Association for the Advancement of Science.

Books

Vocabulary

Lockard I. *Desk reference for neuroscience.* 2nd ed. New York: Springer-Verlag, 1992. An extensive glossary of terminology currently used in the neurosciences.

Dorland's illustrated medical dictionary. 27th ed. Philadelphia: WB Saunders, 1988. A well known, comprehensive medical dictionary.

Anatomy

Barr ML, Kiernan JA. *The human nervous system: an anatomical point of view.* 6th ed. Philadelphia: JB Lippincott, 1993.

DeArmond SJ, Fusco MM, Dewey MM. *Structure of the human brain: a photographic atlas.* 3rd ed. New York: Oxford University Press, 1989.

Haines DE. *Neuroanatomy: an atlas of structures, sections, and systems.* 4th ed. Baltimore: Williams & Wilkins, 1995.

Jennes L, Traurig H, Conn PM. *Atlas of the human brain.* Philadelphia: JB Lippincott, 1995.

Martin JH. *Neuroanatomy: text and atlas.* 2nd ed. Stamford, CT: Appleton & Lange, 1996.

2

Gross Anatomy

HELEN S. COHEN, EdD, OTR, FAOTA

• • •

To understand the structure and function of the nervous system, you must understand some basic concepts and be familiar with the basic layout of the system. Chapter 1 introduced you to some concepts about the nervous system. This chapter introduces the anatomy. Later chapters discuss some of these issues in more depth. Because this book is not meant to be an exhaustive anatomy text, if you are interested in the detailed structure of the system you may want to consult other texts as well. This book discusses structure as it relates to function. You may want to prepare by having a good medical dictionary or glossary available.[1,2]

As you learned in Chapter 1, the nervous system is made up of individual cells. The cells that are specialized for nervous system function are known as **neurons**. Collections of their processes are sometimes called **nerves**.

The nervous system has two large subdivisions: the peripheral and central nervous systems. The **peripheral nervous system** (PNS) includes all parts of the system that are outside of the bony casings of the skull and spinal column. The **central nervous system** (CNS) includes all parts of the system that are within the skull and spinal column. The spinal column encases and protects the **spinal cord**; the skull encases and protects the **brain**. The spinal cord and brain are continuous at the **foramen magnum**, the hole at the base of the skull.

Directions

Anatomy is like geography. Just as places on a map are located with reference to directions, so too are places in the CNS located with reference points and directions. To learn anatomy, you must understand the words that define the cardinal directions. These directions can be confusing because the terms used also refer to directions in the brains of lower animals, whose brains are simpler in structure. During its development, the brain starts out as a fairly straight structure, much like a rat's brain, but bends around as a large amount of material fits into the small confines of the skull (see Chap. 19). Therefore, as shown in Figure 2–1, some directions appear to change.

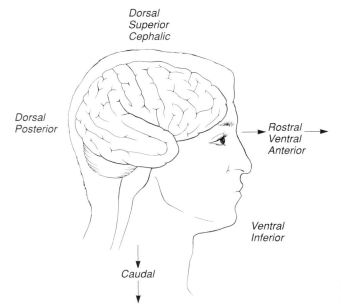

Dorsal
Superior
Cephalic

Dorsal
Posterior

Rostral
Ventral
Anterior

Ventral
Inferior

Caudal

Figure 2–1. Directions in the nervous system in reference to major landmarks.

The standard **anatomical position** is the reference position. Remember that anatomic position refers to an idealized person standing upright, looking straight ahead, with feet and palms facing forward. Starting in one of the lower subdivisions of the brain, the **midbrain** of the **brainstem**, the long axis of the CNS bends forward gradually in higher animals such as primates, including humans. The terms **cephalic** and **caudal** refer to the nose end and the buttocks end, respectively. Caudal actually means the tail end in lower animals with tails. **Rostral** is synonymous with "cephalic." **Dorsal** refers to the back, and **ventral** refers to the front; dorsal also means **posterior** and ventral also means **anterior**. In the most cephalic region of the brain, dorsal means **superior** and ventral means **inferior**. **Medial** means toward the midline, and **lateral**, away from the midline.

The CNS is a three-dimensional structure, with X, Y, and Z axes. To study the system, anatomists make slices of the brain, usually along one of those axes, or in one of the planes defined by those axes. Slices of the brain are known as **sections**. A **sagittal** section has an anterior–posterior cut, and shows either the right or left side of the brain or spinal cord. A sagittal section is usually sliced in the midline; a **parasagittal** section is sliced lateral to the midline.

A **coronal** section has a right–left cut, and shows the dorsal or ventral side. Often, coronal sections are made in the cerebral hemispheres or cerebellum, giving a view across the "top" of the hemispheres.

Central Nervous System

The Spinal Cord

The spinal cord is a long column of **afferent** nerve fibers ascending to carry information to the brain, **efferent** nerve fibers descending to carry commands from the brain, local **interneurons**, and the cell bodies of these neurons. Although it was once thought to be a passive carrier of information, we now know that much **information processing** takes places locally in the spinal cord itself, using **local circuit neurons**. Information from the outside world enters the spinal cord and commands from the CNS exit the spinal cord through **spinal nerves**. Because the spinal cord does not grow to the same length as the spinal column, the bundle of spinal nerves that descends in the spinal column before exiting is called the **cauda equina** (Fig. 2–2).

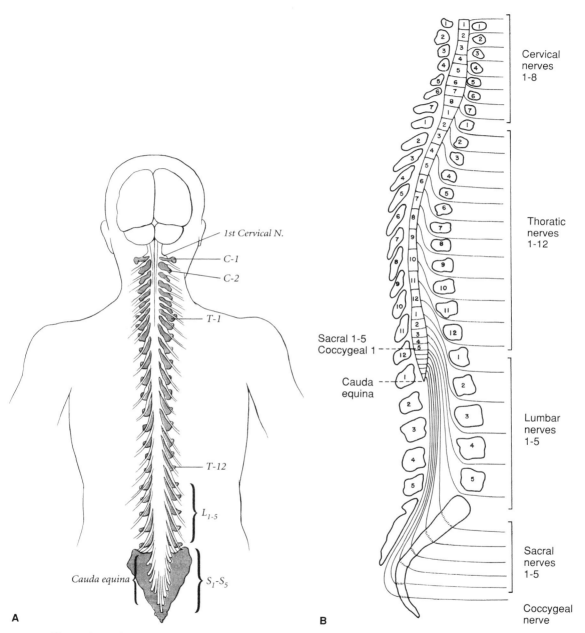

Figure 2–2. The spinal cord and spinal nerves, indicating the various levels of the spinal cord in relation to the vertebrae. **A:** A dorsal view. The vertebrae are shown in gray. The sacral and coccygeal vertebrae are fused. **B:** A lateral view. The corresponding segments of the spinal cord are numbered. (**B** from Barr ML, Kiernan JA. *The human nervous system: An anatomical viewpoint.* 6th ed. Philadelphia: JB Lippincott, 1993. With permission.)

The spinal cord has several subdivisions. The first seven vertebrae of the spinal column are the **cervical** vertebrae. In descending order, the next 12 vertebrae are the **thoracic** vertebrae, followed by the 5 **lumbar** vertebrae, the 5 **sacral** vertebrae, and 1 to 3 **coccygeal** vertebrae. Therefore, the first spinal nerve, which exits between the skull and the uppermost cervical vertebra,

is the first cervical nerve. All other spinal nerves are named for the vertebrae immediately above them.

The sections of the spinal cord corresponding to the spinal nerves and overlying vertebrae are numbered in the same way (see Fig. 2–2B). The area of skin innervated by nerves related to a particular segment of the spinal cord is a **dermatome** (Fig. 2–3). The spinal

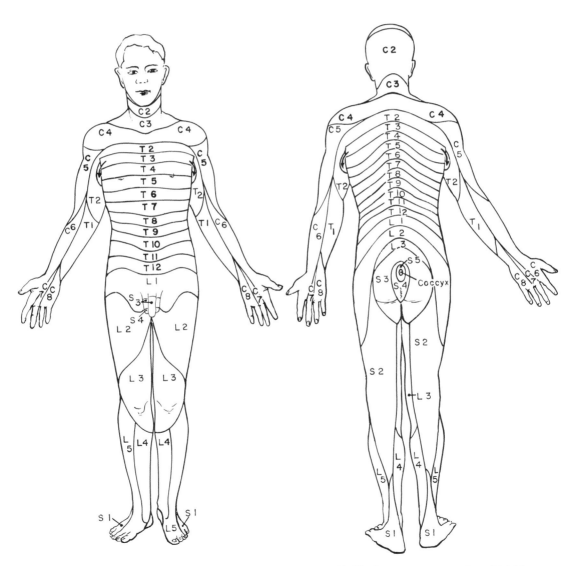

Figure 2–3. Distribution of dermatomes. (Barr ML, Kiernan JA. *The human nervous system: An anatomical viewpoint.* 6th ed. Philadelphia: JB Lippincott, 1993. With permission.)

cord has enlargements in lower cervical and lumbosacral areas known as the **brachial plexus** and **lumbosacral plexus**, respectively. These enlargements are formed by large numbers of nerve cell bodies and processes that collect in those areas. Afferent and efferent nerves in the brachial plexus innervate the upper extremities (the arms); afferent and efferent nerves in the lumbosacral plexus innervate the lower extremities (the legs).

Neurons have particular properties, discussed in Chapter 3. The other cells of the nervous system that support neurons, the **glia**, are discussed in Chapter 5. To understand the gross anatomy of the spinal cord and the brain, however, you should understand something about the relationship between these two cell types. To the naked eye, most neurons and glia are too small to be seen, but large aggregations of them can be observed. Collections of neuron cell bodies appear to be grayish in color. Therefore, areas of the CNS composed primarily of cell bodies are called **gray matter**. Some specialized glia wrap themselves around the processes of many neurons, forming insulating layers. Because the wrappings of glia form fatty layers that are whitish in color, areas composed primarily of neuron processes are called **white matter** (Fig. 2–4).

From the most caudal to the most rostral sections of the spinal cord, the total diameter of the cord increases as nerve cells are added to it. In cross-section, the relative shapes of the white matter and gray matter also change. The central gray matter is sometimes described as having a butterfly shape. Afferent nerves that pierce the spinal cord are bundled together in the **dorsal roots**, with their cell bodies outside the spinal cord in the **dorsal root ganglia**. Efferent nerves that leave the spinal cord are bundled together in the **ventral roots**. The roots are named for the side of the spinal cord they enter or exit (see Fig. 2–4).

Specific layers in the gray matter of the cord are known as laminae, and are discussed in Chapter 13. Specific bundles of processes carry primarily afferent sensory information in the white matter; they are discussed in Chapters 6 through 8. The internal anatomy of the spinal cord is very complex, involving neuron cell bodies, neuron processes, parts of local circuits within each side of the spinal cord and across sides, and parts of longer circuits involving the brain and spinal cord within each side and across sides. Figure 2–5 illustrates some examples.

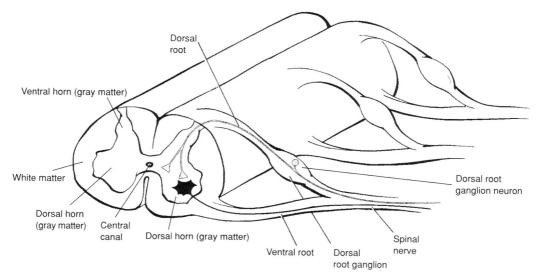

Figure 2–4. A cross-section of the spinal cord. Notice that three segments are included, because three dorsal and three ventral roots are shown. The cell body for the efferent neuron exiting in the ventral root is located in the gray matter. (From Conn PM. *Neuroscience in medicine.* Philadelphia: Lippincott–Raven, 1995; with permission.)

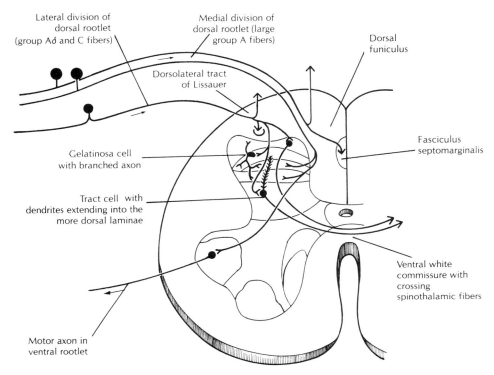

Figure 2–5. A hemisection of the spinal cord showing local circuitry and laminae. (From Barr ML, Kiernan JA. *The human nervous system: An anatomical viewpoint.* 6th ed. Philadelphia: JB Lippincott, 1993; with permission.)

The Brain

Cerebrum and Cerebellum

The brain has several large divisions, illustrated in Figures 2–6 through 2–8. These divisions include the brainstem, with the **medulla oblongata**, the **pons**, and the midbrain; the **diencephalon**, composed of the **thalamus**, **epithalamus** and **hypothalamus**; the **cerebellum**; and the **cerebrum** or the **cerebral hemispheres**. The brainstem and spinal cord, together, are sometimes called the **neuraxis**.

The cerebellum and cerebrum both have three parts. The most superficial part of each structure is known as the **cortex,** which is primarily gray matter or neuron cell bodies. Deep within each structure are groups of cell bodies, the **deep cerebellar nuclei** in the cerebellum and the **basal ganglia** in the

cerebrum. White matter connects the areas of gray matter.

The cerebral cortex is divided into several **lobes**: **frontal**, **parietal**, **temporal**, and **occipital**. The cortex appears wrinkled, with hillocks and grooves, known as **gyri** and **sulci**, respectively. (Those words are the plural forms. The singular forms are **gyrus** and **sulcus**.) Deep sulci are known as **fissures**. Each gyrus and sulcus has a name. For example, the sulcus dividing the **precentral gyrus** of the frontal lobe from the **postcentral gyrus** of the parietal lobe is known as the **central sulcus**, or **fissure of Rolando**. The **parietooccipital sulcus** separates the parietal and occipital lobes. Hiding within the **lateral sulcus**, or **Sylvian fissure**, is a part of the cortex known as the **insula**. The **central fissure** divides the two hemispheres, which are connected by several bundles of fibers. The

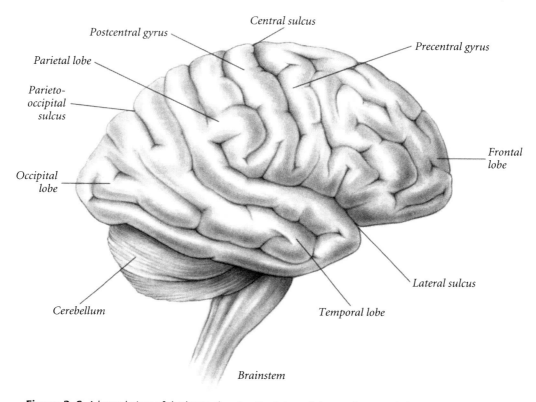

Central sulcus

Postcentral gyrus

Parietal lobe

Parieto-occipital sulcus

Precentral gyrus

Frontal lobe

Occipital lobe

Cerebellum

Lateral sulcus

Temporal lobe

Brainstem

Figure 2–6. A lateral view of the brain showing the lobes of the cerebrum and the cerebellum.

fiber bundles connecting the two cerebral hemispheres include a massive white matter structure known as the **corpus callosum**, and the smaller **anterior** and **posterior commissures**.

The wrinkles in the cortex allow a lot of surface area to be packed into the relatively small, inelastic confines of the skull. Animals lower on the phylogenetic scale have fewer convolutions, and fewer neurons altogether. For example, the rat's brain is **lissencephalic**—it has no gyri and sulci. Instead, it is smooth.

The cortices of the cerebellum and cerebrum include layers of several kinds of cells laid out in regular arrangements. In the cerebellum, the structure of the cortex is remarkably uniform throughout. In the cere-

bral cortex, however, different areas are characterized by different patterns of cell layers and hence different appearances. Neuroanatomists refer to a patch of cortex with a uniformly similar cell pattern as a **cytoarchitectonic area**. Many years ago, Brodmann[3] tried to describe the different cytoarchitectonic areas of the cerebral cortex. He decided on 47 different areas, and gave each one a number. Although much of this information is now outdated, some areas are still identified occasionally by Brodmann's numbers. For example, areas 17, 18, and 19 are all areas concerned with vision, in the occipital lobe. These areas are discussed in more detail in Chapter 11.

(text continued on page 20)

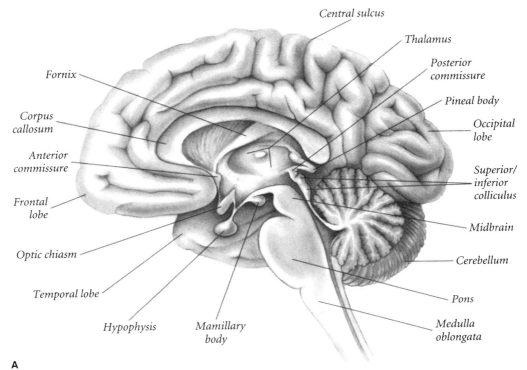

A

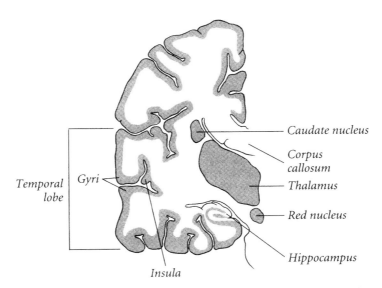

B

Figure 2–7. Lateral and horizontal views of the brain. **A:** A lateral view of the brain showing the parts of the brainstem, the cerebellum, and other major landmarks. **B:** A horizontal section through the cerebrum, showing major landmarks.

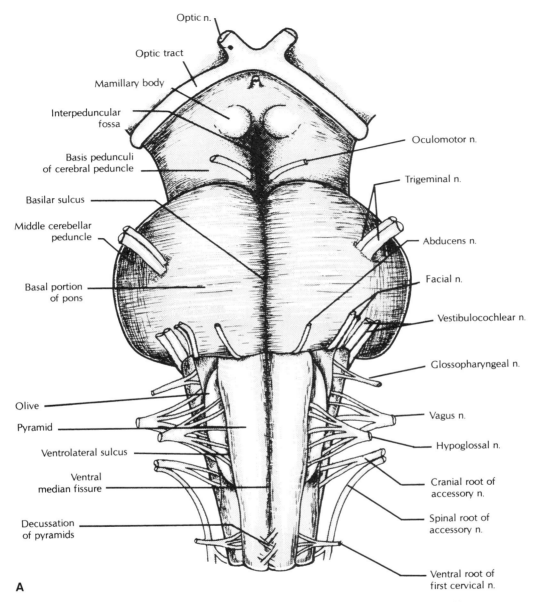

Optic n.

Optic tract

Mamillary body

Interpeduncular fossa

Basis pedunculi of cerebral peduncle

Basilar sulcus

Middle cerebellar peduncle

Basal portion of pons

Olive

Pyramid

Ventrolateral sulcus

Ventral median fissure

Decussation of pyramids

A

Oculomotor n.

Trigeminal n.

Abducens n.

Facial n.

Vestibulocochlear n.

Glossopharyngeal n.

Vagus n.

Hypoglossal n.

Cranial root of accessory n.

Spinal root of accessory n.

Ventral root of first cervical n.

Figure 2–8. The brainstem, showing cranial nerves and major landmarks. **A:** The ventral brainstem. (continued on p. 20)

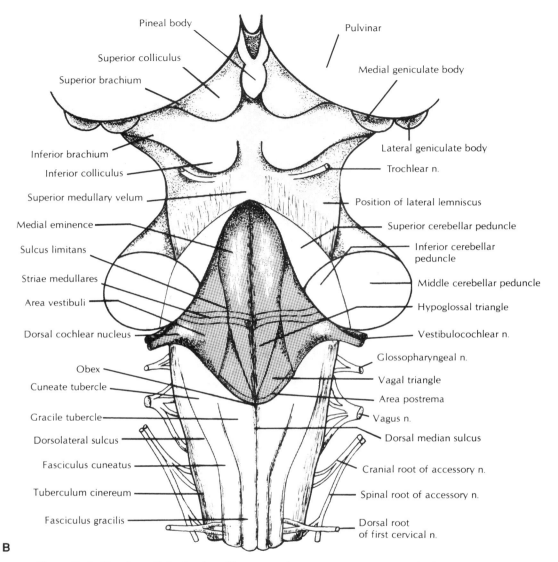

Pineal body
Superior colliculus
Superior brachium
Pulvinar
Medial geniculate body
Inferior brachium
Inferior colliculus
Lateral geniculate body
Trochlear n.
Superior medullary velum
Position of lateral lemniscus
Medial eminence
Superior cerebellar peduncle
Sulcus limitans
Inferior cerebellar peduncle
Striae medullares
Middle cerebellar peduncle
Area vestibuli
Hypoglossal triangle
Dorsal cochlear nucleus
Vestibulocochlear n.
Obex
Glossopharyngeal n.
Cuneate tubercle
Vagal triangle
Area postrema
Gracile tubercle
Vagus n.
Dorsolateral sulcus
Dorsal median sulcus
Fasciculus cuneatus
Cranial root of accessory n.
Tuberculum cinereum
Spinal root of accessory n.
Fasciculus gracilis
Dorsal root of first cervical n.

B

Figure 2–8. (Continued). B: The dorsal brainstem. (From Barr ML, Kiernan JA. *The human nervous system: An anatomical viewpoint.* 6th ed. Philadelphia: JB Lippincott, 1993; with permission.)

The cerebellum, which sits in the **posterior fossa** of the skull, is attached to the brainstem by three **peduncles**,which are composed of afferent and efferent fibers involved in local circuits entirely contained within the brain. The cortex of the cerebellum is also wrinkled and is divided into lobes by fissures. Like the spinal cord and cerebrum, the cerebellum has gray and white areas, shown in Figure 2–9. The function of this structure is somewhat mysterious. It is not essential for maintaining life or for initiating behavior, but rather seems to be involved in "quality control"—in fine-tuning signals generated by other areas.

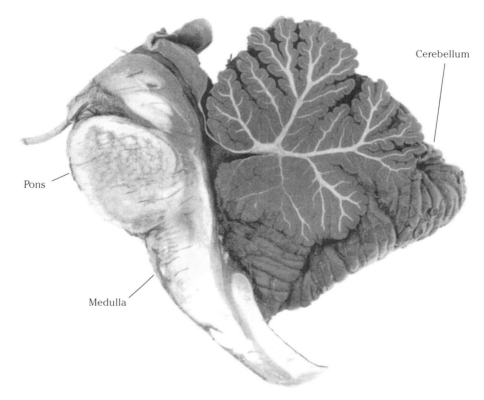

Cerebellum

Pons

Medulla

Figure 2–9. The brainstem and cerebellum. The structures have been sectioned through the midline, showing the *arbor vitae cerebelli* in the vermis, or midline, of the cerebellum. The specimen has been stained to differentiate gray matter from white matter. Notice the separations of the cerebellar lobules. (From Barr ML, Kiernan JA. *The human nervous system: An anatomical viewpoint.* 6th ed. Philadelphia: JB Lippincott, 1993; with permission.)

Other parts of the brain are named for their location or appearance to the original anatomists. For example, the **hippocampus**, a part of the cerebral cortex that is phylogenetically old, is hidden within the Sylvian fissure (see Fig. 2–7B). The Greeks named it for its seahorse shape in cross-section. Similarly, the substantia nigra, in the midbrain, is named for its black appearance. Lesions of the substantia nigra have been implicated in Parkinson's disease. As you read about parts of the brain, remembering the names of structures may be easier if you relate each name to the appearance or function of its area.

Some structures, such as the **caudate nucleus** and the **ventricles**—large internal spaces—can be difficult to image because they do not appear completely in any one section. As the brain develops in the embryo, the neuraxis curves around. The cau-date nucleus separates from the putamen as they are divided by the **internal capsule**, a sheet of white matter. The caudate develops a large head rostrally, with a thinner body and tail that curve around superiorly, posteriorly, and then inferiorly, making a C-shaped structure, as shown in Figure 2–10. Likewise, the overlying lateral ventriclesare curved (Fig. 2–11). Consequently, structures on the superior border of the ventricles are also curved.

The **superior** and **inferior colliculi** are located at the rostral end of the brainstem. The **pineal body**, rostral to the colliculi, is part of the epithalamus. Ventral to the colliculi the **hypophysis**, or pituitary gland, includes both neural and nonneural structures. The neurohypophysis is part of the hypothalamus, as are the **mamillary bodies**. The basal ganglia are a group of structures, the caudate nucleus,

globus pallidus, and **putamen**, which together are called the **striatum**, as well as the **substantia nigra** and the **subthalamic nucleus**. The basal ganglia are located deep within the cerebral hemispheres.

The Brainstem

The phylogenetically oldest part of the brain, the brainstem is the extension of the spinal cord inside the skull (see Fig. 2–8). It is an area of transition between the cerebrum and the spinal cord where many important functions are controlled. In the most caudal region, the medulla oblongata (or simply "medulla"), some descending pathways cross, or **decussate**, in the **pyramids**, named from their roughly triangular shape. Many pathways in the CNS decussate, although the reason is unknown. Rostral to the medulla is the pons, above which is the midbrain. The peduncles that connect the cerebellum to the rest of the brain are connected to the brainstem. The inferior cerebellar peduncle, also known as the **restiform body**, is connected to the medulla; the middle cerebellar peduncle is connected to the pons,

and the superior cerebellar peduncle is connected to the midbrain.

The brainstem contains cell bodies for the cranial nerves, which are like spinal nerves of the brain. It also has afferent and efferent pathways connected with the cerebrum and spinal cord, and many local circuit neurons that perform information processing at each level. The brainstem, which is well protected by its location inside the skull at the base of the brain, contains many centers that control functions essential for life, such as heart rate and breathing.

Cranial Nerves

Just as spinal nerves have efferent and afferent fibers related to parts of the spinal cord some nerves, known as **cranial nerves** (CN), have efferent and afferent fibers related to parts of the brainstem. Because the body is bilaterally symmetric, they are paired. Just like the 31 pairs of spinal nerves, the 12 pairs of cranial nerves have two roles. First, they bring information from the **special senses** and **somatic senses** of the face and head into the brain.

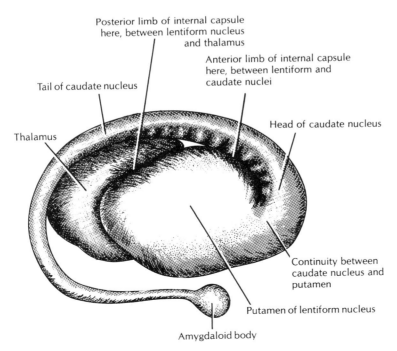

Posterior limb of internal capsule here, between lentiform nucleus and thalamus

Anterior limb of internal capsule here, between lentiform and caudate nuclei

Tail of caudate nucleus

Head of caudate nucleus

Thalamus

Continuity between caudate nucleus and putamen

Putamen of lentiform nucleus

Amygdaloid body

Figure 2–10. The caudate nucleus and putamen in relationship to the thalamus. The internal capsule is absent, but the cleft where it separates the caudate from the thalamus is indicated. (Barr ML, Kiernan JA. *The human nervous system: An anatomical viewpoint*. 6th ed. Philadelphia: JB Lippincott, 1993. With permission.)

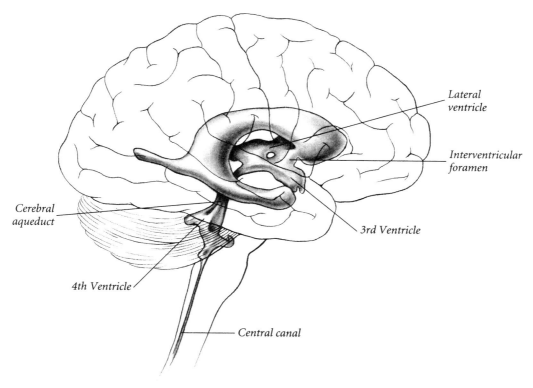

Figure 2–11. The ventricles of the brain, from a lateral view, looking through the brain. The ventricles are spaces, not solid structures.

Special senses are senses with unique receptors located on the head in specific places. These senses include hearing (see Chap. 9), the sense of head motion or equilibrium (see Chap. 10), vision (see Chap. 11), and smell, taste, and the chemical sense (see Chap. 12). Second, they send commands out to the muscles and glands of the head and neck to control behavior. Some nerves are mixed, and carry both sensory and motor signals in different parts of the nerve. They are arranged logically in the brainstem, in vertical columns, according to function. For example, all of the somatic efferents are arranged with their nuclei located ventrally, near the midline of the brainstem (see Fig. 19–9). Table 2–1 lists the cranial nerves.

The cranial nerves are usually classified in seven groups. The special somatic afferents carry information from the special sensory organs of the head: the eye, nose, tongue, and ear. The inner ear contains two sensory organs, the cochlea for hearing and the vestibular labyrinths for detection of head movement. The special somatic afferents include CN II and VIII. The general somatic afferents carry information from the epithelia of the face and mouth, including CN V, IX, and X. The special visceral afferents, for taste and smell, include CN I, VII, IX, and X. The general visceral afferents, carrying sensation from the internal organs, include CN IX and X. The somatic efferents carry motor commands to the striated muscles of the eyes and tongue, which are derived from myotomes. These nerves include CN III, IV, VI, and XII. The special visceral efferents, which carry signals to muscles derived from the branchial arches, control the muscles involved with chewing, facial expression, and speech. The general visceral efferents carry motor commands

			TABLE 2–1
			The Cranial Nerves

Name	Roman Numeral	Type	Function
Olfactory	I	Special visceral afferent	Sense of smell
Optic	II	Special somatic afferent	Sense of vision
Oculomotor	III	1. General somatic motor 2. General visceral motor	1. Four of six extraocular muscles of the eye 2. Intrinsic muscles of the eye
Trochlear	IV	General somatic motor	Superior oblique muscle of the eye
Trigeminal	V	1. General somatic afferent 2. Special visceral motor	1. Input from the skin, mucous membranes, and muscles of the head, and from the meninges 2. Muscles for chewing and the tensor tympani of the middle ear
Abducens	VI	General somatic motor	Lateral rectus muscle of the eye

Facial	VII	1. Intermediate division
		  a. Special visceral afferent
		  b. General somatic afferent
		  c. General visceral motor
		2. Special visceral motor
			1a. Sense of taste
			1b. Skin of the pinna of the ear
			1c. Glands of the face and throat
			2. Muscles of facial expression, stapedius muscle of the middle ear

Auditory (also known as cochlear or vestibulocochlear)	VIII	Special somatic afferent	1. Cochlear branch: sense of hearing 2. Vestibular branch: sense of head position
Glossopharyngeal	IX	1. General somatic afferent 2. General visceral afferent 3. Special visceral afferent 4. General visceral motor 5. Special visceral motor	1. Skin of the pinna 2. Mucous membranes of the head 3. Sense of taste 4. Parotid gland 5. Striated muscles of the throat
Vagus	X	1. General somatic afferent 2. General visceral afferent 3. Special visceral afferent 4. General visceral motor 5. Special visceral motor	1. Meninges, and skin of the pinna 2. Some internal body structures 3. Sense of taste 4. Muscles of the gut, respiration, and heart 5. Striated muscles of the throat
Spinal accessory	XI	Special visceral motor	Primarily sternocleiodomastoid and upper portions of trapezius
Hypoglossal	XII	General somatic motor	Muscles of swallowing

These nerves are listed in rostral to caudal order. By convention they may be indicated either by name or by Roman numeral (e.g., CN III). You may want to use a mnemonic to remember the cranial nerves in order, such as Old Opticians Often Try To Acquire Fair And Glorious Violets Some How (adapted from a mnemonic taught by W. F. McNary, PhD, to his students at the Tufts University–Boston School of Occupational Therapy.) Adapted from Martin JH, Neuroanatomy text and atlas. *2nd ed. Stamford, CT: Appleton and Lange, 1996. With permission.)

to the smooth muscles and glands. These nerves include CN III, VII, IX, and X (see Fig. 2–8).

Support Systems

Inside its armor of bone, the soft, gelatinous nervous system is protected from contusion and infection by tough membranes called **meninges**, and cushioned by **cerebrospinal fluid**,which is formed in theventricles, shown in Figure 2–11. Cerebrospinal fluid is an important part of the circulatory system of the CNS. The CNS is also nourished by complex arterial and venous systems that bring in fresh blood and remove depleted blood and waste products (Figs. 2–12 and 2–13). These support systems of the brain are very important; they are discussed in more detail in Chapter 5.

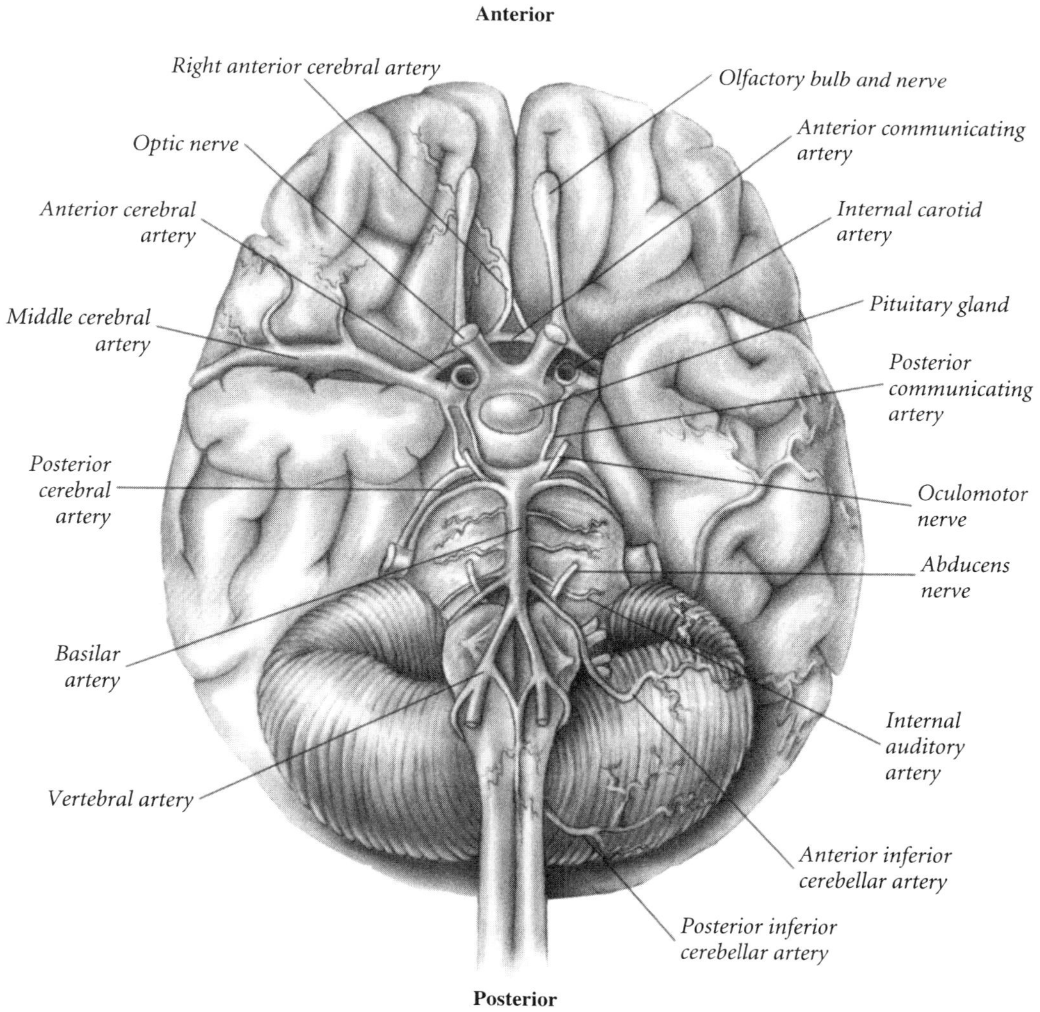

Figure 2–12. Ventral view of the arterial supply to the brain.

Anterior

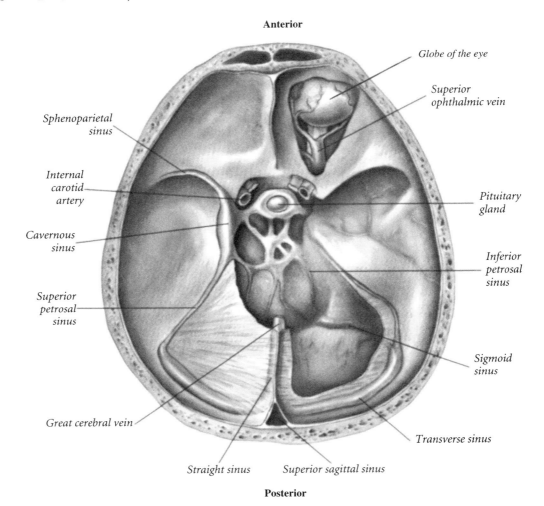

Globe of the eye

Superior ophthalmic vein

Sphenoparietal sinus

Internal carotid artery

Cavernous sinus

Superior petrosal sinus

Great cerebral vein

Pituitary gland

Inferior petrosal sinus

Sigmoid sinus

Transverse sinus

Straight sinus   *Superior sagittal sinus*

Posterior

Figure 2–13. Ventral view of the venous drainage of the brain. (This view is the same as in Fig. 2–12.)

Clinical Correlations

When a patient comes into the clinic with a lesion in a particular part of the CNS or PNS, you must understand the location of the lesion and the function of the damaged area to understand the patient's problems. For example, therapists see many "stroke" victims. A stroke, from the expression "stroke of God," refers to a **cerebrovascular accident** (CVA), caused by either an occlusion or a hemorrhage. An occlu-sive CVA occurs when a blood vessel is blocked, often by the build-up of atherosclerotic plaque or by the presence of a clot that has arrived through the circulation from another part of the body. A hemorrhagic CVA occurs when a blood vessel is broken, as when an aneurysm bursts, or when the pressure in the vessel causes it to burst owing to hypertension. In either case, the loss of blood supply causes an **infarction** in the area fed by that vessel, and the cells die.

The classic CVA patient seen in a rehabilitation center has a lesion from occlusion or hemorrhage of the middle cerebral arteries, manifested by stereotyped unilateral motor disorders, with impaired language or visual perception, depending on which side of the brain the lesion occurred, and often with impaired cognition. To understand such a syndrome, the astute practitioner must understand the pathways of the arterial circulation and the functions of the various areas of the brain.

Less critical situations, where the blood supply is reduced but not completely cut off, are called **transient ischemic attacks** (TIAs). When experiencing a TIA, the person may feel weak or temporarily paralyzed, may have a temporary loss of language, or may be confused. These and other symptoms are caused by **ischemia**, or temporary loss of blood to an area. Ischemia occurs when the blood supply is reduced, from damage to blood vessels caused by diabetes, malformation of the blood vessels, trauma to the vessels during a head injury, or reduction in the internal diameter of the vessels due to arteriosclerosis.

From your understanding of the cranial nerves, you can now understand why audiometric testing is sometimes used to assess brainstem function. CN V and VII control muscles of the middle ear, and CN VIII carries afferent signals about the sense of sound. Therefore, the function of those nerves and their related areas in the brainstem is involved in auditory reflexes that can be tested objectively. This type of testing is important for patients who may be otherwise nonresponsive.

Patients sometimes complain of apparently unrelated symptoms, but a knowledge of basic anatomy, as you have gained from this chapter, may help you to understand them. For example, many patients with traumatic brain injury complain of reduced appetite or reduced smell or taste. Because you know that CN I, VII, and IX send information about smell and taste to the brain, you can understand why a blow to the head might cause this problem.

Similarly, you can now understand why damage to the spinal cord at different locations causes different sensory and motor problems. A lesion at one level may cause a pattern of sensory impairment that differs from the pattern caused by a lesion at another level. An asymmetric lesion, as in **syringomyelia**, may cause sensory loss at one level and motor loss at a different level. To understand the impairments and the subsequent functional limitations, you must understand the anatomy of the spinal cord.

REFERENCES

1. *Dorland's illustrated medical dictionary.* 27th ed. Philadelphia: WB Saunders, 1988.
2. Lockard I. *Desk reference for neuroscience.* 2nd ed. New York: Springer-Verlag, 1992.
3. Brodmann K. *Vergleichende Lokalisationslehre der Grosshimrinde in ihren Prinzipien dargestellt auf Grund des Zellenbaus.* Leipzig: Barth, 1909.

3

Fundamental Elements of the Nervous System 1: The Neuron

DAVID L. SOMERS, PhD, PT
F. RICHARD CLEMENTE, PhD, PT

• • •

In the previous chapter, you learned about the gross anatomy of the nervous system. In this chapter, you will learn about the smallest functional unit of the nervous system, the **neuron.** Above all else, neurons are communication machines. They spend their lives passing information from one neuron to another so that their host can perceive, interpret, and behave within the world. As you might expect, given their role as information couriers, neurons are morphologically and biochemically designed for this purpose. Most neurons have one portion that is designed to receive and process information, a second portion that is designed to move information rapidly, and a third portion that is designed to deliver information to another neuron. In this chapter, you will learn about the features of neurons that enable them to be such fine information couriers. In later chapters, you will see how neurons come together to perform distinct functions.

Overview of a Prototypical Neuron

Although the nervous system comprises many different types of neurons, they all have features in common. Figure 3–1 illustrates a prototypical neuron. Neurons usually have a somewhat central, expanded region called the body or **soma,** and numerous projections or processes, the **axons** and **dendrites,** that extend out from the soma. The entire neuron is a three-dimensional structure enclosed by a single semipermeable membrane, the plasma membrane or **plasmalemma** (Fig. 3–2). This semipermeable

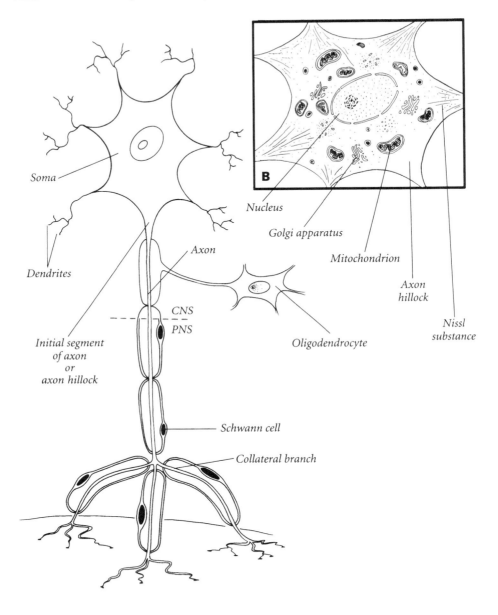

Soma

Dendrites

Axon

CNS
PNS

Initial segment
of axon
or
axon hillock

Schwann cell

Collateral branch

B

Nucleus

Golgi apparatus

Mitochondrion

Axon
hillock

Nissl
substance

Oligodendrocyte

A

Figure 3–1. A: A typical neuron with soma, dendrites, and axon. **B:** Close-up of the soma showing the axon hillock and typical organelles, including the nucleus, Golgi apparatus, Nissl substance, mitochondria. Note that the axon hillock contains no Nissl substance. (Adapted and reproduced with permission from Junqueira LC, Carneiro J, Long JA. *Basic histology.* 5th ed. Norwalk, CT: Appleton & Lange, 1986.)

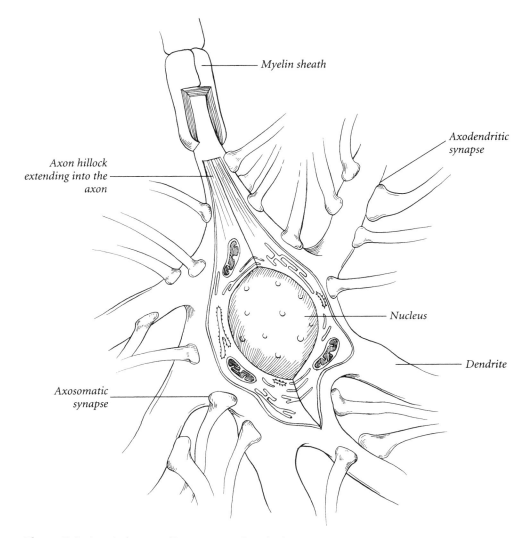

Figure 3–2. A typical mammalian neuron with multiple synaptic contacts. Note the dendrite, axon hillock extending into the axon, nucleus, axodendritic synapse, axosomatic synapse, and myelin sheath. (Adapted and reproduced with permission from Kristic RB. *Ultrastructure of the mammalian cell.* New York/Berlin: Springer-Verlag, 1973.)

membrane selectively regulates the movement of certain substances and ions into and out of the neuron, a function that is central to a neuron's ability to process and move information. The plasmalemma contains the cytoplasm of the neuron, the **neuroplasm,** and various organelles and vesicles.

The neuroplasm of the soma contains the organelles necessary for synthesizing proteins. These or-

ganelles include the nucleus, nucleolus, Golgi apparatus, rough endoplasmic reticulum, and ribosomes. Although these cellular constituents are also found in nonneuronal cells, in neurons they have some distinguishing features. First, the rough endoplasmic reticulum and ribosomes in neurons are collectively known as **Nissl substance,** named after Franz Nissl, the originator of a stain for them. Nissl substance is distributed throughout the neuroplasm of the soma with the exception of a small, tapering region, the **axon hillock** (see Fig. 3–1). The axon hillock is the site of origin for the axon. Second, in neurons some of the synthetic products of these organelles are **neurotransmitters.** Neurotransmitters are chemical messengers released by one neuron to communicate with another neuron. They will be discussed in detail in Chapter 4. Third, the organelles of mature neurons are incapable of orchestrating a division of the cell. Thus, once a neuron is born, it is not able to divide and proliferate.

Two types of processes extend from the soma. The first of these is the axon, a neuronal process that extends toward an anatomic or physiologic target. Neurons usually have only one axon, which is unbranched near its origin. Axons vary in size from 1 to 18 microns (μm) (which is 0.001–0.018 mm) in diameter and from several microns to several feet in length. As an axon approaches its target structure, it may split into numerous terminal branches. Typically, the cytoplasm of axons, or **axoplasm,** does not contain Nissl substance; consequently, proteins cannot be synthesized in axons. Any protein substance required by the axon or at the terminal of the axon must be synthesized in the soma and transported out into the axon. The movement of protein substances from the soma out into the periphery of the axon is accomplished by a mechanism known as **anterograde axoplasmic transport,** a pulsatile or ratchet-like movement along the microtubular skeleton of the axon. Substances that enter through the terminal of the axon can be transported toward the soma in a like manner. This mechanism is called **retrograde axoplasmic transport.**

The second type of process that extends from the soma is a dendrite. Neurons usually have more than one dendrite, and each of these may be highly branched. At least in their proximal portions, dendrites have Nissl substance in their cytoplasm or **dendroplasm,** and they can produce protein substances. Dendrites are usually thinner and shorter than axons, and they are often equipped with small projections or spines that extend from the dendrite into the surrounding neuropil.

Although there are exceptions, most neurons receive information at their dendrites and soma. Here, the information is processed and often passed along to the axon. Axons then rapidly transport the information to their terminals and pass the information on to a target (frequently another neuron).

Classification of Neurons

Neurons are often named or classified for their physical characteristics. Certain neurons, such as giant cortical neurons, are named for their size, whereas others, like the pyramidal neurons of the cerebral cortex, are named for the shape of their somata. One general classification system is based on the number of processes extending from the soma. For example, **bipolar neurons** have two processes, one axon and one dendrite (Fig. 3–3). This type of neuron is commonly found in the neuronal pathways that convey or process information about the special senses (i.e., hearing, vision, smell and equilibrium). **Multipolar neurons** (see Fig. 3–3) are equipped with numerous processes, usually one axon and any number of dendrites. Anterior horn cells of the spinal cord—primary motor neurons—are good examples of multipolar neurons. **Pseudounipolar neurons** (see Fig. 3–3) appear to have only one process that bifurcates. Part of the process extends from a receptor in the periphery to the cell body—the **peripheral process**—and part of the process extends from the cell body toward the axis of the nervous system—the **central process.** Both of these processes function like axons. Dorsal root ganglia cells, the primary sensory neurons of the peripheral nervous system, are pseudounipolar nerve cells.

A functionally more specific classification system for neurons is based on the neurotransmitters used by the neuron for transferring information from one neuron to another. In this system, **cholinergic neurons** use acetylcholine as a chemical messenger, whereas **adrenergic neurons** use epinephrine (adrenaline) and **noradrenergic neurons** use norepinephrine. Other neurons classified as **peptidergic** use peptides as neurotransmitters.

Synaptic Neurotransmission

The nervous system is the communication system of the body. It links all of the other systems of the body and links the internal and external environments. For the nervous system to perform this task, individ-

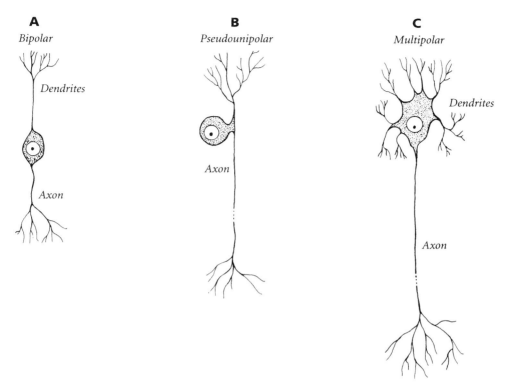

Figure 3–3. Three types of neurons, classified according to the number of processes extending from the soma. (Adapted and reproduced with permission from Cormack DH. *Ham's histology.* 9th ed. Philadelphia: JB Lippincott, 1987.)

ual neurons must communicate with each other. The **synapse** is one point of functional communication or association between two neurons. Synapses can form between virtually any of the various neuronal elements (Fig. 3–4). Two common types of synapses are **axosomatic** synapses, the communication between an axon and a cell body, and **axodendritic** synapses, the communication between an axon and a dendrite. At these synapses, a chemical messenger, or neurotransmitter, is released from the axon of one neuron (**presynaptic element**) and picked up by the dendrite or cell body of another neuron (**postsynaptic element**).

Although a single presynaptic axon is usually limited in the types of neurotransmitters it can release, a host of different transmitters are used by the nervous system (see Chapter 4). The postsynaptic dendrites and soma of a synapse have **receptors** in their plas-malemmas that bind the particular transmitters released by the presynaptic axon. When the neurotransmitter binds to its receptor, a number of responses can occur in the dendrites and soma of the postsynaptic neuron. Such responses are profound and can even include an alteration in the transcription of genes in the postsynaptic cell. Perhaps the most striking alteration a neurotransmitter can produce in the postsynaptic dendrite or soma is one that changes the electrochemical condition of the neuron.

Electrochemical Properties of Dendrites and the Soma

The semipermeable plasmalemma of the dendrites and soma differentially regulates the movement of ions into and out of the neuron. In the resting state (i.e., before a neurotransmitter is released), the plas-

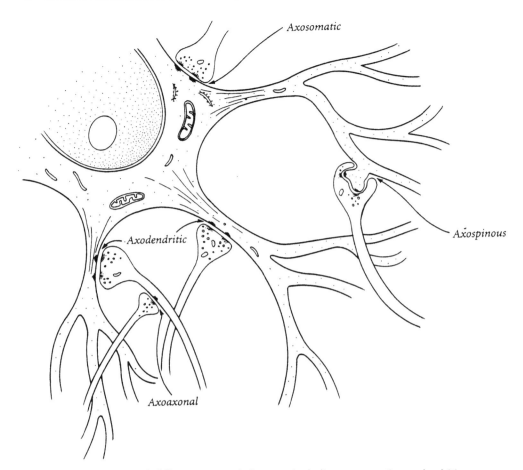

Figure 3–4. Synapses with different neuronal elements, including axosomatic, axodendritic, axospinous, and axoaxonal synapses. (Adapted and reproduced with permission from Bunge R. *Bailey's textbook of histology.* 16th ed. Baltimore: Williams & Wilkins, 1971.)

malemma does not permit the free movement of ions into or out of the cell. Two ions are particularly important to information transfer. The first of these ions is sodium (Na^+), an ion that is not permitted to move across the plasmalemma to any great extent. The second ion, potassium (K^+), is permitted to move with much greater freedom, but it too is subject to some restrictions. Not only is the movement of these two ions influenced by the plasmalemma, but the ions are unevenly distributed across the membrane (Fig. 3–5). The plasmalemma maintains this distribution using a transport mechanism located in the membrane that moves three Na^+ ions out of the dendrites and soma while simultaneously moving two K^+ ions into the neuron. In part because of the action of this **sodium–potassium** pump, an electrical gradient develops with a greater positive charge outside of the plasmalemma. The uneven distribution of ions across the plasmalemma produces a net charge, so the neuron is said to be polarized. The resting membrane potential of -60 to -80 millivolts (mV) means the inside of the neuron has a relatively negative charge compared with the outside of the neuron (see Fig. 3–5).

The action of the sodium–potassium pump also causes a chemical concentration gradient to develop

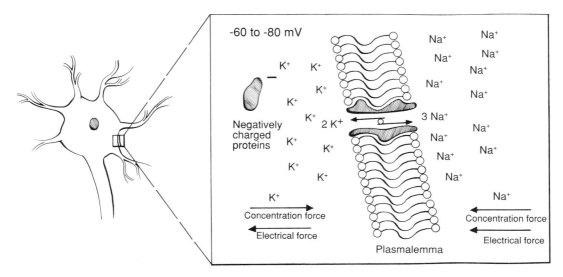

Figure 3–5. Electrochemical condition of a prototypical neuron. The box represents the resting electrochemical conditions found in the plasmalemma throughout the dendrites and soma of a neuron. The channel in the center of the membrane is an energy-consuming sodium–potassium pump that maintains the distribution of these ions across the membrane. The intracellular environment is shown to the left of the bilaminar membrane, the extracellular environment to the right.

across the plasmalemma of the dendrites and soma. The concentration of Na^+ ions is greater outside the dendrites and soma than inside the neuron (see Fig. 3–5). Both the electrical and concentration gradients favor moving Na^+ into the dendrites and soma. The concentration of K^+ ions, however, is higher inside the dendrites and soma than outside the neuron. Therefore, the concentration gradient forces potassium ions out of the cell while the electrical gradient holds them inside the cell. In fact, these two forces are almost but not quite equal when the membrane is at rest.

Although Na^+ and K^+ are vital to information transfer, the plasmalemma regulates other ions as well. Some of these ions, like calcium (Ca^{++}), are restricted in their movement and are maintained at a high concentration outside of the cell. Others, like chloride, are permitted to move more freely across the membranes of dendrites and the soma.

Postsynaptic Responses to Synaptic Neurotransmission

When a neurotransmitter is released from a presynaptic axon terminal and binds to its receptor on a post-synaptic neuron, the resting electrochemical condition of the postsynaptic dendrites and soma can be altered. This alteration is most directly achieved by changing the permeability of the postsynaptic plasmalemma to ions. For example, the neurotransmitter could cause the dendrite or soma to allow more cations (positively charged ions), such as Na^+, to cross the membrane into the neuron. This flow of positive ions into the dendrites or soma decreases the potential difference between the inside and outside of the neuron. That is, the inside of the dendrites or soma becomes more positive after the release of the transmitter than it was before the release of the transmitter (i.e., at rest). This change in membrane permeability then depolarizes the postsynaptic neuron. Alternatively, the postsynaptic membrane could become less permeable to cations or more permeable to anions (negatively charged ions). This sort of change in permeability produces an even greater potential difference between the inside and outside of the neuron. Then, the inside of the dendrites or soma becomes more negative after the release of the transmitter than it was before the release. In this case, the postsynaptic dendrites and soma become hyperpolarized.

Depending on the receptor expressed by the post-synaptic membrane, the release of neurotransmitter can produce either **depolarization** or **hyperpolarization** of the dendrites or soma. If the postsynaptic membrane permeability changes so that a net increase in positive charge moves into the neuron, then the cell will begin to depolarize. This depolarization of the postsynaptic membrane is known as an **excitatory postsynaptic potential** (EPSP; Fig. 3–6). Conversely, if the permeability changes result in a net increase in the negative charge that enters the postsynaptic neuron, then the cell will begin to hyperpolarize, or become more negative than it was at rest. This type of hyperpolarizing synaptic event produces an **inhibitory postsynaptic potential** (IPSP; see Fig. 3–6).

Postsynaptic potentials in dendrites and the soma are transient changes in the postsynaptic membrane potential that are characterized by several features. Postsynaptic potentials travel decrementally; that is, as they move along the postsynaptic membrane, there is an inverse relationship between distance traveled and amplitude and between time traveled and amplitude. Therefore, as the distance traveled or the time elapsed from the original postsynaptic potential increases, the influence of the postsynaptic potential on the postsynaptic membrane decreases.

Integration of Postsynaptic Responses to Neurotransmission

At any given time, the dendrites and soma can receive EPSPs and IPSPs simultaneously from the axons of thousands of other neurons. The responses of the target dendrites and soma are determined by the net effect of all of the incoming potentials. The target dendrites and soma electrically sum the incoming potentials and assume a new electrochemical condition. If the net excitatory influence is greater, then the dendrites and soma depolarize, and the inside of the cell becomes more positive. If the net influence is inhibitory, the target neuron hyperpolarizes and the inside of the cell becomes more negative.

Because postsynaptic potentials travel decrementally, integration of these potentials by a target neuron depends on both temporal and spatial factors. When a target neuron receives an EPSP, its membrane depolarizes. This change in membrane potential is transient, and with time the membrane begins to return to resting levels. If the target neuron re-

ceives a second EPSP at the same location, an additional depolarization of the membrane occurs. The net effect from the two EPSPs depends on how much the target neuron has recovered from the first EPSP when it receives the second EPSP. This summation of EPSPs is called **temporal summation** because the net effect is directly time dependent (Fig. 3–7A). The target dendrites and soma carry out this same integration process when they receive multiple IPSPs or a combination of EPSPs and IPSPs in the same location but at different times.

The target dendrites and soma are also capable of **spatial summation**, integrating multiple postsynaptic potentials that arrive simultaneously but at different locations on the neuron (see Fig. 3–7B). Both EPSPs and IPSPs are caused by the movement of electrical charges (ions) across the membrane. If multiple EPSPs arrive at the target neuron at the same time but at different locations on the cell, the effects of the ion flow are summed, resulting in greater depolarization of the neuron. Similarly, if multiple IPSPs reach the target neuron at the same time but at different locations on the cell, the effects of the ion flow are additive. Because EPSPs and IPSPs result from ion flow in opposite directions across the membrane, if multiple EPSPs and IPSPs arrive at the target neuron simultaneously but at different locations, they too will be additive and produce little or no net change in membrane potential.

The electrical integration of incoming information to the dendrites and soma of a neuron allows post-synaptic neurons to process huge amounts of information. This processing is vital to the function of the nervous system. Without it, something as simple as localizing a pinprick on the skin would be impossible. Such processing, however, is meaningful only if a neuron can pass on the product of its work to another neuron or physiologic target. To do this, the dendrites and soma use the axon, the portion of the neuron that rapidly carries the processed information from the soma to the next neuronal or physiologic target.

Development of an Action Potential

Located in the plasmalemma at the initial segment of the axon, or axon hillock, are many protein channels for Na^+ and K^+. The concentration of these channels is higher here than in any other region of the dendrites or soma. Under resting conditions,

(*Text continues on p. 39*)

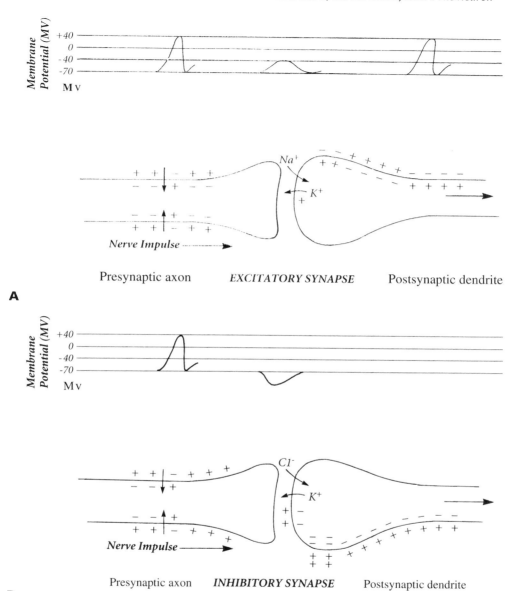

Figure 3–6. A: Synaptic transmission that produces an excitatory postsynaptic potential (EPSP). **B:** Synaptic transmission that produces an inhibitory postsynaptic potential (IPSP). Note the changes that occur in the membrane potential. The EPSP leads to an eventual action potential along the postsynaptic axon.

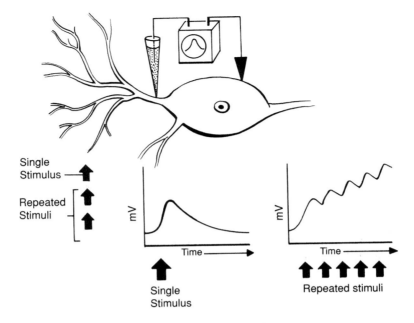

A   TEMPORAL SUMMATION

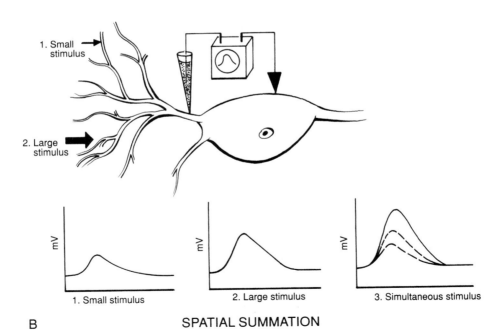

B   SPATIAL SUMMATION

Figure 3–7. Integration of action potentials by individual neurons: **A:** Temporal summation. **B:** Spatial summation. (Adapted and reproduced with permission from Schauf C, Moffett D, Moffett S *Human physiology.* St. Louis: Times Mirror/Mosby, 1990.)

these channels are closed so that Na$^+$ and K$^+$ are not permitted to flow through them. Because the electrochemical condition of the axon is similar to that of the dendrites and soma, at rest Na$^+$ ions are highly concentrated outside the axon hillock, K$^+$ ions are highly concentrated inside the hillock, and the inside of the hillock is negative relative to the outside (-60 to -80 mV).

When the electrical integration of incoming information to the dendrites and soma is such that a critical amount of depolarization occurs in the axon hillock, the Na$^+$channels located there respond by opening. In general, the membrane of the axon hillock must become 10 to 20 mV less negative than the membrane potential of a neuron at rest before Na$^+$ channels begin to open in earnest (Fig. 3–8A). When this amount of depolarization occurs—an event called **threshold** depolarization—the opening of the Na$^+$ channels causes a significant influx of Na$^+$ into the axon hillock. The rush of positive ions into the axon reverses the resting membrane potential and the inside of the axon hillock almost immediately changes its membrane potential from a negative (-55 to -60 mV) to a positive ($+25$ to $+35$ mV)

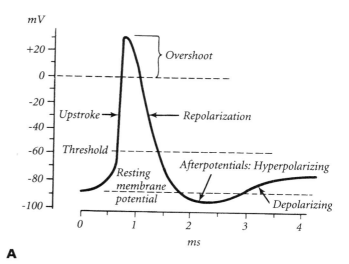

A

Figure 3–8. A: Changes in the neuronal membrane potential during the action potential cycle. (Adapted and reproduced with permission from Schmidt, RF, Thews G, eds. *Human physiology.* New York, Berlin: Springer- Verlag, 1983.) **B:** Changes in ion conductance across the neuron plasmalemma during an action potential cycle. Note the relationship between the change in ion conductance and the curve of the action potential cycle. (The unit mmho/cm² is a unit of measure for membrane resistance.) (Adapted and reproduced with permission from Hodgkin AL. Ionic movements and electrical activity in giant nerve fibers. *Proceedings of the Royal Society of London [Biology]* 1958; 148:1)

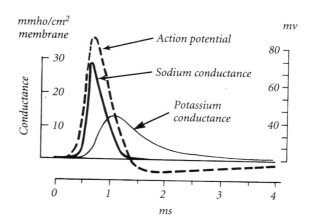

B

value. This explosive change in ion conductance across the axon hillock plasmalemma with the subsequent dramatic reversal of the membrane potential constitutes an **action potential** (see Fig. 3–8A).

The increased Na^+ conductance peaks at approximately the peak of the action potential and rapidly decreases to resting levels (see Fig. 3–8B). Almost immediately after they are opened, the Na^+ channels are closed and no additional Na^+ enters or leaves the axon hillock. At approximately the same time that the Na^+ channels close, the K^+ channels open, and K^+ ions begin to move out of the axon hillock. At this point, more K^+ ions are leaving the axon than there are Na^+ ions entering it. The result of this ion flow is that the membrane potential begins to decrease and approaches the resting membrane potential; the membrane is repolarizing (see Fig. 3–8A). K^+ conductance peaks at about the midpoint of the **repolarization** phase and persists for a much longer period of time than does the increased Na^+ conductance (see Fig. 3–8B). Eventually no more Na^+ ions move into the axon hillock, but K^+ ions continue to leave, causing the membrane potential to drop below resting levels (-100 mV). When the membrane potential drops below resting levels, the axon hillock is said to be hyperpolarized (see Fig. 3–8A). As hyperpolarization occurs, the K^+ channels close in the axon hillock. Because Na^+ and K^+ channels are now closed, the conductance of these ions returns to normal resting levels. The resting membrane potential is then reestablished by the sodium–potassium pump.

When the threshold membrane potential is reached in the axon hillock, the sequence of component phases of the action potential begins and the axon hillock passes through all of the phases. Thus, an action potential is an "all-or-none event"; once triggered, it continues until its completion.

During the period of the action potential, the axon hillock is less responsive to other stimuli. The Na^+ channels are inactivated for a period of time immediately after the peak of Na^+ conductance. At this point, no Na^+ ions move into or out of the axon hillock. During this **absolute refractory period**, the axon hillock cannot be stimulated to fire another action potential regardless of the magnitude of the stimulus. The absolute refractory period limits the number of action potentials a neuron can discharge over a given period of time. Shortly after the absolute refractory period, the Na^+ channels gradually become activated and K^+ conductance nears its peak as the axon hillock plas-

malemma begins to repolarize. At this point, the initial segment of the axon enters the **relative refractory period**. During the relative refractory period, fewer than normal activated Na^+ channels are available. If stimulated to open, however, the number of activated channels is sufficient to allow adequate Na^+ conductance to move the membrane potential to threshold and trigger another action potential. To open enough of these available Na^+ channels, the magnitude of the stimulus received at the axon hillock must be greater than the magnitude of the stimulus that can normally trigger an action potential.

Propagation of the Action Potential

Once an action potential occurs at the axon hillock (Fig. 3–9A), it moves without fail toward the axon terminal. This progression is caused by Na^+ ion diffusion within the axoplasm of the neuron and the presence of voltage-sensitive Na^+ and K^+ channels in the axon cell membrane. As the Na^+ ions diffuse within the axoplasm down the axon (away from the axon hillock), they depolarize a new segment of axon cell membrane. This depolarization is sufficient to move the membrane potential past threshold in this new segment of the axon. Because the plasmalemma of this segment contains a high concentration of voltage-sensitive Na^+ and K^+ channels, a threshold depolarization opens the channels, producing the familiar electrical signature of an action potential (see Fig. 3–9B). In this way, the action potential is completely renewed at a segment of axonal membrane that is closer to the axon terminal.

What happens to the Na^+ ions that enter at this new segment? Some of the Na^+ diffuses through the axoplasm back toward the axon hillock, and some of it diffuses further down the axon. When the Na^+ diffuses closer to the axon hillock, axonal membrane that contains refractory Na^+ channels depolarizes (see Fig. 3–9B). Because these channels are unresponsive to the depolarization caused by the diffusing Na^+, the change in membrane potential here does not affect the channels. When the Na^+ diffuses down the axon, however, it depolarizes membrane containing Na^+ and K^+ channels that are fully capable of opening and renewing the action potential. They do so, and the action potential is now renewed at a segment of the axon that is closer still to the axon terminal (see Fig. 3–9C). This process repeats all the way down the axon cell membrane un-

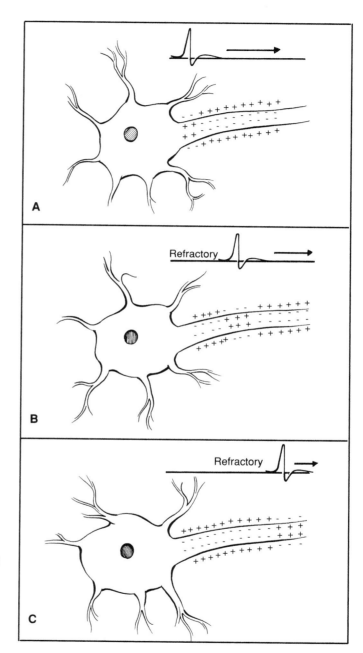

Figure 3–9. Propagation of an action potential. **A–C:** Images of the same neuron over time. The action potential starts at the axon hillock in **(A)** and proceeds away from the cell body in **(B)** and **(C).** In each panel, the electrical condition of the entire axon is depicted above the cell. Notice how, over time **(A–C),** the action potential, indicated by $++$ inside and $--$ outside, moves away from the cell body, leaving refractory channels behind it.

til it reaches the axon terminal. Because an action potential is an all-or-none event and is constantly renewed, the action potential that arrives at the axon terminal is identical to the original action potential started at the axon hillock.

The speed of propagation or **conduction velocity** of an action potential depends primarily on the diameter of the axon and the presence of a **myelin** sheath. The relationship between the diameter of an axon and the internal resistance that it imposes to local current flow is inverse. Larger-diameter axons impose less internal resistance to local current flow, so the adjacent areas of their membranes can be driven to threshold more quickly than in smaller axons. Therefore, the greater the diameter of the axon, the faster the conduction velocity.

Myelin is an insulating lipid that invests axons of various sizes. Specialized glial cells—Schwann cells in the peripheral nervous system and oligodendrocytes in the central nervous system—produce this substance. (These and other glial cells are described in Chapter 5). In both the peripheral and central nervous systems, myelin surrounds axons in multilayered segments that are separated by small areas of bare axon membrane, the **nodes of Ranvier** (Fig. 3–10). The myelin segments act as electrical insulators and significantly increase the resistance to ion flow across the covered portions of the membrane. Unlike the membrane under the myelin segments, the membrane at the nodes of Ranvier is rich in Na^+ and K^+ channels and retains the normal electrical properties that allow voltage-dependent ion flow. Therefore, action potentials do not occur along the myelinated segments but do occur at the nodes.

As an action potential propagates along a myelinated axon, it demonstrates **saltatory conduction** (see Fig. 3–10). The action potential moves from one node of Ranvier to the next, depolarizing only the areas of membrane at the nodes. Because less of the total membrane is depolarized during saltatory conduction, the local current flow travels some distance along the membrane before triggering the next action potential. Therefore, saltatory conduction increases the conduction velocity of an action potential.

The Axon Terminal and Release of Neurotransmitters

Ultimately, an action potential reaches the end of an axon. The Na^+ and K^+ channels located there orchestrate the familiar depolarization–repolarization sequence that is characteristic of all action potentials. The end of the axon, or **terminal bouton**, releases neurotransmitters in response to the arriving action potential. In this way, the information carried on the axon passes on to another dendrite or soma through release of a chemical messenger.

The terminal bouton and the dendrite or soma on which the bouton is releasing neurotransmitter form an intimate connection called a synapse (Fig. 3–11). The terminal bouton is the presynaptic or **afferent element** of the synapse. It usually contains membrane-bound vesicles of neurotransmitter substances, some of which are released with the arrival of the action potential. The process receiving this chemical message is the postsynaptic or **efferent element**. It usually has receptors for the released neurotransmitters in its membrane so that it can respond to the presynaptic element. Therefore, the presynaptic and postsynaptic elements are highly specialized for the transfer of information across the synapse. The presynaptic and postsynaptic elements are separated by a

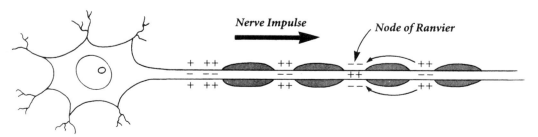

Figure 3–10. Saltatory conduction of an action potential along a myelinated axon. Myelin segments, separated by nodes of Ranvier, encase the axon.

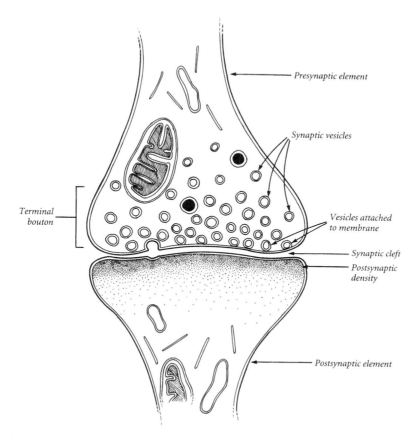

Presynaptic element

Synaptic vesicles

Terminal bouton

Vesicles attached to membrane

Synaptic cleft

Postsynaptic density

Postsynaptic element

Figure 3–11. A typical synapse, including presynaptic element, postsynaptic element, synaptic cleft, terminal bouton, synaptic vesicles, vesicles bound to the presynaptic membrane, and postsynaptic density.

small space (20–30 nm [10^{-6} mm]) or **synaptic cleft**. Although the synaptic elements are not in direct contact with each other, their relative positions are kept constant by intercellular filaments. These intercellular filaments span the synaptic cleft and are enmeshed in the ground substance and filaments of the **postsynaptic density** (see Fig. 3–11).

When the action potential arrives in the terminal bouton, it starts a cascade of events that leads to the release of neurotransmitters at the synapse (Fig. 3–12). The first step in this cascade is the opening of voltage-dependent Ca^{++} channels in the axon terminal. Because the extracellular space has a high concentration of Ca^{++}, the opening of these channels permits Ca^{++} to rush into the terminal. The in-

creased intracellular concentration of Ca^{++} influences several proteins that are found in most presynaptic axon terminals. These proteins can be divided into three functional classifications:

1 The first class of protein helps the synaptic vesicles dock and fuse with the axon terminal membrane.[1,2] This group of proteins directs the neurotransmitter-laden synaptic vesicles to the right position and readies them to fuse with the axon terminal membrane. This part of the process is complete before the action potential depolarizes the axon terminal.

2 Once the vesicles are docked and prepared for fusion, a second class of proteins seems to

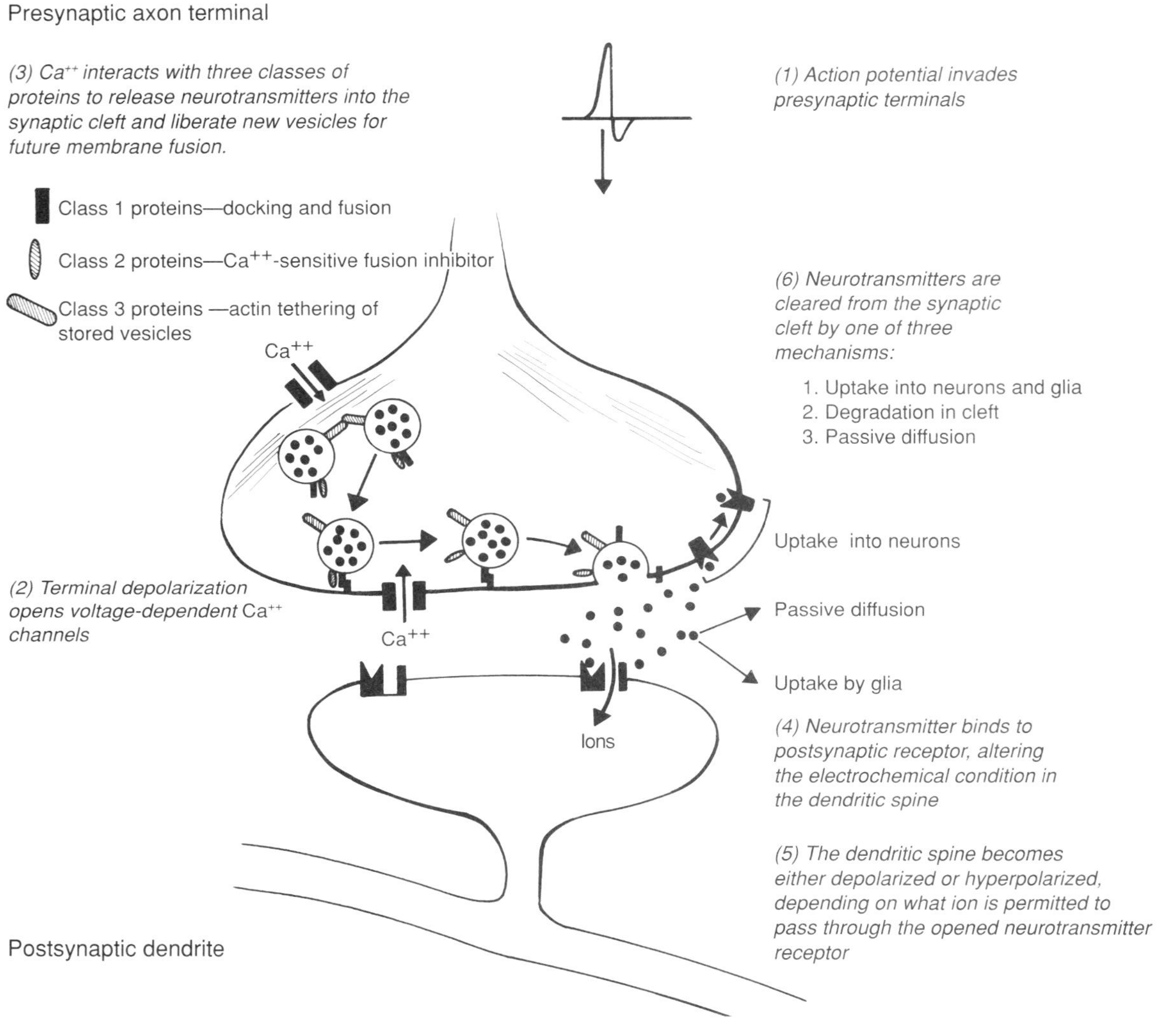

Presynaptic axon terminal

(3) Ca^{++} interacts with three classes of proteins to release neurotransmitters into the synaptic cleft and liberate new vesicles for future membrane fusion.

▮ Class 1 proteins—docking and fusion

▯ Class 2 proteins—Ca^{++}-sensitive fusion inhibitor

▱ Class 3 proteins —actin tethering of stored vesicles

Ca^{++}

(1) Action potential invades presynaptic terminals

(6) Neurotransmitters are cleared from the synaptic cleft by one of three mechanisms:

1. Uptake into neurons and glia
2. Degradation in cleft
3. Passive diffusion

Uptake into neurons

Passive diffusion

Uptake by glia

(2) Terminal depolarization opens voltage-dependent Ca^{++} channels

Ca^{++}

Ions

(4) Neurotransmitter binds to postsynaptic receptor, altering the electrochemical condition in the dendritic spine

(5) The dendritic spine becomes either depolarized or hyperpolarized, depending on what ion is permitted to pass through the opened neurotransmitter receptor

Postsynaptic dendrite

Figure 3–12. The steps in synaptic neurotransmission. Italicized descriptions chronologically depict the passage of information from the axon terminal of one neuron to the dendritic spine of another.

inhibit the completion of the fusion process until the concentration of Ca^{++} increases in the axon terminal.[3] As Ca^{++} levels rise, the inhibition over the first class of proteins is removed and the fusion process continues. The vesicle and axon terminal membranes fuse, and the synaptic vesicle releases its neurotransmitter into the synaptic cleft.

3 The third class of proteins helps retrieve new synaptic vesicles from a storage area so that the release process can be repeated. The storage area is a network of actin filaments (a cytoskeletal protein). This third class of proteins tethers synaptic vesicles to this network and to each other.[4] When Ca^{++} enters the axon terminal, these proteins probably release the synaptic vesicles from their storage site in the actin network, now making them eligible to dock with the axon terminal membrane. In this way, synaptic vesicles are constantly made available for docking and fusion with the axon terminal membrane. Because emptied synaptic vesicles are recycled, as long as neurotransmitter molecules are available, the process can occur repeatedly.

Once neurotransmitters are in the synaptic cleft, they bind to postsynaptic receptors present in the cell membrane of the dendrite or soma involved in the synapse (see Fig. 3–12). This binding can produce many different responses, including an alteration in the permeability of the postsynaptic membrane to ions and the subsequent development of an EPSP or IPSP. Synaptic communication is now largely complete. One neuron, having received information at its dendrite or soma, processed that information, sent it down its axon as an action potential, and passed the information on to another neuron through the release of a chemical messenger.

Termination of Synaptic Communication

Axon terminals receive a constant barrage of action potentials. If each of these potentials is to have an effect on the next neuron, then the impact of any one action potential on a postsynaptic neuron must be of finite duration. For the most part, synaptic communication occurs for a brief period of time because neurotransmitters are removed from the synaptic cleft in three ways (see Fig. 3–12). First, some axon terminals and glial cells have a protein in their membranes that binds to the transmitter and then dumps the substance back into the respective cell. Often the same axon terminal that released the neurotransmitter picks it up so that it can be reused by the axon terminal. The neurotransmitters dopamine, aspartate, and glutamate are usually removed from the synaptic cleft in this fashion.[5-7] Second, many synaptic clefts contain enzymes that degrade neurotransmitters, rendering them inactive at their receptors. The neurotransmitter acetylcholine and the peptide neurotransmitters[8] are usually removed this way. Third, all neurotransmitters can passively diffuse out of the synaptic cleft. Regardless of how the transmitter is removed from the cleft, the chemical messenger is no longer available to bind with its receptor, and the synaptic communication is ended.

Not all synapses occur between axon terminals and the dendrites (axodendritic) or soma (axosomatic) of another neuron. Some axons synapse with other axons (**axoaxonic synapses**; see Fig. 3–4). In these synapses, the presynaptic and postsynaptic elements are axons. Often, axoaxonic synapses serve a modulatory function. In other words, the presynaptic axon modulates the postsynaptic axon. Figure 3–4 shows an axoaxonic synapse just before the postsynaptic axon synapses on the dendrite of a third neuron. Therefore, the axoaxonic synapse may modulate how information is passed to the dendrite of this third neuron.

Nonsynaptic Neurotransmission

Synaptic neurotransmission is not the only form of communication used by the nervous system. Some neurons are electrically coupled instead of being coupled by the release of a chemical messenger. Figure 3–13 illustrates a prototypical electrical coupling between two neurons. In most cases, the plasmalemmas of the two neurons involved are closely approximated at the area of coupling. Although the membranes themselves do not fuse, they form a contact with one another called a **gap junction**. In the gap junction, protein channels (**connexons**) present in the plasmalemma of each of the neurons precisely align themselves, creating an open pore between the two cells. This pore is large enough to permit the movement of many kinds of molecules back and forth between the neurons involved. Among the molecules that can pass through the pores are ions. Because ions can move freely between the cytoplasm of the two cells, when one neuron is depolarized by a sudden influx of positive ions (Neuron 1 in Fig. 3–13), the depolarization is immediately passed to the second neuron (neuron 2 in Fig. 3–13). The opposite would be true if Neuron 2 was to be depolarized first.

As you can imagine, if two or three cells were so joined, they might all become depolarized almost simultaneously. In fact, simultaneous depolarization occurs between neurons in several brain regions where synchronized depolarization is useful. For example, neurons in the hypothalamus that release hormones into the blood stream may have gap junctions between them,[9,10] presumably so that a surge of hormone is released when the coupled cells are depolarized.[11] Amazingly, the electrical couplings between neurons appear to be quite plastic. Although gap junctions have not been identified between these particular cells, the membranes of some hypothalamic neurons become intimately juxtaposed

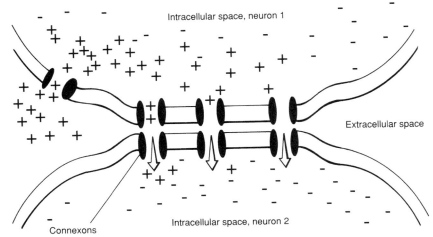

Figure 3–13. Two neurons whose cell membranes are electrically coupled. A cation channel has opened in neuron 1, and the ensuing depolarization is moving across the pores of a gap junction to depolarize neuron 2. The passage of information through electrical couplings is faster than through synapses.

when hormone release is necessary—for example, to orchestrate milk let-down in a nursing mother.[12,13] When the child is weaned, the presumed electrical coupling between the neurons is broken[12,13] and will reform should the mother begin to nurse again.

Neurons can also communicate another way. Sometimes neurons release neurotransmitters as if participating in a synapse, but the apparent postsynaptic element has no receptor for the released neurotransmitter. Instead, the receptor is found on another neuron at some distance from the presumed presynaptic element.[14,15] The neurotransmitter must diffuse through extracellular space before encountering its postsynaptic target. This kind of communication is called **parasynaptic neurotransmission** to distinguish it from classic synaptic neurotransmission.

Clinical Correlations

You now understand that a neuron has portions that receive and process information (dendrites and the soma), a portion that rapidly moves information (axon), and a portion that delivers information to another neuron (axon terminal or terminal bouton). Disease or dysfunction in any of these portions affects behavior. Your appreciation of the neuron

will help you understand the underlying mechanisms of neurologic disorders and their therapeutic interventions.

Alzheimer's disease is one example of a pathologic process that affects the receptive and information-processing portion of neurons. This disease is characterized by a progressive dementia and by the death of neurons that use acetylcholine in the brain.[16] Many cholinergic neurons participate in the formation of spatial memories,[17] a type of memory that people with Alzheimer's disease seem to lose early in the course of the syndrome. One therapeutic strategy to reverse or slow the dementia is to replace the missing acetylcholine pharmacologically. Unfortunately, this strategy has proven unsuccessful, probably because these patients' neurons have diminished responses to acetylcholine. A diminished response is partly the product of membrane changes in the dendrites and somata of neurons that normally respond to acetylcholine.[18] Thus, disease-induced alterations in the dendritic and somal cell membranes of neurons impair the ability of these cells to receive and process information passed through acetylcholine neurotransmission.

The axon is also a target of several categories of diseases. One such category is demyelinating disease, one of the most common of which is multiple sclerosis (MS). Most often, MS first appears during the third or fourth decade, more often in women. This disease is characterized by areas of demyelination or **plaques** that occur throughout the nervous system, especially the central nervous system. The visual system appears to be especially sensitive to plaque formation, whereas the peripheral nervous system in general demonstrates little involvement. Although the exact mechanism of MS is unknown, the plaques probably form after some type of viral infection. An alteration in the body's immune system (major histocompatibility proteins) may cause it to attack central nervous system myelin.[19] Regardless of the cause for demyelinization, nerve fibers that cross a plaque region lose their myelin. The loss of myelin seriously impairs the function of a given neuron and disrupts the rapid transduction of information down an axon. The type and severity of the symptoms demonstrated by a patient with MS are related to the number and location of the demyelinated areas.

The axon is not only the target of disease, but is the target of some anesthetic agents. For example, lidocaine (Xylocaine), an anesthetic that is commonly used for local nerve blocks and for topical **anesthesia**, prevents the conduction of an electrical potential along an axon. These local anesthetics stabilize the plasma membrane of the neuron and inhibit the movement of Na^+ ions into the cell.[20] Small, unmyelinated neurons are more susceptible to the effects of these agents than larger, or myelinated neurons.

Finally, the synapse can also be impaired. Presynaptically, botulin toxin can target the proteins in the axon terminal that help synaptic vesicles dock and then fuse to the cell membrane. This toxin, a product of *Clostridium botulinum* that is frequently found in poorly preserved canned foods, cleaves these proteins and thus prevents neurotransmitter release.[2] As you might expect, ingestion of botulinum toxin leads to weakness and paralysis. Typically, the weakness starts in the muscles that move the eye, spreads to jaw and throat muscles, and later occurs in the muscles of the extremities. As you will learn later in this book, the muscles of the eye, jaw, and throat are innervated by neurons from the brainstem (cranial nerves). The muscles of the extremities are innervated by neurons from the spinal cord.

A disease that affects the postsynaptic element is myasthenia gravis. This autoimmune disease disrupts the transmission of neural impulses across the **neuromuscular junction**. Such a disruption causes impaired function of skeletal muscle. Symptoms commonly seen with this disease are postexercise fatigue, double vision (diplopia), drooping eyelids (ptosis), facial droop, impaired chewing and swallowing, and impaired ventilation. The manifestations of the disease stem from the body's failure to recognize postjunctional acetylcholine receptors as "self." Because these receptors are seen by the body as foreign substances, the immune system produces antibodies against them. The antibodies bind with the postjunctional receptors and render them ineffective. With the receptors blocked by antibodies, acetylcholine cannot bind with an appropriate receptor, diminishing transmission across the neuromuscular junction. The decreased transmission across the neuromuscular junction prevents the postjunctional muscle membrane from depolarizing sufficiently to trigger an action potential, thus limiting the functional capabilities of the muscle.

Even the termination of synaptic neurotransmission can be impaired. The addictive drug, cocaine, appears to interfere with the uptake of the neurotransmitter dopamine.[21] Normally, this neurotransmitter is cleared from the synaptic cleft by uptake into the same neurons that release dopamine. Cocaine seems to prevent this uptake, elevating the concentration of dopamine in the synaptic cleft. The continued presence of dopamine in the cleft probably gives rise to the addictive highs sought by drug addicts. Amphetamines may act in this way, too. The final stage of synaptic neurotransmission can also be interrupted therapeutically. In people who have myasthenia gravis, blocking the enzyme that degrades acetylcholine in the synaptic cleft can increase the concentration and longevity of acetylcholine there, allowing more time for neuronally released acetylcholine to interact with impaired postsynaptic muscle acetylcholine receptors. The result is an amelioration of the pervasive weakness characteristic of the disease.

REFERENCES

1. Lledo PM, Johannes L, Vernier P, et al. Rab3 proteins: key players in the control of exocytosis. *Trends Neurosci* 1994;17:426–431.
2. Söllner T, Rothman E. Neurotransmission: harnessing fusion machinery at the synapse. *Trends Neurosci* 1994; 17:344–348.
3. Littleton JT, Hugo BJ. Synaptogamin controls and modulates synaptic vesicle fusion in a Ca^{2+}-dependent manner. *Trends Neurosci* 1995;18:177–183.

4. Trifaró J-M, Vitale ML. Cytoskeletal dynamics during neurotransmitter release. *Trends Neurosci* 1993;16:466–471.

5. Henn FA, Hamberger A. Glial cell function: uptake of transmitter substances. *Proc Natl Acad Sci U S A* 1971; 68:2686–2690.

6. Hertz L. Functional interactions between neurons and astrocytes: I. turnover and metabolism of putative amino acid transmitters. *Prog Neurobiol* 1979;13:277–323.

7. Cooper JR, Bloom FE, Roth RH. *The biochemical basis of neuropharmacology.* New York: Oxford University Press, 1986:245–247.

8. McKelvy JF, Blumberg S. Inactivation and metabolism of neuropeptides. *Annu Rev Neurosci* 1986;9:415–435.

9. Yamazaki S, Inouye ST, Kuroda Y. TTX-resistant Ca^{2+} oscillation in cultured hypothalamus: similarity to the mammalian circadian pacemaker. *Neuroreport* 1995;6: 1306–1308.

10. Matesic DF, Germak JA, Dupont E, et al. Immortalized hypothalamic luteinizing hormone-releasing hormone neurons express a connexin 26-like protein and display functional gap junction coupling assayed by fluorescence recovery after photobleaching. *Neuroendocrinology* 1993;58:485–492.

11. Purves D, Augustine GJ, Fitzpatrick D, et al. *Neuroscience.* Sunderland, MA: Sinauer Associates, Inc., 1997:85–87.

12. Theodosis DT, Poulain DA. Oxytocin-secreting neurons: a physiological model for structural plasticity in the adult mammalian brain. *Trends Neurosci* 1987;10:426–430.

13. Theodosis DT, Poulain DA. Activity-dependent neuronal–glial and synaptic plasticity in the adult mammalian hypothalamus. *Neuroscience* 1993;57:501–535.

14. Cuello AC. Nonclassical neuronal communication. *Fed Proc* 1983;42:2912–2922.

15. Herkenham M. Mismatches between neurotransmitter and receptor localization in brain: observations and implications. *Neuroscience* 1987;23:1–38.

16. Davies P, Maloney AJF. Selective loss of central cholinergic neurons in Alzheimer's disease. *Lancet* 1976;2:1403.

17. Berger-Sweeney J, Heckers S, Mesulam M-M, et al. Differential effects on spatial navigation of immunotoxin-induced cholinergic lesions of the medial septal area and nucleus basalis magnocellularis. *J Neurosci* 1994; 14:4507–4519.

18. Roth GS, Joseph JA, Mason RP. Membrane alterations as causes of impaired signal transduction in Alzheimer's disease and aging. *Trends Neurosci* 1995;18:203–206.

19. Williams KC, Ulvestad E, Hickey WF. Immunology of multiple sclerosis. *Clin Neurosci* 1994;2:229–245.

20. Ciccone CD. Local anesthetics. In: Ciccone CD, ed. *Pharmacology in rehabilitation.* 2nd ed. Philadelphia: FA Davis Company, 1990:147–157.

21. Baiter M. New clues to brain dopamine control, cocaine addiction. *Science* 1996;271:909.

Fundamental Elements of the Nervous System 2: Neurotransmitters

WILLIAM F. SEWELL, PhD

What Is a Neurotransmitter?

The primary means by which cells communicate with each other is with chemicals. Hormones released into the blood from endocrine glands can signal billions of other cells in the body within seconds. Pheromones are released into the atmosphere to signal other organisms. Perhaps the most intricate use of intercellular chemical signaling, however, is in the nervous system, where a single neuron can communicate with another neuron by releasing a chemical **neurotransmitter**. As the name implies, a neurotransmitter transmits information from a neuron to another cell. Neurotransmitters generally act over very short distances and are released at points called synapses, where neurons are in very close apposition. The process of neurotransmitter release and action at a synapse is called chemical synaptic

49

transmission. The overwhelming majority of synapses in the brain transmit information chemically, although synaptic transmission is mediated electrically in rare cases.

The use of chemical transmission by the nervous system makes the process vulnerable to interference by drugs. Indeed, most of the drugs that affect the nervous system do so by altering the process of synaptic transmission. Knowledge of neurotransmitters also provides a very important tool for understanding how the brain works. The use of drugs that can selectively block or stimulate one or another neurotransmitter is a very powerful tool to understand and modify brain function. Also, because different populations of neurons can use different neurotransmitters, we can use knowledge of a neuron's neurotransmitter to identify certain neuronal populations anatomically.

How Do Neurotransmitters Work?

Neurotransmitters are synthesized by neurons, stored in vesicles at nerve terminals, and released when neurons are depolarized. After the neurotransmitter is released into the synaptic cleft (the narrow gap between two adjacent neurons), it binds to a **receptor** located at the synapse on the receiving neuron (Fig. 4–1). The receptor is simply a large protein whose structure includes a binding site for the neurotransmitter. When the neurotransmitter binds to the receptor, the receptor changes its shape. This change in shape (called a **conformational change**) evokes a change in the physiology or chemistry of the postsynaptic cell. Different receptors produce different changes, but only two broad classes of receptors are known. Receptors that allow ions to pass through the membrane are classified as **ionotropic receptors**. The other class of receptors evokes a chemical change in the cell. Because the chemical changes are mediated by a mobile intracellular protein called a G-protein, these receptors are called **G-protein–coupled receptors**.

The ionotropic receptors actually form a channel in the membrane through which ions can pass. This flow of ions changes the membrane potential of the cell, producing excitation or inhibition. The channels are normally closed and are opened by the binding of the neurotransmitter to the receptor.

The G-protein–coupled receptors initiate a wide-ranging series of chemical changes in the cell mediated through G-protein. These changes can include activation or deactivation of enzymes and changes in the conductance of ion channels. G-proteins get their name because they contain a guanosine triphosphate (GTP) binding site that is activated by the neurotransmitter receptor. The several different kinds of G-proteins produce different kinds of responses in cells. All G-protein–coupled neurotransmitter receptors are structurally similar.

Many Different Neurotransmitter Chemicals

Not all neurons use the same neurotransmitter, and a surprisingly large number of different chemicals have been identified as serving putative roles as neurotransmitters. We can group them into three broad classes of compounds: fast neurotransmitters, **neuropeptides**, and nontraditional transmitters (Fig. 4–2).

Most fast (i.e., moment-by-moment) communication between neurons is mediated by small molecules often related to amino acids. These compounds include acetylcholine, catecholamines (norepinephrine, epinephrine, and dopamine), gamma-aminobutyric acid (GABA), glycine, and excitatory amino acids. For the millisecond-by-millisecond transfer of information from neuron to neuron, we might expect really to need only two neurotransmitters—one to excite and one to inhibit—but in fact at least a half-dozen different neurotransmitters have been identified that perform these functions. No hard-and-fast rule defines whether a given neurotransmitter is necessarily excitatory or inhibitory; the receptor for the transmitter determines whether it is excitatory. Some generalizations, however, are useful as long as one keeps in mind that they are only generalizations.

Fast Neurotransmitters

Neurotransmitters that act on receptors that form cation channels tend to be excitatory because opening cation channels usually allows more Na+ than any other ion into the cell, and Na+ entry usually depolarizes the cell. Transmitters that have cation channel ionotropic receptors include acetylcholine and the excitatory amino acids. Neurotransmitters that act on ionotropic receptors that form chloride chan-

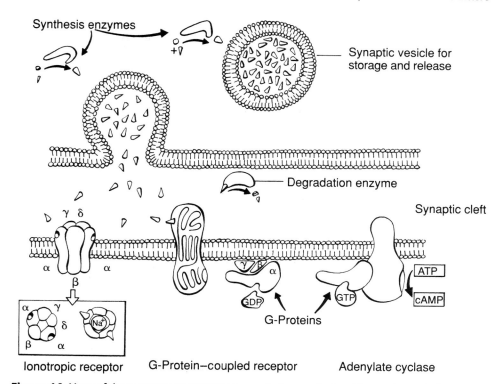

Figure 4-1. Many of the processes in synaptic transmission are depicted here schematically. Neurotransmitter is usually synthesized in the cytosol of a presynaptic neuron and packaged into a synaptic vesicle for release. Release of the synaptic vesicle involves fusion of the synaptic vesicle with the presynaptic membrane of the neuron. Entry of calcium ions into the neuron is necessary for vesicular release of the transmitter. Typically, calcium enters through voltage-sensitive calcium channels that are activated by depolarization of the neuron with an action potential. Once released, the neurotransmitter diffuses across the synaptic cleft to interact with receptors on the postsynaptic neuron. Both ionotropic and G-protein–coupled receptors are indicated here, although both types of receptors would not necessarily be present at a single synapse. Ionotropic receptors form gated ion channels in the membrane from five subunits. The channel is normally closed and opens when the transmitter binds to the receptor. Entry of ions through the channel changes the membrane potential of the cell. G-protein–coupled receptors are characterized by an extracellular binding site for neurotransmitter, an intracellular binding site for a G-protein complex, and an amino acid chain that runs back and forth through the membrane seven times. The G-protein has three subunits, termed alpha, beta, and gamma. The gamma subunit is activated by the neurotransmitter receptor. The activated gamma subunit dissociates from the rest of the complex and diffuses to target sites elsewhere on the membrane. Activation of the gamma subunit is achieved by phosphorylation of guanosine diphosphate (GDP) to form guanosine triphosphate (GTP). Each of the many different types of G-protein has its own specific target protein. In the case shown schematically here, the target is a membrane-bound enzyme called adenylate cyclase. This enzyme, when activated by the G-protein, catalyzes the formation of cyclic adenosine monophosphate (cAMP). When the G-protein activates adenylate cyclase, GTP returns to GDP, which in turn inactivates the G-protein. ATP, adenosine triphosphate.

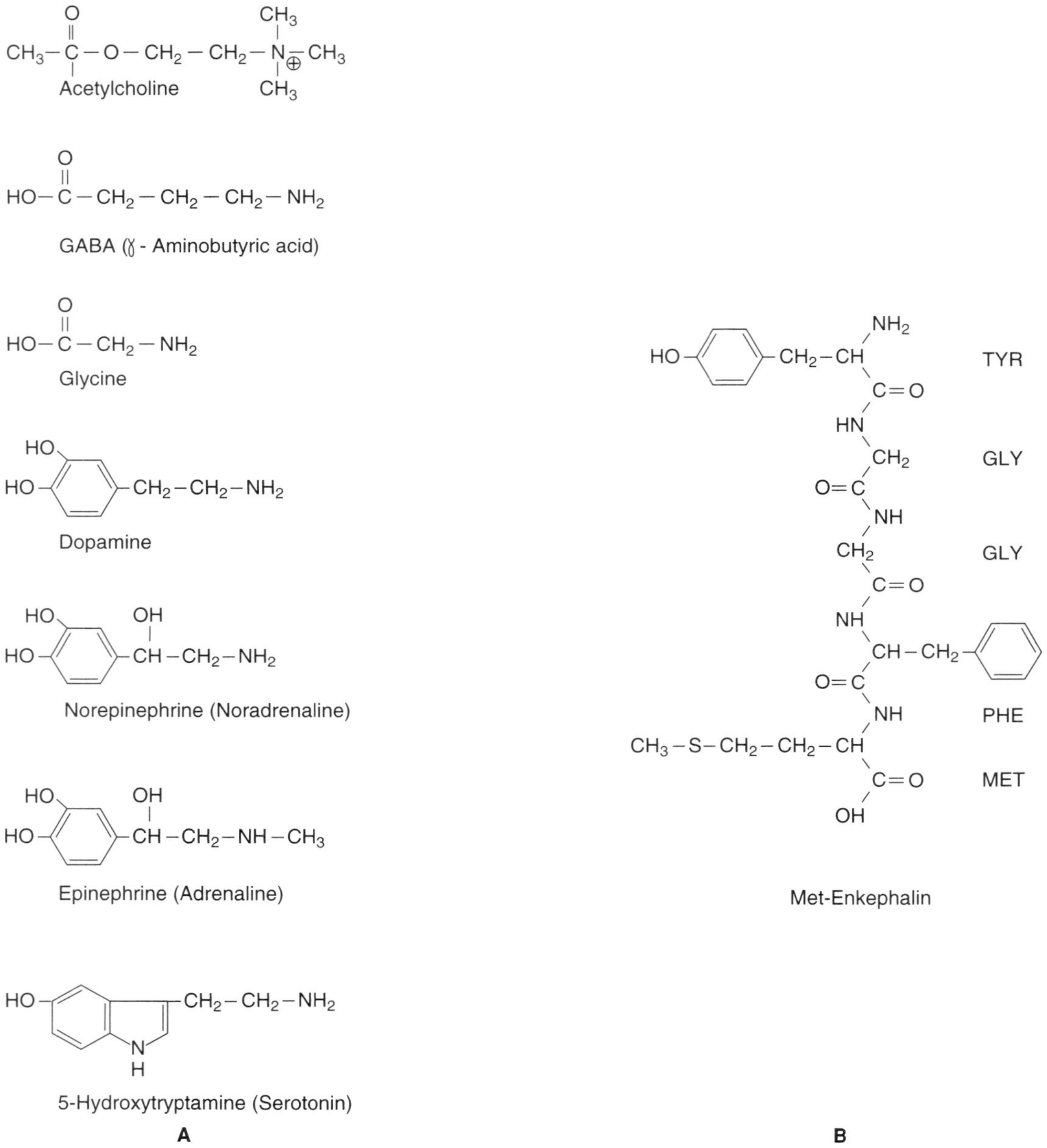

Figure 4-2. A: The chemical structures of several transmitters are shown. Note that the fast neuro-transmitters tend to be relatively small compounds, about the size of amino acids. **B:** Peptides are much larger, comprising amino acids strung together with peptide bonds. The example shown, met-enkephalin, is a very small peptide, with only five amino acids. Calcitonin gene-related peptide, by contrast, contains 37 amino acids. The nontraditional transmitters include an exceedingly small volatile compound, nitric oxide, which can cross cell membranes, and a number of compounds that are derivatives of compounds that make up cell membranes, such as the eicosanoids.

nels tend to be inhibitory. Chloride channels are present in some types of GABA and glycine receptors; thus, GABA and glycine often serve as inhibitory neurotransmitters, especially in the central nervous system. Almost all of these fast transmitters also have G-protein–coupled receptors. The specific action of a G-protein–coupled receptor on a cell depends on which type of G-protein is activated by the neurotransmitter receptor.

Neuropeptides

The peptides form a second class of neurotransmitter compounds. Peptides are similar to proteins in that they are composed of amino acids strung together, but they generally contain a smaller number of amino acids (from a few to a few dozen amino acids). Dozens of neuroactive peptides have been identified, including the endorphins, calcitonin gene-related peptide, and substance P. Peptides have time courses on the order of seconds or longer, and their actions are often to modulate, rather than mediate, synaptic transmission between neurons. All neuropeptide receptors identified so far appear to be G-protein–coupled receptors.

Nontraditional Neurotransmitters

Finally, a variety of chemicals used by neurons to communicate with other cells do not fit into the traditional view of neurotransmitters in that they are not necessarily released at the synapse and can influence many surrounding neurons. One group includes small, volatile molecules that are generated by breakdown of larger amino acids and rapidly diffuse across cell membranes, producing effects on nearby neurons by directly activating second messenger systems in receptive neurons. Included in this class are nitric oxide and carbon monoxide. Because these compounds readily diffuse through cell membranes, communication can take place anywhere along the neuron, but may not be as discrete as other forms of transmission. Another example is a family of compounds called **eicosanoids**, which are related to fatty acids. These compounds are often generated from membrane phospholipids secondary to transmitter activation, and can affect adjacent cells. An example of a class of eicosanoids is the prostaglandins. Related to the eicosanoids is a group of compounds called **cannabinoids**, a series of endogenous compounds related to fatty acids that interact with receptors for the cannabinoids (active compounds in marijuana). Receptors for these compounds have been identified, as well as several endogenous ligands. The mechanisms of release and the specific role of these compounds are not well understood, and are not covered further in this chapter.

Storage and Release of Neurotransmitters

Neurotransmitters are usually stored in, and released from, small vesicles in the nerve terminal. Vesicular storage allows sequestration of relatively high concentrations of the neurotransmitter. Neurotransmitters are released from the vesicles when the nerve terminal is depolarized, as when an action potential traveling down an axon reaches the nerve terminal. Depolarization of the nerve is a voltage change that activates voltage-dependent calcium channels that in turn open to allow calcium to enter the nerve terminal. The entry of calcium triggers fusion of the membrane of the synaptic vesicle with the plasma membrane of the nerve terminal; this action allows the neurotransmitter stored in the vesicle to diffuse into the synaptic cleft.

Neurotransmitter Receptors

Neurotransmitter receptors may be divided into two large families: those that form ion channels gated by the neurotransmitter (ionotropic receptors), and those that are coupled to G-proteins such that neurotransmitter binding initiates a series of chemical reactions in the cell to produce an effect.

Ionotropic Receptors

The ionotropic receptors are composed of different subunits that associate with one another to form ion pores. Ionotropic receptors have been identified for acetylcholine, GABA, glycine, and excitatory amino acids. In fact, receptors for acetylcholine, GABA, and glycine appear to be members of a superfamily of receptors. The amino acid sequences of the receptors are similar enough to one another to suggest they evolved from each other relatively recently.

Most ionotropic receptors appear to have five subunits and are thus said to be pentameric. With GABA, glycine, and nicotinic acetylcholine receptors, the neurotransmitter binding site is on the alpha subunit. The biophysical and pharmacologic properties of the whole receptor depend on the specific subunit composition of the receptor.

G-Protein–Coupled Receptors

Receptors that do not directly form ion channels evoke an action through a group of regulatory proteins, called G-proteins, that are intricately associated with the receptor. All of the G-protein–coupled neurotransmitter receptors are structurally similar to one another and all contain a sequence of amino acids that form seven transmembrane segments: that is, they cross from the inside to the outside of the membrane seven times. Because of this arrangement, they are sometimes called 7TM receptors. These receptors have a site on the outside of the cell that can bind the neurotransmitter and a site on the inside of the cell that can bind to and activate the regulatory G-protein. A G-protein–coupled receptor has been identified for almost every fast neurotransmitter, and all of the receptors identified so far for peptides are G-protein coupled. These receptors are not in general as fast as the ionotropic receptor because several chemical interactions within the cell must take place before the action of neurotransmitter binding is apparent.

Neurotransmitter binding to the receptor produces activation of the receptor-coupled G-protein by converting guanosine diphosphate on the G-protein to GTP. The activated G-protein leaves the receptor to bind to another effector protein. Each cell contains many more G-protein molecules than receptors, allowing each receptor molecule to activate large numbers of G-proteins. This mechanism allows even very small numbers of neurotransmitter molecules interacting with only a fraction of the available receptors to produce very large responses.

Activated G-proteins then bind to another effector protein within the cell. G-proteins have several different forms, each of which has a specificity for different effector proteins. For example, the G_s G-protein stimulates adenylate cyclase, whereas G_i inhibits it. Adenylate cyclase is an enzyme that generates, from adenosine triphosphate, the cell signal molecule, cyclic adenosine monophosphate (cAMP), which regulates many other cellular processes. G_o activates potassium channels. G_q activates phospholipase C, an enzyme that triggers several other processes in the cell by breaking down constituents of the cell membrane to form inositol triphosphate and diacylglycerol.

Individual Fast Neurotransmitters

Acetylcholine

Acetylcholine, one of the first neurotransmitters to be identified, is the major neurotransmitter used in the peripheral nervous system. Contraction of voluntary (skeletal) muscle is initiated when the motor neuron releases acetylcholine onto the muscle. Because the neuromuscular junction is very accessible for experimental analysis, acetylcholine is the best understood of the neurotransmitters. Acetylcholine is also the predominant transmitter released at all autonomic ganglion cells and by parasympathetic nerve terminals. In addition, acetylcholine is used as a neurotransmitter in some parts of the central nervous system, although it cannot be considered a major brain neurotransmitter. Cells that contain acetylcholine are scattered throughout the nervous system. Many **cholinergic** neurons are found in the basal forebrain and project diffusely throughout the brain. Figure 4–3 depicts a hypothetical acetylcholine synapse.

Acetylcholine is synthesized in the cytosol of the nerve terminal. The completed molecule is transported into synaptic vesicles, where it is stored until release. Acetylcholine is synthesized by an enzyme (choline acetyltransferase) that joins together acetyl-coenzyme A (CoA) and choline. Both choline and acetyl-CoA are very common chemicals found throughout the body, but acetylcholine is made only in neurons that use it as a neurotransmitter. Indeed, the enzyme choline acetyltransferase can be used as a marker for neurons that release acetylcholine.

Acetylcholine is released and diffuses across the synaptic cleft to the postsynaptic neuron, where it acts on cholinergic receptors. Cholinergic receptors are divided into two broad classes: **nicotinic** and **muscarinic**. Nicotinic receptors were so named because the drug nicotine (found in tobacco) could stimulate these receptors. Nicotinic receptors are ionotropic; they form ion channels. Muscarinic receptors were named because the drug muscarine (present in the poisonous mushroom, *Amanita muscaria*) could selectively stimulate these receptors. Muscarinic receptors are all G-protein–coupled receptors.

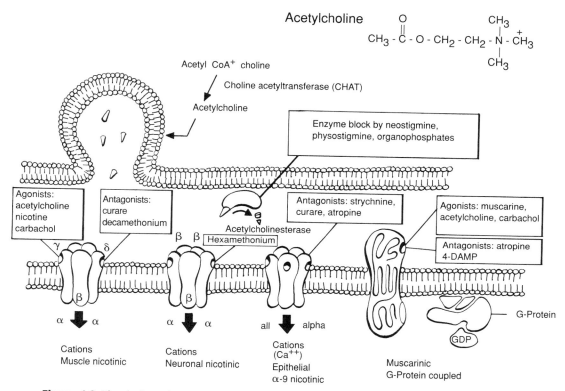

Figure 4-3. The cholinergic synapse is schematically depicted here (although as with all of these examples, different cholinergic receptors are not likely to be found at the same synapse). Acetylcholine differs from other known transmitters in that a highly active enzyme in the synapse (acetylcholinesterase) destroys the acetylcholine soon after it is released. This enzyme can be blocked with the drugs neostigmine and physostigmine. All of the cholinergic receptors are activated by acetylcholine and carbachol (an esterase-resistant acetylcholine analog). Relatively selected agonists and antagonists exist for each of these receptors, and are indicated in the diagram. dAMP, deoxyadenosine monophosphate; GDP, guanosine diphosphate.

Each nicotinic receptor is composed of five subunits that form a cation-permeable pore through the membrane. Five broad types of subunits have been identified, although not all five types are present in all receptors. These types have been called alpha, beta, gamma, delta, and epsilon. Each of these five types often has several variants; for example, at least nine types of the alpha subunit and at least four different beta subunits have been identified. These subunits come together in different ways to form two major different types of nicotinic receptors. The **muscle nicotinic receptor** is found on muscle and is composed of one each of all five subtypes of receptor. The **neuronal nicotinic receptors** are composed of only alpha and beta subunits. Some neuronal receptor subtypes contain only alpha subunits. The acetylcholine binding site appears to be on the alpha subunit.

Enzymatic degradation removes acetylcholine from the synapse. The enzyme **acetylcholinesterase** breaks acetylcholine into the compounds choline and acetic acid, neither of which has much activity on cholinergic receptors. Choline and acetic acid are taken back up by cells and metabolized. Acetylcholinesterase is made by a large number of cells and secreted into the extracellular space. It can be found in places where acetylcholine is not used as a neurotransmitter. For that reason, its presence cannot be used as an indicator of a cholinergically transmitting synapse. Drugs that inhibit cholinesterase, such as neostigmine and physostigmine, have been useful in treating disorders, such as myasthenia gravis, in which a boost in cholinergic transmission is desirable.

Gamma-Aminobutyric Acid

The strongest evidence that GABA serves as a neurotransmitter comes from experiments in the lobster, where GABA is a neurotransmitter in inhibitory motor neurons. The advantage of using crustaceans in this work is that the individual neurons are large enough to allow neurochemical and pharmacologic approaches to be integrated at the cellular level. Because GABA was the most potent inhibitory substance found in extracts of lobster motor neurons, and because it was found to be concentrated in the inhibitory motor neurons, a convincing case could be made that GABA is an inhibitory neurotransmitter. In the mammalian central nervous system, GABA is also primarily inhibitory. Some of the fundamental elements of a GABAergic synapse are depicted in Figure 4–4.

Gamma-aminobutyric acid is a very small molecule easily produced in the cytosol of the cell by metabolism of the amino acid glutamate with the enzyme glutamate decarboxylase. This enzyme is present in high concentrations in inhibitory neurons. GABA is stored in synaptic vesicles for release into the synaptic cleft. Two types of GABA receptors have been identified. The GABA$_A$ receptor is a pentameric ion channel that is permeable to chloride ions. Two subunits have been identified (alpha and beta) that can bind GABA.

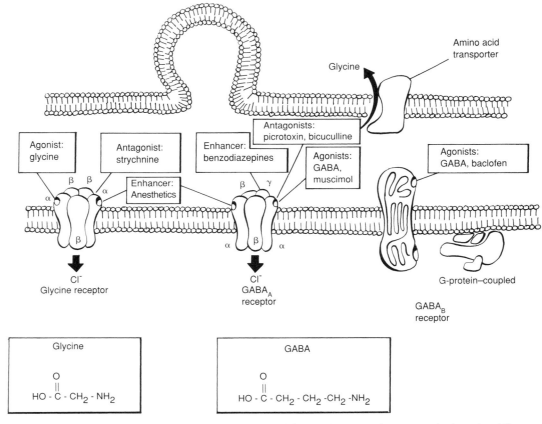

Figure 4-4. A schematic diagram of the generally inhibitory GABAergic (gamma-aminobutyric acid) and glycinergic synapses. Glycine and GABA receptors are drawn together here for convenience, but are not normally present at the same synapse.

The alpha subunit has a binding site for the benzodiazepine class of tranquilizers. The GABA$_B$ receptor is apparently a G-protein–coupled receptor, although the receptor has not yet been cloned.

Glycine

Another transmitter with an inhibitory role is glycine (see Fig. 4–4). A common amino acid, glycine is distinctly localized in different parts of the brainstem. It is not synthesized by neurons; instead, it is taken up from the extracellular fluid by neurons that require it. It is probably stored in vesicles for release, although this process has not yet been demonstrated directly.

The glycine receptor, like the GABA and acetylcholine receptors, is a pentameric ion channel that is selective for chloride. Two subunits have been identified. The alpha subunit contains the glycine binding site, whereas the beta subunit is a determinant of channel conductance. Because the ion channel is selectively permeable to chloride, glycine is in general inhibitory in its action. A drug that potently blocks the glycine receptor is strychnine. In the past, strychnine was often used as rat poison and killed by producing convulsions, an action consistent with blocking inhibitory transmission in the brain.

Catecholamines (Norepinephrine, Epinephrine, and Dopamine)

Three metabolically related compounds—epinephrine, norepinephrine, and dopamine—serve as neurotransmitters in both the brain and peripheral nervous system. They are called **catecholamines** because their chemical structure contains a catechol (dihydroxyphenyl) group. Epinephrine and norepinephrine are also known as adrenaline and noradrenaline, respectively. In the peripheral nervous system, epinephrine is often released from the adrenal gland as a hormone (having widespread actions in the body), whereas norepinephrine is more locally released from sympathetic nerve fibers (see Chapter 15 for a description of the sympathetic division of the autonomic nervous system). Both norepinephrine and dopamine are used as neurotransmitters in the central nervous system. Catecholaminergic synapses are depicted in Figure 4–5.

All three catecholamines are produced by subsequent modifications of the amino acid, tyrosine. Tyrosine is converted to DOPA (dihydroxyphenylalanine), which is converted to the neurotransmitter dopamine by an enzyme called DOPA decarboxylase. Dopamine, once produced, is taken up into synaptic vesicles, where it is stored until it is released by dopaminergic neurons in the brain. In neurons that use norepinephrine, the dopamine in the synaptic vesicles is further modified to produce norepinephrine by an enzyme (dopamine-beta-hydroxylase), which sits on the inside surface of the vesicle. Epinephrine is produced from norepinephrine by the removal of a methyl group from the norepinephrine. All three neurotransmitters are released from the vesicles in which they are stored.

Norepinephrine is released by sympathetic nerve fibers of the autonomic nervous system (see Chapter 15). In the central nervous system, it is mostly used by neurons in the locus ceruleus, which innervates widespread regions of the brain. Dopaminergic neurons in the brain are found in the hypothalamus and midbrain. A population of dopaminergic neurons that are involved in movement control arise in the substantia nigra and project to the basal ganglia. Even though epinephrine acts on the same receptors as norepinephrine, it is usually considered a hormone because it is released from the adrenal glands into the blood.

All known catecholamine receptors are G-protein–coupled receptors. Dopamine acts on separate receptors, but norepinephrine and epinephrine usually act on the same receptors, called adrenoceptors, which have two broad classes called alphas and beta. Although all adrenoreceptors are G-protein coupled, they differ in the type of G-protein that mediates their action in the cell. Within each category are numerous subtypes, distinguished from each other by their amino acid sequences and by their drug-binding characteristics.

At least five dopamine receptors have been cloned and the genes for four of them have been localized. They are in general coupled either to G$_s$- or G$_{i/o}$-proteins. Selective antagonists are available for four of these receptors.

Termination of action of the catecholamines involves several different processes, including reuptake of the transmitters into the nerve terminal, where an enzyme called monamine oxidase removes the amine group, and simple diffusion away from the synapse. An extraordinary number of drugs have been developed that interfere with almost every facet of metabolism and action of the catecholamines. Drugs such as cocaine and amphetamines can block reuptake of the transmitter into the synapse, resulting in prolonged action of the trans-

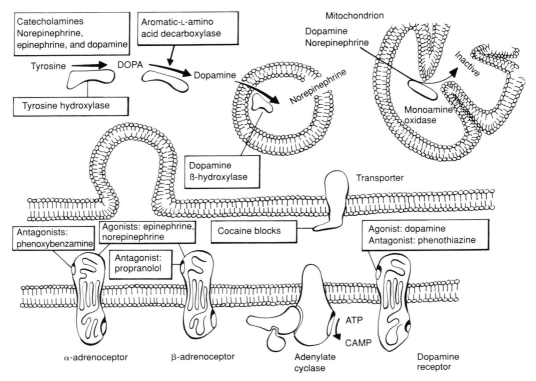

Figure 4-5. Catecholamines. Dopamine is synthesized in the cytosol ultimately from the amino acid tyrosine and packaged into vesicles for release. Neurons that use norepinephrine generate it from dopamine in the vesicle with the enzyme dopamine-beta-hydroxylase. All adrenoreceptors identified so far are G-protein coupled. ATP, adenosine triphosphate; cAMP, cyclic adenosine monophosphate; DOPA, dihydroxyphenylalanine.

mitter. Many antidepressant drugs act by interfering with the metabolism of these transmitters. Administration of a transmitter precursor, L-DOPA, is very effective in ameliorating early signs of Parkinson's disease.

Excitatory Amino Acids

Most excitatory transmission in the brain is probably mediated by glutamate or a related "excitatory amino acid." The difficulty in establishing whether this excitatory amino acid is glutamate is compounded by the ubiquitous presence of glutamate throughout the brain and its widespread role in basic metabolism. Other endogenous substances that are transmitter candidates include aspartate, *N*-acetylaspartyl glutamate, and homocysteine. In spite of the lack of strong evidence for the identity of the

transmitter, the receptors on which this excitatory amino acid acts have been well characterized both at the molecular and pharmacologic levels; they are often called "glutamate receptors."

As with many other neurotransmitter receptors, both ionotropic and G-protein–coupled receptors have been identified, and each receptor has several subtypes (Fig. 4–6). Over a dozen different subunits are grouped together in different ways to form these receptors. At least three different ionotropic receptors are named after agonists that can interact with them with some selectivity. All are pentameric.

1 AMPA receptors are composed of glutamate receptor subunits GR_1 through GR_4 and have the property of desensitizing very rapidly to the presence of an agonist. Receptors that contain the GR_2 receptor subunit have a low permeability to calcium.

2 Kainate receptors contain glutamate receptor subunits GR_5 through GR_7 and KA_1 and KA_2, and do not readily desensitize in the presence of an agonist.

3 NMDA receptors are composed of subunits NR_1 and NR_2, several isoforms of which have been found.

NMDA receptors are especially interesting because their physical properties suggest they may play a role as coincidence detectors. These ionotropic receptors do not open simply on binding of agonist. To open, they must also be depolarized by the neuron in which they are located. Thus, they open when two or more inputs to the cell are active, one that releases transmitter on the receptor and another that can depolarize the cell. When open, NMDA receptors have a high permeability to calcium, and calcium is an important and ubiquitous intracellular signaling chemical.

Another excitatory amino acid subtype is the metabotropic (*or* G-protein–coupled) glutamate receptor, of which several subtypes have been identified. These receptors are coupled to G-proteins and, as with many other G-protein–coupled receptors, contain the 7TM segment. Eight different metabotropic receptor subtypes have been cloned.

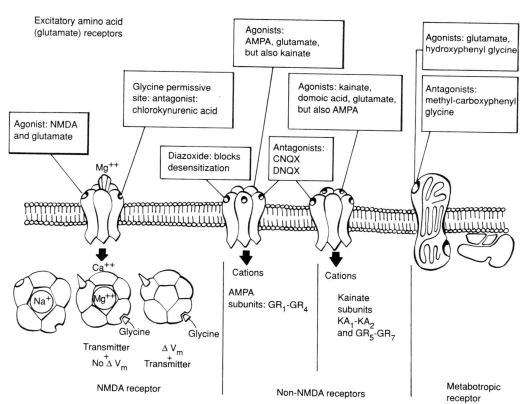

Figure 4-6. Glutamate receptor subtypes are depicted schematically here. The (NMDA) receptor is interesting because it requires both a change in membrane potential (ΔV_m) and the presence of the transmitter to be activated. Some examples of agonists and antagonists for each of the receptor types are indicated on the diagram. DNQX, 6,7-Dinitroquinoxaline-2,3-dione; CNQX, 6-Cyano-7-nitro-quinoxaline-2,3,-dione.

Drugs have been developed to block glutamate receptors, but they do not in general have high specificity. The AMPA and kainate receptor can be blocked by quinoxalinediones (CNQX and DNQX). NMDA receptors can be blocked by raising the extracellular magnesium concentration to the millimolar range. Magnesium normally sits in the ion pore to block conduction unless the cell is depolarized, which ejects the magnesium. Raising the extracellular magnesium concentration, however, can change the kinetics so that it is difficult to open the pore with depolarization. The NMDA receptor also has a site that binds glycine. Bound glycine is necessary for the receptor to respond to NMDA. The drug chlorokynurenic acid can block this permissive glycine site.

Miscellaneous

A number of substances have been hypothesized to serve as neurotransmitters, but either their roles are not well understood or they do not appear to be major neurotransmitters. These substances include histamine, 5-hydroxytryptamine (also called serotonin and 5-HT), adenosine triphosphate, and adenosine. Histamine and 5-HT are found in only a very small number of neurons, with very diffuse projections throughout the brain. 5-HT is involved in regulation of sleep–wake cycles. Histamine-containing neurons are found almost exclusively in some neurons of the hypothalamus and project throughout the brain to innervate not only neurons, but glia and blood vessels.

Neuropeptides

Neuropeptides are larger molecules than the fast neurotransmitters and are made up of amino acids strung together with peptide bonds. Peptides are stored in and released from vesicles in the nerve terminal. Peptide-containing vesicles coexist with, and are larger than, the vesicles containing fast transmitters. Peptides are formed in the same way that proteins are formed; they are encoded by DNA and transcribed through production of RNA. The peptides are synthesized near the nucleus of the cell in the endoplasmic reticulum, packaged into vesicles in the Golgi apparatus, and then transported to the nerve terminal. The neuropeptides are produced from larger precursor peptides, and often multiple peptides can be produced from a single precursor.

When released from the neuron, peptides probably act on any nearby neurons with receptors for the peptide. The peptide receptors identified so far all appear to be G-protein–coupled receptors with the 7TM segment structure. Peptides are in general extremely potent, probably because of the nature of the G-protein–coupled receptor, in which a small number of peptide molecules bound to the receptor for a relatively long time can activate a large number of G-proteins. The time course for action of peptides is relatively slow, on the order of hundreds of milliseconds to tens of seconds, because the peptides are large molecules that diffuse slowly and act through G-proteins.

The number of peptides found in neurons and known to be neuroactive is very large. The receptors for most of these candidates have not yet been identified, but it is only a matter of time until most are known. Receptors that have been identified include those for opioid peptides, neurotensin, substance P, and bombesin. Notable examples of drugs that affect a peptide receptor are the narcotics, morphine and heroin, which bind to and activate receptors for the peptide enkephalin. The action of both the peptide and the narcotics leads to relief from pain.

Clinical Correlations

Almost all of the therapeutic drugs for the nervous system act through neurotransmitters or their receptors. A striking example is in the treatment of patients with Parkinson's disease with L-DOPA. Parkinson's disease is a clinical syndrome characterized by tremor, muscle rigidity, and bradykinesia (slowness of movement) and is caused by degeneration of dopaminergic neurons in the substantia nigra. L-DOPA, a precursor to the synthesis of dopamine, can restore function in this disease by boosting production of dopamine in the remaining dopaminergic neurons. Another example is the drug morphine, which produces analgesia by activating receptors for the peptide enkephalin. Diazepam (Valium; Roche Laboratories, Nutley, NJ), chlordiazepoxide (Librium; Roche Laboratories), and the other benzodiazepine tranquilizers act by enhancing the effect of GABA on GABA receptors. Stimulant drugs, such as cocaine and amphetamines, can enhance the effects of catecholamines by preventing their clearance from the synapses. See *Goodman and Gilman's The Pharmacological Basis of Therapeutics* for many more examples.

BIBLIOGRAPHY

Alberts B, Bray D, Lewis J, Raff M, Roberts K, Watson J. *Molecular biology of the cell*. 3rd ed. New York: Garland Publishing Inc., 1994.

Alexander SPH, Peters JA. 1997 Receptor and ion channel nomenclature supplement: 8th ed. Elsevier: *Trends Pharmacol Sci*.

Gilman AF, Rall TW, Nies AS, Taylor P, eds. *Goodman and Gilman's the pharmacological basis of therapeutics*. 8th ed. New York: Pergamon Press, 1990.

Hall Z, ed. *An introduction to molecular neurobiology*. Sunderland, MA: Sinauer Associates, 1992.

Nicholls JG, Martin AR, Wallace BG. *From neuron to brain*. 3rd ed. Sunderland, MA: Sinaur Associates, 1992.

5

Fundamental Elements of the Nervous System 3: Circulation and Nonneural Cells

SHEILA A. MUN-BRYCE, PhD, OTR/L

Every activity you do each day, whether sleeping, eating, or studying, requires interaction and modulation by your nervous system. You become more aware of the importance of your nervous system when sudden mishaps occur during routine activities, such as narrowly escaping a collision with the car in front of you as you drive to work, or cutting yourself as you prepare dinner. When you cut your finger, the pain receptors send signals that are transduced and integrated with other sensory information in your nervous system. These transmitted signals govern resultant movement, such as pulling your finger away from the painful stimulus. Similarly, interaction and modulation within the nervous system control your movements and activities as you interact with your daily environment.

Although the neuron is in general considered the key element of the nervous system, several nonneuronal components are critically involved in every aspect of nervous system activity. The properly functioning nervous system requires an adequate blood supply and circulatory system, a protective **blood–brain barrier** system, and a multifunctional **neuroglia** population. The transduction, integration, and transmission of signals between the brain and the rest of the body requires a high level of energy production. The nervous system relies on its cerebrovascular and cerebrospinal fluid (CSF) systems for the continuous delivery of energy-rich substances such as glucose and the removal of metabolic by-products. In addition, the nervous system requires a consistent internal environment so that proper signaling and

63

neuronal activity can occur. The nervous system is protected from systemic fluctuations by the blood–brain barrier. This barrier system regulates the exchange of substances between the blood and the neuronal environment even though chemical concentrations in the blood change. Finally, neurons and neuroglia engage in constant, complementary interactions for signal processing and transmission during human development, injury or disease, and recovery. This chapter focuses on the structure and physiology of nervous system components other than the neuron. We examine the crucial roles of these nonneuronal components during normal functioning and in common disease processes seen in the recovering client.

Circulatory Systems of the Central Nervous System

Homeostasis is a regulatory process that restricts variability in a system to maintain a constant internal environment. The nervous system is maintained at a constant, nonfluctuating level so that efficient signal detection and transmission can occur. This homeostatic environment is achieved in part by regulating the continuous supply of oxygen, glucose, nutrients, and ions and the removal of metabolic byproducts such as carbon dioxide. Two major circulatory systems in the central nervous system (CNS) that modulate the delivery of nutrients and removal of waste are the cerebrovascular system and the CSF system. A unique attribute of the nervous system that contributes to its consistent internal milieu is the blood–brain barrier, which restricts the movement of elements in and out of the neuroenvironment.

Blood Supply of the Nervous System

Although an average human brain weighs approximately 3 pounds, it uses 20% of the body's oxygen at rest, an indication of the brain's high metabolic rate. Uninterrupted delivery of oxygen and glucose to the brain is essential because storage of these resources in the CNS is minimal. Low levels of glucose in the brain can result in dizziness, cognitive disorders, disorientation, convulsions, and unconsciousness. The cerebrovascular system is designed to meet the high energy demands of the CNS. This vascular system has a relatively high blood flow rate, and contains countless **anastomosing** vessels and collateral blood vessels at all levels of the CNS. Regulation of blood flow depends on several factors, including arterial pressure, neuronal activity, and local metabolic conditions that affect pH and oxygen and carbon dioxide concentrations.

The brain receives its blood supply through two main arterial groups, the **internal carotid arteries** and the **basilar artery**, shown in Figure 5–1. The left and right internal carotid arteries branch off from the left and right common carotid arteries, respectively, in the anterior portion of the neck. The basilar artery is formed by the joining of the left and right vertebral arteries at the midline of the pontomedullary junction. The **vertebral arteries** arise at the posterior region of the neck, from the subclavian arteries, and enter the skull through the foramen magnum. The bilateral internal carotid arteries and basilar artery anastomose at the base of the brain, forming the **circle of Willis**. Each segment of the circle of Willis is named according to its proximity, allowing easy localization of the site of vascular injury in a clinical situation. For example, the **anterior cerebral branches** of the internal carotid arteries form the anterior portion of the circle and are connected by a segment called the **anterior communicating artery**. The posterior communicating branches of the internal carotid arteries form the lateral portion of the circle of Willis, and join with the **posterior cerebral branches** of the basilar artery to complete the posterior portion of the circle.

Table 5–1 summarizes the major arteries of the brain and the regions they supply blood to. Several arteries arise from the circle of Willis and provide blood supply to all surface areas and deep structures of the brain. Some of the larger vessels include the **middle cerebral artery**, a major branch of the internal carotid artery that supplies blood to the surface and different layers of each brain hemisphere, and the **superior cerebellar artery**, which arises from the basilar artery and supplies blood to the surface and various layers of the cerebellum.

Blood supply to the spinal cord is provided primarily by the **anterior spinal artery**, two **posterior spinal arteries**, and two **vertebral arteries**. The anterior spinal artery travels along the midline of the spinal cord, whereas the posterior spinal arteries run laterally along both sides of the spinal cord. The bilateral vertebral arteries, which arise from the

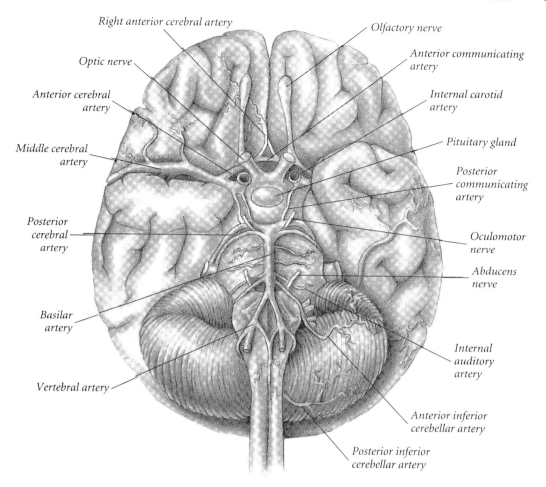

Figure 5-1. Ventral view of the arteries supplying blood to the brain. The brain is well vascularized by many vessels that anastomose and the collateral circulation that occurs at several levels of the central nervous system. The largest example of cerebral anastomosis is the circle of Willis at the base of the brain.

subclavian artery, provide blood supply to the cervical region of the spinal cord, and traverse into the cranium to form the basilar artery.

Most of the blood flow from the heart to the brain enters the circle of Willis and can flow in either direction within this vascular ring, providing a redundancy in the brain's blood supply. Blood vessel branching and anastomoses promote collateralization of blood supply at all levels of the brain, including the meninges and brain parenchyma. When blockage occurs in a cerebral artery, such as that

caused by a stroke or cerebrovascular accident, the ability of other vascular routes to maintain necessary blood flow to the ischemic region often determines the extent of brain tissue damage and subsequent neurologic symptoms. Recent advances in the early treatment of stroke with tissue plasminogen activator (TPA) are based on the degradation of fibrin clots that are formed in a blocked cerebral artery, so that blood flow can be restored.

The measurement of cerebral blood flow is a reliable marker of regional activity and injury in the

TABLE 5–1

Cerebral Arteries and Brain Regions Supplied

Artery	Site of Origin (Where Artery Arises)	Brain Region Supplied
Middle cerebral artery	Internal carotid artery	Insula, claustrum, lateral regions of the cerebral hemispheres, inferior occipital poles to the temporal poles, globus pallidus, putamen, caudate, superior internal capsule, corona radiata, lateral orbital, inferior frontal gyrus
Anterior cerebral artery	Internal carotid artery	Orbital gyrus, olfactory bulb and tract, optic nerves, optic chiasm, anterior hypothalamus, septum pellucidum, medial anterior commissure, fornix columns, anteroinferior corpus striatum, head of the caudate nucleus, putamen, anterior internal capsule, superior and medial frontal gyrus, precentral and postcentral gyri, paracentral lobule, anterior precuneus, superior parietal lobule
Posterior communicating artery	Internal carotid artery	Optic tract and posterior optic chiasm, posterior hypothalamus, cerebral peduncle, anterior and ventral nuclei of thalamus
Anterior choroidal artery	Internal carotid artery	Choroid plexus, optic tract, internal capsule genu and posterior limb, medial globus pallidus, piriform cortex, temporal lobe uncus, hippocampal and dentate gyri, caudate tail, posteromedial amygdaloid body, cerebral peduncle, substantia nigra, red nucleus, subthalamus, ventral anterior and ventral lateral nuclei of thalamus, lateral geniculate body, optic radiations
Posterior cerebral artery	Basilar artery	Tectum , cerebral peduncles, thalamus, hypothalamus, subthalamus, geniculate bodies, pulvinar, quadrigeminal plate, perineal gland, choroid plexus, fornix, inferior region of temporal lobe, parietooccipital lobe, lingual and cuneate gyri
Posterior inferior cerebellar artery	Vertebral or basilar artery	Choroid plexus of fourth ventricle, lateral and posterior medulla, occipital region of cerebellar hemisphere
Anterior inferior cerebellar artery	Basilar artery	Middle cerebellar peduncle, cerebellar hemisphere
Superior cerebellar artery	Basilar artery	Midbrain, pons, superior and middle cerebellar peduncles, dentate nucleus, cerebellar hemisphere
Middle meningeal artery	External carotid artery	Dura mater, trigeminal ganglion
Meningohypophyseal trunk	Internal carotid artery	Incisura, tentorium, dura, ethmoid, cribriform plate, frontal sinus, falx cerebri
Anterior and posterior meningeal branches	Vertebral artery	Dura, foramen magnum, falx cerebelli

brain. Changes in the rate of cerebral blood flow are reliable indices of neuronal activity, brain metabolism, and local brain function. For example, in the medial temporal cortex, regional blood flow increases with voluntary intent to perform a memory task; regional blood flow rises further as the task is executed. In contrast, portions of the brain show significant metabolic depression in patients diagnosed with organic dementia such as Alzheimer's disease. Noninvasive techniques such as positron emission tomography, computed tomography, and magnetic resonance imaging (MRI) have expanded our understanding of blood flow regulation and functional activity in the nervous system.

Cerebrospinal Fluid Circulation

In addition to its vascular supply, the CNS contains a second circulatory system that is composed of **cerebrospinal fluid**. CSF circulates around brain and spinal cord tissues, and is important in protecting and sustaining the CNS. The meninges and CSF protect the CNS by suspending and cushioning the brain and spinal cord within the skull cavity and vertebral column. CSF cushions the soft neural tissues from normal impact against their bony confines. The CSF also transports nutrients to brain cells and removes metabolic waste through the interstitial fluid that circulates around every cell in the CNS. In this way, the composition of CSF is instrumental in maintaining the steady state of the nervous system.

Cerebrospinal fluid is virtually protein free and has a different chemical composition than blood plasma. Compared with plasma, CSF has lower glucose, potassium, and calcium levels, but higher sodium, magnesium, and chloride levels. The nervous system expends a lot of energy to maintain the ionic concentration of the CSF, which, in turn, ensures a stable environment for proper neuronal functioning. Alterations in CSF composition, such as an increase in protein content or a decrease in glucose concentration, are evident in many CNS diseases.

The total volume of CSF in the adult nervous system is approximately 100 to 125 ml (4 ounces). It is replaced entirely three to four times a day. Production of CSF occurs primarily at the **choroid plexuses**, which are located in the ventricles of the brain. The choroid plexuses are composed of ependymal cell-lined capillaries that invaginate the **pia mater** layer of the meninges.

Once CSF is secreted from the choroid plexus of the **lateral ventricles**, it circulates through the interventricular **foramina of Monro**, and fills the **third ventricle**. CSF then flows into the fourth ventricle, and through the connecting **cerebral aqueduct of Sylvius** to the **foramina of Magendie and Luschka**. CSF then flows into the **subarachnoid space**, the central spinal canal, and the cisterna magna space surrounding the spinal cord (Fig. 5–2).

The subarachnoid space is the region between two of the meningeal layers, the **arachnoid** and **pia mater**. These thin membranes have many blood vessels and closely follow the surface of the brain and spinal cord. CSF in the subarachnoid space flows primarily upward around the cerebral hemispheres. It is then reabsorbed into the venous blood system at the **superior sagittal sinus** by **arachnoid villi**. These arachnoid villi penetrate the third meningeal layer, the **dura mater**, which is a thick membrane that covers and protects the CNS. The dura mater contains sinus cavities that collect venous blood destined for return to the heart.

A pathologic increase in CSF volume, due to slowed or blocked CSF circulation, can cause enlarged ventricles and compressed brain tissue, which is constrained by the rigid, nonyielding skull. Viral or bacterial invasion into the nervous system can alter CSF composition. Under normal conditions, CSF does not contain red or white blood cells. During neural infection or inflammation, immune cells (white blood cells) are recruited to fight the invading pathogens and dispose of dead cells and tissue. The resulting increase in cells and debris alters CSF viscosity and can impede its flow rate. This pathophysiologic event is seen in bacterial meningitis and hydrocephalus, two diseases that are prevalent in children and elderly. Dysfunctional CSF reabsorption or obstructed CSF circulation can result in irreversible neuronal injury and brain damage. Neurologic damage can manifest as mental retardation and various learning disabilities, depending on the severity of the CSF-related disorder.

Cerebrospinal fluid sample assays are reliable indicators of nervous system dysfunction. These samples can readily be obtained by lumbar puncture. High levels of circulating inflammatory mediators and blood-borne proteins have been found in CSF samples of patients diagnosed with meningitis and septic shock. Similarly, patients experiencing acute episodes of multiple sclerosis show high levels of matrix metalloproteinases in their CSF samples.

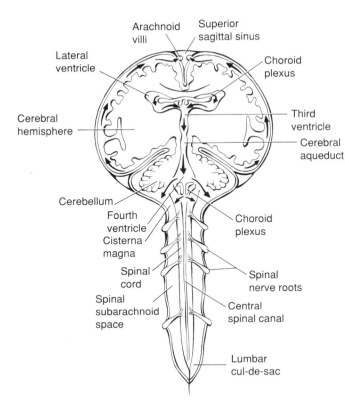

Figure 5-2. Posterior view of the cerebrospinal fluid circulation of the central nervous system. As cerebrospinal fluid is produced at the choroid plexuses in the cerebral ventricles, it circulates down around the spinal cord and up around the cerebral hemispheres.[2] (From Rosenberg GA, Wolfson LI. Disorders of brain fluids and electrolytes. In: Rosenberg RN, ed. *Comprehensive neurology.* New York: Raven Press.

These enzymes have been linked with myelin degradation and blood–brain barrier breakdown. In this latter study, patients treated with the steroid methylprednisolone showed a significant drop in metalloproteinase content of assayed CSF samples, coupled with a decrease in blood–brain barrier breakdown as detected by gadolinium-enhanced MRI.

The Blood–Brain Barrier

Although the composition of our blood fluctuates according to what we eat, the emotions we experience, and other factors in our daily lives, the nervous system must preserve a constant internal environment. Because neuron signal transduction is propagated through ion gradients and electrical impulse conduction, the nervous system needs to be shielded from systemic fluctuations that could impair these gradients and electrical activity.

As discussed earlier, a high blood flow rate and redundant circulatory systems ensure the continuous delivery of oxygen and nutrients to all levels of the brain and spinal cord. The movement of substances that enter and leave the neuronal environment, however, must also be regulated to achieve proper functioning. Structural and physiologic barriers separate blood from the CNS. Functionally unique components of the cerebral blood vessel wall exclude the movement of certain substances in and out of the nervous system. These components make up a physiologic barrier that is known as the blood–brain barrier. Similar restrictive interfaces between the rest of the body and the CNS include the blood–nerve barrier, the blood–CSF barrier, and the blood–retinal barrier.

The blood–brain barrier acts as a physical and enzymatic shield to help maintain homeostasis in the CNS. Endothelial cells that line the blood vessel walls in the body are separated by gap junctions. These gap junctions allow the free exchange of ions, proteins, and nutrients in and out of the vessel. In the CNS, however, the endothelial cells that line the walls of blood vessels have tight junctions that restrict the movement of ions, proteins, and nutrients in and out of the vessel. Other barrier components, **astrocytes**, **pericytes**, and the **basal lamina**, provide a further restrictive defense against the infiltration of blood-borne substances that penetrate the endothelial cell layer (Fig. 5–3). As a result of this exclusive barrier, nonlipid substances such as glucose, amino acids, and other nutrients depend on active transporters that use the energy substrate adenosine triphosphate (ATP) to enter the brain. These active transporters require energy-generating mitochondria, which are more numerous in endothelial cells lining the brain's blood vessels than in endothelial cells of other organs.

Although the blood–brain barrier restricts the movement of various substances across the nervous sys-

tem interface, it is not a barrier to migrating cells. The amount of white blood cells, or leukocytes, in the intact nervous system is minimal. During infection or inflammation, however, increased migration of leukocytes across the blood–brain barrier results in elevated levels of these cells in the CNS. Metastasizing tumor cells are also believed to access the CNS compartment by migrating across the blood–brain barrier. Both leukocytes and tumor cells secrete proteinases, enzymes that break down proteins, which probably allows the cells to migrate across the blood vessel.

Not all parts of the brain are shrouded by a blood–brain barrier. At the areas surrounding the ventricles of the brain, including the pituitary gland, pineal gland, subfornical organ, area postrema, choroid plexus, and the median eminence of the hypothalamus, the blood has direct access to the brain environment. The **ependymal cells**, also called tany-

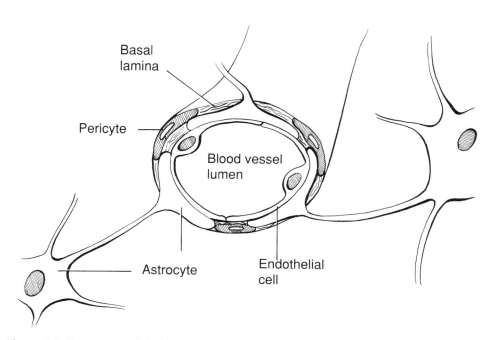

Basal
lamina

Pericyte

Blood vessel
lumen

Astrocyte

Endothelial
cell

Figure 5-3. Components of the blood–brain barrier, which separates the systemic blood circulation from the nervous system compartment. Tight junctions exist between the endothelial cells that line the lumen of the blood vessel. An extracellular matrix basal lamina surrounds the endothelial cells and anchors astrocytes and pericytes, which function as an additional defense against blood-borne substances.

cytes, line the capillaries and ventricles in these regions, forming a blood–CSF barrier. The ventricular surface of these ependymal cells contains microvilli that aid in CSF flow. Neurons in these areas sense systemic alterations in hormone levels and other blood-borne chemical messengers, and can respond to these alterations. The apical tight junctions between ependymal cells prevent the movement of substances between the blood and the rest of the neuronal environment.

Opening of the blood–brain barrier or leakage of blood-borne substances at the blood–brain barrier has been linked to damage and disease in the CNS. Barrier opening can be detected both by histologic examination of CNS tissue and by physiologic measurements. Electron microscopy of brain tumor tissue biopsy specimens illustrates the presence of **fenestrations** and **vesicles** in capillary endothelial cells. Fenestrations and vesicles are normal in blood vessels of other systemic organs, but are absent in most brain capillary endothelia. Clinically, blood–brain barrier breakdown can be monitored in patients suffering from brain trauma, hemorrhagic stroke, or multiple sclerosis using computed tomography or MRI scans. Leakage of an intravenously injected contrasting agent, such as gadolinium, across a damaged blood–brain barrier can be detected using MRI techniques, and is a reliable indicator of CNS injury (Fig. 5–4).

Many pharmaceutical companies are focusing on ways to control the opening and closing of the blood– brain barrier. Because the blood–brain barrier restricts the entry of blood-borne substances, many potentially therapeutic drugs cannot access the nervous system environment to combat diseases or cancerous tumors. In the future, progres-

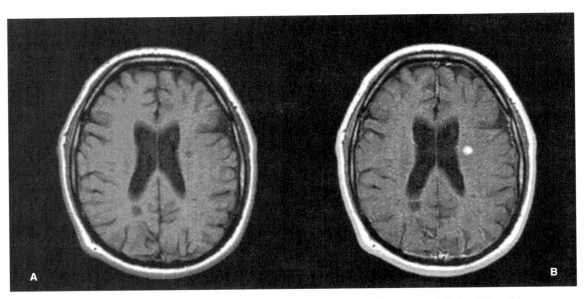

Figure 5-4. Magnetic resonance imaging (MRI) techniques, such as these pregadolinium **(A)** and gadolinium-enhanced **(B)** images, are used to detect focal lesions in patients with clinical signs of multiple sclerosis. MRI abnormalities, showing up as bright areas on the gadolinium-enhanced MRI, are often strong indicators of blood–brain barrier breakdown. The darker, hypointense area in the lower left part of the brain is most likely a lesion from an earlier episode of multiple sclerosis. (Courtesy of Drs. C. Ford and W. Brooks, Department of Neurology and the Center for Non-invasive Diagnosis, University of New Mexico, Albuquerque, New Mexico.)

sive disorders such as Alzheimer's or Parkinson's disease may be retarded or cured if therapeutic access to the brain through the blood–brain barrier can be regulated.

Neuroglia

The concept of neuroglia has changed dramatically since it was initially observed in the 19th century and characterized as nonneuronal "nerve glue." Neuroglia, originally described as connective tissue that supports neurons, outnumber neurons by at least 10-fold and constitute the microenvironment of the nervous system. Much of the evidence suggesting that glial cells are more than connective tissue surrounding neurons comes from neurotransmitter studies. Receptors for many of the neurotransmitters, including glutamate, gamma-aminobutyric acid (GABA), and acetylcholine, have been detected on glia. The release of GABA, an inhibitory transmitter, into the synaptic cleft results in an influx of chloride and a hyperpolarization (inhibition) of postsynaptic neurons. Simultaneously, in the same synaptic cleft, GABA causes an efflux of chloride, resulting in the depolarization (excitation) of glial cells. This reciprocal interaction between neuron and glia may promote an ionic homeostasis in the synaptic cleft region, allowing quicker recovery for the next synaptic event. Neuroglia also buffer local concentrations of potassium and neurotransmitters by taking up excesses of these substances from the extracellular spaces of the CNS.

The interconnection and mutual reliance of neurons and glia in nervous system development, disease, injury, and recovery are now widely accepted and are areas of intense research. There are four major types of glial cells: astrocytes, oligodendrocytes, microglia, and ependymal cells. Ependymal cells were discussed briefly in the section on the Blood–Brain Barrier.

A transient population of neuroglia, called **radial glia**, are present during the prenatal period of the developing brain. As these glial cells migrate from the ventricular zone to the cortical surface of the developing brain, they set up a scaffolding network that is used to guide migrating neurons to their targeted destination. Because of their importance in the developing nervous system, damage to the radial glia could lead to abnormal neuronal migration, resulting in developmental brain disorders such as seizures and cerebral palsy. Radial glial cells are believed to transform later into astrocytes, oligodendrocytes, and other types of neuroglia in the CNS. Radial glial cells are discussed in more detail in Chapter 19.

Astrocytes

Astrocytes were named for their starlike processes and appearance in histologic studies of the CNS (Fig. 5–5). Two general populations of astrocytes have been identified based on their physical characteristics and regional specialization: Type 1 are protoplasmic astrocytes, which have a clearer cytoplasm and are found primarily in gray matter regions; Type 2 are fibrous astrocytes, which have more glial filaments and are situated primarily in white matter regions. More significantly, the function of astrocytes varies according to their cytoplasmic and membrane composition and their CNS proximity.

Astrocytes have multiple functions that are regionally specific. They regulate neurons and the surrounding environment. Recent findings demonstrate that astrocytes secrete various growth factors and immune-related cytokines that have clinical significance in wound healing and recovery from nervous system injury. When injury occurs in the CNS, blood-borne factors cross the damaged blood–brain barrier and activate astrocytes. Astrocytes respond by proliferating and migrating to the injured site. During this process, known as **reactive gliosis**, neuroglia release several neurotrophic growth factors. These growth factors are instrumental in regulating the development of glial scars and regenerative neuronal sprouting. Chapter 21 discusses this process further. Certain diseases, such as multiple sclerosis, epilepsy, and acquired immunodeficiency syndrome (AIDS) dementia are characterized by dense glial scars that often are a result of reactive astrocytes. These fibrous scars build up at sites where myelin and neurons have degenerated. Functional regeneration of the neuron or glia at these sites is poor because these scars appear to impair astrocytic properties.

Scientists have drawn on the ability of astrocytes to secrete growth factors as a therapy to facilitate nerve tissue regeneration after injury or degeneration. Such therapies include amplifying the effect of

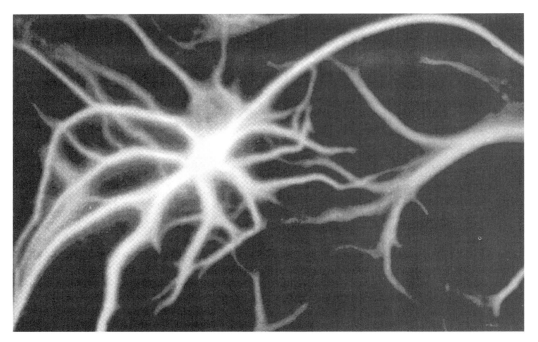

Figure 5-5. The starlike appearance of these astrocytes is enhanced by immunostaining with glial fibrillary acidic protein antibody. These astrocytes were grown in cell culture. (Courtesy of Drs. L. A. Cunningham and G. A. Rosenberg, Departments of Neurology and Pharmacology, University of Mexico, Albuquerque, New Mexico.)

growth factors that appear to stimulate axonal regeneration. This therapeutic approach involves the implantation of fetal astrocytes that are genetically engineered to secrete growth factors and neurotrophins into the degenerated or injured site. The extent and location of injury, as well as the timing of therapeutic intervention during the healing and recovery stages, add to the complexity of implementing these novel treatments.

Oligodendrocytes and Schwann Cells

Similar to astrocytes, the function of **oligodendrocytes** varies according to their location and physical traits. Satellite oligodendrocytes are in general confined to gray matter regions and are in close proximity to neuron surfaces. The interfascicular oligodendrocytes are the myelinating cells of the CNS. Oligoden-

drocytes are very responsive to signaling and alterations in the CNS microenvironment. They are especially vulnerable to injury during developmental periods of axon myelination. The myelinating process can continue well into the second decade of life.

Membranes of CNS oligodendrocytes and **Schwann cells** of the peripheral nervous system form the myelin sheaths that surround nerve axons. These multiple layers of myelin give the characteristic white appearance to neuronal tracts in the brain and spinal cord; hence the name "white matter." As you learned in Chapter 3, the tightly wrapped myelin sheath, shown in Figure 5–6, acts as an insulator of electrical impulses along the axon, facilitating the conduction of signals along a neuron. An oligodendrocyte can myelinate several internodes of different axons in the CNS simultaneously. The cell body of the oligodendrocyte is usually distant from its myelinating processes. In contrast, a Schwann cell ensheaths only

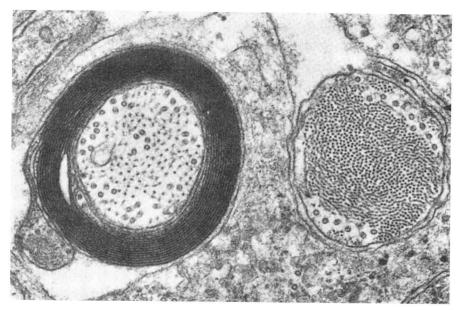

Figure 5-6. Electron microscopy of the compact myelin membrane of an oligodendrocyte ensheathing a nerve axon (left) and a cross-sectional view of an astrocyte process (right). (From Raine CS, *Basic neurochemistry.* 4th ed. New York: Raven Press, 1989, used by permission.)

one internode of an axon, and its cell body remains close to this internode.

The involvement of Schwann cells of the peripheral nervous system in nerve axon regeneration has been well documented. Schwann cells are very resilient to most injuries and diseases. Mitosis, the process of cell division and growth, occurs readily after local trauma. In addition, Schwann cells are able to migrate and phagocytose myelin debris, then stimulate new myelin formation. Regeneration of Schwann cell myelin can be detected 1 week after initial loss.

In comparison, because one oligodendrocyte myelinates several central nerve axons, damage to an oligodendrocyte often results in multiple sites of demyelination. This fact, coupled with their low regenerative capacity and slow mitotic rate, renders these glial cells particularly vulnerable to disease or injury. Demyelinating diseases such as multiple sclerosis cause widespread focal lesions on oligodendrocytes, leading to degenerated signal transduction in the CNS.

Oligodendrocytes are also very susceptible to toxic substances and infection. Fetal alcohol syndrome is often characterized by delays in motor and CNS development. Results from studies on animals exposed to alcohol during the final 2 weeks of gestation showed abnormally developed oligodendrocytes and poor responsiveness to neurotransmitters in newborn animals.

Injured neurons in the adult CNS of several species, including humans, are not known to regenerate on their own. The presence of glial cells in the regeneration of severed or crushed nerve axons is significant in the rehabilitation of a spinal cord injury. Although it is unlikely that they are the sole factors inhibiting neuronal regeneration, components of myelin and oligodendrocytes have been shown to block the growth of neurites in the CNS. Similarly, the developmental period at which neurons lose their ability to regenerate seems to coincide with the initial appearance of oligodendrocytes and the onset of myelination. Blocking the molecules found on the surface of myelin and oligodendrocytes that inhibit neurite outgrowth has been examined as a possible treatment strategy for regeneration of spinal cord injuries, especially when coupled with a regime of neurotrophic factors.

The extracellular matrix surrounding glia may also regulate the growth or inhibition of regenerating axons. A novel approach to axonal regrowth involves the tissue engineering of a three-dimensional tube seeded with growth factors, extracellular matrix components, and even Schwann cells. A neurotrophin-enriched tissue microenvironment is created in these synthetic conduits that physically bridges the gap created by severed axons. These guidance chambers are designed to facilitate regrowth of neuronal axons.

Microglia

Microglial cells are the link between the nervous system and the immune system. Microglia are part of the **mononuclear phagocyte system**, which includes bone marrow monoblasts, monocytes in the blood, and macrophages. These neuroglia probably migrate into the nervous system before the formation of the blood–brain barrier and are the resident macrophages of the CNS. Similar to macrophages in the body, microglia engulf and digest pathogens and debris at the site of injury.

In the normally functioning brain, microglia are at a resting state. They become active and mobile at the onset of injury or disease to the CNS. Microglia have been observed to migrate to the area of insult and exhibit macrophage-like traits, including the engulfing and disposal of invading antigens and wound debris. These glial cells may also play a homeostatic role in the nervous system by phagocytosing cellular debris resulting from normal wear and tear.

More recently, microglia have been implicated in regulating the destructive, tissue-damaging effects of many CNS inflammatory diseases, including ischemic stroke, AIDS, and epilepsy. When injury or disease transforms microglia into their reactive state, these neuroglial cells secrete factors that are meant to defend the system against infection or injury. Extensive secretion of these factors has been shown to be toxic to neurons. One area of research focuses on inhibiting the secreted toxins in efforts to prevent extensive nerve tissue damage.

Clinical Correlations

Understanding nervous system circulation is essential when providing rehabilitative treatment for many neurologic injuries and diseases. The location and extent of the injury often determine functional prognosis and the behavioral symptoms that the client will exhibit. In both ischemic and hemorrhagic stroke, the blood supply to specific regions of the brain is compromised. An ischemic stroke occurs as a result of an occluded blood vessel, and a hemorrhagic stroke is due to a ruptured vessel. The diagnosis of a stroke is usually described by the blood vessel that was affected. Knowledge of the blood circulation in the nervous system enables allied health professionals to determine appropriate treatment modalities.

Why should therapists be interested in neuroglial cells? A primary reason is the concept of neuroplasticity. As therapists, most of the goals we set with our clients focus on learning a new skill that has not been adequately developed, or relearning an essential ability that has been lost by injury or disease. This learning and relearning is inherently dependent on the neuroplasticity of the brain, spinal cord, and peripheral nervous system. Studies have shown that the neuroglia are key components regulating the activity-dependent neuroplasticity of the CNS. "Plasticity" in this context refers to modulating synapse formation to establish neuronal contacts, as well as the efficient release and uptake of synaptic messengers, the neurotransmitters. The size of the neuron body, its number of synaptic contacts, and the amount of neurotransmitters synthesized can be altered in an activity-dependent manner.

As you learned earlier in this chapter, glial cells are the major component of the CNS and exert a regulatory effect on neurons. Glial cells can effectively influence the physical properties and functions of neurons, including neuronal regeneration and synaptic responsiveness to transmitted signals, and can establish permanent physical changes in the neuron. All these factors implicate therapeutic, purposeful activity as an essential component of functional recovery from nervous system injury or disease. In other words, recovery from brain injury requires the purposeful activities implemented by the therapist, which facilitate activity-dependent changes in the neuronal environment.

The cerebral circulation and neuroglia exert a definite impact on the neuron and nervous system, especially during dysfunctional events, as summarized in

<table>
<tr><td></td></tr>
</table>

TABLE 5-2

Possible Dysfunctions of Nonneural Components

Nervous System Component	Dysfunction	Resultant Disorders
Cerebral blood supply	Blood clots/plaques, hemorrhage, vessel wall aneurysm	Cerebrovascular accident (stroke), atherosclerosis
Cerebrospinal fluid	Bacterial or viral invasion, blocked cerebrospinal fluid circulation, enlarged ventricles	Bacterial meningitis, septic shock, viral infection, hydrocephalus, learning disabilities
Blood-brain barrier and meninges	Inflammation-related barrier opening, bacterial or viral invasion	MS, bacterial meningitis, viral infection, encephalitis, other central nervous system infections
Neuroglia	Aberrant glial cell production, glial cell damage	Nervous system tumors, cerebral palsy, seizures, Guillain-Barré syndrome, MS

MS, multiple sclerosis.

Table 5–2. Our understanding of the dynamic interactions between these nonneuronal elements and neurons continues to develop as more basic science studies are correlated with behaviorally related clinical research. Modulating the nervous system microenvironment—that is, the neuroglia and the blood–brain barrier system–may be essential for neuronal regeneration and improved recovery of function after injury or disease.

REFERENCES

1. Cohen H. *Neuroscience for rehabilitation*. Philadelphia: JB Lippincott, 1993.
2. Rosenberg GA, Wolfson LI. Disorders of brain fluids and electrolytes. In: Rosenberg RN, ed. *Comprehensive neurology*. New York: Raven Press, 1991.
3. Raine CS. Neurocellular anatomy. In: *Basic neurochemistry*.4th ed. New York: Raven Press, 1989.

section two

SENSORY SYSTEMS

6

Somatic Senses I: The Anterolateral System

S. ESSIE JACOBS, PhD, OTR
DEBORAH L. LOWE, PhD

**Sensory Receptors for the
Anterolateral System**

Thermoreceptors

Nociceptors

Primary Afferent (or First-order) Neurons

*Termination of Primary Afferent Fibers in the
Dorsal Horn of the Spinal Cord*

Gate Control Theory of Pain

Clinical Correlations

Transcutaneous Electrical Nerve Stimulation

Referred Pain

Anterolateral System Pathways

The Spinothalamic Tract

The Spinoreticular Tract

Damage to the Anterolateral Pathway

The Trigeminal Pathways

**Clinical Correlations:
Thalamic Pain Syndrome**

Cerebral Cortex

Primary and Secondary Somatosensory Cortex

Descending Pathways Involved in Pain Modulation

Clinical Correlations

Pain Perception

Phantom Limbs

• • •

Sensory information ascends from the spinal cord to the higher levels of the central nervous system for processing by two major pathways: 1) the anterolateral system and 2) the dorsal column system. This chapter addresses the anterolateral system, the major route by which pain and temperature information is transmitted. It also makes a minor but functionally significant contribution to our perception of touch that provides some secondary tactile information to the input primarily provided by the dorsal column system. This redundancy of touch information means that, even in the face of dorsal column system damage, a person can continue to appreciate tactile sensation from the skin. This redundancy, however, is not usually the case for information about pain and temperature—that is, damage to the anterolateral system results in marked decreases in the perception of pain and temperature. In this chapter, we take you systematically through the process by which stimuli carried in the anterolateral system work their way from the peripheral tissue through the spinal cord, and then, along one of the anterolateral system pathways, to the higher-level centers where the stimulus is perceived.

Sensory Receptors for the Anterolateral System

The anterolateral system originates from axons of sensory neurons in the spinal cord, but these neurons are far from the sites where receptors in our skin, muscles, joints, and viscera (e.g., stomach, heart, lung) detect pain and temperature. You should understand how information that will ultimately be carried by anterolateral system pathways reaches these spinal cord neurons in the first place.

The presence of sensory receptors that are selectively sensitive to specific stimuli facilitates our ability to discriminate varied types of cutaneous sensations. This specificity of the sensory receptors depends primarily on the structure of the peripheral ending of the primary sensory neuron. Although the structures of peripheral receptors that convey different qualities of touch vary considerably, thermal sensitivity and pain sensation are both activated by free, unencapsulated nerve endings, called **thermoreceptors** and **nociceptors**, respectively. Although the sensory endings for these two modalities appear similar, the receptor membranes around them have different response properties that account for their specificity.

Thermoreceptors

Our skin is exquisitely sensitive to minute changes in temperature. The ability to appreciate temperature changes depends primarily on the skin's thermoceptors. Receptors for hot and cold are separate, and these receptors are not distributed uniformly across the skin. Rather, areas of skin approximately 1 mm wide respond to either cold or hot. Normal skin temperature is 34°C. Application of a cold stimulus

(10°–33°C) to a cold receptor results in an increased firing rate of the afferent fiber; exposing the skin innervated by a cold receptor to temperatures slightly above a neutral skin temperature results in a decreased firing rate. Warmth receptors respond within the range of 32°C to 45°C. Extremes in temperature (below about 5°C and above 45°C) are perceived as noxious stimuli and therefore are not carried by thermoreceptors, but rather by nociceptors.

Nociceptors

Nociceptors respond preferentially to noxious stimuli. Nociceptive sensory endings are free nerve endings located in skin, muscle, joints, and viscera that serve as the body's warning system about stimuli that either cause or threaten to cause damage. Each nociceptor is specifically activated by one of several types of sensory input, including 1) mechanical (or cutaneous), 2) thermal, and 3) polymodal. Mechanical nociceptors are excited by mechanical stimuli that damage the skin, and therefore serve as pain receptors, not mechanoreceptors. Thermal nociceptors, as indicated previously, are different from thermoreceptors because they are activated by temperature extremes. As with thermoreceptors, the free nerve endings conveying heat are different from those conveying cold. Polymodal nociceptors are activated by several different forms of noxious stimuli, including mechanical, thermal, or chemical.

Primary Afferent (or First-order) Neurons

All sensory receptors from the body have their somata in **dorsal root ganglia** neurons. These cells, the first in line to receive information from the periphery, are therefore called **first-order neurons**. Their morphology is unique in that they are pseudounipolar, having an axon process that divides into two branches, one extending into the periphery and another, central branch that extends into the spinal cord (Fig. 6–1). The terminal of the peripheral branch transduces stimulus energy from a sensory receptor. The signal is then transmitted as an action potential along the peripheral branch and its continuation in the central branch. Together these branches are referred to as the **primary afferent fiber**. The primary afferent fiber terminates on a sensory neuron

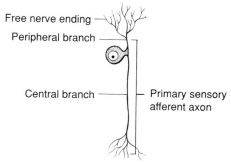

Free nerve ending

Peripheral branch

Central branch

Primary sensory afferent axon

Figure 6–1 An example of a pseudounipolar neuron found in the dorsal root ganglion.

in the dorsal horn of the spinal column (second-order neuron). Sensory information from the head and neck is conveyed in a similar manner, but through a cranial nerve with its primary sensory neuron in the brainstem. This **trigeminal pathway** is discussed later in this chapter.

Two types of primary afferent fibers convey pain and temperature to the spinal cord: A-delta (Aδ) fibers and C fibers. These fibers can be classified according to:

1 Conduction velocity of the action potential along the fiber to the central nervous system

2 Aspects of the stimulation that must be present to evoke a response (e.g., intensity, duration, quality)

3 Characteristic responses of the nociceptor to natural stimuli (e.g., slow vs. fast adaptation)

Aδ fibers are lightly myelinated, relatively fast-conducting, small-diameter fibers, propagating an action potential at a rate of 5 to 30 m/second (which is substantially slower than the nonnociceptive, large-diameter A-alpha (Aα) and A-beta (Aβ) fiber velocities. C fibers are unmyelinated, small-diameter fibers that are slow conducting, conveying information to the spinal cord at a speed of about 1 m/second.

Aδ fibers are stimulated by low-threshold, superficial receptors that are functionally associated with pain that has a sharp, pricking quality. This type of pain can be localized on the body surface and diminishes quickly. It has been called **fast pain** as well as **initial** or **first pain**. The unmyelinated C fibers are stimulated by high-threshold receptors. C fibers convey diffuse, persisting pain that we experience as aching, throbbing, burning pain that is poorly localized. It has been labeled **slow pain** or

delayed or **second pain**. Many people find this type of pain almost intolerable, compared with the initial stabbing pain conducted by Aδ fibers that can often precede slow pain. Thermal nociceptors for cold are connected to the spinal cord by Aδ fibers, whereas painful sensations arising from heat result in C fiber activation. Finally, polymodal nociceptors responding to a variety of stimulus energies (chemical, mechanical, and very hot or cold) are associated with C fibers.

Termination of Primary Afferent Fibers in the Dorsal Horn of the Spinal Cord

Fibers destined for both the dorsal column and anterolateral pathways segregate as they enter the spinal cord. As they pass through the zone of Lissauer, which lies immediately outside the dorsal horn, the large-diameter Aα and Aβ fibers carrying touch and proprioceptive information to the dorsal columns occupy a medial position; the small Aδ and C primary nociceptive afferents are laterally positioned. In general, the pathways carrying these stimuli remain segregated as they ascend through the central nervous system en route to the cortex.

The Aδ and C fibers that provide the predominant sensory information conveyed by the anterolateral pathways divide as they enter the spinal cord. Axonal branches ascend and descend as far as four segments from the segment of entry as part of the **dorsolateral tract of Lissauer**. Axons in this tract send collateral fibers into sensory neurons in the dorsal horn of the spinal cord. The dorsal horn cells that receive afferent input from primary sensory afferents are called **second-order sensory neurons**. The primary afferent Aδ and C fibers make different synaptic connections in the dorsal horn, which results in the division of the anterolateral system into the **spinothalamic** and **spinoreticular** pathways.

The dorsal horn of the spinal cord has six anatomically defined cell layers, or laminae (Fig. 6–2). These laminae do not have distinct borders, nor do the cells within them perform the same functions. Function may be related to the morphology of the dendritic arborizations rather than the location of the cell bodies themselves. An appreciation of the organization of afferent input to the dorsal horn laminae is fundamental for understanding clinical syndromes related to pain. As you will see, neurons in the dorsal horn of any lamina do not act as simple

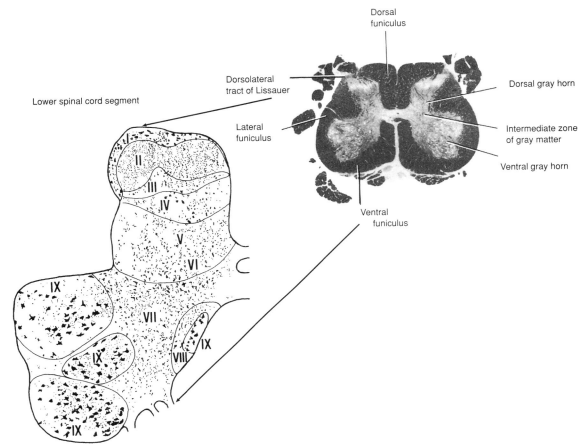

Figure 6-2. Schematic showing the laminae of a lower spinal cord segment. Inset is a photomicrograph of a segment in cross-section in which dark areas contain fiber tracts; light areas contain cell bodies (Weigert's stain, original magnification, 27). (Schematic adapted and reproduced with permission from Willard FH. *Medical neuroanatomy: a problem-oriented manual with annotated atlas.* Philadelphia: JB Lippincott, 1993:27. Photomicrograph adapted and reproduced with permission from Barr ML, Kiernan JA. *The human nervous system: an anatomical viewpoint.* 6th ed. Philadelphia: JB Lippincott, 1993:72.

conduits of information from the periphery to the cortex. Instead, they receive and integrate information from other laminae and pathways before relaying their information to higher centers. Later, we discuss how dorsal horn neurons are influenced by information descending from higher centers.

Lamina I is the dorsal-most part of the dorsal horn. Neurons in this lamina respond to sharp, prickling pain and cold relayed by Aδ nociceptors and Aδ

thermoreceptors, respectively. Axons of these lamina I neurons cross the midline of the spinal cord in the **ventral commissure** and ascend as part of the spinothalamic pathway. These neurons are called **projection neurons** because they have long axons that relay information from one region of the central nervous system to another. Sensory information is also conveyed from lamina I neurons to the more ventral lamina V neurons through a series of synaptic connections onto **interneurons** with short, locally projecting axons. Unlike projection neurons that have long axons, interneurons have short axons and synapse on neighboring neurons. Finally, lamina I is the termination site for **second-order axons** carrying C fiber diffuse pain-related information whose neurons lie in lamina II.

Lamina II (also known as the **substantia gelatinosa**) has neurons that are primarily activated by C fiber nociceptors, thermoreceptors, and mechanoreceptors conveying noxious mechanical and thermal stimuli. Innocuous mechanical information from Aδ and even Aβ fibers excites some lamina II neurons, although this input from Aδ and Aβ fibers appears to occur through indirect, polysynaptic projections. As noted earlier, some lamina II neurons send axons that terminate on lamina I and conduct mainly C fiber thermal nociceptive information to the contralateral spinothalamic tract. Most of the lamina II neurons send axons that reenter the tract of Lissauer to terminate a few segments higher or lower in the spinal cord. Through a series of synaptic connections onto interneurons, this information is conveyed from lamina II to lamina V projection neurons. The diffuse, burning pain information is then conveyed from lamina V across the midline to the contralateral spinoreticular pathway. Lamina II axons, themselves, probably do not send direct contributions to ascending sensory pathways. Rather, through local connections with lamina I and lamina V (by interneurons), lamina II neurons act as a first-line defense for determining if sensory inputs are conveying painful sensations.

Laminae III and IV neurons respond to cutaneous Aδ mechanoreceptors as well as collaterals of large-diameter Aβ primary afferent neurons conveying light touch. Most of the second-order Aβ axons relaying light touch information project to the dorsal columns; some fibers cross to contribute to the contralateral spinothalamic pathway. These laminae also contain interneurons that integrate sensory information and excite projection neurons in lamina V.

Laminae V and VI lie in the ventral portion of the dorsal horn. In a manner similar to lamina I, cutaneous nociceptive Aδ primary afferent fibers synapse directly onto second-order projection neurons in lamina V, which then send axons across to the contralateral spinothalamic tract. Some Aβ fibers carrying touch information send collaterals that terminate in lamina VI and contribute to the light touch component of the anterolateral pathway. The C fiber pain and temperature information that terminated in lamina II is conveyed by a series of synapses to projection neurons in lamina V, which then carry the information across the midline to the contralateral spinoreticular tract.

In summary, the projection neurons of laminae I and V contribute the greatest number of fibers to the anterolateral pathways. The other laminae (i.e., laminae II–IV) function primarily as integration centers for sensory information. Sensory information is thus evaluated and, as we show later, modulated before being relayed to the projection neurons in laminae I and V. Afferent fibers from visceral structures are also important in nociception. Through connections with dorsal horn neurons, visceral and somatic afferents in the same spinal segments can become associated and produce referred pain (see section on Clinical Correlations).

Gate Control Theory of Pain

The gate control theory of pain[1] (Fig. 6–3) was proposed as a conceptual model to explain the neural mechanisms associated with pain. This theory also suggested that specific psychological mechanisms (i.e., the gate) might influence a person's perception of pain. Melzack and Wall[1] postulated that at those places in the dorsal horn where the large and small afferents come into contact, the large, myelinated Aα and Aβ (touch and proprioception) fibers exert inhibitory control over the small, unmyelinated C (pain) fibers. The balance between the myelinated and unmyelinated afferent fiber activity at these sites of convergence could therefore modulate the signal to the higher brain centers. Descending control mechanisms are also important in pain control and are discussed later in the chapter.

The gate control theory involves the following classes of dorsal horn cells: 1) C fiber afferents, 2) nonnociceptive A fibers, 3) inhibitory interneurons, and 4) dorsal horn projection neurons that convey pain to the ascending spinothalamic tract of the anterolateral system when activated. Nociceptive C fiber activity is relayed to the spinothalamic tract by axons from contralateral spinal cord projection neurons. The projection neuron is normally inhibited by the interneuron, which is spontaneously active. That is, the normal activity of the inhibitory interneuron acts on the projection neuron to reduce the intensity

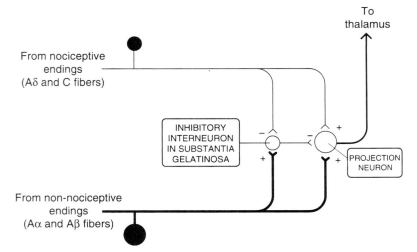

Figure 6-3. Simple illustration of the gate control theory of pain. Nonnociceptive sensory fibers stimulate the inhibitory interneurons, whereas nociceptive afferents inhibit them. An increase in nonnociceptive input reduces the rate of firing of the spinothalamic tract neurons. (Adapted and reproduced with permission from Barr ML, Kiernan JA. *The human nervous system: an anatomical viewpoint.* 6th ed. Philadelphia: JB Lippincott, 1993:299.

of the painful input from C fibers. In theory, the C fiber inhibits the activity of the interneuron, thereby releasing the projection neuron from the inhibitory suppression. This "opening of the gate" results in enhanced perception of pain being transmitted to higher brain structures. In contrast, the nonnociceptive A fiber excites the inhibitory interneuron, and in this way tries to suppress or "close the gate" on pain perception. So, when you rub the place on your body that you have just bruised, you are stimulating the Aα and Aβ nonnociceptive afferent fibers to ease the discomfort.

The gate control theory of pain is being tested with laboratory research. It remains the most important working model used by pain investigators.

Clinical Correlations

Transcutaneous Electrical Nerve Stimulation

Responses to and perceptions of acute and chronic pain are functions of the sensitivity of Aδ and C afferents and the excitability of neurons in the nociceptor–pain pathways. Alterations in sensitivity or excitability of afferents or sensory neurons can result in seemingly paradoxic responses. One response is a general increase in the sensitivity to previously nonnoxious subthreshold stimuli, resulting in pain. The other response is a decreased sensitivity or analgesia

that renders the person unresponsive to previously noxious stimuli.[2] **Transcutaneous electrical nerve stimulation (TENS)** capitalizes on the electrical properties that result in analgesia to suppress pain. This effect is achieved through the use of repetitive electrical stimulation applied over peripheral nerves, trigger points, acupuncture points, or dermatomes from which the painful sensations arise.[3]

The electrical properties of receptor and neuronal membranes determine their sensitivity and excitability. Altering these electrical properties with externally applied current is the scientific basis for treatment of acute and chronic pain with TENS. The quality of the electrical stimulation that TENS provides can be varied by altering stimulus frequency, intensity, and waveform.[4]

Two types of TENS are most commonly used. Conventional TENS uses low-intensity (two to three times the sensory threshold) and high-frequency (60–100 Hz) stimulation. Acupuncture-like TENS uses high-intensity (more than three times the sensory threshold) and low-frequency (2–4 Hz) stimulation.[3] As yet, neither type has been shown to be more efficacious, so the therapist and patient must empirically determine the optimal settings (frequency, intensity, waveform) and regimen (electrode placement, period of stimulation, activity during stimulation).

The analgesia produced by conventional TENS probably occurs through peripheral mechanisms; acupuncture-like TENS has been shown to work through central and peripheral mechanisms.[3] The central mechanism involves stimulation of endorphin production.[5] Endorphins are naturally occurring and act as endogenous analgesics. TENS may produce analgesia through two different peripheral mechanisms. One mechanism involves a reduction of conduction velocity and the amplitude of the compound action potential of the fast-conducting Aα and Aβ fibers and the slow-conducting Aδ and C fibers, thus effectively suppressing nonnoxious and noxious input to the central nervous system.[6] The other mechanism involves presynaptic suppression of Aδ and C input by Aα and Aβ input[3] (see section on Gate Control Theory of Pain).

Transcutaneous electrical nerve stimulation is only part of a treatment program for patients with acute and chronic pain. A full program of normal functional activities must be used in conjunction with TENS so that normal use can be restored to the affected part once the pain has been reduced or relieved.

Referred Pain

Referred pain sensations result from the extensive convergence of visceral and somatic inputs on the same neurons at various levels of the central nervous system. Pain that begins as a deep, dull, poorly localized sensation becomes referred to more superficial regions of the body (e.g., muscle, joint, skin), usually in the same dermatome. In the case of visceral disease, pain can be experienced in regions remote from the affected organ.[7] Afferent activity triggered in C fibers by injury or inflammation in the viscera can induce an increased state of excitability in sensory neurons, especially second-order neurons in the dorsal horn. This convergence of visceral and nociceptive inputs can alter how the neurons process normal afferent input from the referred (somatic) area.[8] In effect, the higher centers cannot discriminate the source of the painful stimuli, so it is experienced in nonvisceral tissue. Referred pain is most commonly experienced in muscle, but may also involve subcutaneous tissue and skin. It can also be accompanied by an increased sensitivity to painful stimuli (hyperesthesia) and a decreased pain threshold (secondary hyperalgesia) in the referred zone.[7,8]

The patient who is experiencing a myocardial infarction reports referred pain sensations radiating through the chest wall, left axilla, and inside of the left arm. These regions are affected because cardiac and cutaneous fibers travel in spinal cord segments T1 through T5 and converge on the same dorsal horn neurons.[8] Referred pain can also have a somatic source. For example, in myofascial pain syndrome, pain originates from trigger points that are hyperirritable spots in a band of skeletal muscle or fascia, resulting from overuse or misuse.[9]

Anterolateral System Pathways

As its name implies, the anterolateral system pathways are located in the corresponding quadrant of the spinal cord, more properly referred to as the ventrolateral quadrant. Two major ascending sensory pathways in the ventrolateral quadrant, the spinothalamic tract and the spinoreticular tract, convey pain, temperature, and some light touch impulses, relayed from the periphery to the spinal cord through Aδ and C fiber afferents. They originate from axons of second-order neurons in the contralateral dorsal horn (Fig. 6–4). A small number of axons remain ipsilateral as they ascend. Among the structures in which the fibers in these tracts terminate are the brainstem reticular formation and the thalamus.

The Spinothalamic Tract

This tract originates predominantly from projection neurons in laminae I, IV, and V (see Fig. 6–4). This pathway conveys Aδ inputs carrying sharp pain and cold, and C fiber thermoceptive input. In addition, some dorsal horn cells that receive light touch information from large-diameter Aα and Aβ input convey this information to the spinothalamic tract. This contribution of tactile input to the spinothalamic tract protects against complete loss of tactile sensation after lesions of the dorsal column.

The fibers in this tract are arranged in an orderly fashion, with input from the caudal-most spinal cord segments (i.e., sacral and lumbar) occupying the most lateral position, and rostral segments a medial position (Fig. 6–5). Structures that demonstrate this preservation of the periphery are said to be **somatotopically organized**. This feature can be important for clinical diagnosis, although the organization of the anterolateral system tracts is cruder than that of the dorsal column–medial lemniscus tract.

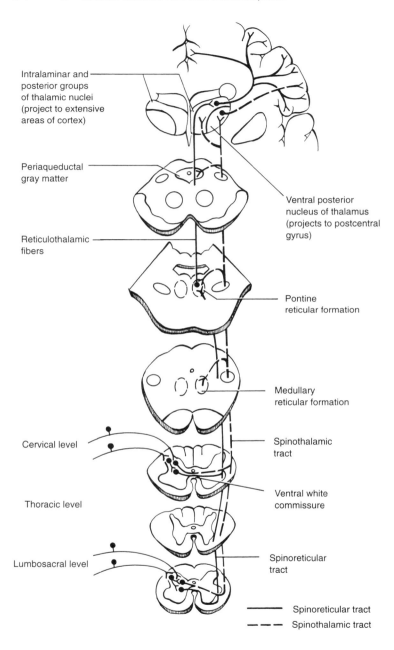

Intralaminar and posterior groups of thalamic nuclei (project to extensive areas of cortex)

Periaqueductal gray matter

Reticulothalamic fibers

Cervical level

Thoracic level

Lumbosacral level

Ventral posterior nucleus of thalamus (projects to postcentral gyrus)

Pontine reticular formation

Medullary reticular formation

Spinothalamic tract

Ventral white commissure

Spinoreticular tract

——— Spinoreticular tract
- - - - Spinothalamic tract

Figure 6–4. Ascending pathways for the appreciation of pain. The spinothalamic tract is shown as a dotted line and the spinoreticular tract is shown as a solid line. (Adapted and reproduced with permission from Barr ML, Kiernan JA. *The human nervous system: an anatomical viewpoint.* 6th ed. Philadelphia: JB Lippincott, 1993:301.)

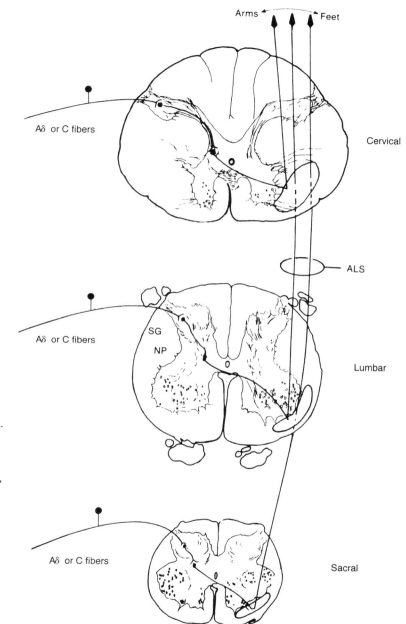

Figure 6–5. Diagram of the somatotopic arrangement of afferent fibers in the anterolateral system pathway (ALS). (**Source:** Small primary afferent fibers, Aδ or C fibers, from the periphery. **Function:** ALS carries pain, temperature, and crude touch conveyed by source fibers. **Laterality:** Sensory information crosses the midline at the segmental level). (Adapted and reproduced with permission from Willard FH. *Medical neuroanatomy: a problem-oriented manual with annotated atlas.* Philadelphia: JB Lippincott, 1993:39.

The spinothalamic tract and the dorsal column–medial lemniscal tract, which conveys information about discriminative touch and proprioception, move closer together as they ascend to the thalamus. By the time they reach the midbrain, the two tracts are apposed, but their fibers remain segregated. Both the spinothalamic and medial lemniscal tracts terminate in the **ventral posterior lateral (VPL) nucleus** of the thalamus, where they continue to maintain their separation (Fig. 6–6). The information in both of these tracts remains somatotopically organized in their progression from the periphery to the VPL and finally to somatosensory areas of the cortex. In this way, the VPL acts as a relay station, rapidly and accurately passing information to the cerebral cortex.

Although the VPL is the termination site of all dorsal column information before its transmission to the somatosensory cortical regions, it is one of several thalamic nuclei receiving pain, temperature, and light touch information. Nevertheless, this innervation of VPL neurons by the spinothalamic tract, with the information in turn relayed in an organized manner to the somatosensory cortex, is essential to our ability to perceive and localize painful stimuli.

Additional terminations of the spinothalamic tract include the small, centrally located **intralaminar nuclei of the thalamus**. The axons of these thalamic nuclei make widespread connections throughout the cerebral cortex that are not somatotopically organized. In this way, pain and temperature information is conveyed from the thalamus to a wider area of the cerebral cortex than the specific somatosensory cortical regions to which the dorsal column system projects.

The Spinoreticular Tract

This tract conveys the dull, burning pain associated with C fiber afferents to widespread regions of the brainstem reticular formation (see Fig. 6–4). This tract arises following a series of synapses in the dorsal horn by which information passes from lamina II neurons to projection neurons in the deep laminae. Although some fibers remain uncrossed, the information conveyed in this tract is largely from the contralateral spinal cord. The spinothalamic tract also contributes collateral branches to the spinoreticular tract as it progresses through the brainstem. In this manner, afferents conveying different types of sensory information make connections with neurons in the reticular formation. This convergence of sensory information onto individual reticular formation neu-

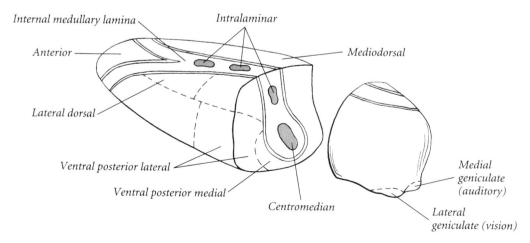

Figure 6–6. Oblique view of the left thalamus, showing the major somatosensory thalamic nuclei. The posterior nuclear complex is not delineated in the drawing. (Adapted and reproduced from Kelly JP. Anatomical basis of sensory perception and motor coordination. In: Kandel ER, Schwartz JH, eds. *Principles of neural science.* 2nd ed. New York: Elsevier, 1985 [which has been assigned to Appleton & Lange, Norwalk, CT].)

rons contributes to their diversity of function; it is also a factor in their being considered an important relay station in the ascending nonspecific system. Cells in the reticular formation project axons that ultimately terminate in a nonsomatotopic manner on the intralaminar nuclei of the thalamus. These intralaminar thalamic nuclei project to wide areas of the cerebral cortex. This diffuse pathway is most likely involved in the awareness of pain and the affective responses to the painful stimulus; its widespread distribution suggests it does not contribute to discriminating the location from which the pain is arising.

Damage to the Anterolateral Pathway

After hemisection of the spinal cord, a dramatic difference between the anterolateral and dorsal column systems is evident from the marked loss of tactile sense ipsilaterally, which is mediated by the dorsal column system, and a loss of pain and temperature contralaterally due to damage to the anterolateral system. Specific consequences of unilateral anterolateral pathway damage include contralateral loss of pain and temperature sensation beginning one or two segments below the site of fiber interruption; light touch is essentially intact as long as the dorsal columns are not affected.

The Trigeminal Pathways

Sensory innervation of the face is primarily supplied by the **trigeminal nerve** (**cranial nerve V**), which enters the brain at the level of the pons. Additional structures innervated by the trigeminal nerve include the mouth, the outer two thirds of the tongue, and the dura mater covering the brain. In a similar manner to the spinal cord, the trigeminal nerves are primary afferent axons whose cell bodies lie in the **trigeminal ganglia**, the cranial nerve equivalent of the dorsal root ganglia.

The trigeminal nerve has two groups of primary afferent fibers: large-diameter, myelinated Aα and Aβ afferents and small-diameter Aδ and C fiber afferents. The Aα and Aβ afferents convey discrete, localizable information about tactile input to the face and head, and proprioceptive input to the jaw. Information from these primary afferents is ultimately conveyed by the dorsal column system. We focus our attention on the Aδ and C fiber primary afferents carrying pain and temperature sensation through the anterolateral system.

The second-order neurons for pain and temperature impulses from the face are located in the pars caudalis of the **spinal trigeminal (spinal V) nucleus**, a structure that is continuous with the cervical spinal cord and that most closely resembles the dorsal horn. Because these second-order neurons are situated below the level of entry of the primary afferent fiber, the trigeminal nerves must first descend to make synaptic connections onto them. These descending primary trigeminal afferents are somatotopically organized. During this descent, primary afferent fibers from cranial nerves VII (facial nerve), IX (glossopharyngeal), and X (vagus) enter the trigeminal nerve tract, carrying input from areas around the ears, nose, and pharynx.

Neurons of the spinal trigeminal nucleus project to the **ventral posterior medial (VPM) nucleus** by way of the **trigeminothalamic tract** and to intralaminar thalamic nuclei by way of the **trigeminoreticulothalamic tract**. The trigeminothalamic tract is comparable with the spinothalamic tract. Trigeminothalamic projections arise in the spinal trigeminal nucleus, most of them cross in the lower brainstem reticular formation, and, during the decussation, some collaterals are projected to nuclei in the reticular formation. Most of these second-order trigeminal axons ascend in the contralateral anterolateral pathway to terminate in the VPM nucleus. In the VPM nucleus, the somatotopic organization of the sensory information from the contralateral face is retained. Some fibers from this tract project onto the intralaminar thalamic nuclei, which then sends projections to widespread areas of the cortex.

Trigeminoreticulothalamic tract projections convey diffuse, poorly localized pain and temperature information. Like the spinoreticular pathway with which it can be compared, the second-order axons terminate on third-order neurons in the reticular formation, which project to the intralaminar nuclei of the thalamus.

Lesions of the spinal trigeminal nerve result in diminished or absent pain and temperature sensation in the head and face regions innervated by this nerve. Tactile sensation, however, remains relatively unaffected because the dorsal column system conveying tactile information travels by a different route to second-order neurons in the brainstem.

Clinical Correlations: Thalamic Pain Syndrome

Several of the numerous thalamic nuclei receive afferent information from the anterolateral tracts originating from the contralateral body and then relay it to the cortex. This sensory information includes pain, thermal and mechanical sensations, and proprioception. Thalamic lesions therefore result in disturbances of sensation on the side of the body contralateral to the lesion. The sensory disturbances include pain resulting from nonnoxious stimuli (allodynia), abnormally decreased sensitivity to stimuli (hypoesthesia), diminished sensitivity to pain (hypoalgesia), abnormally exaggerated responses to painful stimuli (hyperpathia, hyperalgesia), and abnormally negative responses to sensations produced by normal stimuli (dysesthesia).[10,11] An example of dysesthesia is when tactile contact of a patient's clothing creates unpleasant or painful sensations. The most common causes of thalamic lesions are intracerebral hemorrhages or infarctions, but thalamic lesions can also be caused by insults from multiple sclerosis, trauma, and surgical complications.[10]

The exact nature of the sensory modalities affected by thalamic lesions differs depending on the nuclei involved. Patients diagnosed with **thalamic pain syndrome** most often have lesions in the intralaminar nuclei of the thalamus, a region in which nuclei specific for pain and temperature sensation have been identified.[12] Neurons in lamina I of the dorsal horn relaying input from the Aδ and C nociceptive fibers project to these nuclei through both the spinothalamic and spinoreticular tracts of the anterolateral system. Patients experiencing thalamic pain syndrome demonstrate somatosensory deficits and report poorly localized, spontaneous burning and crushing pain.

There is no single mode of therapy that effectively treats patients with thalamic pain syndrome. Narcotics are of little help and neuroablative procedures have very poor results. Deep brain stimulation of the thalamus and periaqueductal gray regions has led to some limited success in relieving chronic pain, but this technique is still experimental and should be pursued with caution. The best news is that, after months, most patients have some clinical improvement regardless of the treatment they receive.[13] In the interim, therapists should encourage patients to maintain mobility in the joints around the area of altered sensitivity.

Cerebral Cortex

Primary and Secondary Somatosensory Cortex

Complex processing of somatosensory information ultimately occurs at the level of the cerebral cortex. The **primary somatosensory cortex (S-I),** located in the postcentral gyrus within the parietal cortex, contains a sensory representation of the body that is somatotopically organized. At the lateral end of the postcentral gyrus, buried in the lateral sulcus, is the **secondary somatosensory cortex (S-II).** This region is also somatotopically organized, but in a sequence different from that of S-I.

Sensation is both discriminative and affective. Sensory information conveyed to S-I and S-II by the ventroposterior nuclei (both VPL and VPM) enables discrimination of stimulus properties, such as locality and intensity. This information is then integrated to develop perceptions about the sensory experience (e.g., size, shape). The thalamocortical projection to S-I is quite dense, whereas that to S-II is less substantial. S-II also receives input from other thalamic nuclei. More important, S-II requires input from S-I to process sensory information. Animal experiments in which S-II has been deactivated, either surgically or pharmacologically, have indicated that this region is not essential for somatic discrimination. Damage to S-I, however, results in contralateral loss of tactile discrimination and stereognosis (recognition of an object's size and shape by touch alone). Pain and temperature sensation, however, remain intact after postcentral gyrus damage.

Pain is a major factor in the affective experience of sensation. Pain manifests itself in many forms that often defy localization; interpretations or clinical evaluations of its intensity often cannot be isolated from an understanding of the person who is experiencing the pain.

Descending Pathways Involved in Pain Modulation

Dorsal horn cells can be inhibited from conveying nociceptive information to higher centers by a number of regions of the brain (Fig. 6–7). Among these are the cerebral cortex, the reticular formation of the medulla, and the periaqueductal gray, the region surrounding the cerebral aqueduct. Similar to the gate control theory proposed by Melzack and Wall,[1]

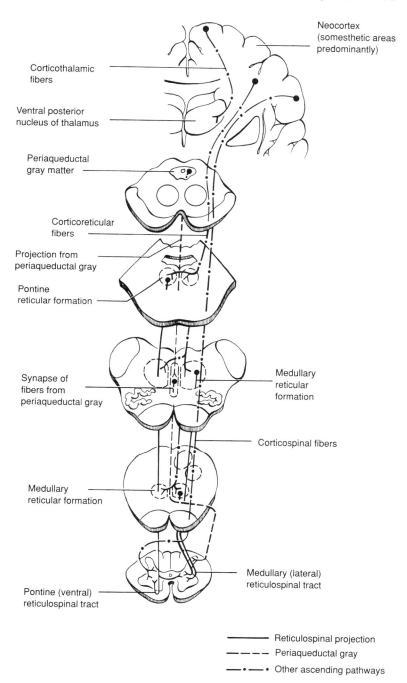

Figure 6–7. Descending pathways that modulate the transmission of sensory information from the spinal cord to the cerebral cortex. Reticulospinal projections are shown as the solid line; the descending tract from the periaqueductal gray is the dotted line; other descending pathways are indicated by the dot–solid line. (Adapted and reproduced with permission from Barr ML, Kiernan JA. *The human nervous system: an anatomical viewpoint.* 6th ed. Philadelphia: JB Lippincott, 1993:309.

Labels in figure:

Neocortex (somesthetic areas predominantly)

Corticothalamic fibers

Ventral posterior nucleus of thalamus

Periaqueductal gray matter

Corticoreticular fibers

Projection from periaqueductal gray

Pontine reticular formation

Synapse of fibers from periaqueductal gray

Medullary reticular formation

Corticospinal fibers

Medullary reticular formation

Medullary (lateral) reticulospinal tract

Pontine (ventral) reticulospinal tract

——————— Reticulospinal projection

– – – – – Periaqueductal gray

– • —— • Other ascending pathways

descending fibers from these areas inhibit transmission from nociceptive afferent fibers to projection neurons by acting on inhibitory interneurons in the dorsal horn. The descending pathways exert this inhibitory control selectively on nociceptive afferents, leaving tactile inputs unaffected.[14] This finding is clear evidence that nociceptive sensory information flow is not a static, unidirectional process. That is, brainstem and cortical structures are heavily involved in determining whether the information received in the spinal cord from the periphery will ascend.

Higher centers do not change noxious inputs entering from the periphery because higher centers cannot inhibit peripheral receptors from transducing noxious stimuli that occur in the environment (or viscera). Rather, descending signals from higher centers converge on input from the periphery at the site of the dorsal horn to influence the transmission of this noxious information. By exciting the inhibitory interneurons on which C fiber and nonnociceptive A fiber inputs converge, these descending pathways can either dampen the intensity of noxious information or inhibit it altogether. This mechanism has similarities with the gate control theory. An example of this mechanism is reduction of background sensory information when you need to pay attention to a specific sensory source.

Clinical Correlations

Pain Perception

The perception of pain is a complex phenomenon dependent on the nature of the physiologic stimuli activating sensory receptors as well as the affective state of the person.[15,16] Sensory receptors that relay information to subcortical and cortical regions of the nervous system by the anterolateral pathways respond to specific stimuli, as described previously. A given stimulus, however, does not always elicit the same response in the same person. In addition, each person's responses are a function of not only the quality of the stimulus but of that person's affective state. In other words, perception of pain is highly individual. Furthermore, **pain thresholds**, the point at which a stimulus is first perceived as painful, and **pain tolerance**, the amount of pain a person can bear, differ between individuals. Factors influencing these differences are psychological stress,[16] prior experience with the stimulus,[15] the modality with which

the stimulus is administered,[15,17] gender,[18] motivation, attitude, and disease state.[19]

The therapist must be aware that the experience of pain is a subjective matter that cannot be expressed in scientific or medical terminology because it has a highly emotional component. The challenge for the therapist is to be sensitive to the physical and emotional factors contributing to a patient's condition when implementing therapeutic intervention.

Phantom Limbs

A **phantom limb** is experienced when sensory and motor sensations arise from an appendage that is not physically present or is no longer capable of transmitting information from the periphery to higher centers because of nerve root avulsion or transection of the spinal cord.[20] The sensations experienced include pressure, temperature, itching, and cramping, among others. A diverse population of patients experiences these phenomena, including those with congenital limb deficiencies,[21,22] amputations,[23] and spinal cord injuries.[20] These sensations are not always unwelcome; the phantom limb is as "real" to the person experiencing it as any intact appendage, but phantom sensations become problematic and even debilitating when they manifest themselves as pain. Preoperative pain in a limb often predisposes patients to the development of phantom pain. Many amputations are performed because of painful, life-threatening infections. Alleviating the pain before surgery can significantly reduce the incidence of phantom limb pain.

Phantom limb pain is most commonly experienced by amputees. Up to 80% of amputees experience varying degrees of phantom pain.[20] The trauma associated with amputation may precipitate the development of phantom pain. Amputation involves a significant amount of peripheral nerve damage; as these nerves regenerate, they form neuromas that are spontaneously active. This spontaneous activity is relayed to the dorsal horn neurons, inducing hyperexcitability in second-order neurons. The signals generated by the dorsal horn neurons are relayed to areas of the cortex by the spinothalamic tract, where they are perceived as painful. In other words, the changes that occur at the periphery induce local changes in the activation pattern of the dorsal horn neurons. These local changes in turn alter the normal activation pattern in the thalamus and cortex.[20,24] In this manner, all levels of the nervous system participate in a chain of events, the consequence of which is an altered representation of sensory information in the nervous system and, ultimately, altered sensory perception. Attempts to control phantom pain include preoperative prevention and postoperative management using adrenergic, opioid,[25] and serotonergic agonists,[26] glutamatergic and sodium channel antagonists,[27] and local anesthetics.[25,28,29]

A controlled study by Jahangiri and colleagues[25] of patients undergoing lower limb amputation demonstrated the effectiveness of a combination of opioid and adrenergic agonists and a local anesthetic in preventing the development of phantom limb pain. Pavy and Doyle[28] used direct infusion of a local anesthetic into the sciatic nerve both before a below-the-knee amputation and then for 96 hours after surgery successfully to prevent phantom pain in one high-risk patient.

In those patients for whom preoperative management is not successful or is not an option, postoperative management is the only alternative. Successful management of phantom limb pain has been shown with the sodium channel blocker mexiletine,[27] the serotonergic agonist calcitonin,[26] and the glutamatergic antagonist ketamine.[29] These treatment regimens usually involve daily use of the prescribed drug, making management of phantom limb pain a lifetime challenge.

REFERENCES

1. Melzack R, Wall PD. Pain mechanisms: a new theory. *Science* 1965;150:971–979.
2. Woolf CJ. Central mechanisms of acute pain. In: Bond MR, Charlton JE, Woolf CJ, eds. *Proceedings of the VIth World Congress on Pain*. New York: Elsevier, 1991:25–34.
3. Levin MF, Christina W, Hui-Chan Y. Conventional acupuncture-like transcutaneous electrical nerve stimulation excite similar afferent fibers. *Arch Phys Med Rehabil* 1993;74:54–60.
4. Taylor DN, Katmis JJ, Lorenz K, Ng Y. Sine-wave auricular TENS produces frequency-dependent hypesthesia in the trigeminal nerve. *Clin J Pain* 1993;9:216–219
5. Sjölund BH, Eriksson MBE. The influence of naloxone on analgesia produced by peripheral conditioning stimulation. *Brain Res* 1979;173:295–301.
6. Ignelzi RJ, Nyquist JK. Direct effect of electrical stimulation on peripheral nerve evoked activity: implications in pain relief. *J Neurosurg* 1976;45:159–165.
7. Giamberardino MA, Vecchiet L. Visceral pain, referred hyperalgesia and outcome: new concepts. *Eur J Anaesthesiol* 1995;12(Suppl 10):61–66.
8. Mense S. Spinal mechanisms of muscle pain and hyperalgesia. In: Vecchiet L, Albe-Fessard DG, Lindblom U, eds. New trends in referred pain and hyperalgesia, vol. 7. New York: Elsevier, 1993, 25–35.
9. Auleciems LM. Myofascial pain syndrome: a multidisciplinary approach. *Nurs Pract* 1995;20:18–28.
10. Wessel K, Vieregge P, Kessler C, Kompf D. Thalamic stroke: correlation of clinical symptoms, somatosensory evoked potentials, and CT findings. *Acta Neurol Scand* 1994;90:167–173.
11. De Salles AAF, Bittar GT. Thalamic pain syndrome: anatomic and metabolic correlation. *Surg Neurol* 1994;41:147–151.
12. Craig AD, Bushnell MC, Zhang ET, Blomqvist A. A thalamic nucleus specific for pain and temperature sensation. *Nature* 1994;372:770–773.
13. Likavec MJ. Central pain. In: Raj PP, ed. *Practical management of pain*. New York: Year Book Medical Publishers, Inc., 1986:217–223.
14. Skevington SM. Biological mechanisms of pain. In: Skevington SM, ed. *Psychology of pain*. New York: John Wiley & Sons, 1995:8–23.
15. Rainville P, Feine JS, Bushnell MC, Duncan GH. A psychophysical comparison of sensory and affective responses to four modalities of experimental pain. *Somatosens Mot Res* 1992;9:165–177.
16. Sheps DS, Ballenger MN, De Gent GE, et al. Psychophysical responses to a speech stressor: correlation of plasma beta-endorphin levels at rest and after psychological stress with thermally measured pain threshold in patients with coronary artery disease. *J Am Coll Cardiol* 1995;25:1499–1503.
17. Gruener G, Dyck PJ. Quantitative sensory testing: methodology, applications and future directions. *J Clin Neurophysiol* 1994;11:568–583.
18. Ellermeier W, Westphal W. Gender differences in pain ratings and pupil reactions to painful pressure stimuli. *Pain* 1995;61:435–439.
19. Boven RW, Johnson KO. A psychophysical study of the mechanisms of sensory recovery following nerve injury in humans. *Brain* 1994;117:149–167.
20. Melzack R. Phantom limbs. *Sci Am* 1992;266:120–126.
21. Saadah ESM, Melzack R. Phantom limb experiences in congenital limb-deficient adults. *Cortex* 1994;30:479–485.
22. Weinstein S, Sersen EA, Vetter RJ. Phantoms and somatic sensation in cases of congenital aplasia. *Cortex* 1964;1:276–290.
23. Smith J, Thompson JM. Phantom limb pain and chemotherapy in pediatric amputees. *Mayo Clin Proc* 1995;70:357–364.
24. Kaas JH. The reorganization of sensory and motor maps in adult mammals. In: Gazzaniga MS, ed. *The cognitive neurosciences*. Cambridge: MIT Press, 1995:51–71.
25. Jahangiri M, Bradley JWP, Jayatunga AP, Dark CH. Prevention of phantom pain after major lower limb ampu-

tation by epidural infusion of diamorphine, clonidine and bupivacaine. *Ann R Coll Surg Engl* 1994;76:324–326.

26. Jaeger H, Maier C. Calcitonin in phantom limb pain: a double-blind study. *Pain* 1992;48:21–27.

27. Davis RW. Successful treatment for phantom pain. *Orthopedics* 1993;16:691–695.

28. Pavy TJG, Doyle DL. Prevention of phantom limb pain by infusion of local anaesthetic into the sciatic nerve. *Anaesth Intensive Care* 1996;24:599–600.

29. Nikolajsen L, Hansen CL, Nielsen J, Keller J, Arendt-Nielsen L, Jensen TS. The effect of ketamine on phantom pain: a central neuropathic disorder maintained by peripheral input. *Pain* 1996;67:69–77.

7

Somatic Senses 2: Discriminative Touch

SHARON L. JULIANO, OTR, PhD
DEBRA F. McLAUGHLIN, PhD

• • •

This chapter describes the major components of discriminative touch, from the skin to the cerebral cortex. One of the most important elements of the path mediating discriminative touch is the **dorsal column** pathway. The dorsal columns are large and have often been described as the most important sensory pathway carrying information about sensation of the body into the central nervous system (CNS). The main fiber bundle travels without synapsing in the spinal cord and up to the dorsal column nuclei (DCN) in the medulla. At this point, the dorsal column fibers synapse and decussate, and the pathway continues on to the thalamus as the **medial lemniscus**. The recipient nucleus in the thalamus projects to somatosensory regions of the cerebral cortex. Despite their size and obvious significance as a major ascending pathway, a clear definition of the function of the dorsal columns has proved elusive. This lack of definition arises because many of the deficits associated with injury to the dorsal column pathway are transient; the problems that persist are subtle and difficult to define. Current thinking describes its main function as discriminative touch: to distinguish between different types of stimuli to the skin, including detection of such features as direction, intensity, and frequency. Another factor contributing to the difficulty in defining dorsal column function is that it acts as a conduit for a number of other pathways, both ascending and descending, that join and ascend or descend for various distances. The dorsal columns can therefore be distinguished as several entities. One is the major ascending conduit that carries somatosensory information to the DCN and on to higher centers by way of the medial lemniscus. The second is the fiber system that receives ascending information at many different levels, which subsequently leaves the dorsal columns and either terminates in the spinal cord or continues to ascend in a different pathway. The third set of fibers descends in the dorsal column, carrying information from higher centers. The dorsal column pathway, therefore, is a composite bundle composed of many fiber systems that enter either from lower levels or from higher centers. Many of the fibers running in the dorsal columns do not contribute to the system that eventually makes its way to the DCN, thalamus, and the cerebral cortex, but consist of axons that enter the pathway, travel for short distances, and then leave for another destination. (Note that the dorsal columns are often called the "posterior columns.")

Peripheral Receptors, Nerves, and Their Physiology

The receptors mediating discriminative touch are located in the skin. The skin is our largest sensory organ, forming a receptor sheet of about two square yards. This immense sheet provides a protective covering for the body, enables detection of noxious (tissue-damaging) events, enables recognition and use of objects, and records all forms of touch, including pressure, vibration, tickle, itch, and qualities such as wetness and smoothness. Touch serves as a universal means of communication, as exemplified by handshakes, embraces, or caresses.

Innocuous physical contact with the skin causes mechanical alteration or deformation detected by specialized receptors in the dermal layers. These receptors, called **mechanoreceptors**, lie either superficially near the epidermis or deep in the dermis (Fig. 7–1). The types of mechanoreceptors are similar for both hairy and smooth (glabrous) skin, with the exception of **hair follicles** and their smooth skin counterparts, **Meissner's corpuscles**. Hairy skin covers most of the body, except for the palmar, plantar (underside of the foot), and vermilion (lip) surfaces. Nonhairy skin is more sensitive with regard to touch and discriminative capacity than hairy skin,

consistent with the use of smooth skin for sensory exploration.

Mechanoreceptors lie in the collagenous dermis and in the epidermis, surrounded above by dead epidermal cells (stratum corneum) and below by subcutaneous tissue (containing adipose and connective tissue). The epidermis forms the sheet that covers the external surface of the body (see Fig. 7–1). It extends into the dermis as folds, and the dermis protrudes into the epidermis in finger-like projections. As epidermal cells mature, they become flattened and move outward into the keratin-rich outermost layer (stratum corneum), where they lose cytoplasmic content and eventually slough off. The epidermis is renewed roughly every 2 months. Skin layers vary in thickness over the body surface, with facial skin thickness measuring roughly 0.5 mm and plantar surface skin measuring 10 times thicker. The plantar and palmar surfaces contain a thick, highly keratinous epidermis, giving these surfaces a relatively thicker epidermis than that of hairy skin (see Fig. 7–1).

Mechanoreceptors and Afferent Fibers

Low-threshold mechanoreceptors in hairy and glabrous skin have specialized, encapsulated nerve endings associated with functionally specific peripheral nerve fibers, or units. Low-threshold mechanoreceptors are activated by light, nonpainful tactile stimuli, whereas high-threshold, unencapsulated (free) nerve endings transduce intense, potentially tissue-damaging sensory events. Tactile stimulation elicits a generator potential in the nerve ending. When the generator potential reaches a threshold level of activation, an action potential is generated in the axon that innervates the receptor, initiating the propagation of the impulse to the CNS. Touch-sensitive fibers conduct impulses at rapid rates, and fall into the beta fiber category, indicating that these fibers have conduction velocities in the 30- to 70-m-per-second range and wide diameters (6 to 12 micrometers [μm]) because of Schwann cell myelination.[1]

Functional properties of nerve fibers are characterized using microelectrodes to record from individual axons within nerve bundles, such as the median and ulnar nerves of the hand and forearm. Using this approach, axons are classified based on their temporal and spatial properties. Classification of temporal properties is based on whether the fiber exhibits a

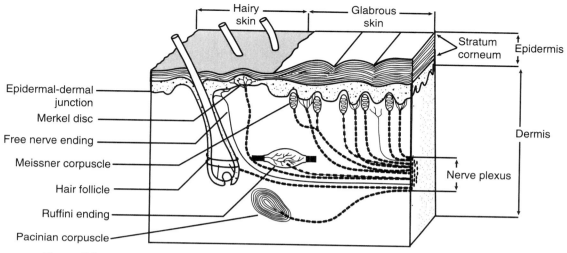

Figure 7–1. Location and morphology of mechanoreceptors in a vertical cross-section of skin. Nerve fibers are shown contacting specialized receptors and free nerve endings. The nerve plexus continues proximally to join one of the peripheral nerve trunks. (Modified and used by permission from Martin JH. *Neuroanatomy: Text and atlas.* 2nd ed. Stamford, Connecticut: Appleton and Lange, 1996. Figure 5-4, p. 133.)

transient or sustained response to a tactile stimulus. Some fibers respond only when a tactile stimulus is first applied to the skin (onset), but not during maintained contact; these fibers also discharge when the stimulus is removed from the skin (offset). The axons responding only to the onset and offset of mechanical deformation of the skin are classified as **rapidly adapting** (RA), indicating that they quickly adapt to an object in contact with the skin. Other nerve fibers discharge when a tactile stimulus is applied and continue to respond during the stimulus presentation. Fibers of this type are called **slowly adapting** (SA).

Classification of spatial properties is based on the amount of skin innervated by a single unit. A single nerve fiber distributes to a specific region of the skin; this region, or the spatial extent of skin that activates the nerve fiber, is called the **receptive field** of that unit. Nerve fibers fall into two broad categories of receptive field size: large and small. Units with large receptive fields are also called "diffuse" because the borders of the input zone from the skin are often difficult to define. Receptive fields of diffuse

fibers sometimes cover entire fingers or as much as half the palmar surface. Units with small receptive fields are referred to as "punctate" because the receptive field borders are sharply defined.

Nerve fibers can therefore be defined using a combination of receptive field size (the spatial properties) and adaptation rate (the temporal properties). Using the two types of temporal responses with the two types of spatial attributes, four classes of fiber types have been described: SAs with small receptive fields (SA type I), SAs with large receptive fields (SA type II), RAs with small receptive fields (RA type I), and RAs with large receptive fields (RA type II; Table 7–1).

The functional properties of the peripheral nerves (i.e., the adaptation rate and receptive field size) are associated with the morphologic features of the specialized receptors in the dermis and epidermis (see Table 7–1). For instance, RA type II peripheral fibers, or RAII, match the properties of an encapsulated receptor referred to as the **Pacinian corpuscle**; therefore it is thought that RAII fibers innervate the Pacinian corpuscle.

TABLE 7-1

Classes of Cutaneous Sensory Units in the Hand

Peripheral Afferent Characteristics					Receptor Characteristics			
Peripheral Fiber Type	Response Properties	Receptive Field Size	Activation Threshold	Adequate Stimulus	Sensation Evoked	Associated Receptor	Receptor Shape	Fiber : Receptor Ratio
Slowly adapting type I	Continued discharge	Small; 2–8 mm diameter, containing zones of maximal sensitivity	Low, 5 g/mm²*	Deformation of skin	Light, uniform pressure, like a watercolor brush against the skin	Merkel's disc	Dome-shaped complex, containing up to 30 specialized Merkel's cells	1 fiber: 3–4 complexes
Slowly adapting type II	Continued discharge	Large; several centimeters, with area of maximal sensitivity under 2 mm diameter	Moderate, 10 g/mm²	Skin stretch; joint movement	No conscious experience	Ruffini ending	Thinly lamellated, fluid-filled capsule; elongated parallel to skin surface	1 fiber: 1 receptor
Rapidly adapting type I	Transient discharge	Small; 2–8 mm diameter, containing zones of maximal sensitivity	Low, 4 g/mm²	Rapid skin displacement	Buzzing, wobbling, or flutter	Meissner's corpuscle	Small capsule; elongated perpendicular to skin surface	1 fiber: 15–20 receptors
Rapidly adapting type I	Transient discharge		Low	Displacement of hair shaft	?	Hair follicle	Epidermally derived follicle, elongated perpendicular to skin surface	
Rapidly adapting type II	One to two impulses per transient	Large; several centimeters	Low, 4 g/mm²	High-frequency mechanical transients; most sensitive to vibration at 200–300 Hz	Buzzing, flutter	Pacinian corpuscle	Lamellated, onion-like capsule, elongated parallel to skin surface	1 fiber: 1 receptor

* A 5 g/mm² threshold is comparable with the pressure generated by a human hair pushed against the skin.

Pacinian Corpuscle

The Pacinian corpuscle is the largest sensory end or-gan in the body (approximately 0.5 mm wide and 1.0 mm long). It is the most deeply situated of the spe-cialized receptors. Each corpuscle consists of ap-proximately 70 layers assembled in an onion-like fashion on the end of a peripheral nerve fiber (see Fig. 7–1). The corpuscle transduces only high-frequency components of touch sensations and is unresponsive to sustained deformation of the skin, consistent with the functional characteristics of RA nerve fibers (see Table 7–1). The Pacinian corpuscle is thought to be associated with RAII units, which have large receptive fields: the corpuscle is located deep in the skin and has its long axis oriented paral-lel to the surface of the skin, enabling it to detect sensory input from relatively wide areas. The Pacin-ian corpuscle has one of the lowest thresholds for ac-tivation (4 g/mm^2, less than the pressure generated by a human hair pushed against the skin). Each Pacinian corpuscle is innervated by its own periph-eral nerve fiber—that is, the ratio of nerve axon to re-ceptor is 1 : 1 (see Table 7–1). In human **microneu-rographic** studies, electrical stimulation of isolated RAII peripheral fibers elicits a sensation described as "buzzing" or "flutter."[2] When the microelectrode is used to record from RAII fibers rather than to stimu-late the fibers, RAIIs were found to respond at the stimulus presentation rate, up to rates as rapid as 400 stimuli per second. RAII fibers are maximally sensi-tive to stimulus rates of 200 to 300 presentations per second. Entrainment at such high rates of stimula-tion indicates that RAIIs, and Pacinian corpuscles, exhibit high temporal resolution.

Meissner's Corpuscle

Meissner's corpuscle is superficially located at the epidermal–dermal junction within the folds, and in close apposition to epidermal cells (see Fig. 7–1). A small capsule forms the end organ of Meissner's cor-puscle, and each ending is thought to be innervated by RAI peripheral units. This association implies that Meissner's corpuscle displays discharges that adapt rapidly and small receptive field sizes. These recep-tive units have low activation thresholds, and share their innervation fiber with as many as 20 additional Meissner's corpuscles. Electrical stimulation of RAI fibers in humans evokes sensations of buzzing, wob-bling, and flutter. RAI fibers, however, prefer stimula-tion rates in the range of 20 to 40 presentations per second. Thus, RAIs linked to Meissner's corpuscles have somewhat lower temporal resolutions than RAIIs and Pacinian corpuscles.

Merkel's Disc

Merkel's disc lies near the epidermal–dermal junc-tion. Each receptor is a complex of specialized cells, numbering as many as 30 cells per complex. Up to four Merkel's cell complexes may be innervated by collaterals of an individual peripheral afferent. These afferents are larger-diameter, myelinated fibers and have the functional characteristics of SAI mechano-receptive units, that is, afferent discharges are sus-tained during indentation of the skin and receptive field sizes are spatially confined to a small area. Mild electrical stimulation of SAI fibers in humans elicits a sensation of light pressure, like the experience of a watercolor brush against the skin (see Table 7–1).

Ruffini Ending

The **Ruffini ending** is located deep in the dermis of the skin, although more superficially than the Pacin-ian receptor. The receptor is lamellated, fluid-filled, and anchored to surrounding tissue by collagen. This interaction with surrounding tissue and its mor-phologic resemblance to other receptors found near tendons and joints suggest that the Ruffini ending is a stretch receptor. The morphologic features of the receptor are consistent with the physiologic proper-ties of SAII afferents, which respond maximally to tactile stimulation of a spatially confined area of skin but also respond to skin stretch outside this area of maximal sensitivity. Like the Pacinian receptor, there is a one-to-one innervation ratio for the Ruffini end-ing and its afferent. Electrical stimulation of individ-ual SAII afferents, however, fails to elicit a conscious experience (see Table 7–1).

Joint Receptor

Joint receptors are located in the joint capsule, and are present as four different types. Type I joint re-ceptors are functionally and structurally similar to Ruffini endings; type II to Pacinian corpuscles; and type IV to free nerve endings. The third type of joint receptor resembles a sensory apparatus that responds to muscle tension, called the Golgi tendon organ. This diversity of morphologic features is consistent with the role of joint receptors in the perception of objects by touch, a sensory capacity referred to as "haptics."

Discriminative Touch as a Function of Receptor Specialization

Mechanoreceptors are specialized to respond best to specific characteristics of a tactile stimulus, as discussed previously and shown in Table 7–1. These anatomic and functional specializations led investigators to propose that each receptor responds only to specific stimulus characteristics, a principle referred to as the specificity theory. An alternate theory, the pattern theory, has also been proposed. This theory holds that a receptor responds to many different stimulus features, but more vigorously and selectively to some features than to others. Thus, keep in mind that although mechanoreceptors are exquisitely sensitive to light, nonpainful touch, they can also be activated by other stimulus modalities, such as warmth, cold, or pain.

The study of tactile perception in humans and other primates has focused largely on the hand—more specifically, on the glabrous surface of the hand. Discriminative capacity, tactile exploration, and object recognition have been extensively studied for the glabrous skin, but little is known about these faculties in hairy skin. Several studies have also examined the sensibilities of the face, often conducted by those interested in dental research or in speech.

The fingers and the face, including the tongue, have received the most attention in the study of sensory thresholds and tactile acuity. Women have lower sensation thresholds (i.e., are more sensitive) than men for all body regions tested. The tongue has the lowest sensation threshold (highest sensitivity) followed by the tip of the nose, the lips, the cheeks, the forehead, and then the fingertips. Similarly, **two-point discrimination**, which measures the ability to detect whether a stimulus touches two points on the skin rather than a single point, is most acute on the tongue, followed by glabrous skin of the fingertips, then the lips, cheeks, and tip of the nose. Tactile acuity, as measured in a two-point discrimination task, is largely governed by the packing density of mechanoreceptive units with small receptive fields, namely SAIs and RAIs[3] (Fig. 7–2A). In contrast, SAIIs and RAIIs have large receptive fields and low innervation densities in the fingers and probably do not contribute to two-point discrimination thresholds (see Fig. 7–2B). Although the fingertips are by far the most densely innervated and sensitive parts of the glab-

rous hand, for the face, the most sensitive region is the perioral region (around the mouth). The receptive field sizes and innervation densities for SAIs and RAIs are comparable on the fingertips and perioral region.

Various types of stimuli have been used to assess the role of different mechanoreceptors in discriminative touch. These stimuli typically mimic attributes of touch, such as roughness, as experienced when touching sandpaper, a wire mesh, or corduroy. The stimulus surfaces are typically systematically arranged or regularly spaced to facilitate evaluation and quantification of the responses.[4] Raised, or embossed, alphabets and dots (such as used in reading Braille) have been used as stimuli in experiments where an electrode records the activity of individual SAI or RAI peripheral afferents (microneurographic recording). Experiments of this type reveal which features of the stimulus are detected and encoded by each afferent.[5] These studies show that SAI responses match the stimulus features remarkably well, RAIs match less well, and RAIIs nearly completely fail to reveal any of the stimulus features (Fig. 7–3). Perceptual aspects of these sensory experiences have also been investigated. The density of raised dots produces a perception of roughness that varies with dot spacing. Participants perceive both closely spaced and widely spaced dots as smooth, whereas intermediately spaced dots are perceived as rough.

Our skin receptors respond to touch delivered in either of two ways: passive or active touch. In passive touch, a tactile stimulus is placed on the skin, whereas active touch entails exploration of the object or environment, and ongoing feedback to the somatosensory system from both the touch and joint receptors.[6] In studies using object identification tasks with raised or embossed stimuli, performance was comparable under passive and active conditions. Performance is comparable, however, only so long as the stimuli are raised a sufficient distance above the background surface. For example, a dot raised 10 μm (1/100,000 m) high can be detected when pressed against the skin (passive touch), whereas a dot raised only 1 μm can be detected when the finger is actively pressed against the dot (active touch), indicating that active touch conveys more sensory information. Studies using small metal cookie cutters shaped like a star, a triangle, and so forth, indicate that active exploration led to higher

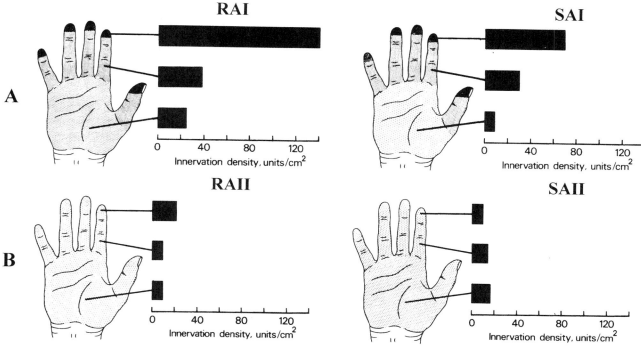

Figure 7–2. Average innervation of slowly adapting and rapidly adapting peripheral fibers within different regions of glabrous skin. Shown are innervation densities of mechanoreceptors with *(A)* small receptive fields and *(B)* large receptive fields. Each dot drawn on the palm represents a single sensory unit innervating the skin area. Histograms give the density of innervation in the following three skin regions: the fingertip, remaining parts of the finger, and the palm. RAI, rapidly adapting type I; RAII, rapidly adapting type II; SAI, slowly adapting type I; SAII, slowly adapting type II. (Modified and used by permission from Vallbo AB, Johansson RS. Properties of cutaneous mechanoreceptors in the human hand related to touch sensation. *Hum Neurobiol,* 1984;3:3–14. Figure 2C, p. 6 and Figure 3C, p. 8.)

identification accuracy than the passive condition, where a cookie cutter was pressed and rotated against the fingertips. Accuracy is improved during active touch because information from mechanoreceptors is combined with information about the location of the hand and the relative positions of the fingers.

Deficits in Sensory Processing

Many people have sensory deficits derived from alterations at the receptor level. Mild deficits occur during the normal aging process. Deficits may also arise because of skin disorders and diseases, or through damage incurred in a person's occupation. Injury to the skin or peripheral nerve can also lead to persistent alterations in sensory processing.

As we age, subtle changes occur in our tactile sensibilities. In elderly people, discriminative capacities are in general worse than in young adults, although detection of these changes typically requires examination using carefully controlled, near-threshold stimuli. In discrimination tasks, such as two-point discrimination, the size of the change, or difference threshold, increases 1% every year from

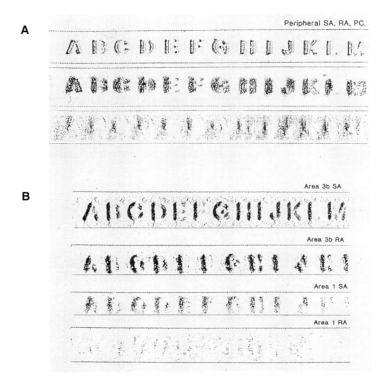

Figure 7–3. Evoked responses reconstructed from primary afferents and cortical neurons. **A:** Evoked responses for typical SA, RA, and PC fibers to patterned stimulation. PC, Pacinian corpuscle. **B:** Evoked responses reconstructed from five single SA cortical neurons in area 3b of awake monkey. Each embossed letter was repeatedly scanned across the receptive field of the nerve fiber or cortical neuron. Each grouping of responses comprises a set of rasters resulting from repetitive parallel scans of the stimulus across the receptive field, with the stimulus shifted vertically by 0.2 mm between each scan. (Reproduced with permission from Pons TP. Representation of form in the somatosensory system. *Trends in neuroscience,* Vol. II. New York, Elsevier, 1988:374.)

approximately 20 to 80 years of age. These losses are more pronounced in the extremities (e.g., on the fingertip and big toe) than on more proximal body sites, such as the very acute lip and tongue. Deterioration of acuity in the extremities may adversely affect manual skills such as grasping.

More severe sensory deficits occur in diseases and because of injury. Discriminative capacities show marked deterioration in diabetes, lead poisoning, leprosy, vibration-induced neuropathy, vitamin B_{12} deficiency, carpal tunnel syndrome, and other clinical conditions. Deficits typically manifest as numbness, paresthesia, and elevated touch-pressure thresholds. Compared with normal adults, people with these clinical symptoms are less accurate and have longer latencies on object and texture identification tasks. In some cases, people with sensory deficits cannot detect even potentially tissue-damaging, painful events. Clinicians routinely monitor at-risk patients for threatening changes in tactile detection thresholds.

Organization of the Dorsal Columns in the Spinal Cord

The nerves that carry sensory impulses enter the spinal column through the dorsal roots. The fibers carrying discriminative touch ascend in the dorsal columns. The dorsal columns are large and lie in the dorsal funiculus of the spinal cord; they extend the length of the spinal cord. The receptors and nerve fibers discussed previously contribute to this ascending bundle. The fibers that comprise the major ascending pathway (i.e., those that eventually contribute to the medial lemniscus) enter the pathway through the sensory dorsal roots. The large, heavily myelinated fibers segregate toward the medial part of the root and enter directly into the dorsal columns without synapsing in the gray matter of the spinal cord itself.

This large fiber bundle is divided into two smaller pathways, the fasciculus gracilis and the fasciculus cuneatus (Fig. 7–4). The axons that enter the spinal cord from the lower portion of the body, including fibers from sacral, lumbar, and half of the thoracic segments (T12–T7), shift medially and form the fasciculus gracilis. The term *gracilis* means slender or graceful, to convey the thin and slender nature of this pathway. Axons that enter the spinal cord from the upper half of the body (i.e., those arriving from the cervical and half of the thoracic segments [C1–T6]) remain in a relatively lateral position and form the fasciculus cuneatus. The word *cuneiform* means wedge shaped, to describe the relative shape of the pathway and its associated nucleus (the nucleus cuneatus). These pathways remain distinct and separate throughout the length of the spinal cord until their termination on the respective DCN, the **nucleus gracilis** and **nucleus cuneatus**, which are found in the lower part of the medulla (see Fig. 7–4). The fasciculus gracilis extends the entire length of the spinal cord, because fibers at the lowest levels enter the dorsal columns and carry information to the nucleus gracilis. The fasciculus cuneatus, however, is present only from T6 to its termination in the medulla at the nucleus cuneatus, because it is formed by axons entering at a higher level (see Fig. 7–4).

Precision of Topography in the Spinal Pathway, Dermatomal Distribution

The dorsal columns display a precise organization in terms of the somatotopic or topographic organization in the pathway itself[7] (Fig. 7–5). Fibers at the lowest levels of the spinal cord (i.e., caudal and sacral) travel in the most medial portion of the fasciculus gracilis and remain in this position during their ascent. Fibers entering at lumbar levels position themselves immediately lateral to the sacral fibers; the thoracic fibers are positioned lateral to the lumbar fibers. A similar organization occurs in the fasciculus cuneatus, so that the T6 axons are positioned the most medial in this pathway and the C1 fibers are the most lateral. Thus, the organization of the ascending fiber bundles display a precise somatotopy that contributes to the topographic representation of

the body surface at different levels of the CNS. Despite this exact arrangement of the dorsal columns, there is evidence that the ascending axons sort themselves into a more precise somatotopic arrangement as they rise. Several researchers describe a reshuffling of the ascending fibers so that by the level of the DCN the receptive cells are organized in a somatotopic pattern rather than a dermatomal pattern[8,9] (Fig. 7–6). This means that rather than the DCN possessing an organization that represents the strips of skin in a given **dermatome**, clusters of cells in the nuclei respond to stimulation of specific body parts (such as fingers). In fact, the DCN are organized in a highly morphologic manner so that each digit is represented in a given cluster of cells.[10,11]

This exact topographic organization remains in the pathway as it continues to higher levels of the CNS. Because the medial lemniscus is beltlike as it ascends toward the thalamus, the body organization shifts its orientation en route to higher levels, but the relationship of one segment to another remains consistent (see Fig. 7–4).

Path to the Somatosensory Cortex

The dorsal columns terminate in the DCN, the nucleus cuneatus and nucleus gracilis, which are located in the lower portion of the medulla. The fibers that terminate in these nuclei are first-order fibers and differ from the axons in the other ascending pathways because they do not synapse in the spinal gray (see Fig. 7–4).

After synapsing in the DCN, the axons of neurons from DCN cells form the internal arcuate fibers of the medulla decussate and then form the medial lemniscus. By the time the medial lemniscus terminates in the thalamus, the spinothalamic tract joins this pathway and much of the ascending somatosensory information is consolidated. The medial lemniscus has a winding course through the brainstem and terminates in the ventral posterior lateral (VPL) nucleus of the thalamus. The somatotopic organization of the ascending fiber bundle is preserved throughout its course. Therefore, after the dorsal column axons terminate in the DCN, the most medial axons (i.e., the lumbar and sacral) decussate by way of the internal arcuate fibers and take a ventral position in the lower medulla. The fibers that terminate in successively more lateral positions in the nucleus gracilis and cuneatus decussate and apply themselves to increasingly more

(text continues on page 104)

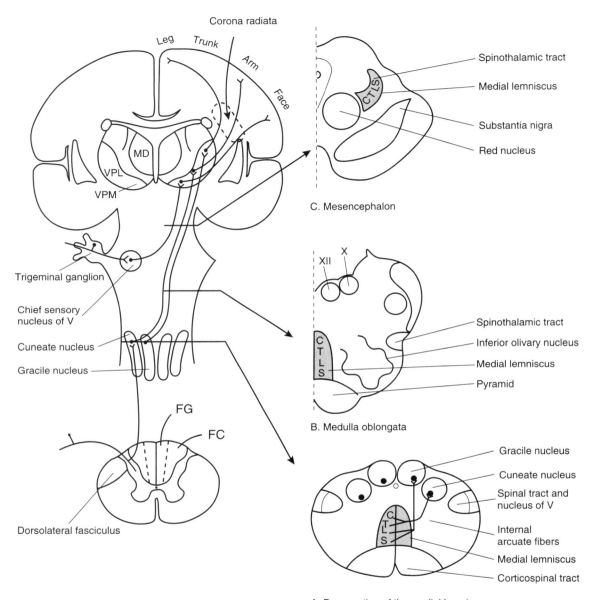

Figure 7–4. Pathways for tactile, vibratory, and proprioceptive impulses from the face and body. **A–C:** Cross sections showing the decussation of the medial lemniscus (*A*), and the position of the medial lemniscus in the medulla oblongata (*B*) and mesencephalon (*C*). C, cervical; FC, fasciculus cuneatus; FG, fasciculus gracilis; L, lumbar; MD, mediodorsal nucleus; VPL, ventral posterior lateral nucleus; VPM, ventral posterior medial nucleus; S, sacral; T, thoracic. (Used by permission from Heimer L. *The human brain and spinal cord: Functional neuroanatomy and dissection guide.* 2nd ed. New York: Springer-Verlag, 1995, Figure 9-5, p. 209.)

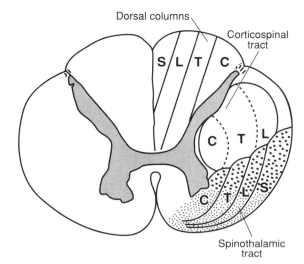

Figure 7–5. Location and somatotopic organization of spinal cord pathways at the level of the lower cervical region. *Large dots* represent fibers concerned with temperature and pain; *small dots,* fibers carrying touch and pressure impulses. C, cervical; L, lumbar; S, sacral; T, thoracic. (Used by permission from Willis WD, Coggeshall RE. *Sensory mechanisms of the spinal cord.* New York: Plenum Publishing Corp., 1978. Figure 5-2, p. 172.)

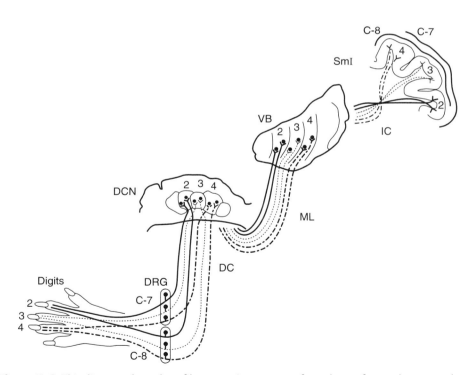

Figure 7–6. This diagram shows how fiber resorting accounts for a change from a dermatomal to a somatotopic organization in the dorsal column pathway. DRG, dorsal root ganglion; DC, dorsal column; DCN, dorsal column nuclei; ML, medial lemniscus; VB, ventrobasal complex of thalamus; IC, internal capsule; SmI, sensorimotor area I. (Used by permission from Willis WD, Coggeshall RE. *Sensory mechanisms of the spinal cord.* New York: Plenum Publishing Corp., 1978. Figure 6-4, p. 205.)

dorsal levels in the medulla. As the medial lemniscus ascends through the brainstem, the pathway swings laterally in the pons so that more rostral regions of the body are represented medially (i.e., the upper extremities) and lower regions of the body are represented in a lateral position (see Fig. 7–4). Finally, at midbrain levels, the ascending bundle swings into its final position for termination in the thalamus, so that the lower extremities are located dorsally and the upper extremities are found ventrally. The medial lemniscus is also joined by fibers from the trigeminothalamic tract, which carries sensory information from the head. After synapsing in the VPL nucleus of the thalamus, axons of cells in this nucleus travel through the corona radiata into specific sensory regions of the cerebral cortex (see Fig. 7–4). The most important of these are the primary somatosensory area and the secondary somatosensory area, which both receive information from the dorsal columns by the DCN and the VPL nucleus. This is the point where the somatic sensory information reaches consciousness. The somatotopic organization is preserved in the primary and secondary somatosensory areas by the familiar homunculi, which are found in both these neocortical areas.

Trigeminal Component

The previously described pathway carries information only from the body and the back of the head. Information from the face reaches the thalamus and primary **somatosensory cortex** by a slightly different route. This information travels by the trigeminal nerve (one of the 12 cranial nerves) into the brainstem, where it distributes fibers containing specialized sensory information to specific portions of the trigeminal nuclear complex. The trigeminal nuclear complex extends from the medulla to the midbrain and consists of three nuclear groups that receive ascending somatic sensory information corresponding to the information ascending in the spinal cord. The trigeminal fibers containing information similar to that carried in the dorsal columns, described as discriminative touch, travel to the principal, or chief, sensory nucleus of the **trigeminal complex**, which is located primarily in the pons. After synapsing in the principal trigeminal nucleus, the axons eventually join the medial lemniscus and travel to the thalamus. Once reaching the thalamus, the trigeminal axons synapse in the ventral posterior medial (VPM) nucleus. The VPM is immediately adjacent and medial to the VPL nucleus; together they are often called the ventral basal complex. Neurons in the VPM nucleus project to the somatosensory cortex and contribute to the well known topographic pattern by supplying sensory information about the face and head (see Fig. 7–4).

Other Components of the Dorsal Column System

As indicated previously, in addition to the fibers that do not synapse in the spinal gray and continue to the DCN, the dorsal columns contain other components. The dorsal column–medial lemniscal pathway is credited with housing fibers that serve discriminative touch for the body and extremities. In the course of projecting to brainstem nuclei, primary afferent fibers often begin their path through the dorsal columns but also send collateral projections to cells in the spinal cord. Spinal cord cells that receive this input, in turn, submit their own projections to brainstem nuclei, thereby providing redundancy of sensory information to the more central centers.[12] Although some of this redundant input is carried in the dorsal columns, much of it is carried in other spinal tracts of the spinal cord, which explains the residual sensory capacities that remain when the dorsal columns are interrupted. Because information regarding the modality of touch is carried in a number of ascending sensory pathways, this sensation often persists, despite large lesions of the spinal cord.

Low-threshold mechanoreceptive units send their collaterals primarily to cells of laminae III and IV (nucleus proprius) and lamina V of the spinal cord **dorsal horn** (Fig. 7–7). Recipient dorsal horn cells then make postsynaptic contributions to at least three ascending pathways: the dorsal columns, the dorsolateral fasciculus, and the anterolateral system (also called the spinothalamic tract). The size of the contributions to these pathways varies as a function of spinal segment level. For instance, less than 40% of cervical-level input to the dorsal columns originates from dorsal horn cells (without first synapsing in the spinal cord), whereas as much as 85% of thoracic-level contributions to the dorsal columns comes directly from dorsal horn cells.[13] Fibers traveling in the dorsolateral fasciculus exhibit RA characteristics and respond to hair follicle deflection and to light touch. Evidence suggests that these fibers

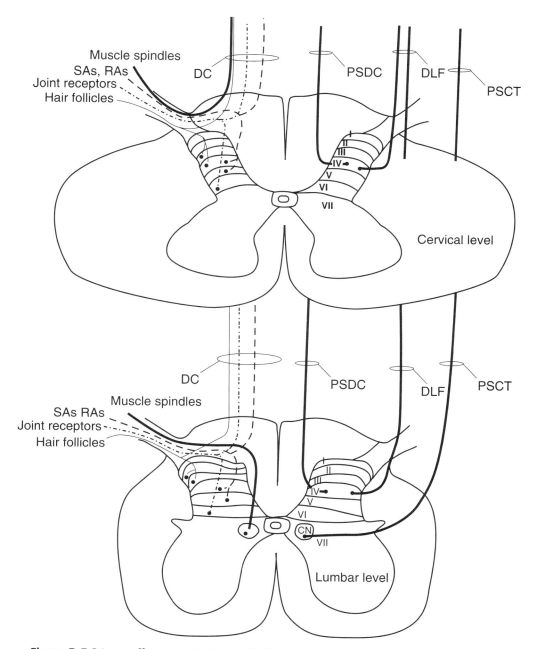

Figure 7–7. Primary afferent terminations and cells of origin of the postsynaptic ascending pathways. The *left side* shows terminations of slowly adapting (SA), rapidly adapting (RA), hair follicle, and joint receptor afferents into specific laminae of the dorsal horn. Primary afferents from muscle spindles terminate in Clarke's nucleus (CN). The *right side* shows the location of dorsal horn cells that contribute to the ascending pathways, i.e., the postsynaptic dorsal columns (PSDC), dorsolateral fasciculus (DLF), and the posterior spinocerebellar tract (PSCT). DC, dorsal column.

branch, or bifurcate, to terminate in both the DCN in the medulla and in the lateral cervical nucleus at cervical level C1–C2.

A large group of fibers that travel for some distance in the dorsal columns are those of the spinocerebellar pathway (see Fig. 7–7). These axons originate from **muscle spindles** and supply information about muscle position to the cerebellum. Axons that originate from lower segmental levels of the spinal cord enter the dorsal columns through the dorsal horn cells and ascend until L2. At this point, these large-diameter fibers synapse in **Clarke's nucleus**, which is found in the intermediate zone of the spinal gray at segmental levels L2–T2. After synapsing, the fibers form the spinocerebellar pathway and continue on ipsilaterally to the cerebellum. At segmental levels above T2, the large-diameter fibers supplying muscle spindles enter the dorsal columns and ascend until the brainstem, where they encounter and synapse in the accessory cuneate nucleus, the upper limb equivalent of Clarke's nucleus. From there, the cuneocerebellar pathway is formed, which projects to the cerebellum (see also Chaps. 8 and 13).

Functions of the Dorsal Column Pathway

The dorsal columns have classically been considered as a pathway of discriminatory sensation, that of "discriminative touch." If an animal or person suffers a lesion of the dorsal columns, an immediate impairment is observed in the awareness of stimuli and in the ability to localize a stimulus delivered to the affected region. These relatively severe deficits are transitory, however, and it appears that substantial capacity for discriminating sensations can be carried by other ascending pathways that receive information from cells in the dorsal horn, such as the spinothalamic and the dorsolateral pathways.[14,15] Important and enduring deficits persist after dorsal column lesions, however, which are manifested in both sensory and motor capacities. Although it is possible for subjects to detect stimuli to the skin, and even to localize where the stimuli were delivered after lesions involving the dorsal columns, they cannot distinguish features, such as direction, intensity, or frequency. This inability to detect the qualitative and quantitative nature of stimuli suggests that interruption of the dorsal columns may interfere with the ability to code features of somatic

sensations.[16] Studies of evoked potentials in the somatosensory cortex after a lesion of the dorsal column find that although neurons in the somatosensory cortex respond to tactile stimulation, the ability to follow repetitive stimulation and respond to changes in the nature of the stimulation deteriorates.[17]

The integrity of the dorsal columns also appears necessary for precise and refined movements. Sensory input from the dorsal columns provides important feedback to motor pathways that together produce smooth and coordinated fine movements. This feedback probably consists of a number of features and is most evident for movements that involve fine coordination of the upper limb. The most important loss after interruption of the dorsal columns (particularly the fasciculus cuneatus) is probably the diminution of sensory feedback to the motor cortex, which results in poor execution of fine motor activities. After a lesion involving the fasciculus cuneatus, monkeys were impaired in the ability to use their fingers for fine grasps. They rarely used their fingers for manipulations that involved fine opposition, and never used multiarticular patterns of flexion and extension; rather, more crude patterns of flexion and extension were observed.[18,19]

Another function attributed to this pathway is the awareness of the position of our limbs in space, or **proprioception**. It is not clear whether this aspect of dorsal column function is due to the fibers that traverse the entire pathway to the DCN, or if the proprioceptive capacity is due to fibers that enter and leave the fiber bundle, and contribute to other pathways and aspects of discrimination. A major fiber system that travels incompletely in the dorsal columns and may contribute to the proprioceptive capacity is the fiber system headed for either the dorsal nucleus of Clarke or the accessory cuneate nucleus (see Fig. 7–7). These axons supply receptors involved with sensing muscle and joint position as well as the amount of stretch and tension in joints and in muscles. This information eventually terminates in either the dorsal nucleus of Clarke (for axons entering the spinal cord from sacral to C8 levels) or the accessory cuneate nucleus (for axons entering the spinal cord above C8) and continue on to contribute information to the cerebellum (primarily through either the spinocerebellar tract or the cuneocerebellar tract). In the case of muscle spindle information from the upper limb, its entire trajectory through the spinal cord is within the fasciculus cuneatus. Although technically these axons are part of the spinocerebellar or cuneocerebellar system, they run for substantial distances within the dorsal columns. A lesion involving this level of the dorsal columns, therefore, is likely to produce an impairment of position sense (see also Chap. 8).

The dorsal columns have often been thought to mediate a multitude of sensations, some of which are represented in redundant ascending pathways. A function often lost with a lesion involving the dorsal columns is stereognosis; this is the ability to detect the form, shape, and identity of objects through the use of sensory exploration. Although the dorsal columns certainly contribute to this sensory ability, stereognosis is probably a more complex function that involves integration of multiple sensory pathways at the level of the cerebral cortex.

Clinical Correlations

Several classic syndromes involve modalities that ascend through the dorsal columns. In some instances, these diseases involve not the dorsal columns themselves but the dorsal roots, thereby interrupting the large-diameter fibers headed for the dorsal columns. It is in fact rare to encounter an isolated dorsal column injury or disease, but damage to these pathways usually occurs in conjunction with other pathways or inputs, leading to losses more devastating than those particular to the dorsal columns. One of these syndromes is **tabetic syndrome** (or tabes dorsalis); it is often a result of neurosyphilis, but can also be caused by diabetes mellitus. This syndrome affects the dorsal roots or dorsal root ganglia and thus interferes with the axons projecting into the dorsal columns, but may involve other ascending fibers as well. This syndrome leads to an ataxic gait as well as poor position sense and diminution of two-point discrimination.

Another classic syndrome is the **Brown-Sequard syndrome**. This syndrome occurs after a hemisection of the spinal cord, which may result from such causes as a vascular insult or a knife wound. Major deficits that result from this damage include 1) ipsilateral loss of lower motor neuron function at the level of the lesion, 2) ipsilateral loss of upper motor neuron function below the level of the lesion, 3) ipsilateral loss of dorsal column function below the

level of the lesion, and 4) contralateral loss of spinothalamic sensation (pain and temperature) below the level of the lesion.

Cortical Functions Associated With Dorsal Column–Medial Lemniscal Input

Anatomy and Function of Primary Somatosensory Cortex

Tactile input is conveyed from the thalamus to the primary somatosensory cortex, which occupies the anterior portion of the parietal cortex (Fig. 7–8). In primates, including humans, the somatosensory cortex consists of four distinct anatomic regions, as classified by Brodmann; these are areas 3a, 3b, 1, and 2 (see Fig. 7–8). Area 3a is the most rostral area and area 2 is the most caudal. Brodmann divided the neocortex into regions defined by the appearance and packing density of the cells. In area 3b of the somatosensory cortex, which receives the heaviest projection from the thalamus, the cortical layer that contains the densest projection (layer 4) consists of densely packed, small neurons called granule cells. Brodmann's anatomic distinctions are accompanied by functional specializations; each of the four somatosensory areas receives input from a specific subset of the receptor family that contributes to the dorsal columns.

The most rostral portion of the somatosensory cortex is cytoarchitectonic area 3a, which primarily receives input from receptors that monitor muscle tension and muscle length. Recent evidence suggests that area 3a may also mediate pain. Although all the somatosensory areas receive a strong projection from the thalamus, area 3b receives the densest thalamic input; area 3b is just caudal to area 3a. Cortical neurons with SA and RA characteristics have been recorded in area 3b. Cortical neurons in area 3b show similar encoding patterns for raised dots and embossed letters as demonstrated in SAI and RAI peripheral afferents (see Fig. 7–3). Similarly, RAI cortical neurons have been identified based on their ability to respond to repetitive stimuli presented at rates comparable with those of RAI mechanoreceptive units.[20] Area 1 lies caudal to area 3b, and receives

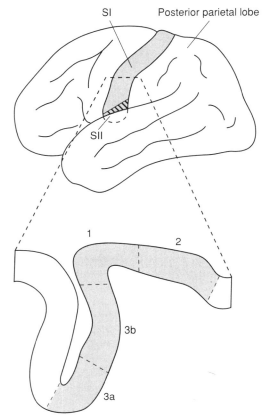

A. Somatosensory cortices

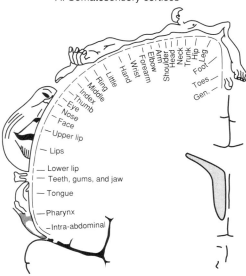

B. Sensory homunculus

Figure 7–8. Somatosensory cortex, cytoarchitecture and homunculus. **A:** The primary somatosensory cortex (SI) is located in the postcentral gyrus (dotted region) and in the depth of the central sulcus (shown magnified). It corresponds to Brodmann's areas 3 (3a, 3b), 1, and 2. A secondary sensory area is located in the upper portion of the lateral fissure (SII, shown hatched and with a dashed line). **B:** Within primary somatosensory cortex, parts of the body are represented in relation to that part's importance in somatic sensation rather than to its size. Large areas of cortex are devoted to the lips, thumb, and fingers, as shown here, and to the genitals, as recently described by WE Bradley, DF Farrell, and GA Ojemann in *Somatosens Mot Res* 1998, vol. 15. (Used by permission from Heimer L. *The human brain and spinal cord: Functional neuroanatomy and dissection guide.* 2nd ed. New York: Springer-Verlag, 1995. Figure 9-7, p. 211.)

substantial input from area 3b. Area 1 cells have more complex receptive field properties than those of area 3b, suggesting that cells in area 1 reflect input convergence. The most caudal portion of primary somatosensory cortex is area 2, which receives input predominantly from joint receptors. The projection zones of SAIIs and RAIIs are not entirely clear. Area 2 joint receptor specialization supports it as a candidate for SAII termination. Recent evidence suggests that RAII-like cortical cells reside in the secondary somatosensory cortex, lateral to the primary somatosensory cortex.

Experimental and clinical evidence confirms the functional specialization of the four cytoarchitectonic areas of the primary somatosensory cortex. This phenomenon has been shown by inactivating localized regions of the sensory cortex and measuring the behavioral consequences. For instance, ablation of, injury to, or inactivation of specific cytoarchitectonic areas led to behavioral deficits related to the functional specialization of that area. Before experimental manipulation and using only tactile cues, a monkey trained to retrieve small pieces of food embedded in small wells in a wooden block is able to detect the presence of the food and successfully extract it from the well. After inactivation of area 3b, the monkey reaches into the wells but is unable to detect the presence of the food. With experimental manipulation of area 2, and leaving the other cytoarchitectonic areas intact, however, the monkey can detect the food but cannot make the coordinated finger movements necessary for extraction.[21]

Topography in the Primary Somatosensory Cortex

Somatic receptive fields are mapped onto the somatosensory cortex as a distorted homunculus, or image of a person (see Fig. 7–8). The lower extremity is located the most medially, dipping into the paracentral lobule, followed by the trunk, the upper extremity, and the face, located the most lateral. The regions of skin that contain the densest peripheral innervation are the most heavily represented in the cortex. Researchers have found that each cytoarchitectonic area in the somatosensory cortex (i.e., areas 3a, 3b, 1, and 2) contains separate representations of the body. This arrangement allows different modalities to be completely represented at the level of the cortex.

Although maps of the body surface were once thought to be relatively inflexible and static, we now know that sensory cortical representations are fluid and dynamic. Representations of specific body parts expand or contract depending on the modified input. Since the mid-1980s, researchers have demonstrated that after the removal of a specific sensory input, such as after amputation of a digit, or a nerve lesion, the remaining normally innervated skin regions expand their representation in the somatosensory cortex. More recently, investigators have learned that expansions, or changes in peripheral representation, occur after increased or altered use of a digit or other body part. These changes can be rapid or occur over a long time. An example of a relatively rapid change has been shown to occur in people with syndactyly (webbed fingers), who have maps of the hand in the somatosensory cortex that reflect peripheral input from fused fingers. After surgery to correct for this problem, the cortical maps rapidly remodel to reflect distinct digits.[22] Dramatic long-term changes have been demonstrated in animals living with lesions of the cervical dorsal roots for many years. In this situation, representation of the face invades cortical territory previously dedicated to the upper limb to an extent not previously seen in short-term deprivations.[23] These experimental findings have been replicated to some degree in people with upper limb amputations, who have been found to report sensation on the face after stimulation to the stump of the amputated limb.[24]

The factors that produce these changes probably involve a number of mechanisms. For example, the changes occurring rapidly most likely reflect a shift in the balance of excitation and inhibition. Also, rapid changes are often described as reflecting the uncovering of so-called "silent synapses" (see Chap. 21).

REFERENCES

1. Light AR, Perl ER. Peripheral sensory systems. In: Dyck PJ, Thomas PK, eds. *Peripheral neuropathy*. 3rd ed. Vol 1. Philadelphia: WB Saunders, 1993:149–165.
2. Johansson RS, Vallbo A. Tactile sensory coding in the glabrous skin of the human hand. *Trends Neurosci* 1983;6:27–32.
3. Vallbo A, Johansson RS. Properties of cutaneous mechanoreceptors in the human hand related to touch sensation. *Hum Neurobiol* 1984;3:3–14.
4. Johnson KO, Hsiao SS. Neural mechanisms of tactual form and texture perception. *Ann Rev Neurosci* 1992; 15:227–250.

5. Phillips JR, Johnson KO, Hsiao SS. Spatial pattern representation and transformation in monkey somatosensory cortex. *Proc Natl Acad Sci U S A* 1988;85:1317–1321.

6. Heller MA, Schiff W, eds. *The psychology of touch*. Hillsdale, NJ: Lawrence Erlbaum Associates, 1991.

7. Willis WD, Coggeshall RE. *Sensory mechanisms of the spinal cord*. New York: Plenum, 1978.

8. Pubols BH, Welker WI, Johnson JI. Somatic sensory representation of forelimb in dorsal root fibers of raccoon, coatimundi, and cat. *J Neurophysiol* 1965;28:312–341.

9. Whitsel BL, Petrucelli LM, Sapiro G, Ha H. Fiber sorting in the fasciculus gracilis of squirrel monkeys. *Exp Neurol* 1970;29:227–242.

10. Florence SL, Wall JT, Kaas JH. The somatotopic pattern of afferent projections from the digits to the spinal cord and cuneate nucleus in macaque monkeys. *Brain Res* 1988;452:388–392.

11. Florence SL, Wall JT, Kaas JH. Somatotopic organization of inputs from the hand to the spinal gray and cuneate nucleus of monkeys with observations on the cuneate nucleus of humans. *J Comp Neurol* 1989;286: 48–70.

12. Rustioni A, Weinberg R. The somatosensory system. In: Bjorklund A, Hokfelt T, Swanson LW, eds. *Handbook of chemical neuroanatomy. Vol. 7: Integrated systems of the CNS, part II*. Amsterdam: Elsevier Science, 1989:219–321.

13. Giuffrida R, Rustioni A. Dorsal root ganglion neurons projecting to the dorsal column nuclei of rats. *J Comp Neurol* 1992;316:206–220.

14. Vierck CJ Jr. Tactile movement detection and discrimination following dorsal column lesions in monkeys. *Exp Brain Res* 1974;20:331–346.

15. Vierck CJ Jr, Favorov O, Whitsel BL. Neural mechanisms of absolute tactile localization in monkeys. *Somatosens Mot Res* 1988;6:41–61.

16. Vierck CJ Jr, Cohen RH, Cooper BY. Effects of spinal lesions on temporal resolution of cutaneous sensations. *Somatosens Res* 1985;3:45–56.

17. Makous JC, Friedman RM, Vierck CJ Jr. Effects of a dorsal column lesion on temporal processing within the somatosensory system of primates. *Exp Brain Res* 1996; 112:253–267.

18. Glendinning DS, Cooper BY, Vierck CJ, Leonard CM. Altered precision grasping in stumptail macaques after fasciculus cuneatus lesions. *Somatosens Mot Res* 1992; 9:61–73.

19. Leonard CM, Glendinning DS, Wilfong T, Cooper BY, Vierck CJ. Alterations of natural hand movements after interruption of fasciculus cuneatus in the macaque. *Somatosens Mot Res* 1992;9:75–89.

20. Mountcastle VB. Central nervous mechanisms in mechanoreceptive sensibility. In: Darian-Smith I, ed. *Handbook of physiology: the nervous system, III*. Bethesda, MD: American Physiological Society, 1984: 789–878.

21. Hikosaka O, Tanaka M, Sakamoto M, Iwamura Y. Deficits in manipulative behaviors induced by local anesthetics of muscimol in the first somatosensory cortex of the conscious monkey. *Behavior Res* 1985; 325:375–380.

22. Mogliner A, Grossmann JA, Ribary U, et al. Somatosensory cortical plasticity in adult humans revealed by magnetoencephalography. *Proc Natl Acad Sci U S A* 1993;90:3593–3597.

23. Pons TP, Garraghty PE, Ommaya AK, Kaas JH, Taub E, Mishkin M. Massive cortical reorganization after sensory deafferentation in adult macaques. *Science* 1991; 252:1857–1860.

24. Ramachandran VS, Rogers-Ramachandran D, Stewart M. Perceptual correlates of massive cortical reorganization. *Science* 1992;285:1159–1160.

8

Somatic Senses 3: Proprioception

LYNETTE A. JONES, PhD

• • •

Our ability to know where our limbs are in space when they have moved and our ability to know the forces generated by muscles comes from receptors found in muscles, skin, and joints. Collectively, these sensory perceptions are known as our kinesthetic or proprioceptive capacities. Taken literally, **kinesthesia** means a sense of movement, but the word is now used to refer to both the senses of movement and of limb position. The word, **proprioception**, was introduced by the English physiologist, Charles Sherrington, and comes from the Latin *proprius*, meaning "one's own," and refers to the sensory processes involved in the conscious appreciation of posture and movement. "Proprioception" is often used interchangeably with "kinesthesia."

In this chapter, the properties of mechanoreceptors in muscle are first described together with the pathways involved in transmitting information from these receptors to the cerebral cortex. The characteristics of the proprioceptive system are then reviewed in the context of psychophysical studies in which the relations between movements or forces applied to a limb and the perception of these events have been documented. Finally, the role of proprioceptive signals in perception is considered from the perspective of studies of people who have had a limb amputated, and of people with peripheral sensory neuropathies in whom proprioceptive input is either deficient or absent.

Muscle Receptors

Information about changes in muscle length and force arises from three types of **mechanoreceptors** found in muscle, as illustrated in Figure 8–1. Two of these sensors are stretch receptors, known as the primary and secondary spindle receptors because they are found in **muscle spindles**. The spindles are elongated structures ranging from 4 to 10 mm in length that are composed of bundles of small intrafusal

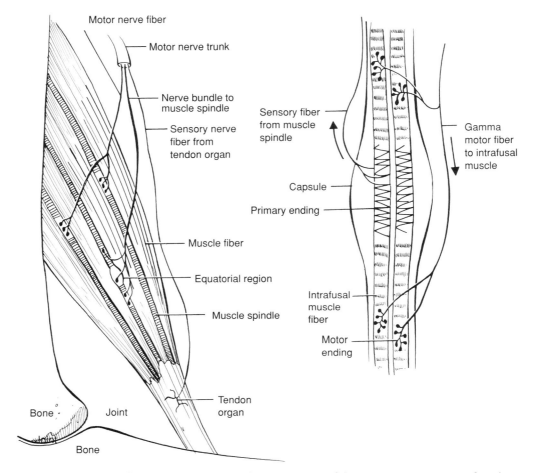

Figure 8–1 A simplified diagram illustrating the arrangement of the main sensory receptors found in a typical muscle. The proportions in the drawing on the left are highly distorted. A muscle fiber is usually 0.1 mm in diameter and a muscle spindle, which consists of a bundle of intrafusal muscle fibers, is even thinner. (From Merton PA. How we control the contraction of our muscles. *Sci Am* 1972;226: 30–37, with permission of the illustrator's estate and *Scientific American*.)

muscle fibers. They lie parallel to the **extrafusal fibers**, the force-producing component of muscle, and attach at both ends to either the extrafusal fibers or to muscle tendons. Each spindle normally has one or two primary sensory receptors innervated by Group Ia (large myelinated) afferent fibers and one to five secondary sensory receptors which are innervated by Group II afferent fibers. Muscle spindles have their own motor innervation through the fusimotor or gamma system.[1,2] Some spindles are also innervated by skeletofusimotor fibers that project to both extra-fusal and intrafusal muscle fibers. Gamma motor neurons are situated among the alpha motor neurons in the anterior horn of the gray matter of the spinal cord. The cell bodies of gamma motor neurons are smaller than those of alpha motor neurons, and their axons are more slowly conducting (10–40 m/second).

One function of the fusimotor system is to regulate the sensitivity of muscle spindles. The two types of fusimotor axons, dynamic and static, are named for the effects of axonal stimulation on the responses of primary and secondary spindle receptors during muscle stretch. Stimulation of a dynamic fusimotor axon does not excite secondary receptors but does result in a small increase in the firing rate of primary spindle receptors when the muscle is held at constant length, and has a very marked effect on the dynamic component of their response to stretch (Fig. 8–2). When a static fusimotor axon is stimulated, both primary and secondary receptors are excited, but the sensitivity of the primary receptor to the dynamic phase of the ramp stretch diminishes with this type of excitation.[3]

The number of spindles in human muscles varies depending on the function of the muscle, and has been estimated to range from 34 for the first dorsal interosseus, an intrinsic muscle of the hand, to 320 in the biceps brachii, an elbow flexor.[4] Some human muscles such as the digastric (a facial muscle in-

volved in chewing and swallowing) appear to have no spindles.[5] When expressed in terms of the number of spindles per gram of mean weight of adult muscle, higher spindle densities are generally found in muscles involved in fine movements, such as the distal finger muscles, and in the maintenance of posture. Unlike the tactile sensory system, in which higher densities of mechanoreceptors (e.g., in the fingertips) are clearly associated with superior tactile acuity,[6] for the proprioceptive system higher spindle densities do not appear to be associated with superior proprioceptive acuity.

Because of their position in muscle, spindles are specifically responsive to changes in muscle length. Both primary and secondary spindle receptors respond to changes in muscle length, but primary spindle receptors are much more sensitive to the velocity component of a lengthening contraction, and

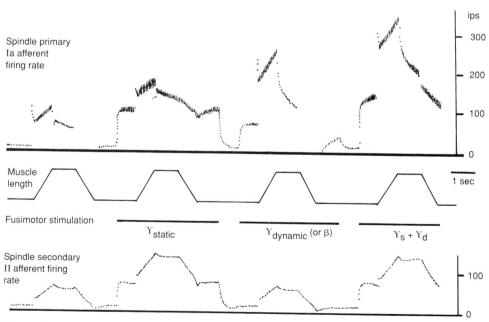

Figure 8–2. Schematic summary of the firing rate responses of primary and secondary spindle receptors to length changes with and without concomitant fusimotor stimulation. The firing rates illustrated are typical of displacements of about 10% of rest length and velocities of 0.05 rest length/second. The horizontal bars indicate periods of fusimotor stimulation at 100/second ips, impulses per second. (From Prochazka A. Proprioceptive feedback and movement regulation. In: Rowell L, Shepherd JT, eds. *Handbook of physiology. Section 12. Exercise: regulation and integration of multiple systems.* New York: Oxford University Press, 1996, with permission of the author and the American Physiological Society.)

increase their discharge rates considerably as the velocity of the stretch increases. Primary spindle receptors are, however, highly nonlinear and their discharge rates depend on several factors, including the recent contractile history of the muscle, the length of the muscle, the actual velocity with which the muscle changes length, and the activity of the fusimotor system. Secondary spindle receptors show much less dynamic responsiveness and have a more regular discharge rate than primary receptors at a constant muscle length.[7] The higher dynamic sensitivity of primary spindle receptors is consistent with the idea that they signal the velocity and direction of muscle stretch or limb movement, whereas the secondary spindle receptors provide the central nervous system with information about static muscle length or limb position. The discharge rates of muscle spindle receptors are not, however, simply a function of changes in muscle length, but also reflect the activity of the fusimotor system. To decode these afferent signals, the central nervous system must have access to the level of fusimotor activity so that it can distinguish changes in discharge rates that are proprioceptively significant from those that are a consequence of fusimotor activity. This decoding could be accomplished by a simple subtractive mechanism, as proposed by McCloskey et al.[8] and depicted in Figure 8–3.

The third type of mechanoreceptor found in muscle is the **Golgi tendon organ**, an encapsulated receptor about 1 mm long and 0.1 mm in diameter, normally found at the junction between the muscle tendon and a small group of extrafusal muscle fibers (see Fig. 8–1). The receptor is therefore said to be "in series" with this group of extrafusal muscle fibers, is selectively responsive to the forces they develop, and has little or no response to the contraction of other muscle fibers.[9] A single Group Ib axon innervates each tendon organ. In human muscles, the muscular end of each tendon organ receptor is attached to 10 to 20 muscle fibers.[10] Therefore, only a few motor units in a muscle activate a given tendon organ, although the activity of every motor unit is signaled by at least one tendon organ. Because tendon organs are very sensitive to the in-series forces, most tendon organs in a muscle discharge in all but the smallest contraction.[11] The number of tendon organs in different muscles varies considerably, and some muscles such as the lumbrical muscle of the hand do not appear to have any tendon organ receptors. These

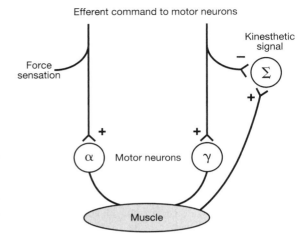

Figure 8–3. The possible sensory roles of corollary discharges in the decoding of spindle afferent input and in the perception of force. (Adapted from McCloskey et al.[8])

receptors are always less frequent and more variable in number than spindle receptors.[12]

Muscle spindle receptors and Golgi tendon organs provide the central nervous system with information about the static length of muscles, the rate at which the length changes, and the forces muscles generate. Based on this information, people can detect movements generated by their limbs, perceive changes in limb position, and estimate the weights of objects they support. Sensory information about changes in limb position and movement also arises from other sources, in particular receptors in the skin and joints. One of the continuing themes in research on proprioception has been to identify the nature of the information that comes from each of these sources. In addition to these peripheral discharges, some evidence suggests that central feedback pathways provide information that is used in decoding spindle afferent signals and in the perception of force. These pathways are described in the section on force perception.

Cortical Projections

For many years, investigators thought that muscle afferent fibers did not project to the cerebral cortex because surface cortical potentials could not be recorded during peripheral stimulation of muscle afferent fibers.[13] The small size and relative inaccessibility of the muscle afferent fiber projection area (area 3a) in the somatosensory cortex may explain the difficulty in detecting these potentials. In the 1960s, inputs from muscle spindle receptors were shown to project to the contralateral somatosensory cortex[14]; in 1984, electrophysiologic recordings demonstrated that Golgi tendon organ afferents also projected to the somatosensory cortex.[15]

The central pathways for proprioceptive inputs are different for the upper and lower limb (Fig. 8–4). For the upper limb, the central processes of dorsal root ganglion cells, the first-order neuron, enter the spinal cord and form the **dorsal columns**, where they ascend without synapsing in the **dorsal column–medial lemniscal system** to the medulla. On entering the spinal cord, these fibers are situated medial to the dorsal horn, but as they ascend they are pushed in a more medial direction by fibers entering at successively more rostral levels. Not all of these primary afferent fibers reach the medulla; some terminate at spinal levels and are known as **propriospinal fibers**. Other fibers in the dorsal columns are ascending axons of dorsal horn neurons and are therefore second-order cells; these fibers terminate in the dorsal column nuclei. In addition, some descending fibers in the dorsal columns arise in the dorsal column nuclei and terminate somatotopically in the cord.

At higher spinal levels, the dorsal columns are divided into two bundles or fascicles of axons: the **gracile fascicle** and the **cuneate fascicle**. The gracile fascicle ascends medially and includes fibers from the ipsilateral sacral, lumbar, and lower thoracic segments, whereas the cuneate fascicle ascends laterally and contains fibers from the upper thoracic and cervical segments. In the medulla, these axons synapse on the gracile and cuneate nuclei, which are known collectively as the **dorsal column nuclei** and are second-order neurons.

In the dorsal column nuclei, axons have two patterns of termination: 1) a cluster region that mainly receives input from the distal parts of the body, and 2) a reticular zone that receives more proximal inputs, predominantly from second-order afferents. The dorsal column nuclei also receive input from afferent fibers in the cerebral cortex, which is somatotopically organized so that the hand area of somatosensory cortex projects to the cuneate nucleus, whereas inputs from the leg area in the sensory cortex go to the gracile nucleus. These inputs influence

the transmission of impulses from the dorsal column nuclei and appear to be predominantly inhibitory in nature. From the dorsal column nuclei, fibers cross the midline and are now called the **internal arcuate fibers**. After crossing the midline, the fibers ascend through the contralateral lower brainstem as the medial lemniscus and project to the **ventral posterior lateral (VPL) nucleus** of the thalamus. Neurons in the ventral posterior nucleus are third-order afferent neurons whose axons ascend through the posterior limb of the internal capsule to the primary somatosensory cortex, known as S-I. These thalamocortical fibers are said to be "cortically dependent" in that they show retrograde cellular changes or cell loss after ablation of parts of the cerebral cortex.[16] Most of these thalamic nuclei also receive abundant input (corticothalamic fibers) from the same cortical areas to which they project.

The projection of muscle afferents from the lower limb to the somatosensory cortex involves four populations of neurons in contrast to the three sets for the upper limb (see Fig. 8–4). The primary afferent fibers enter the spinal cord from the lumbar and sacral dorsal roots and then bifurcate into ascending and descending branches in the dorsal funiculus. The ascending branch terminates in the **nucleus dorsalis (Clarke's column)**, a column of large cells on the medial side of the dorsal horn from C8 to L3. The neurons in the nucleus dorsalis give rise to axons that ascend ipsilaterally as the **dorsal spinocerebellar tract** in the dorsolateral funiculus. Before entering the inferior cerebellar peduncle, some of the axons give off collateral branches that remain in the medulla. These collaterals end in **nucleus Z**, which lies just rostral to the gracile nucleus in the floor of the fourth ventricle. Cells of nucleus Z give rise to internal arcuate fibers that cross the midline and join the medical lemniscus. Nucleus Z is considered an important relay site for transfer of proprioceptive information to the cerebral cortex because a large proportion of its cells can be activated from the thalamus. From this point, the pathway is the same for the upper and lower limbs, with a synapse in the ventral posterior thalamic nucleus, after which thalamocortical fibers project to the leg area of the sensory cortex.

At all levels of the dorsal column–medial lemniscal system, somatotopy is preserved. In other words, information about a particular sensory modality, such as force or muscle length, and about a specific body region, such as the index finger, is segregated at each level of the system and processed by neurons that

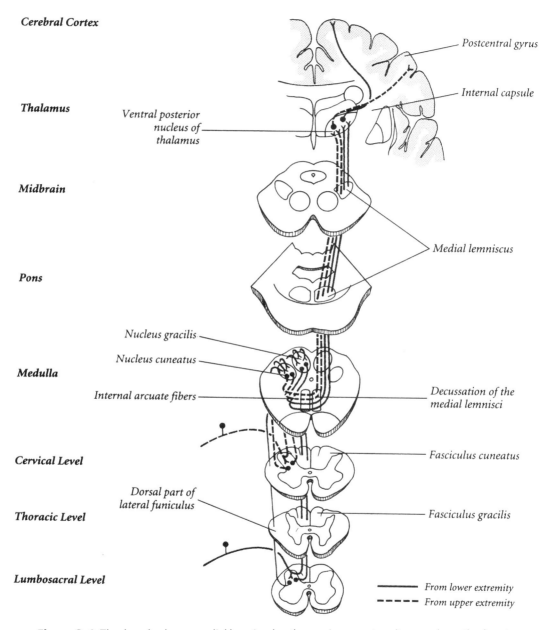

Figure 8–4. The dorsal column–medial lemniscal pathways. Lower extremity proprioceptive input is shown traveling through Clarke's column. (Reproduced with permission from Barr ML, Kiernan JA. *The human nervous system: an anatomical viewpoint.* 5th ed. Philadelphia: JB Lippincott, 1988.)

form separate functional groups. Input from different modalities does not begin to converge until sensory information reaches the somatosensory cortex. The primary somatosensory cortex is located in the postcentral gyrus of the parietal lobe and in the depths of the central sulcus, and is somatotopically organized (see Chapters 6, 7). It comprises four distinct cytoarchitectural regions, designated areas 1, 2, 3a, and 3b, according to the subdivisions of the cortex made by Brodmann. Most of the thalamic fibers terminate in area 3, which then projects to areas 1 and 2. Area 3a receives input from muscle spindle and Golgi tendon organ receptors, as well as joint receptors, whereas area 3b processes information from cutaneous receptors. The input from muscle and joint receptors appears to overlap in area 3a, but is segmented in the subsequent projections to areas 2 and 1. From here, proprioceptive information is transmitted through association fibers to area 5 of the parietal cortex. All of these projections come from the contralateral side of the body, so unilateral removal or damage to the postcentral gyrus is associated with abnormalities in the perception of limb position and movement on the opposite side of the body.[17] This finding indicates that the somatosensory cortex receives no functionally effective ipsilateral projections from proprioceptive afferent fibers.

For many years, the dorsal columns were thought to be solely responsible for carrying information about proprioception in the upper limb. Early knowledge about the function of the dorsal column medial–lemniscal system came from studies of patients with traumatic injuries of the spinal cord or with diseases that affected the spinal cord such as tabes dorsalis, a syndrome associated with the advanced stages of syphilis. These diseases often affected axons in more than one funiculus and the dorsal roots themselves, and sensory testing was often very rudimentary and qualitative. More recent studies indicate that lesions to the dorsal columns cause impairments on tasks involving the spatiotemporal integration of complex tactile information, such as discriminating the direction of a movement across the skin, or identifying the relative locations of two points of stimulation on the skin. Limb position sense, weight discrimination, and thresholds for detecting tactile stimuli are, however, essentially normal in these people, which suggests the existence of pathways outside the dorsal columns that are capable of transmitting proprioceptive information from the upper limb. The effects of circumscribed dorsal column lesions on motor be-

havior indicate which aspects of proprioceptive function may be uniquely conveyed by this pathway. After damage to the dorsal columns, monkeys have deficits in the ability to grasp, in regulating precisely the forces exerted by the hand, and in responding quickly to significant environmental stimuli.[18]

Sensory Basis of Proprioception

Psychophysical studies of the human proprioceptive system have usually focused on three variables: the perception of limb position, limb movement, and force.[19] Much of this research has been concerned with establishing the relative importance of sensory information that arises in receptors in muscles, skin, and joints to kinesthetic perception. These experiments have tried to eliminate the input from one receptor population, for example, by anesthetizing the skin using a local anesthetic or injecting an anesthetic agent into a joint to block joint receptors, and measuring the changes in perception that occur after this temporary loss of sensory input. Perception is then assessed using tasks such as having the experimental subject detect the direction of movements passively imposed on a joint, or match the positions, movements, or forces produced by two corresponding muscle groups on the left and right sides of the body.

Muscle Receptors

The body of evidence accumulated since the early 1970s indicates that no one source of afferent information can be excluded from contributing to proprioception. In the early 1970s, a series of experiments on the effects of muscle tendon vibration on the perception of limb movement demonstrated the importance of feedback from muscle spindle receptors to the perception of limb movement.[20,21] In these studies, a vibrator was applied to the skin overlying the biceps muscle tendon while the vibrated arm was immobilized and subjects were blindfolded. They were asked to indicate any change in the position of the vibrated arm by moving the opposite arm, which was free to move. Goodwin et al.[21] found that vibration of the tendon at a frequency of 100 Hz produced the illusion that the elbow was moving into extension, as if the vibrated muscle were being stretched, and that conversely, vibration of the triceps tendon produced an illusory flexion movement. The illusion persisted after anesthesia of the hand that blocked cutaneous mechanoreceptors normally activated by vibration,[22] but did not occur when the vibrator was placed over the elbow joint. Even when the muscle tendon was located some distance from the joint it moved, such as the wrist flexor tendon in the region of the elbow, illusory movements were always referred to the appropriate joint (wrist) while the perceived position of the adjacent joint (elbow) remained unchanged.[23]

The vibration-induced illusion is primarily a sensation of movement, although a 5- to 8-degree error in the sense of limb position is associated with the illusory movement. The illusion was interpreted as indicating that muscle spindle receptors do contribute to the perception of limb movement and position. This conclusion represented a reversal of the prevailing viewpoint, which emphasized the importance of joint receptors to proprioception. The illusion occurs because of the intense discharge rates of muscle spindle receptors, which are extremely sensitive to vibration. The nervous system interprets this high discharge rate as indicating that the muscle is being stretched. The subsequent finding that the velocity of the illusory movement evoked by vibration depended on both the frequency[24] (Fig. 8–5) and amplitude[25] of stimulation provided additional support for this interpretation. Goodwin et al.[21] further hypothesized that because movement illusions do not occur during the course of normal voluntary motor activities, only those spindle discharges that are inappropriate for the level of activation of the muscle must be perceived. This proposition was supported by the finding that the movement illusion was reduced or eliminated if the vibrator was applied while the muscle was generating a large force.

Illusions induced by vibration have been evoked in postural, facial, and axial muscles. In each situation, subjects experience illusory changes in body motion and posture, as long as visual information about the limb or body orientation is absent.[26–28] The magnitude of the errors in perceived limb position evoked by vibration can be increased by applying the vibrator while the muscle is being stretched. Under these conditions of stimulation, Craske[23] found that subjects often indicated that the limb was in an anatomically impossible position. For example, when the wrist extensor tendon was vibrated, subjects perceived that the hand was so extended that it was almost making contact with the dorsum of the

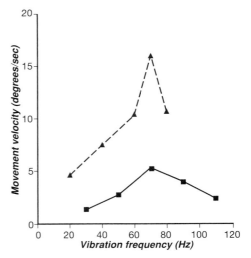

Figure 8–5. Mean angular velocity of illusory movements of the forearm perceived by subjects during vibration of the left biceps tendon at different frequencies (squares), and during alternate vibration of the left biceps and triceps tendons at different frequencies (triangles). In each experiment, the perceived movements were reproduced by the right arm and were recorded using a linear potentiometer. (Data from Roll and Vedel.[24])

forearm. Other investigators have reported similar results. These findings suggest that cortical sensory centers are prepared to extrapolate beyond previous experience on the basis of incoming sensory information, and that the perceptual limits of the sense of position are not set by the anatomic constraints of joint excursion. They also suggest that the sense of limb position is very labile and will readily adapt to changing sensory input. This capacity to modify one's body image may be important to the skilled use of tools, during which they are considered as extensions of human limbs.[19]

Although the vibration-induced movement illusion is subservient to vision, in that it does not occur if subjects can see their arms while the vibrator is applied, interesting interactions occur between visual and proprioceptive sensory signals under degraded viewing conditions, such as in the dark or without full view of the limb. Lackner and Taublieb found that when subjects were asked to fixate on the position of their unseen index finger while the biceps tendon was vibrated, they lowered their direction of gaze.[29] This result indicates that the visual system had interpreted these illusory movements as if they were real movements of the limb. If a light was then affixed to the restrained hand while vibration was applied, subjects not only perceived that their unseen, stationery arm was moving, but perceived that the target light moved in the direction of the perceived movement of the arm, even though they continued to fixate on the stationary target.[30] When part of the limb can be seen, both the apparent displacement and velocity of forearm motion are diminished. Under these conditions, subjects report a dissociation between the visual and proprioceptive locations of a limb, and between the location of adjacent limb segments such as the finger and hand. These findings suggest that the perception of limb position and movement does not simply arise from modality-specific topographic maps, but rather results from interactions between representations in different afferent domains, such as vision, touch, and proprioception.[29]

The results from these studies on the effects of vibration on proprioception led to a reexamination of earlier findings that had been interpreted as suggesting that muscle receptors did not contribute to proprioception. One early result that was contentious was the report that patients whose finger flexor tendons were stretched during carpal tunnel surgery, in which the carpal ligament is sectioned so as to relieve pressure on the median nerve, did not perceive that any movement of the finger had occurred when the muscle was stretched.[31] Matthews and Simmonds[32] replicated this study and found that during surgery patients did experience movements of the finger when the tendon was pulled if they were told to focus on movement of the finger rather than stretch of the muscle, as in the earlier studies. Even when the finger was restrained so that it could not move, patients perceived that it did move if the muscle was stretched. More recently, McCloskey and colleagues repeated this experiment under laboratory conditions and, in a heroic gesture, McCloskey had the tendon of his extensor hallucis longus (big toe) muscle exposed and transected under local anesthetic.[33] Without any visual feedback of the toe's position, McCloskey was able to detect movements imposed on the muscle through the proximal end of the cut tendon, even though the interphalangeal joint of the toe was immobilized. The threshold for detecting a displacement was similar for stretches imposed on the muscle through its exposed tendon and for the intact toe. These results were interpreted as indicating that the information arising from muscle receptors is perceived and is essential to the perception of limb movement.

Joint and Cutaneous Receptors

Several morphologic types of receptor endings have been identified in joint capsules. Based on their similarity to receptors found in other tissues, they have been called **Ruffini endings**, which are found in the joint capsule, **Golgi endings**, located in ligaments of the joint, and **encapsulated paciniform endings**, often found in the fibrous periosteum near articular attachments.[34] Free nerve endings are also found in the joint capsule. The distribution of these receptors is nonuniform in a joint, which may reflect the location of stresses during movement.[35] Joint receptors are innervated by separate nerve branches as well as by branches from nerves supplying adjacent muscles and overlying skin. Most joint receptors discharge near the extremes of movement and typically discharge during both extreme flexion and extension, and so do not provide an unambiguous signal related to joint position. Estimates of the number of receptors firing during the midrange of joint movement in various animal species vary from less than 5%[36] to 18%[37]; some of the receptors identified in the latter study are probably muscle spindle receptors and not from the joint. These response properties suggest that joint receptors may function as limit detectors whose role is to signal extreme positions of the joint and in so doing prevent damage to the joint.[38] This function contrasts to the role of muscle spindle receptors, which appear to be unable to function as limit detectors, given the illusions of impossible limb positions induced by vibration.

Four types of mechanoreceptor have been identified in human glabrous or nonhairy skin, two rapidly adapting receptors identified as the **Meissner corpuscle** and the **Pacinian corpuscle**, and two slowly adapting receptors known as **Merkel cells** and Ruffini endings. Hairy skin contains Merkel cells, which are grouped under visible touch domes, and Ruffini endings, which are usually found around hairs and hair follicle receptors. Pacinian corpuscles are rare in hairy skin and usually occur around joints and tendon sheaths. In the hand, many cutaneous afferents in glabrous skin respond to voluntary finger movements, and most receptors show no directional specificity—that is, they discharge in response to both extension and flexion movements. In contrast, receptors on the back of the hand readily respond to finger movements and show considerable directional specificity. Many of these receptors not only discharge in response to movement of the underlying joint, but signal movements of adjacent joints.[39]

Signals arising from these joint and cutaneous receptors contribute to proprioception, and they appear to be most important for the hand and less critical for more proximal joints such as the knee. The evidence for this statement comes from studies comparing the effects of skin or joint anesthesia on the ability to detect movements imposed on different joints. Gandevia et al.[40] and Ferrell and Smith[41] showed that when inputs from the skin overlying the distal interphalangeal joint of the middle finger and from the joint itself were eliminated after a block of the digital nerve, movement detection thresholds were elevated and there were increased errors when matching the position of the anesthetized finger, as shown in Figure 8–6. The anesthesia does not affect the muscles in the forearm controlling flexion and extension movements of the finger. Subjects were still able to detect movements and match positions of the finger during skin and joint anesthesia, which shows that muscle receptors do provide an important source of proprioceptive information. The impairment in performance indicates, however, that the perception of finger movement and position does depend on afferent input from receptors other than those in the muscle.

When input from only cutaneous receptors is eliminated, finger position is not accurately perceived and the ability to detect finger movements is impaired, as shown in Figure 8–6.[42] Clark et al.[43] showed that the effects of skin anesthesia on movement detection are not limited to the skin surface overlying the joint being moved, but can also occur when other sites on adjacent fingers are anesthetized. This finding is consistent with electrophysiologic data from cutaneous mechanoreceptors in the dorsal surface of the human hand that show that they can respond to skin stimulation applied 70 to 80 mm away from the actual location of the receptors.[39] Based on these observations, it appears that signals arising from cutaneous receptors in the hand can indicate to the central nervous system that a move-

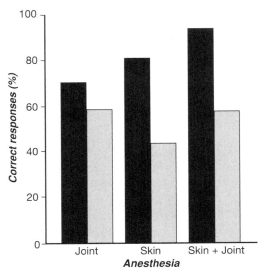

Figure 8–6. The effect of anesthetizing the distal interphalangeal joint of the middle finger, the skin on the tip of the index finger, and both the joint and the skin surrounding the distal interphalangeal joint of the middle finger on the ability to detect 5- or 10-degree displacements imposed on the joint. The *black bars* are the results obtained under control conditions (preanesthesia) and the *gray bars* are the results during anesthesia. (The data on the effects of joint or skin anesthesia are taken from Clark et al.[43] and Clark et al. [The contribution of articular receptors to proprioception with the fingers in humans. *J Neurophysiol* 1989; 61:186–193] respectively, and those for combined skin and joint anesthesia are from Gandevia et al.[40]). (From Jones LA. Proprioception and its contribution to manual dexterity. In: Wing AM, Haggard P, Flanagan JR, eds. *Hand and brain.* San Diego: Academic Press, 1996: 349–362, redrawn with the permission of Academic Press.)

ment has occurred and can be used to interpret signals arising from other sources.

The contribution of signals arising from joint receptors in the hand to proprioception is still subject to debate. Some studies have shown that when a finger joint is anesthetized, there is an impairment in the ability to detect movements imposed on the joint[43] and to match the position of the anesthetized joint.[41] The effects of anesthesia are most evident near the extremes of joint excursion, which is consistent with electrophysiologic data from joint receptors. Recordings of the activity of isolated afferent fibers from finger joints in the human hand indicate that over 80% of joint afferent fibers discharge at the extremes of the range of motion of the joint, and a much smaller percentage are active when the joint is placed in midrange positions.[44]

Studies of people with prosthetic (artificial) joint replacements provide another source of information about the contribution of joint receptors to proprioception. In this procedure the joint, its capsule, and presumably its complement of joint receptors are surgically removed and replaced by an artificial joint. Several months after hip replacement surgery, slow movements of about 1 degree/second can be detected on the operated side, compared with approximately 0.5 degree/second normally,[45] so there is a slight but not significant loss of acuity after hip replacement. After replacement of the metatarsophalangeal joint of the great toe, patients can detect small flexion and extension movements (less than 10 degrees applied manually at 2 to 3 degrees/second) at essentially normal levels of performance.[46] Not only is the detection of passive movements relatively normal in people with prosthetic joints, but also the ability to reproduce movements of specific amplitudes with the artificial joint remains unimpaired.[47] Apparently, whatever information is provided by joint receptors about the speed and direction of joint movement is adequately duplicated by other sensory sources.

In contrast to the results from the hand described previously, skin or joint anesthesia apparently has no effect on the perception of knee position[48] or on the threshold for detecting passive movements of the knee,[49] as illustrated in Figure 8–7. These findings suggest that the hand should be considered unique with respect to the sensory mechanisms underlying the perception of limb movement and position and should not be used as a model of the behavior of more proximal joints.[50] The importance of cutaneous sensory feedback to the perception of finger movements and positions is not surprising in view of the high innervation density of cutaneous mechanoreceptors and the specialization of the hand for tactile exploration and manipulation. This feedback may also be important for proprioception in the hand because of the ambiguity of muscle receptor discharges owing to the multiarticular control of finger joints, with most muscles acting over many joints.

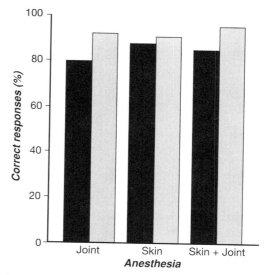

Figure 8–7. The effect of anesthetizing the knee joint, a 150-mm band of skin around the joint, and both the joint and skin on the ability to detect 5-degree changes in the angle of the knee. The *black bars* are the results obtained under control conditions (i.e., preinjection and postinjection) and the *gray bars* the results during anesthesia. The data are taken from Clark et al.[48] (From Jones LA. Proprioception and its contribution to manual dexterity. In: Wing AM, Haggard P, Flanagan JR, eds. *Hand and brain*. San Diego: Academic Press, 1996:349–362, redrawn with the permission of Academic Press.)

Perception of Limb Position and Movement

Under most conditions, when we move our arms or legs we are aware that our limbs have changed position, so we have an awareness of both limb movement and limb position. These two aspects of perception can be separated experimentally by imposing extremely slow movements on a joint (i.e., 1–4 degrees/minute) that result in a change in the position of the joint without the subject having any awareness that a movement has occurred. In these experiments, a single trial may last 5 minutes, at which point the subject simply indicates whether the position of the limb is the same as or different from that at the beginning of the trial. Using this procedure, Clark et al.[51] have shown that people can make

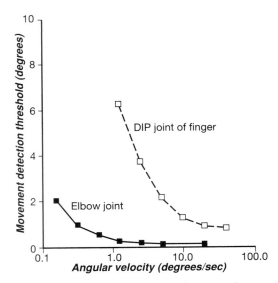

Figure 8–8. Detection thresholds for flexion and extension movements imposed on the elbow joint and the distal interphalangeal (DIP) joint of the finger. (Data from Hall and McCloskey.[53])

grees/second to 1 degree at a movement velocity of 80 degrees/second. The threshold is relatively constant at 1 degree over the velocity range of 10 to 80 degrees/second, as shown in Figure 8–8.[40,53] This region of optimal velocity sensitivity is the one that people use spontaneously when they are asked to make self-paced pointing movements.[53] Movement thresholds decrease significantly if the movement is imposed while the muscles acting on the joint are actively contracting rather than relaxed. For the elbow flexor muscles, the threshold for detecting movements imposed on the elbow joint is more than 10 times smaller if the muscles are contracting when the movement is imposed, and this effect is greater at lower movement velocities, as illustrated in Figure 8–9.[54] This finding indicates that the enhanced level of muscle spindle afferent activity that occurs when a muscle contracts facilitates the detection of a movement.

In contrast to the sense of limb movement, the ability to detect a change in the position of a limb is not affected by the angular velocity of the movement,[51] but does depend on the absolute position of the limb and on the joint moved. Taylor and McCloskey[55] reported that the threshold for detecting a change in the posi-

independent judgments of the position and movement of a limb.

The ability to detect movements of a limb depends on several factors, including the particular joint moving, the velocity of the movement, and the contractile state of the muscles controlling the joint. As Goldscheider[52] noted more than a century ago, proximal joints such as the shoulder or elbow have a greater sensitivity to movement than more distal joints such as the metacarpophalangeal joint in the hand (Fig. 8–8). The superior performance of more proximal joints is not surprising because they move more slowly than distal joints, and rotation of these joints causes a larger displacement of the end-point of the limb than the same angular rotation at a more distal joint. For example, rotation of the shoulder 1 degree moves the middle fingertip of the outstretched arm 13 mm (0.5 in.), whereas a 1-degree rotation of the distal interphalangeal joint of the middle finger moves the fingertip 0.5 mm (0.02 in.).

As the velocity of a movement imposed on a joint increases, so too does the ability to detect the movement. For the distal interphalangeal joint of the middle finger, the threshold for detecting a movement decreases from approximately 8 degrees at 1.25 de-

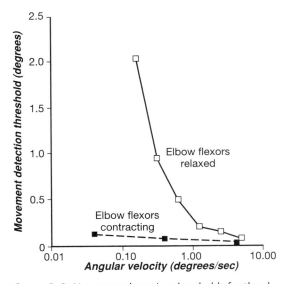

Figure 8–9. Movement detection thresholds for the elbow joint measured when the muscles were relaxed and when they maintained a background contraction. (Data from Hall and McCloskey[53] [relaxed position] and Taylor and McCloskey[54] [active contraction].)

tion of the joints of the hand ranges from 4.4 degrees for the metacarpophalangeal joint, to 6.8 degrees for the proximal interphalangeal joint. These thresholds were obtained using movement velocities of less than 2 degrees/ minute, so subjects could not perceive that their fingers had moved.

The perception of limb position is often evaluated using a matching procedure in which the subject or patient is asked to align the positions of two corresponding joints on the left and right sides of the body in the absence of any visual feedback about limb position. The limits of performance on this type of task are probably imposed by the sensory input, and not by the motor capacity of the subject to achieve the target position,[22] although clearly errors can arise from both sources. This assumption is supported by a finding reported by Head and Holmes[56] in their studies of patients with cerebral lesions that resulted in a loss of position sense and deficits in motor control on the side contralateral to the lesion. These patients found it much easier to move the affected limb to match the position of the normal limb, than to move the normal limb to match the position of the impaired limb.

The errors in matching the positions of two corresponding joints are often surprisingly large in normal, healthy adults. For example, for the proximal interphalangeal joint of the index finger, errors range from 0.75 to 6 degrees over a range of 100 to 175 degrees of finger flexion.[57] Matching accuracy varies with the position of the target limb; subjects tend to be most accurate near the midrange of joint movement.[19] For the knee, ankle, and elbow joints, this position is close to a joint angle of 90 degrees. Acuity is superior for axial muscles compared with limb muscles, as shown by the observation that subjects are able to reposition the trunk in the frontal plane with errors of less than 1 degree.[58] Acuity is also better if subjects move their limbs actively rather than having the experimenter move a limb passively. This result is consistent with the findings on the perception of movement, where it was noted that muscle contraction enhanced the detection of limb movements. With active positioning, the errors in matching the positions of the outstretched arms average 0.6 degree, compared with 2 degrees when the limb is moved passively.[59] These findings attest to the importance of using active movements for evaluating the proprioceptive system, rather than the classic tests in which the limb is passively moved by the clinician.

Perception of Force

Information about the forces generated by muscles arises from at least two sources. First, afferent discharges arising peripherally in Golgi tendon organs signal intramuscular force and therefore provide the central nervous system with information about the forces exerted by muscles. Second, force information could be derived from an internal neural correlate or copy of the motor command (sometimes known as **corollary discharge**) sent to the motor neuron pool in the spinal cord. This signal is probably transmitted to the sensory centers in the brain and may reflect the magnitude of the descending motor signal.[60] These centrally mediated sensations are often termed a **sense of effort**, whereas the peripherally arising sensations are termed a **sense of force** or **tension**.

In the absence of disease or muscle fatigue, the senses of effort and of force provide congruent information—that is, as the motor command increases, so too does the discharge rate of Golgi tendon organs signaling the force of contraction. Under these conditions, distinguishing which of the two sources of force information is used perceptually is not possible. Experiments in which the normal relation between the descending motor command and the discharge of tendon organ receptors is decoupled provide a basis for examining the role of centrally generated and peripherally arising signals in the perception of muscle force.

The results from a number of these experiments indicate that as the motor command sent to a muscle increases, the perceived magnitude of the force of contraction increases correspondingly, even when the force exerted by the muscle remains constant. For example, when subjects are required to estimate the magnitude of a force maintained at a constant amplitude until the point of maximal endurance is reached, the perceived amplitude of the sustained force increases linearly, as shown in Figure 8–10.[61,62] In this situation, as the force is maintained, the neural drive required to generate the force increases as the muscle fatigues. It seems unlikely that the overestimation of force is based on discharges arising from Golgi tendon organs in the muscle because these would remain constant or decrease (if they adapt) while the muscle continued to generate a constant force.

Changes in the perception of force and heaviness are also apparent during other states and conditions

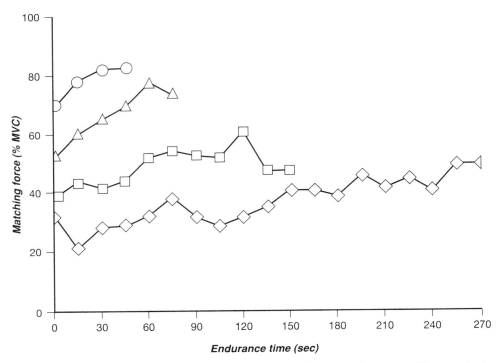

Figure 8–10. The matching forces exerted by the left elbow flexor muscles as one of four constant forces (30% [diamonds], 45% [squares], 60% [triangles], and 75% [circles] of maximum voluntary contraction [MVC]) was maintained by the right elbow flexors until maximal endurance. (From Jones LA. The senses of effort and force during fatiguing contractions. In: Gandevia SC, Enoka RM, McComas AJ, et al., eds. *Fatigue: neural and muscular mechanisms.* New York: Plenum Press, 1995:305–313, redrawn with the permission of Plenum Press.)

that affect the force-generating capacity of the muscle. Weakness or paresis can be induced experimentally by partially blocking transmission at the myoneural junction (motor end-plate) using a neuromuscular blocking agent, such as curare. The forces produced by a muscle weakened by curarization are overestimated in magnitude, as indicated by the amplitude of the forces generated by the corresponding muscle group on the contralateral side of the body.[63] In addition to fatigue and partial curarization, in a number of clinical conditions an increase in the descending motor command is accompanied by a corresponding increase in the perceived amplitude of muscle forces and hence the weight of objects supported by the affected limb (Fig. 8–11). For example, in pa-

tients with cerebellar disease that causes reduced excitability of the spinal motor neuronal pool, larger than normal motor commands are required to achieve any given level of muscle force.[64] This overestimation of force in patients with cerebellar lesions occurs in the presence of normal sensory function, as was first noted by Holmes.[65] He reported that even though there was no difference between the patients' hands in their ability to discriminate weights, most of these people with unilateral cerebellar lesions overestimated the heaviness of weights lifted on the affected side.

Patients with unilateral upper motor neuron paresis who show no evidence of sensory loss in the upper limb also overestimate the forces generated on

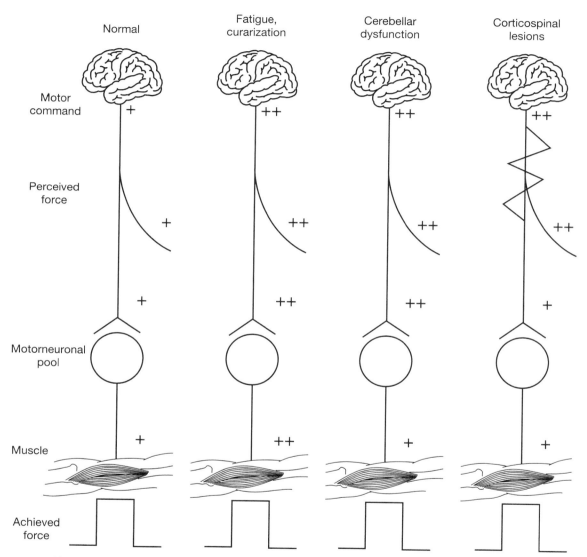

Figure 8-11. Schematic illustration of the relation between the magnitude of the descending motor command and the perceived force exerted under different experimental and clinical conditions. (Adapted from McCloskey et al.[8])

the affected side.[66] The weakness resulting from this type of motor lesion is a consequence of damage to the corticofugal pathways and, possibly, cortical structures. To achieve a normal input to spinal motor neurons, increased neural output along the unaffected pathways would be needed, and this increase is associated with a change in the perceived magnitude of forces. In patients with complete muscular paralysis caused by a cortical lesion, the command to move the paralyzed limb is not accompanied by a sensation of effort or heaviness, and patients are aware that the limb has remained immobile.[67]

The results from these studies indicate that an increase in the motor command sent to a muscle is accompanied by a change in the perceived amplitude of force generated by that muscle. This finding suggests that our perception of force is based on information that is derived centrally rather than from the activity of peripheral receptors in the muscle. Apparently, the central nervous system monitors its own activity in producing muscle contractions, and our perception of force and heaviness derives from this internal monitoring. This conclusion should not be interpreted as dismissing a contribution from peripheral receptors such as the Golgi tendon organ receptors to the awareness of force. Under some conditions, subjects can estimate muscle force when only muscle receptors, presumably Golgi tendon organs, could be providing the guiding signals.[68] Even under normal conditions, peripheral afferent input is required to indicate that the force produced by the muscle is adequate for the task being performed. In addition, reflex inputs from joint, muscle, and skin receptors can inhibit and facilitate spinal motor neurons and, in so doing, influence the magnitude of the centrally generated motor command.

The neural systems involved in transmitting correlates of the descending motor command are unknown, although a number of neuroanatomic pathways have been proposed. Collaterals from corticospinal neurons in the motor cortex have been traced at different levels of the system and, in particular, the reciprocal connections between motor cortex cells and neurons in the primary sensory cortex are one pathway that is capable of transmitting information that could be used perceptually. Because motor cortex cells discharge in proportion to the force of contraction generated in the distal muscles that they innervate,[69] changes in their discharge rates would lead to changes in perceived force if, as the evidence reviewed previously suggests, they are the predominant source of force information.

Clinical Correlations

Phantom Limb Illusions

After amputation of a limb, a person inevitably experiences a **phantom limb**, that is, the illusion that the amputated limb still exists and can change its position in space. Phantom limbs are reported by approximately 95% of amputees who have lost their limbs traumatically (in an accident or as a result of an acute injury), and are usually described as a pleasant tingling sensation associated with the missing body part.[70] Phantom limbs are much less common in patients who have slowly developing limb losses, and occur less frequently when the limb loss is in the first decade of life. The percentage of children who report phantom limb sensations increases as a function of the age at which the limb was amputated,[71] although they have been described in children who were congenital amputees.[72] The less frequent appearance of phantom limbs in young children is probably related to the limited sensory and motor experiences with the limb before its loss.

Phantom limbs are relevant to our understanding of proprioception in that they suggest that an awareness of limb position can be experienced in the absence of any sensory input from a muscle and that sensations of movement can result from centrally generated motor commands. A phantom limb may be perceived to move in two ways. First, when the limb bearing the stump of the limb is moved, the phantom may appear to move with it, although it is not perceived to change its position relative to other limb segments. In this situation, the phantom limb maintains its position with respect to the stump, so its neural representation based on incoming sensory signals is unchanged. Second, the phantom limb may be perceived to move in response to a motor command, and the relative positions of limb segments in the phantom may also move. For this perceived motion to occur, the command to move the limb would have to have perceptual consequences.[26]

The incidence of phantom limbs does not depend on either the level of amputation or on the limb amputated, and they are usually experienced very soon after the amputation.[73] The more distal parts of the limb, such as the fingers, are more strongly perceived than the proximal segments, a finding that is consistent with the cortical representation of the limb, with more extensive representation in the somatosensory cortex of the hand, and in particular the thumb and index finger, than, for example, the wrist or forearm. The perception of the phantom limb changes over time, with the more weakly perceived body segments fading from awareness in what is described as a "telescoping" of the limb.[74] An amputation below the elbow can result in the phantom fingers being perceived as if they were attached to the stump. This phenomenon is probably related to changes that occur in the somatosensory cortex after amputation, during the considerable reorganization of cortical areas that occurs when one part of the cortex is deprived of its sensory input.[75] If an amputee starts wearing a prosthesis, however, the form of the phantom limb changes and the telescoping of the limb is lost as the phantom and prosthetic device become integrated. Under these conditions, the amputee often reports that the limb has returned to its original length.[76]

Most amputees report that they can move certain parts of the phantom limb, although these movements become more difficult with time and may be lost completely 12 to 18 months after the amputation. The movements are always made consciously, do not occur spontaneously, and are almost always accompanied by a contraction of the appropriate muscles in the stump. If the muscles remaining in the stump are denervated, which eliminates the contractions, the ability to move the phantom voluntarily is lost.[76] These findings indicate that the perception of voluntary movements of a phantom limb depends on afferent feedback from the periphery. In other words, a descending motor command cannot produce a conscious awareness of movement in the absence of peripheral sensory feedback. In contrast, the phantom limb itself and its static position do not depend on peripheral feedback because they persist after denervation of the stump and so must arise from neural activity originating in the sensorimotor cortex.

Deafferentation

Another clinical condition that gives a different perspective on how the proprioceptive system functions is deafferentation resulting from a large-fiber sensory neuropathy. In this relatively rare condition, large myelinated fibers in the peripheral nerves are lost, so inputs from muscle and many types of skin receptors are either nonexistent or severely limited. This condition usually results in a complete loss of kinesthesia in the affected limbs and a loss of the senses of touch, pressure, and vibration. Studies of these patients provide a unique opportunity to investigate the contribution of proprioceptive afferents to perception and motor performance. One frequently reported finding from these patients is an impairment in maintaining a constant position of the limb or a constant force output in the absence of visual feedback,[77,78] which attests to the importance of input from peripheral receptors to the maintenance of a stable motor output. For some patients, motor tasks can be mastered by substituting visual for proprioceptive feedback and by concentrating on the activity being performed.[79]

The perceptual abilities of these patients are also profoundly impaired. In the absence of proprioceptive information and without visual guidance, they are capable of making only very gross discriminations.[79,80] In some situations, such as discriminating between weights or matching a movement imposed on an arm, they may be unable to make any judgments because they do not know when a hand-held weight has been lifted[77] or have any awareness of the extent of movement.[79] One deafferented patient, however, was able to match quite accurately a constant force applied to one thumb with a variable force applied to the opposite thumb. No visual feedback of thumb position was provided, but two lights indicated when each thumb had exerted sufficient force to move its respective lever off the backstop.[77] On initial inspection, it appears that in the absence of peripheral feedback, this patient was able to match correctly the motor output to the thumb flexor muscles. Closer examination revealed that the patient may have accomplished the task using other cues, such as timing how long it took for the light to be illuminated and then matching the time intervals rather than the forces exerted. These compensatory strategies are a common feature of the performance of people with sensory loss, who learn to make very effective use of whatever sensory channels are available. The use of subtle visual cues to assist in discrimination is a commonly reported finding, and using vision, weight discrimination thresholds can be similar to those measured in healthy subjects.[79,80] As soon as the visual feedback is eliminated, discrimination deteriorates dramatically, to the extent that it is no longer functionally useful.

Conclusions

The proprioceptive system derives information from receptors in muscles, skin, and joints and uses these sensory inputs to determine where our limbs are in space and the amplitude and velocity of limb movements. Muscle receptors appear to be the predominant source of this proprioceptive information, but receptors in the skin and joints also contribute to these perceptual processes. Their input appears to be especially important for the hand, and in the absence of sensory information from the skin of the hand, and to a lesser extent the finger joints, deficiencies in proprioceptive abilities become apparent. Similar impairments are not found after joint or skin anesthesia of more proximal joints. The latter finding should not be interpreted as dismissing a role for joint and cutaneous receptors at these joints, but as an indication that the information they provide is available from other afferent sources.

The internal monitoring of efferent output has been ascribed two separate roles in the processing of proprioceptive information. First, the perception of force and heaviness appears to be based on corollaries that are derived from the descending motor command and not from signals originating in receptors in the muscle, although the latter do provide a signal of muscle force. The preference for using force information derived from a central rather than peripheral source may serve a protective function, in that by monitoring motor outflow it may be possible to detect imminent failure in the force-generating capacity of the muscle and take corrective action. The monitoring of motor commands has also featured in explanations of the central processing of muscle spindle receptor activity. In this context, corollary discharges have been proposed as a mechanism that the central nervous system could use to enable it to distinguish between afferent activity that results from activity of the fusimotor system from that which reflects an external stimulus. In the absence of corollary discharges, the task of decoding signals from muscle spindle receptors seems extremely arduous, because a change in firing rate may result from an increase in fusimotor activity, a change in muscle length, or both. In many situations, the level of fusimotor activity is probably adjusted to maintain spindle recep-

tor firing at a relatively constant rate, even when the muscle is changing length.[81] The process by which corollary discharges assist in decoding spindle activity is not known, but they appear to be used to distinguish the spindle receptor firing rate that is appropriate for the level of motor activity from that which is inappropriate and therefore of potential proprioceptive importance.

REFERENCES

1. Barker D. The morphology of muscle receptors. In: Hunt C, ed. *Symposium on muscle receptors*. Hong Kong: Hong Kong University Press, 1974:1–190.
2. Boyd IA. The isolated mammalian muscle spindle. *Trends Neurosci* 1980;3:258–265.
3. Hulliger M. The mammalian muscle spindle and its central control. *Rev Physiol Biochem Pharmacol* 1984;101:1–110.
4. Buchthal F, Schmalbruch H. Motor unit of mammalian muscle. *Physiol Rev* 1980;60:90–142.
5. Burke D, Gandevia SC. Peripheral motor system. In: Paxinos G, ed. *The human nervous system*. New York: Academic Press, 1990:125–145.
6. Gandevia SC, Burke D. Does the nervous system depend on kinesthetic information to control natural limb movements? *Behav Brain Sci* 1992;15:614–632.
7. Prochazka A. Proprioceptive feedback and movement regulation. In: Rowell L, Shepherd JT, eds. *Handbook of physiology. Section 12. Exercise: regulation and integration of multiple systems*. New York: Oxford University Press, 1996:89–127.
8. McCloskey DI, Gandevia SC, Potter EK, et al. Muscle sense and effort: motor commands and judgments about muscular contractions. In: Desmedt JE, ed. *Motor control mechanisms in health and disease*. New York: Raven Press, 1983:151–167.
9. Jami L. Golgi tendon organs in mammalian skeletal muscle: functional properties and central actions. *Physiol Rev* 1992;72:623–666.
10. Bridgman CF. Comparisons of structure of tendon organs in the rat, cat and man. *J Comp Neurol* 1980;138:369–372.
11. Houk JC, Crago PE, Rymer WZ. Functional properties of the Golgi tendon organs. In: Desmedt JE, ed. *Spinal and supraspinal mechanisms of voluntary motor control and locomotion*. Basel: Karger, 1980:33–43.
12. Devanandan MS, Ghosh S, John KT. A quantitative study of muscle spindles and tendon organs in some intrinsic muscles of the hand in the bonnet monkey (*Macaca radiata*). *Anat Rec* 1983;207:263–266.
13. Mountcastle VB, Covian MR, Harrison CR. The central representation of some forms of deep sensibility. *Res Publ Assoc Res Nerv Ment Dis* 1952;30:339–370.

14. Landgren S, Silfvenius H. Projection to cerebral cortex of group 1 muscle afferents from the catís hind limb. *J Physiol* 1969;200:353–372.

15. McIntyre AK, Proske U, Rawson JA. Cortical projection of afferent information from tendon organs in the cat. *J Physiol* 1984;354:395–406.

16. Brodal A. *Neurological anatomy*. 3rd ed. New York: Oxford University Press, 1981.

17. Jeannerod M, Michel F, Prablanc C. The control of hand movements in a case of hemianaesthesia following a parietal lesion. *Brain* 1984;107:899–920.

18. Vierck CJ. Interpretations of the sensory and motor consequences of dorsal column lesions. In: Gordon G, ed. *Active touch*. New York: Pergamon Press, 1978:139–159.

19. Clark FJ, Horch KW. Kinesthesia. In: Boff K, Kaufman L, Thomas JP, eds. *Handbook of perception and human performance*. Vol 1. New York: John Wiley & Sons, 1986: 13-1–13-62.

20. Eklund G. Position sense and state of contraction: the effects of vibration. *J Neurol Neurosurg Psychiatry* 1972; 35:606–611.

21. Goodwin GM, McCloskey DI, Matthews PBC. The contribution of muscle afferents to kinaesthesia shown by vibration induced illusions of movement and by the effects of paralysing the joint afferents. *Brain* 1972;95: 705–748.

22. Goodwin GM. The sense of limb position and movement. *Exerc Sport Sci Rev* 1976;4:87–124.

23. Craske B. Perception of impossible limb positions induced by tendon vibration. *Science* 1977;196:71–73.

24. Roll JP, Vedel JP. Kinaesthetic role of muscle afferents in man, studied by tendon vibration and microneurography. *Exp Brain Res* 1982;47:177–190.

25. Clark FJ, Matthews PBC, Muir RB. Effect of the amplitude of muscle vibration on the subjectively experienced illusion of movement. *J Physiol* 1979;296:14P–15P.

26. Jones LA. Motor illusions: what do they reveal about proprioception? *Psychol Bull* 1988;103:72–86.

27. Lackner JR. Some proprioceptive influences on the perceptual representation of body shape and orientation. *Brain* 1988;111:281–297.

28. Lackner JR, Levine MS. Changes in apparent body orientation and sensory localization induced by vibration of postural muscles: vibratory myesthetic illusions. *Aviat Space Environ Med* 1979;50:346–354.

29. Lackner JR, Taublieb AB. Influence of vision on vibration-induced illusions of limb movement. *Exp Neurol* 1984;85:97–106.

30. Lackner JR, Levine MS. Visual direction depends on the operation of spatial constancy mechanisms: the oculobrachial illusion. *Neurosci Lett* 1978;7:207–212.

31. Gelfan S, Carter S. Muscle sense in man. *Exp Neurol* 1967;18:469–473.

32. Matthews PBC, Simmonds A. Sensations of finger movement elicited by pulling upon flexor tendons in man. *J Physiol* 1974;239:27P–28P.

33. McCloskey DI, Cross MJ, Honner R, et al. Sensory effects of pulling or vibrating exposed tendons in man. *Brain* 1983;106:21–37.

34. Zimny ML. Mechanoreceptors in articular tissues. *Am J Anat* 1988;182:16–32.

35. Gandevia SC. Kinesthesia: roles for afferent signals and motor commands. In: Rowell LB, Shepherd JT, eds. *Handbook of physiology. Section 12: Exercise: regulation and integration of multiple systems*. New York: Oxford University Press, 1996:128–172.

36. Clark FJ, Burgess PR. Slowly adapting receptors in cat knee joint: can they signal joint angle? *J Neurophysiol* 1975;38:1448–1463.

37. Ferrell WR. The adequacy of stretch receptors in the cat knee joint for signalling joint angle throughout a full range of movement. *J Physiol* 1980;299:85–99.

38. Proske U, Schaible HG, Schmidt RF. Joint receptors and kinaesthesia. *Exp Brain Res* 1988;72:219–224.

39. Edin BB, Abbs JH. Finger movement responses of cutaneous mechanoreceptors in the dorsal skin of the human hand. *J Neurophysiol* 1991;65:657–670.

40. Gandevia SC, Hall LA, McCloskey DI, et al. Proprioceptive sensation at the terminal joint of the middle finger. *J Physiol* 1983;335:507–517.

41. Ferrell WR, Smith A. The effect of loading on position sense at the proximal interphalangeal joint of the index finger. *J Physiol* 1989;418:145–161.

42. Ferrell WR, Smith A. Position sense at the proximal interphalangeal joint of the human index finger. *J Physiol* 1988;399:49–61.

43. Clark FJ, Burgess RC, Chapin JW. Proprioception with the proximal interphalangeal joint of the index finger. *Brain* 1986;109:1195–1208.

44. Burke D, Gandevia SC, Macefield G. Responses to passive movement of receptors in joint, skin and muscle of the human hand. *J Physiol* 1988;402:347–362.

45. Grigg P, Finerman GA, Riley LH. Joint-position sense after total hip replacement. *J Bone Joint Surg Am* 1973; 55:1016–1025.

46. Cross MJ, McCloskey DI. Position sense following surgical removal of joints in man. *Brain Res* 1973;55:443–445.

47. Kelso JAS, Holt KG, Flatt AE. The role of proprioception in the perception and control of human movement: toward a theoretical reassessment. *Perception Psychophys* 1980; 28:45–52.

48. Clark FJ, Horch KW, Bach SM, et al. Contribution of cutaneous and joint receptors to static knee-position sense in man. *J Neurophysiol* 1979;42:877–888.

49. Barrack RL, Skinner HB, Brunet ME, et al. Functional performance of the knee after intraarticular anesthesia. *Am J Sports Med* 1983;11:258–261.

50. Jones LA. Peripheral mechanisms of touch and proprioception. *Can J Physiol Pharmacol* 1994;72:484–487.

51. Clark FJ, Burgess RC, Chapin JW, et al. The role of intramuscular receptors in the awareness of limb position. *J Neurophysiol* 1985;54:1529–1540.

52. Goldscheider A. Untersuchungen uber den Muskelsinn. *Arch Anat Physiol* 1889;3:369–502.

53. Hall LA, McCloskey DI. Detections of movements imposed on finger, elbow and shoulder joints. *J Physiol* 1983;335:519–533.

54. Taylor JL, McCloskey DI. Detection of slow movements imposed at the elbow during active flexion in man. *J Physiol* 1992;457:503–513.

55. Taylor JL, McCloskey DI. Ability to detect angular displacements of the fingers made at an imperceptibly slow speed. *Brain* 1990;113:157–166.

56. Head H, Holmes G. Sensory disturbances from cerebral lesions. *Brain* 1911;34:102–254.

57. Clark FJ, Larwood KJ, Davis ME, et al. A metric for assessing acuity in positioning joints and limbs. *Exp Brain Res* 1995;107:73–79.

58. Jakobs T, Miller JAA, Schultz AB. Trunk position sense in the frontal plane. *Exp Neurol* 1985;90:129–138.

59. Paillard J, Brouchon M. Active and passive movements in the calibration of position sense. In: Freedman SJ, ed. *The neuropsychology of spatially oriented behavior*. Homewood, IL: Dorsey Press, 1968:37–55.

60. McCloskey DI. Corollary discharges: motor commands and perception. In: Brooks VB, ed. *Handbook of physiology. Section 1: The nervous system*. Vol 2. Bethesda, MD: American Physiological Society, 1981:1415–1445.

61. Jones LA. The senses of effort and force during fatiguing contractions. In: Gandevia SC, Enoka RM, McComas AJ, et al., eds. *Fatigue: neural and muscular mechanisms*. New York: Plenum Press, 1995:305–313.

62. Jones LA, Hunter IW. Effect of fatigue on force sensation. *Exp Neurol* 1983;81:640–650.

63. Gandevia SC, McCloskey DI. Changes in motor commands, as shown by changes in perceived heaviness, during partial curarization and peripheral anaesthesia in man. *J Physiol* 1977; 272:673–689.

64. Angel RW. Barognosis in a patient with hemiataxia. *Ann Neurol* 1980;7:73–77.

65. Holmes G. The symptoms of acute cerebellar injuries due to gunshot injuries. *Brain* 1918;40:461–535.

66. Gandevia SC, McCloskey DI. Sensations of heaviness. *Brain* 1977;100:345–354.

67. Gandevia SC. The perception of motor commands or effort during muscular paralysis. *Brain* 1982;105:151–159.

68. Roland PE, Ladegaard-Pedersen H. A quantitative analysis of sensations of tension and kinaesthesia in man: evidence for a peripherally originating muscular sense and for sense of effort. *Brain* 1977;100:671–692.

69. Evarts EV. Relation of pyramidal tract activity to force exerted during voluntary movement. *J Neurophysiol* 1968;31:14–27.

70. Henderson WR, Smyth GE. Phantom limbs. *J Neurol Neurosurg Psychiatry* 1948;11:88–112.

71. Simmel ML. Phantom experiences following amputation in childhood. *J Neurol Neurosurg Psychiatry* 1962; 25:69–78.

72. Weinstein S, Sersen EA. Phantoms in cases of congenital absence of limbs. *Neurology* 1961;11:905–911.

73. Melzack R. Phantom limbs and the concept of a neuromatrix. *Trends Neurosci* 1990;13:88–92.

74. Riddoch G. Phantom limbs and body shape. *Brain* 1941;64:197–222.

75. Kaas JH, Merzenich MM, Killackey HP. The reorganization of somatosensory cortex following peripheral nerve damage in adult and developing mammals. *Annu Rev Neurosci* 1983;6:325–356.

76. Sunderland S. *Nerve and nerve injuries*. Edinburgh: Livingstone, 1978.

77. Rothwell JC, Traub MM, Day BL, et al. Manual motor performance in a deafferented man. *Brain* 1982;105:515–542.

78. Sanes JN, Mauritz K-H, Dalakas MC, et al. Motor control in humans with large-fiber sensory neuropathy. *Human Neurobiology* 1985;4:101–114.

79. Cole JD, Sedgwick EM. The perceptions of force and of movement in a man without large myelinated sensory afferents below the neck. *J Physiol* 1992;449:503–515.

80. Fleury M, Bard C, Teasdale J, et al. Weight judgment: the discrimination capacity of a deafferented subject. *Brain* 1995;118:1149–1156.

81. Vallbo AB, Hulliger M, Nordh E. Do spindle afferents monitor joint position in man? A study with active position holding. *Brain Res* 1981;204:209–213.

9

Special Senses 1: The Auditory System

SUSAN E. SHORE, PhD

• • •

Hearing occurs through a series of complex transformations of the physical signal known as "sound." These transformations, or **transductions**, begin from the time sound waves impinge on the external ear, or **pinna**. The ear, of course, consists of much more than just the external ear (Fig. 9–1). The pinna extends into a **resonating** canal, the external auditory meatus, which abuts a taut eardrum at the entrance to the **middle ear**. The external ear together with the air-filled middle ear (which contains the three tiniest bones in the body, the **ossicles**) modify the

sound for use by the fluid-filled, coiled part of the inner ear—the **cochlea**. The airborne vibrations from the middle ear are transformed into movements of the membranes on which the sensory cells are located within the cochlear fluids. This motion, in turn, stimulates the sensory hair cells to release a neurotransmitter that excites the auditory nerve (cranial nerve VIII). Without these transformations, we would be unable to hear because the brain cannot respond to mechanical vibrations. The ear, therefore, is a *transducer,* like a microphone. It changes mechanical energy into electrical energy. This chapter describes the very intricate and complex transductions that occur between the sound stimulus at the external ear and the electrical signal that is passed from neuron to neuron until it reaches its final destination, the auditory cortex, where the signal is decoded, and we perceive sound. (For a detailed review of complex signal processing, see Shore.1)

The Physical Stimulus

Sound

The sound we hear is the result of alternating compressions and expansions of air molecules. A mechanical disturbance, such as banging a tuning fork, initiates a wave of displacement that is passed along

131

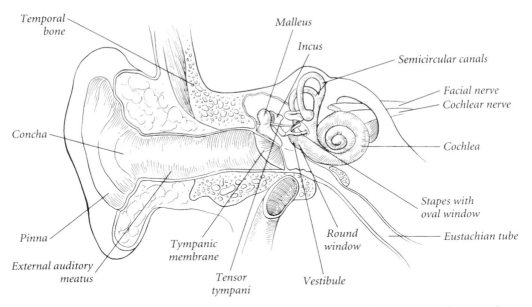

Figure 9–1. The external, middle, and inner ear of the human. (Adapted from Brödel M. Three unpublished drawings of the anatomy of the human ear. Philadelphia: WB Saunders, 1946.)

among the molecules. In the same way, a pebble dropped into water creates waves of disturbance dissipated in a circle surrounding the spot where the pebble submerged—the wave moves, not the pebble. The molecules themselves are alternately pressed closer and farther, vibrating around an average resting place. The **frequency** of the sound is the number of oscillations per second, expressed as hertz (Hz). Frequency is related to the subjective perception of **pitch**—higher frequencies produce higher pitch sensations. The amplitude, or intensity, is the magnitude of the oscillations, and is related to the subjective perception of loudness. The larger the amplitude, the louder the sound appears.

Sounds can be simple (Fig. 9–2A), such as those produced by a tuning fork (e.g., composed of only one frequency component—a pure tone). More commonly, sounds are complex (see Fig. 9–2B), containing more than one frequency component. All naturally occurring sounds are complex. The analysis of sound into its sinusoidal frequency components is called a Fourier or spectral analysis. Waveforms, which show the variation in amplitude of sound

pressure over time (see Fig. 9–2A), can also be represented as plots of the amplitude of each frequency component. These plots are called spectra (see Fig. 9–2A). When two or more frequencies are combined to form a complex signal (see Fig. 9–2B), the spectrum shows more than just the two original frequencies. Other components at higher frequencies also exist. The cochlea can perform a Fourier analysis as it separates a complex sound into its frequency, or spectral components. The auditory nerve maintains this spectral separation. In this chapter, we examine how each level of the auditory system preserves the frequency and intensity information present in the sound.[2]

Impedance

Sound must travel through two different media, air and fluid, in its path toward neural stimulation. Sound travels more readily in the easily compressible medium of air than in the dense, incompressible medium of water. Thus, water has a higher resistance, or **impedance**, than air. More energy is required to move the molecules in a medium of higher impedance. When there is a mismatch in the impedances of two substances through which sound must travel, some of the sound energy is reflected back, which is what would happen if sound were applied directly to the fluid-filled cochlea. If sound waves moved through the air-filled middle ear cavity and impinged directly on the entrance to the cochlea, at the **oval window**, they would not have enough pressure to move the cochlear fluids, which is what happens if the eardrum or **tympanic membrane** is punctured, or the ossicles are damaged and prevented from moving. Instead, in the normal system, the action of the middle ear increases the sound pressure at the oval window and allows for transmission of the energy into the cochlea.[3]

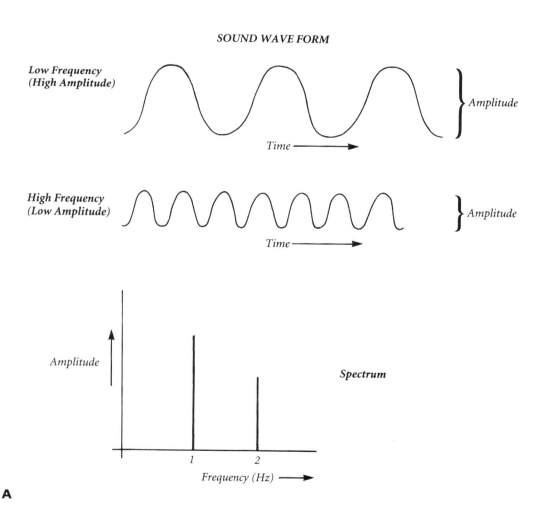

A

Figure 9–2. Sound waves and their spectra. **A:** The waveforms of a low- (top) and a high- (middle) frequency sound, with their respective spectra (bottom). (continued)

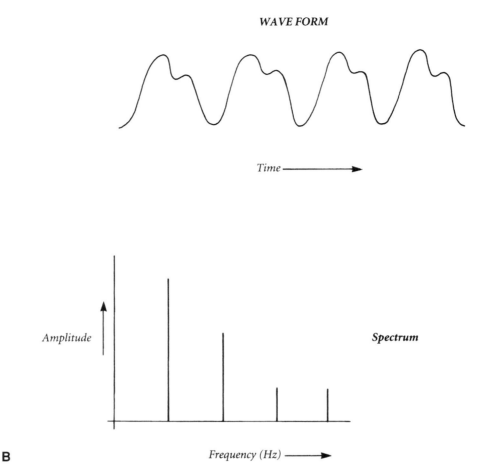

Figure 9–2 (continued). B: The waveform (top) of a complex sound containing the low and high frequencies shown in (A), and its spectrum (below). Note the occurrence of higher frequencies in addition to the original frequency components.

Structure and Function of the Ear

Outer Ear

The outer ear has two major functions: 1) it improves the transfer of sound energy to the eardrum, and 2) it aids in sound localization.

Energy Transfer
The pinna, which includes a resonant cavity, leads into the ear canal or **external auditory meatus**.

The resonant, or amplifying, action of this cavity at frequencies between 2 and 7 kHz results in a selective increase in sound pressure at the tympanic membrane of frequencies important for speech perception.

Localization
Sounds on one side of the head arrive sooner and are more intense at the ear closest to the sound. These time and intensity differences between the two ears provide the major cues for localizing sounds in the horizontal plane. The pinna and **concha** aid in

localizing sounds above, below, in front, and behind. Different frequencies are reduced in amplitude because of these structures, producing a complex spectral modulation that depends on the direction of the sound source. Movements of the head can aid in exploring the subtle cues provided by these modulations.[4]

Middle Ear

The middle ear transfers the airborne sound pressure fluctuations in the external canal to pressure variations in the fluid-filled cochlea of the inner ear. The sound vibrating the tympanic membrane is transmitted to the cochlea by three small bones, or ossicles, the **malleus**, **incus**, and **stapes** (Fig. 9–3). The handle of the malleus attaches to the tympanic membrane, whereas the other end is joined rigidly to the incus. Therefore, movement of the tympanic membrane causes the malleus and incus to move as a unit. The force of this movement is passed to the stapes, which is attached to the oval window, a membrane that forms a flexible entrance to the cochlea. The middle ear acts as a matching device between 1) low-impedance air and high-impedance fluids, and 2) the large area of the tympanic membrane and the small area of the oval window.

The middle ear uses two major physical principles to achieve the increase in pressure at the oval window required to move the cochlear fluids. Most important, the area of the tympanic membrane is 20 to 30 times greater than the area of the oval window. Therefore, the same force concentrated on each membrane means a greater pressure (pressure equals force/unit area) at the oval window. Also, the actual force at the tympanic membrane is increased by the time it reaches the oval window because the rela-

tively long malleus and short incus form a lever that increases the force in the direction of the cochlea.

The resulting gain in pressure measured at the oval window can be represented in a graph as a function of frequency, known as the **middle ear transfer function**. It has the characteristics of a **bandpass filter**. That is, it increases steadily up to a maximum around 1 kHz, followed by a steeper decrease above 2 kHz. The low-frequency fall-off is caused by the elasticity of the tympanic membrane and middle ear muscle ligaments; greater force is required for low frequencies to overcome these elasticities to produce movement. The high-frequency fall-off is caused primarily by middle ear mass; it is more difficult to move the ossicles at high frequencies.

Middle Ear Muscles

Two small muscles are attached to the ossicles: the **tensor tympani**, to the malleus, and the **stapedius** muscle to the stapes. They modulate energy transmission by the ossicles. When the muscles contract, the stiffness of the ossicular chain increases. This change reduces the transmission of sounds, primarily those below 1 kHz. The muscles contract in response to loud sounds, tactile stimulation of the head, or gross muscle movement. The middle ear muscles may operate primarily to protect the ear from loud, damaging sounds. They may also perform more subtle, frequency-specific functions, such as selectively diminishing low-frequency sounds to aid in perception of complex sounds, such as speech.[5]

Inner Ear

Embedded deep in the temporal bone, the auditory part of the inner ear consists of a coiled, bony labyrinth, the cochlea, within which is located a mem-

Figure 9–3. The three middle ossicles—the malleus, incus and stapes—transmit airborne vibrations from the tympanic membrane to the entrance to the cochlea, the oval window. (Adapted and reproduced with permission from Pickles JO, ed. *An introduction to the physiology of hearing.* 2nd ed. New York: Academic Press, 1988.)

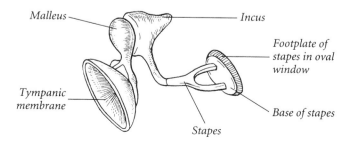

branous, fluid-filled sac, the **cochlear duct** or **scala media**. On either side of the scala media are found the **scala tympani** below and the **scala vestibuli** above (Fig. 9–4). The fluid within the scala media, **endolymph**, has a chemical composition similar to that of intracellular fluid. In contrast, the fluid in the scala tympani and scala vestibuli, **perilymph**, is more like extracellular fluid and cerebrospinal fluid in its composition. The high potassium concentration in the scala media is maintained by an active pump located in secretory cells in the lateral wall of the cochlear duct, the **stria vascularis**. The contrasting high sodium concentration in the perilymph-

containing scalae sets up an electrochemical gradient between the scala media and the other two scalae. This gradient results in electrical potentials across the **hair cells**, causing them to depolarize and release a neurotransmitter.

The function of the cochlea is more easily understood if we imagine it uncoiled (Fig. 9–5A). Near the oval window, at its base, the cochlea is wider than at its apex. The membranous cochlear duct within (see Fig. 9–5B) contains the **basilar membrane**, on which rest the sensory hair cells that are the transducer organs. The basilar membrane together with the **organ of Corti** makes up the cochlear partition.

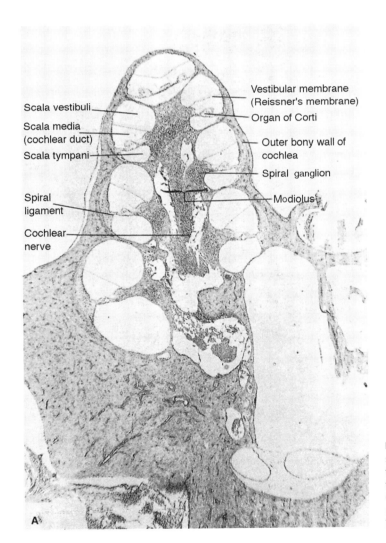

Scala vestibuli

Scala media
(cochlear duct)

Scala tympani

Spiral
ligament

Cochlear
nerve

Vestibular membrane
(Reissner's membrane)

Organ of Corti

Outer bony wall of
cochlea

Spiral ganglion

Modiolus

A

Figure 9–4. Cross-section of the cochlear scalae. **A:** Cross-section of the spiral. Note the scala vestibuli, scala media, and scala tympani. (Adapted from Jennes, Traurig, Conn. *Atlas of the human brain.* Philadelphia: Lippincott–Raven Publishers, 1995:158.) (continued)

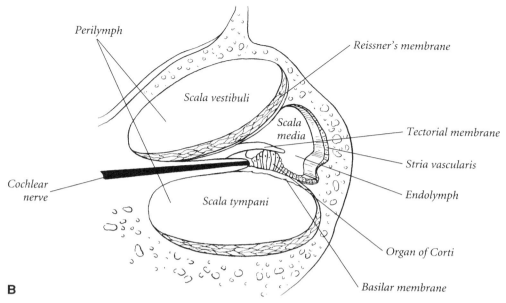

Figure 9–4 (continued). B: Magnified view of the cochlear scalae. (Adapted and reproduced with permission from Fawcett DW. *A textbook of histology.* 11th ed. Philadelphia: WB Saunders, 1986;348.)

In contrast to the cochlea, which is wider at the base and narrower at the apex, the basilar membrane is wider at its apex and becomes gradually more narrow toward its base. It is also more flaccid in the apex and becomes gradually stiffer toward the base. This physical gradation has important implications for the mechanical processes that occur before transduction. When the footplate of the stapes, embedded in the oval window, moves in and out, it produces alternating increases and decreases in pressure in the perilymph surrounding the cochlear duct. Because fluid cannot be compressed, the increase in pressure causes a displacement of the cochlear partition from its resting position and initiates a wave of displacement that always travels from the base to the apex (see Fig. 9–5A; Fig. 9–6).

The gradation in stiffness of the basilar membrane from the base to the apex is responsible for the direction of the traveling wave. It is also responsible for the Fourier analysis mentioned earlier, which takes place in the cochlea. Like a violin string in which shorter and stiffer strings vibrate better at higher frequencies than longer, flaccid strings, so the cochlear partition vibrates "better" to high frequencies at its base and to low frequencies at its apex. For high frequencies, the traveling wave shows a peak in its displacement toward the base, whereas for lower frequencies, the peak is toward the apex. Thus, frequencies are separated into different places along the cochlear partition. The hair cells and, in turn, the auditory nerve fibers that line up along the length of the basilar membrane maintain this "place" frequency code by responding mostly when the place they are innervating is maximally displaced. So, for high frequencies, the hair cells and nerve fibers innervating the basal end of the cochlea respond best, and for lower frequencies those innervating the apical end respond best (see Fig. 9–6). Thus, auditory hair cells and nerve fibers are "tuned" to a best or **characteristic frequency**, which is that frequency to which they are most sensitive. They also respond to other frequencies above and below the best frequency. All the frequencies to which a hair cell or auditory nerve fiber responds define the **response area** or **tuning curve** of the hair cell or nerve fiber.

The auditory system appears to have a safety factor, a second way in which it codes frequency. In addition to setting up a traveling wave, a particular stimulus frequency causes many points along the membrane to vibrate at the exact frequency of stimulation. The hair cells or nerve fibers, then, fire in time to the cycles or phases of the stimulating sound

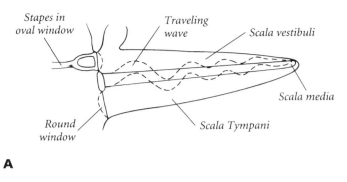

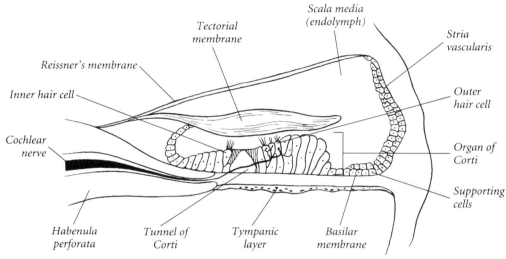

Figure 9–5. A: The cochlea in its uncoiled state. **B:** Magnified cross-section of scala media showing the organ of Corti. (Adapted and reproduced with permission from Davis H. Biophysics and physiology of the inner ear. *Physiol Rev,* 1957;39:1–49.)

waves. This so-called "phase locking" is limited in frequency to 1,000 Hz in auditory nerve fibers, which is the upper limit of neural firing because of the refractory state of the neuron.

Transduction

To understand how the vibration of the cochlear partition is translated into neural firing patterns, we must examine the structure of the scala media, which is bounded by the basilar membrane on one side and by ***Reissner's membrane*** on the other (see Fig. 9–5B). These two membranes separate the endolymph-containing scala media from the perilymph-containing scalae, tympani, and vestibuli, which

are joined by a small opening, the **helicotrema**, at the apical end of the cochlea. The transducer elements, the hair cells, are contained in the highly specialized organ of Corti, which rests on the basilar membrane. The two types of hair cells, inner and outer, are named for their positions with respect to the tunnel of Corti. One row of inner and three rows of outer hair cells are surrounded by supporting cells that lend rigidity to the whole organ of Corti. Each hair cell gives rise to hairs, or **stereocilia**, of different lengths at its apical end, the tallest of which, in the case of the outer hair cells, is firmly embedded in a gelatinous mass, the **tectorial membrane**, which covers the organ of Corti. Outer hair

A

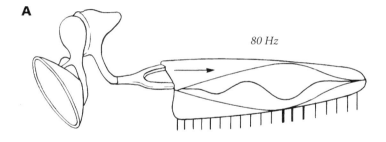

80 Hz

B

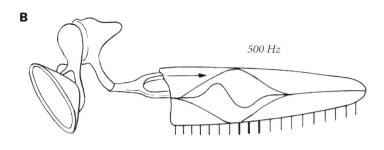

500 Hz

C

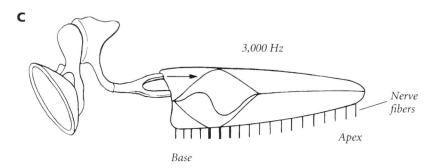

3,000 Hz

Nerve fibers

Apex

Base

Figure 9–6. The displacement of the cochlear partition and the envelopes of traveling waves produced by three different frequencies. The peaks of the traveling waves occur basally for higher and apically for lower frequencies, stimulating different sets of nerve fibers.

cells can be distinguished by their characteristic "W"-shape, formed by their cilia (Fig. 9–7). The inner hair cell cilia are not actually embedded in the tectorial membrane, but rest in a groove on its undersurface.

Humans have approximately 3,500 inner and 11,500 outer hair cells in each ear. Although fewer in number, inner hair cells contact as many as 20 auditory nerve fibers, but the more numerous outer hair cells contact only six nerve fibers. The functional implication of this convergent–divergent system is that synaptic transmission in the inner hair cell–auditory nerve synapse is more secure and faster than in the outer hair cell–auditory nerve synapse. Therefore, the inner hair cells, although fewer in number, are the true sensory transduc-

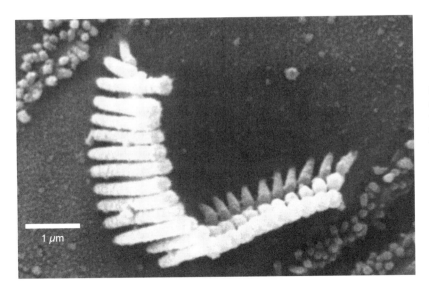

Figure 9–7. Stereocilia from a single cochlear outer hair cell, from an adult gerbil. Note the characteristic "w" formation of the cilia. On the right side of the bundle note the three rows of cilia, which are graduated in length, with tallest cilia lower-most and shortest cilia upper-most in the figure. (Photomicrograph courtesy of Yehoash Raphael, PhD, Kresge Hearing Research Institute, The University of Michigan, Ann Arbor, Michigan.)

ers that pass information up to second-order neurons of the cochlear nucleus in the brainstem. The outer hair cells modulate the responses of auditory nerve fibers contacting inner hair cells. By shortening their length, outer hair cells can reduce the amount of stimulation of the inner hair cells.[6]

Stimulation of the Hair Cells

When the basilar membrane and organ of Corti move up and down, the tectorial membrane, which is attached only at one end, moves out of phase with the basilar membrane and causes the hairs to bend. Bending of the hair cells causes ion channels in the hairs to be opened. The electrical potential in scala media of +80 mV, and the potential in the inner hair cell of −45 mV at rest, add up to a potential difference across the stereocilia of +125 mV. This potential difference causes K^+ ions to move down their concentration and electrical gradients to enter the open channels and depolarize the hair cell. Movement in the opposite direction causes hyperpolarization of the hair cell. This alternating depolarization and hyperpolarization of the hair cells, or **receptor potential**, can be recorded from the cochlea with an electrode. This potential is also called the **cochlear microphonic** because it mimics the incoming sound. The hair cell depolarization in turn causes the release of a neurotransmitter into the synaptic cleft at the base of the hair cell. This change in turn depolarizes cranial nerve VIII fibers.

Outer hair cells modulate the way inner hair cells activate auditory nerve fibers in a manner not yet fully understood. Outer hair cells differ from inner hair cells, both in their mode of stimulation and in their innervation pattern. Because outer hair cell stereocilia are embedded in the tectorial membrane, whereas inner hair cells are not, outer hair cells are stimulated directly and inner hair cells are stimulated by fluid movement produced by movement of the cochlear partition. Outer hair cells can contract and shorten their length, the process that is believed to modulate the stimulation of inner hair cells. The fibers connecting outer hair cells are unmyelinated and are called Type II fibers. They also terminate in the cochlear nucleus, but their function is still unknown.

Additional modulatory input to the cochlea comes from efferent fibers called the olivocochlear bundle that originate in the superior olivary complex and terminate on outer hair cells. They influence the way outer hair cells modulate inner hair cell excitation. Their overall effect is to improve signal-to-noise levels and protect the ear from acoustic overstimulation.[7,8]

Auditory Nerve

Type I auditory nerve fibers are bipolar neurons, with their cell bodies, spiral ganglion cells, located in the cochlea. The peripheral, unmyelinated processes of these cell bodies synapse with the hair cells, and the central, myelinated (for Type I) processes synapse with cells in the cochlear nucleus. Recordings from individual Type I auditory nerve fibers demonstrate that they are activated by sounds in a highly organized manner. As with hair cells, each fiber is sharply tuned, in that it responds best to one frequency, with gradually decreasing responses to frequencies on either side of this best or characteristic frequency. Figure 9–8 shows typical tuning curves, or response areas, obtained from auditory nerve fibers with different characteristic frequencies. The sound pressure required to elicit an increase in firing rate is plotted against the different frequencies that activated the nerve. The frequency selectivity of the auditory system can be approximated by the sharpness of these tuning curves. The sharper or narrower the tuning curve, the more frequency-selective the fiber.

Auditory nerve fibers also preserve frequency information by firing in phase with cycles of the stimulus below 1 kHz, a rate above which neurons cannot fire because of their refractory periods. This so-called **phase locking** can be illustrated by plotting a fiber's firing rate during one cycle of the stimulus, which demonstrates that the responses cluster at a certain point during the stimulus cycle.

In addition to providing information about stimulus frequency, firing rate can provide information about the excitation state of the fiber. Typically, auditory nerve fibers show rapid firing at the stimulus onset, followed by a rapid decrease in firing that levels off to a steady-state level. This change in firing rate can be shown by plotting firing rate during the entire stimulus in the form of a **poststimulus time histogram** (Fig. 9–9). The response decrement results

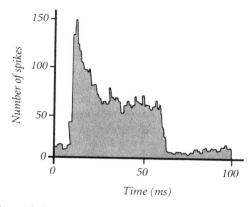

Figure 9–9. Poststimulus time histogram showing a typical firing pattern of one auditory nerve fiber in response to a tone burst. An initial burst of firing is followed by a gradual decrement to a steady firing level. (Adapted and reproduced with permission from Kiang NYS. *Discharge patterns of single fibers in the cat's auditory nerve.* Research Monograph #35. Cambridge, MA: MIT Press, 1965.)

from depletion of neurotransmitter in the hair cell–auditory nerve synapse, and is called **adaptation**. When a neuron is adapted, it is less excitable. Therefore, a given array of auditory neurons will show different degrees of adaptation because neurons closer to the basal end of the cochlea are stimulated first, and those closer to the apex are stimulated later. The diverse adaptation states may provide important information to higher centers about the excitation pattern across the whole array of fibers. It may also partly determine how the array responds to a com-

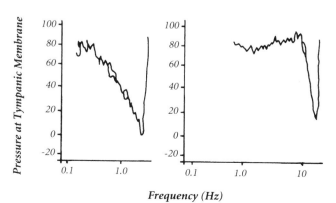

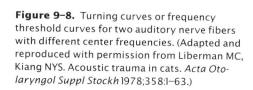

Figure 9–8. Turning curves or frequency threshold curves for two auditory nerve fibers with different center frequencies. (Adapted and reproduced with permission from Liberman MC, Kiang NYS. Acoustic trauma in cats. *Acta Otolaryngol Suppl Stockh* 1978;358:1–63.)

plex signal such as speech, which contains more than one frequency component.

In addition to the contrasts produced in this manner, one tone, although itself excitatory, can reduce the responses elicited by a second tone close in frequency to the first. This phenomenon, called **two-tone suppression**, is a result of nonlinear properties of cochlear mechanics. It is also observable in inner hair cell responses. Different frequency components in a complex signal can suppress one another in this manner. Another important aspect of the signal is its intensity. As intensity increases, more of the basilar membrane is activated and thus more fibers respond. Individual fibers also respond more vigorously as the signal intensity is raised, increasing their firing rate.

Clinical Correlations

Much research has concentrated on the development of cochlear prostheses for patients who have lost hair cells. These devices are designed to provide direct electrical activation to the auditory nerve fibers. Stimulating electrodes are placed in the scala tympani of the cochlea and are controlled by a computerized device, worn in much the same way as a conventional hearing aid. Varying degrees of success have been obtained with cochlear implants, depending on many factors, including the age of the patient, the amount of surviving nerve fibers, the age at which the hearing loss occurred, and the patient's ability to make use of the electrical stimulation.

More than 2,000 profoundly deaf people in the United States have been helped by prosthetic stimulation. Those patients who do not have surviving auditory nerves may benefit from prosthetic stimulators placed directly in second-order auditory neurons of the cochlear nucleus. This approach is relatively new and still requires further research and development, but potentially it could benefit patients such as those with acoustic neuromas, which render the auditory nerve nonfunctional.[9,10]

Central Pathways

Figure 9–10A shows the ascending auditory pathway from the auditory nerve to the auditory cortex. Each level is discussed in a separate section.

Brainstem Pathways

Cochlear Nucleus

The frequency information present in the firing patterns of auditory nerve fibers is preserved in neurons of the cochlear nucleus, located in the rostral medulla. As the fibers enter the cochlear nucleus, they divide at the nerve root (see Fig. 9–10B) into ascending and descending branches that innervate the anteroventral, posteroventral, and dorsal regions of the cochlear nucleus (AVCN, PVCN and DCN, respectively). Because the nerve divides, each frequency is represented in each of the nuclei. At the same time, auditory nerve fibers contact individual neurons in each nucleus with unique synaptic arrangements for further processing of incoming information in each nucleus. The ventral cochlear nucleus has four major cell categories, named according to their shapes: spherical bushy, globular bushy, stellate, and octopus cells. Some neurons have synapses on their somata, resulting in fast transmission to the axon. Other neurons have synapses on their dendrites, with slower transmission to the axons.

The spherical bushy cell, found mainly in the AVCN, is contacted on its cell body by large, calyx-type endings from one or two auditory nerve fibers. This arrangement makes for a very secure synaptic contact and results in a "primary-like" response pattern and tuning curve very similar to that seen in auditory nerve fibers. Globular bushy cells, found in the caudal AVCN and PVCN, receive several synaptic connections from auditory nerve fibers, also on their cell bodies. They have a "primary-notch" pattern of response, similar to the primary-like, but with a small gap in the time pattern after the initial peak. Stellate cells, found mainly in the PVCN, receive numerous nerve endings primarily on their dendrites, and respond to sounds with a rhythmic pattern, or "chopper response," which is unrelated to the stimulus frequency. Octopus cells receive input from many auditory nerve fibers with widely varying characteristic frequencies that terminate on their long dendrites. This multiple synaptic convergence is reflected in their wide tuning curves. They respond vigorously to the beginning of the stimulus with an "onset" response, followed by either no further response or a low-level response to the remainder of the stimulus. This pattern is probably produced by strong excitation, followed by inhibition.

In the DCN, the major neuron type projecting out of the nucleus is the fusiform cell. It receives audi-

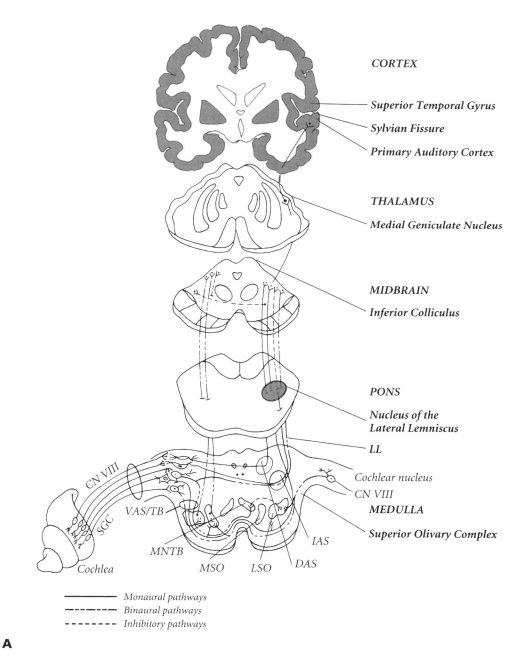

CORTEX

Superior Temporal Gyrus

Sylvian Fissure

Primary Auditory Cortex

THALAMUS

Medial Geniculate Nucleus

MIDBRAIN

Inferior Colliculus

PONS

Nucleus of the
Lateral Lemniscus

LL

Cochlear nucleus

CN VIII

MEDULLA

Superior Olivary Complex

CN VIII

SGC

VAS/TB

Cochlea

MNTB

MSO

LSO

DAS

IAS

——————— Monaural pathways

––––––– Binaural pathways

- - - - - - - Inhibitory pathways

A

Figure 9–10. A: The ascending auditory pathway from the cochlea to the auditory cortex. Monaural and binaural pathways are mostly excitatory. Some inhibitory pathways are indicated. (continued)

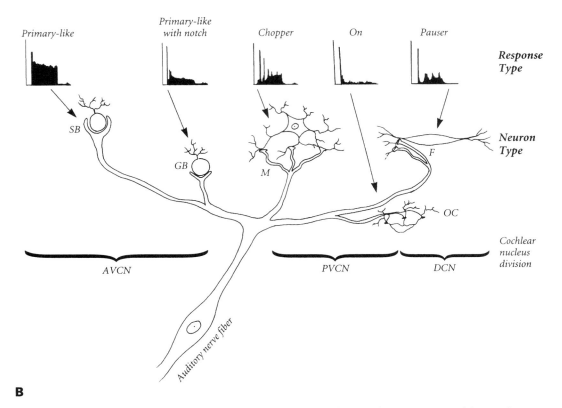

B

Figure 9–10 (continued). B: The neurons of the cochlear nucleus are diverse in terms of their auditory nerve input, their dendritic patterns, and their subsequent response types. AVCN, anteroventral cochlear nucleus; CN, cranial nerve; DAS, dorsal acoustic stria; DCN, dorsal cochlear nucleus; F, fusiform cell; GB, globular bushy cell; IAS, intermediate acoustic stria; LL, lateral lemniscus; LSO, lateral superior olivary complex; M, multipolar cell; MNTB, medial nucleus of the trapezoid body; MSO, medial superior olivary complex; OC, octopus cell; PVCN, posteroventral cochlear nucleus; SB, spherical bushy cell; SGC spinal ganglion cells; VAS/TB, ventral acoustic stria/trapezoid body.

tory nerve endings on its soma and dendrites and responds with a "pauser" or "build-up" response. As the name suggests, it shows an initial sharp peak in the response, followed by a pause and a gradual resumption of the response (see Fig. 9–10B).

The different types of responses from each kind of neuron in the cochlear nucleus result from the complex synaptic arrangements of auditory nerve fibers, and also of other neurons, within and outside of the cochlear nucleus.[11,12] Many of the inputs from other parts of the brain onto these cells are inhibitory and may alter long-term responses of these neurons, in addition to contributing to their response patterns. The different cell types, after modifying incoming auditory

nerve responses, pass each new pattern, in parallel pathways, to higher auditory centers (see Fig. 9–10A). Bushy cells convey information that is a good representation of their own input to the superior olivary complex through the **ventral acoustic stria**. Octopus cells project greatly modified information by the **intermediate acoustic stria** to the **lateral lemniscus**, and send a small branch to the superior olivary complex. Fusiform cells also convey highly processed information to the **inferior colliculus** by way of the **dorsal acoustic stria**. Thus, one pathway, arising from the ventral cochlear nucleus, preserves much of the information contained in auditory nerve responses and conveys it to the superior olivary complex, where it is used to localize sounds in space. The other pathway, arising from both the DCN and the PVCN, conveys highly modified information to higher auditory centers, where it is integrated with input from the superior olivary complex.[13,14]

Superior Olivary Complex

The superior olivary complex is a group of nuclei essential for the localization of sounds in space. It consists of three main nuclei (see Fig. 9–10A): the lateral superior olivary complex (LSO), the medial superior olivary complex (MSO), and the medial nucleus of the trapezoid body. The major nuclei are surrounded by a group of smaller, periolivary nuclei (not shown), named for their positions in relation to the larger nuclei. The periolivary groups, together with some cells in the LSO, exert descending control over the cochlea and cochlear nucleus through feedback pathways.

The LSO is an "S"-shaped nucleus that receives excitatory input directly from bushy cells in the ipsilateral AVCN, and inhibitory input indirectly from bushy cells in the contralateral AVCN through the medial nucleus of the trapezoid body. Therefore, cells in the LSO are called "EI" cells. They are excited by ipsilateral sound stimulation and inhibited by contralateral sound stimulation. These cells are excited best by high frequencies, which, because of their short wavelengths, tend to be reflected off the head, and thus attenuated in the ear that is directed away from a sound source. LSO neurons are specialized to detect this intensity difference between the two ears and, in this way, to provide information regarding the sound source.

Neurons in the MSO, in contrast, receive direct excitatory input from bushy cells on both sides and respond best to low-frequency stimulation. When low frequencies impinge on the head, the wavelength is large enough that it is not reflected, but rather arrives later at the ear farther away from the sound source. Information about the time of arrival of sounds at each ear therefore provides cues for the direction of the sound source. Bushy cells in the AVCN, because of their secure synapses from eight nerve fibers, provide accurate timing information about the sound, which is then passed on to MSO cells, which, in turn, are sensitive to the phase (timing) of the sounds. MSO cells, in fact, have a **characteristic delay**, so that they respond best to a particular time difference between sounds presented at the two ears. This characteristic delay is unique to a particular cell in the same way that characteristic frequency is unique to

a cell. Thus, different MSO cells provide information about different delays between the ears that reflect the position of the sound source.[15]

Clinical Correlations: Assessment of Auditory Brainstem Centers

The clinical evaluation of the integrity of auditory nerve and brainstem centers is a relatively new area where research has made much progress. Two commonly used tests of centers caudal to the inferior colliculus are the **auditory brainstem response** (ABR) and the acoustic reflex. The ABR is used to assess the synchronous neural discharges of the auditory nerve and brainstem nuclei in response to sound. It is elicited by short-duration tones, or clicks, presented repeatedly while electroencephalographic activity is recorded with scalp electrodes. The recorded activity is time-locked to the stimulus, so that five discrete waves are recorded corresponding to the sequential activation of the auditory nerve (waves I and II) and the auditory tracts in the pons (waves II, IV, and V). Brainstem lesions can result in abnormalities in the time of occurrence of each successive wave in the ABR, or in the absence of some waves. The ABR may also be affected by peripheral hearing loss, as assessed by standard audiologic tests such as audiograms. These factors must be taken into account when interpreting the ABR.

The acoustic reflex refers to the reflex contraction of the stapedius muscle after presentation of an intense sound. Activation of the reflex requires an intact system, including the middle ear, cochlea, auditory nerve, and caudal brainstem. Testing of the acoustic reflex can be accomplished by an audiologist or a physician during routine testing of middle-ear function using an impedance-measuring device. These tests, together with behavioral tests, can yield a high degree of success in identifying brainstem lesions.[16]

Inferior Colliculus

Information from all auditory brainstem nuclei must pass through the **inferior colliculus** on the way to its final destination, the **auditory cortex**. This important integrating center consists of a central portion, which is the main auditory relay center, and an external portion, which is involved with integration of auditory information with somesthetic input. The central nucleus is a complicated structure, laminated like an onion, with different layers formed by its dendrites and incoming afferent axons. The targets of these afferent inputs from the contralateral DCN and both superior olivary complexes are segregated into different groups in this structure. The tonotopic organization found at lower levels of the auditory brainstem is maintained in the central nucleus, with similar characteristic-frequency cells arranged in laminae across the nucleus. The frequency responses of these cells are diverse, ranging from broad to very narrow tuning. The broadly tuned units reflect input from other neurons with heterogeneous characteristic frequencies, whereas the narrowly tuned units derive their characteristics from other processes, such as lateral inhibition. The presence of very sharply tuned units at higher levels of the auditory system reflects the high-frequency resolving power of the auditory system. Complex interactions occur between excitation and inhibition at this level, and are also present to a lesser extent in the DCN. Therefore, these neurons may respond especially well to certain types of signals, particularly those that change in time, such as amplitude- or frequency-modulated sounds. Sounds that have biologic significance, such as animal calls and human speech, are made up of elements that vary rapidly over time and frequency.

Just as the complex processing begun in the DCN is reflected, and perhaps refined, in the inferior colliculus, so the binaural processing begun in the superior olivary complex is modified in binaurally sensitive cells in the central nucleus. In some species, such as the barn owl, detailed maps of auditory space can be demonstrated spatially across the nucleus. Very little is known about the integration of information from the ipsilateral and bilateral systems, but it may result in the ability to encode complex sounds while recognizing their direction in space.

The inferior colliculus is also involved in certain reflexes such as the startle reflex, and reflex turning of the head toward a sound source. These reflexes are mediated by the pericentral and external nuclei. Descending projections from the inferior colliculus to the DCN and other parts of the brainstem are involved in modulating the ascending information on its way to the cortex.[17]

Auditory Cortex

The inferior colliculus sends projections through the **medial geniculate nucleus**, which is the thalamic relay center, to the temporal lobe, where the auditory cortex rests in the sylvian fissure (see Fig. 9–10A). The auditory cortex has been divided into a primary region, a secondary region, and other association areas. Multiple thalamic relay pathways innervate these different regions, the most specific being the ventral medial geniculate nucleus to primary auditory cortex. The relationship of these areas to speech and language areas is discussed later in this book.

The precise tonotopicity shown at lower levels of the auditory system has been shown only to a limited extent in the auditory cortex in anesthetized animals. It is not evident in unanesthetized animals. The responses of individual cells vary greatly. Some units are sharply tuned, some have bimodal tuning, and some are very broadly tuned, with variable thresholds. Most units can be inhibited, some by sounds with the same characteristic frequency and others by diverse frequencies. Many units do not respond to sound and some respond only to specific complex sounds, such as frequency-modulated sounds with specific rates and directions of frequency change. Some cells respond only to novel stimuli. Cells in awake and behaving animals show greater responsiveness.

Like the superior olivary complex and inferior colliculus, the auditory cortex has cells that are excited by both ears (EE cells), or, more commonly, excited by the contralateral ear and inhibited by the ipsilateral ear (EI). This finding suggests that these cells code sound direction. They are organized in columns perpendicular to columns of cells with similar characteristic frequencies. Many of the cells are sensitive to time differences between the two ears and show characteristic delays of the kind described in cells of the superior olivary complex.

Like cells at lower levels, some cortical cells are also sensitive to intensity differences between the two ears, showing optimal responses to a particular intensity difference. Other cells, however, do not respond to stationary stimuli but are sensitive to movement in a particular direction. These responses result from a complex integration of excitatory and inhibitory inputs. Each cortex represents sound sources predominantly on the contralateral side of the head.

The responses of neurons in the auditory cortex are enhanced and become more stable when the animals are involved in a task that demands alertness and attention. In addition to the superior temporal lobe, other areas, such as the posterior-inferior frontal lobe, the inferior parietal lobe, and the corpus callosum, also show responsiveness to auditory stimuli.

Behavioral studies in which performance is tested before and after cortical lesions have resulted in contradictory findings. A consistent finding, however, has been that performance of a variety of difficult auditory tasks was upset by these lesions, although easy tasks were unaffected. In addition, damage to the primary auditory cortex resulted in deficits in localization. Even though information about cues of interaural time and intensity differences are extracted at lower levels of the auditory system, the auditory cortex appears to be responsible for the completion of sound localization.[18–20]

The major functions of the auditory cortex may thus be summarized as follows:

1 Analysis of complex sounds
2 Localization of sounds
3 Selective attention to specific sounds in certain positions
4 Discrimination of temporal auditory patterns
5 Performance of difficult auditory tasks

Clinical Correlations: Assessment of the Higher Auditory Centers

Information about the integrity of cortical auditory centers can be obtained from both electrophysiologic and behavioral data. The middle and late auditory-evoked potentials are recorded in response to auditory signals in much the same way as are ABR evaluations. The difference arises in the latency of the peaks. For middle latency responses, several negative and positive waves occur in the response after the ABR, up to approximately 70 milliseconds after the sound is presented. The most prominent peak in the middle latency responses probably originates in the primary auditory cortex. The late auditory evoked response occurs several hundred milliseconds after the sound, and is most successfully elicited by novel sounds. It reflects cognitive processing of auditory information. In addition, because of the complex integration that must take place between the different cerebral centers, assessment of the function of the auditory cortex requires the additional use of an array of behavioral studies that are more sensitive to cortical lesions than are electrophysiologic tests used alone. To assess the auditory system fully, a combination of electrophysiologic and behavioral tests should be used.

REFERENCES

1. Shore SE. Coding of complex signals in the peripheral auditory system. *Seminars on Hearing* 1986;7:65–85.
2. Davis H. Biophysics and physiology of the inner ear. *Physiol Rev* 1957;35:1–49.
3. Pickles JO, ed. *An introduction to the physiology of hearing.* New York: Academic Press, 1988.
4. Shaw EAG. The external ear. In: Keidel WD, Neff WD, eds. *Handbook of sensory physiology.* Vol 5/1. Berlin: Springer-Verlag, 1974:455–490.
5. Dallos P. *The auditory periphery.* New York: Academic Press, 1973.
6. Brownell WE, Bader CR, Bertrand D, de Ribaupierre Y. Evoked mechanical responses of isolated hair cells. *Science* 1985;227:194–196.
7. Warr WB, Guinan JJ, White JS. Organization of the efferent fibers: the lateral and medial systems. In: Altschuler RA, Bobbin RP, Hoffman DW, eds. *Neurobiology of hearing: the cochlea.* New York: Raven Press, 1986: 333–348.
8. Wiederhold ML. Physiology of the olivocochlear system. In: Altschuler RA, Bobbin RP, Hoffman DW, eds. *Neurobiology of hearing: the cochlea.* New York: Raven Press, 1986:349–370.
9. Kiang NYS. *Discharge patterns of single fibers in the cat's auditory nerve.* Research Monograph #35. Cambridge, MA: MIT Press, 1965.
10. Evans EF. Cochlear nerve and cochlear nucleus. In: Keidel WD, Neff WD, eds. *Handbook of sensory physiology.* Vol 5/2. Berlin: Springer-Verlag, 1975:1–108.
11. Shore SE, Helfert RH, Bledsoe SC Jr, Altschuler RA, Godfrey DA. Descending projections to the guinea pig cochlear nucleus. *Hear Res* 1991;52:255–268.
12. Shore SE, Helfert RH, Bledsoe SC Jr, Altschuler RA, Godfrey DA. Connections between the cochlear nuclei in the guinea pig. *Hear Res* 1992;62:16–26.
13. Cant NB, Morest DK. The structural basis for stimulus coding in the cochlear nucleus. In: Berlin CI, ed. *Hearing sciences: recent advances.* San Diego: College Hill Press, 1984:371–421.
14. Young ED. Response characteristics of neurons of the cochlear nuclei. In: Berlin CI, ed. *Hearing sciences: recent advances.* San Diego: College Hill Press, 1984: 423–460.
15. Brugge JF. An overview of central auditory processing. In: Popper AN, Fay RR, eds. *The mammalian auditory pathway: neurophysiology.* New York: Springer-Verlag, 1992:1–33.
16. Musiek FE, Baran JA. Assessment of the human central auditory system. In: Altschuler RA, Bobbin RP, Clopton BM, Hoffman DW, eds. *Neurobiology of hearing: the central auditory system.* New York: Raven Press, 1991: 411–438.
17. Aitkin L. Properties of central auditory neurons of cats

responding to free-field acoustic stimuli. In: Syka J, Masterton RB, eds. *Auditory pathway: structure and function*. New York: Plenum Press, 1987:335–348.

18. Aitkin LM, Gates GR, Phillips SC. Responses of neurons in the inferior colliculus to variations in sound source azimuth. *J Neurophysiol* 1984;52:1–17.

19. Jenkins WM, Merzenich MM. Role of cat primary auditory cortex for sound localization behavior. *J Neurophysiol* 1984;52:819–847.

20. Aitkin LM. *The auditory cortex: structural and functional bases of auditory perception*. London: Chapman & Hall.

10

Special Senses 2: The Vestibular System

HELEN COHEN, EdD, OTR, FAOTA

• • •

Did you ever slip on icy pavement or a wet floor, feel your head whip back, and then catch yourself just before falling? If so, you used your vestibular system to maintain your balance. Did you ever walk on the grass or drive on a bumpy road while watching something in front of you? If so, you used your vestibular system to maintain a stable gaze so you could see clearly while you were moving. Did you ever stand in an elevator or in a room with no window and then look up, knowing that over your head was up and under your feet was down? If so, you used your vestibular system for spatial orientation.

The vestibular system is responsible for an esoteric sense that the average person is unaware of having and learns about only when it becomes deranged. The

last of the special senses to be discovered,[1] the vestibular system detects head movement. The nervous system uses that information for four tasks: 1) to help control balance through the generation of postural reflexes that keep the head erect, 2) to see clearly while moving by keeping the eye pointed toward a desired target, 3) to facilitate spatial orientation by signaling the direction of gravity and keeping track of short-distance changes in position, and 4) to prepare for "fight or flight" in an emergency.

Peripheral Structures

Gross Anatomy

As you learned in the previous chapter, the "ear" comprises three compartments: the external, middle, and inner ears. The middle and external ears are important for the auditory system but not for the vestibular system. The inner ear, however, hidden deep inside the temporal bone behind the medial wall of the middle ear, contains a space known as the **vestibule**, from which the vestibular system takes its name. The cochlea is anterior to the vestibule; the bony **semicircular canals** of the **vestibular labyrinth** are posterior to it. The bony canals and the vestibule contain the membranous labyrinth with the sensors for the vestibular system. The vestibule contains two sacs, collectively known as the **otoliths**.

149

Thin tubes connect one sac, the **saccule**, with the cochlea and with the other sac, the **utricle**. The utricle connects to the three membranous semicircular canals.[2] You cannot see these structures by peering into the external or middle ear with an otoscope. They are accessible only by drilling into the temporal bone (one of the hardest bones in the body) or by removing the stapes to view the otoliths behind it (Fig. 10–1).

The three semicircular canals, arranged approximately at right angles to each other, include the **horizontal canal**, also called the **lateral canal**, and the vertically oriented **anterior** and **posterior canals**, also known as the **superior** and **inferior canals**, respectively. With the head in anatomical position, the horizontal canal is actually tilted 25 degrees above the earth-horizontal. Tilting the head down (i.e., downward **pitch**) brings the lateral canals into alignment with the earth-horizontal, a position usually assumed while walking. The two posterior canals point toward the nose and the two anterior canals point away from it, so that they form

contralateral pairs: the right anterior and left posterior canal (RALP) and the left anterior and right posterior canal (LARP). Because of this arrangement, rotating your head as if looking from left to right (**yaw**) stimulates both lateral canals. When you turn your head approximately 45 degrees toward the left and then make a pitch rotation up or down, the LARP pair is selectively stimulated. Likewise, when you turn your head toward the right 45 degrees and then make a pitch rotation, the RALP pair is stimulated. Pitch rotation of the head with your nose pointed forward, **roll** rotation, or rotation in any other plane in space stimulates at least one pair of canals (Fig. 10–2A).

The sensory surfaces of the otoliths are also oriented approximately, but not completely, at right angles to each other. The palm-shaped sensory surface of the utricle is oriented approximately horizontally; the S-shaped sensory surface of the saccule is oriented approximately vertically. Unlike the canals, which are sensitive to rotation or angular translation, the utricles are sensitive to linear translation (e.g.,

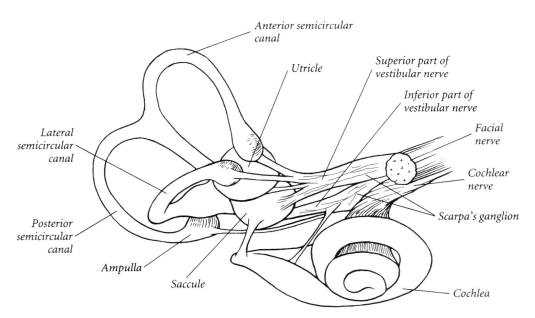

Figure 10–1. The vestibular labyrinth, including the semicircular canals and otoliths. (Adapted from Brödel M. *Three unpublished drawings of the human ear.* Philadelphia: WB Saunders, 1946.)

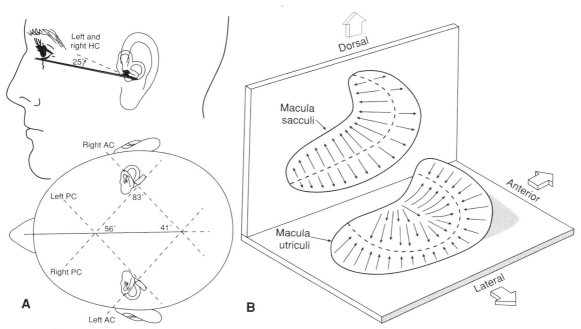

Figure 10–2. Orientation of the receptor surfaces in the vestibular labyrinth in the head. **A:** Orientation of the semicircular canals within the head. HC, horizontal canal; PC, posterior canal; AC, anterior canal. (From Furman JM, Cass SP. *Balance disorders: A case study approach.* Philadelphia: FA Davis, 1996. Used by permission.) **B:** Orientation of the otolith maculae in the head. Note that the receptor surfaces are curved. The *dotted line* represents the striola. The direction of *arrows* indicates the direction of hair bundle deflection that causes excitation. The orientation vectors are different in the two otoliths. (From HO Barber, CW Stockwell. *Manual of electronystagmography.* 2nd ed. St. Louis: CV Mosby Company, 1980.

moving up/down or straight ahead). Because the sensory surfaces are slightly curved, the otoliths are actually sensitive to linear translation in any direction (see Fig. 10–2B).

As you learned in Chapter 9, fluids bathe the membranous labyrinths inside and out. Perilymph surrounds the canals and otoliths, cushioning them from the bony surround. Endolymph fills the interior of these structures. Endolymph has a high specific gravity and viscosity, and is low in sodium and high in potassium. Perilymph has a low specific gravity and viscosity, and is high in sodium and low in potassium. These differences in concentrations are important during signal transmission.

The canals and otoliths have specialized receptor areas (Fig. 10–3): the **ampullae** in the semicircular canals and the **maculae** in the otoliths. As in the cochlea, specialized hair cells from which cilia protrude cover the receptor surfaces. In each ampulla, the hair cells sit on a tiny hillock, the **crista**; therefore, the other name for the ampulla is the **crista ampullaris**. The eight-sided groups of **stereocilia** protrude into an inverted gelatinous cup, the **cupula**, which covers the entire area. The cilia are graduated in height toward the tallest cilium, the **kinocilium** (Fig. 4). The maculae contain similar groups of hair cells, but the **otolithic membrane** replaces the
(text continues on page 154)

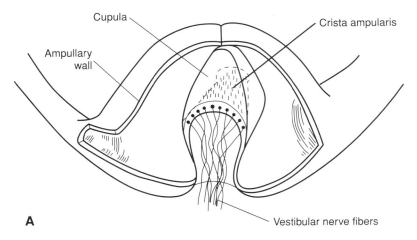

Cupula

Crista ampularis

Ampullary
wall

Vestibular nerve fibers

A

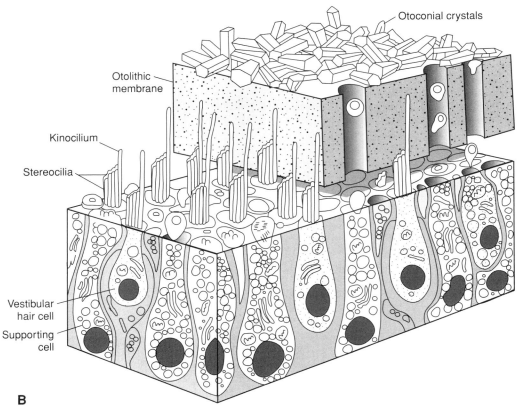

Otoconial crystals

Otolithic
membrane

Kinocilium

Stereocilia

Vestibular
hair cell

Supporting
cell

B

Figure 10–3. Anatomy of the receptor surfaces in the vestibular labyrinth. **A:** The ampulla of a canal. Note the cilia protruding from the crista into the cupula. **B:** The macula of an otolith. (Part B from Furman JM, Cass SP. *Balance disorders: A case study approach.* Philadelphia: FA Davis, 1996. Used by permission.)

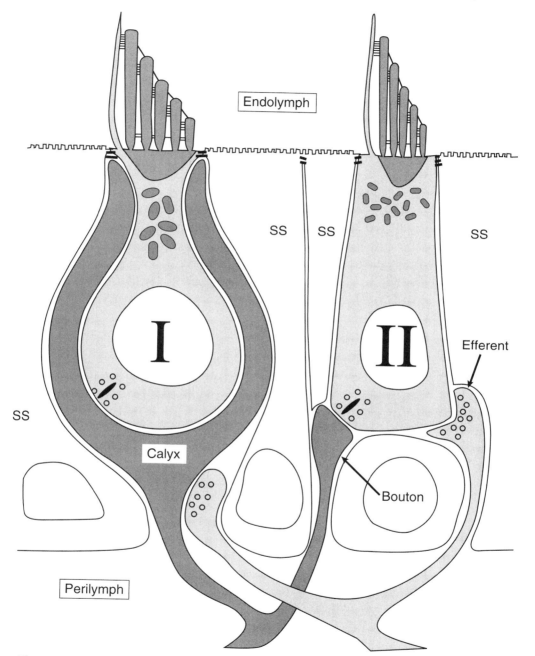

Figure 10–4. Hair cells and their innervation. The hair bundles are bathed in endolymph; the basal ends of the hair cells are bathed in perilymph. Note the different types of afferent nerve endings on type I and type II hair cells. Note also that efferents synapse on the type II cells directly but not on type I cells. I, type 1 hair cell; II, type II hair cell; SS, supporting cells. (From Eatock RA. Stimulus processing in vertebrate hair cells. In: Meza Ruiz G, ed. *Neurobiologica de los systemas sensoriales.* Mexico City: Universidad Nacional Autonoma de Mexico, 1995.)

cupula. The otolithic membrane is really a layer of tiny calcium carbonate crystals, the **otoconia**, imbedded in a protein matrix (see Fig. 10–3B). This arrangement parallels the auditory system, where the cilia of inner hair cells protrude into the tectorial membrane.

Remarkably, the labyrinths and many of the central pathways have changed little over the course of vertebrate evolution. For example, goldfish have vestibular systems that are similar to humans in their overall organization,[3] although details of innervation patterns differ across species.[4] Furthermore, the size of the labyrinth is not directly related to the size of the animal.[5] For example, although a horse weighs approximately 2000 times more than a guinea pig, the internal radius of the horse's semicircular canal is approximately 0.19 mm, and the internal radius of the guinea pig's canal is approximately 0.11 mm. Considering the vast difference in the size of their heads, the similarity in the size of their canals is remarkable. The labyrinth is large enough to obtain the necessary information, but no larger.

Hair Cells

The vestibular system also resembles the auditory system in having two types of hair cells: type I and type II (see Fig. 10–4). Type I hair cells have globular or flask-shaped bases and have been shown to have several subtypes;[6] type II cells have cylindrical bases. At their apical (top) ends, fine filaments called **tip links** connect the stereocilia (Fig. 10–5). In a process known as **mechanoelectrical transduction**, the input or **adequate stimulus** (i.e., head acceleration) is translated by mechanical deflection of the hair cell bundle into classical electrochemical transmission (see Chap. 3) at the basal end of the hair cell.

Gated Spring Model
Just as neurons have a random level of firing that causes a certain level of background "noise," so the ionic channels in the hair bundle have a random level of opening and closing. Therefore, the channels always have some probability of being open. When the hair bundle bends toward the kinocilium, more ionic channels at the tip links open and ions, primarily K^+ and some Ca^{++}, are exchanged. This influx of ions causes the cell membrane to depolarize. The tip links act as elastic "springs" that open or shut the channels. At rest, the spring is somewhat stretched, so that bending the hair bundle reduces the stretch

on the spring, either by opening the "gate" to the channel as the bundle bends toward the kinocilium, or by closing the gate further as the bundle bends away from the kinocilium.[7,8]

Mechanical transduction is very fast, although the mechanism is not very precise. Precision in detecting the direction of head movement is increased as the orientation directions of hair bundles vary. Precision in detecting the amplitude of head movement is increased with cells that have different response characteristics and with a fine-tuning mechanism in the innervation patterns of different hair cells.

Innervation
As with other receptor cells in other sensory systems, hair cells have afferent and efferent innervation. Type I hair cells communicate with a single afferent; type II hair cells communicate with several afferent

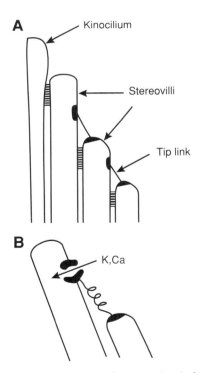

Figure 10–5. Close-up view of the apical end of the hair cell bundle. **A:** Note the tip links between adjacent stereocilia. **B:** When the cilia bend, the tip link relaxes and the transduction channel opens. (From Eatock RA. Stimulus processing in vertebrate hair cells. In: Meza Ruiz G, ed. *Neurobiologica de los systemas sensoriales.* Mexico City: Universidad Nacional Autonoma de Mexico, 1995.)

endings. Efferents coming from the vestibular nuclei innervate several hair cells. The pattern of innervation, both afferent and efferent, as well as the pattern of hair cell arrangement, differs in different parts of the sensory surface. Hair cells and their related nerve endings are arranged in concentric microzones. The zones differ with respect to the density of type I and type II hair cells, the most common subtypes of afferent synapses, and the characteristics of the efferent innervation from the vestibular nuclei that form part of an early feedback mechanism. Each microzone has somewhat different physiologic properties that may be involved in early signal processing.[9,10]

Functional Principles

The vestibular labyrinth works on the principles of Newton's law of inertia: an object in motion stays in motion and an object at rest stays at rest until acted on by an unbalanced outside force. In other words, the system is unaffected by movement at a constant velocity; it responds only to changes in velocity, that is, acceleration. For example, when you sit still in a stationary automobile, you move at 0 degrees/second velocity. When you start the car and move forward, you accelerate—the car changes velocity. When the car accelerates, moving forward, you feel as if you are being thrust backward into the seat. Actually, because of its inertia, your body remains in its original position as the car moves forward around you, with the result that your body seems to move backward. Eventually, the directed outside force of the car pulls your body along.

In the same way, the endolymph in the semicircular canals and the otoconia in the otoliths act as inertial masses. When you turn your head, the endolymph maintains its inertial position while your head moves around it, effectively moving the endolymph backward inside the canals. The cupula bends backward, bending the cilia of the hair cells. When you move linearly (e.g., when the car moves forward), the otoconial membrane maintains its inertial position, too, effectively sliding backward over the underlying cilia, which bend backward. In both cases, bending the cilia starts the transduction process described previously.

Any changes in movement of the head, including weight shifts to adjust posture, stimulate the vestibular end organs. Because the semicircular canals are perpendicular to each other, rotating the head

through any plane in space stimulates one or more of the canals. Furthermore, the head has a pair of labyrinths, one on either side, and the canals work in pairs. Rotating the head in the horizontal plane stimulates both lateral canals, one in a positive direction and the other in a negative direction (i.e., exciting one set of hair cells and the vestibular nerve on one side and inhibiting those on the other side). Because of the orientation of the vertical canals, stimulation of the anterior canal on one side stimulates the posterior canal on the other side. Therefore, pitching the head upward or downward to the left stimulates the LARP pair of canals; pitching the head up or down to the right stimulates the RALP pair.

The otoliths also work in pairs. Kinocilia in each macula are oriented about a line, the **striola**, that divides each macula roughly in half and serves as an orientation vector. Bending the cilia toward or away from the striola is excitatory or inhibitory, depending on the otolith organ. The saccule responds mostly to vertical acceleration, such as the stimulation from an elevator ride, and the utricle responds mostly to horizontal acceleration, such as the forward motion of a car. Gravity, which exerts a constant linear acceleration, acts on the otoconial membrane of the saccule to bend the underlying cilia down somewhat. This input from gravity is important for spatial orientation. (Imagine how you would feel if this pull of gravity was not present, which is the situation in space. The otoliths would become unloaded, and you would no longer have a sense of "up.") When you tilt your head and hold it in a new position, the otolithic membrane maintains its new inertial position so that the cilia do not return to their original position as long as the head is tilted. Therefore, the otoliths also signal the direction of gravity and changes in head position away from that direction.

Central Pathways

The vestibular portion of cranial nerve (CN) VIII, which innervates the vestibular labyrinth, has two parts. The superior vestibular nerve innervates the anterior and horizontal canals and the utricle. The inferior vestibular nerve innervates the posterior canal and the saccule. The cell bodies for both parts are located in **Scarpa's ganglion**. Unlike many ganglia, Scarpa's ganglion is diffuse rather than compact, making it difficult to lesion completely during surgical procedures. (Although annoying for the surgeon, this arrangement might make it difficult to lose vestibular function altogether, which may have some survival value.)

Vestibular Nuclei and Cerebellum

Proximal to Scarpa's ganglion, the vestibular nerve enters the brainstem and travels to the **vestibular nuclei**. This group of at least a dozen nuclei includes several large structures, the superior vestibular nucleus (SVN), the medial vestibular nucleus (MVN), the lateral vestibular nucleus (LVN), which is also called **Deiter's nucleus**, and the inferior vestibular nucleus, also known as the descending vestibular nucleus (Fig. 10–6). The smaller "Y" nucleus is also important in receiving primary vestibular afferent fibers, particularly from the otoliths. The other small nuclei are included in this complex if anatomic studies have shown direct connections with the labyrinths or if electrophysiologic studies have shown them to respond within a short time period to electrical stimulation of the vestibular nerve.

Anatomical studies are usually performed with dyes or radioactive tracers (described in Chap. 16) that are put into the neuron and transported down the axon to the terminal bouton, sometimes across synapses to be taken up by the next neuron. In this way, the projections of a nerve to a nucleus or group of nuclei can be mapped. Physiologic studies are usually performed by stimulating the vestibular nerve or by giving the animal a well defined vestibular stimulus, such as yaw rotation in darkness of 0.5 Hz ± 30 degrees/second, while recording the responses of individual neurons with electrodes placed in the extracellular spaces around the neurons. The electrical potentials generated by neurons (see Chap. 3) can be recorded and used to develop a physiologic map of a nucleus.* Thus, both anatomical and physiologic studies contribute to our understanding of the structure of this area.

---

*The brain's electrical potentials can be recorded visually, as tracings on an oscilloscope or computer screen, or they can be recorded auditorially, as the sounds of different neurons. Each type of neuron and each area of the central nervous system has unique visual patterns and sounds. If you have an artistic rather than computational temperament and you are having difficulty relating to the science in this book, try to imagine your brain as the compilation of thousands of neural line drawings or as a complex counterpoint or neural polyphony.

Some afferents entering the vestibular nuclei maintain their spatial distribution. Signals from the otoliths go primarily to the "Y" nucleus, the MVN, and descending nucleus. Signals from the semicircular canals go directly mostly to the MVN and SVN. A few fibers go to the LVN. A large input also projects directly to the vestibular parts of the cerebellum, particularly the **nodulus** and ventral **uvula**. More signals from the otoliths than from the semicircular canals take this route. A few fibers project to the flocculus. From the **vestibulocerebellum**, secondary afferents go to the vestibular nuclei, many to the LVN. In summary, the SVN receives signals only from the semicircular canals, the descending nucleus receives signals mostly from the otoliths, and the LVN receives both kinds of signals, but most of its inputs have been processed elsewhere, first. The MVN receives mostly primary afferents, from the otoliths and the canals. Figure 10–6 illustrates this rather complicated arrangement.

Physiologic studies of the behavior of individual neurons recorded one at a time while the nerve is stimulated electrically or while the animal is rotated passively indicate several different types of primary and secondary vestibular neurons, such as regularly firing and irregularly firing primary afferents. Within the vestibular nuclei, the input from primary afferents is modified by complex inputs from polysynaptic pathways,[11] so that once a signal is received in the vestibular nuclei it is processed further. Anatomic studies support the idea of different subtypes of vestibular neurons, and confirm the existence of complex patterns of connectivity among local interneurons, within the vestibular nuclear complex.[12]

The vestibular nuclei receive some information from other sensory systems. The most important of these inputs comes from the visual system. The accessory optic tract, an offshoot of the optic tract described in Chapter 11 on vision, synapses with neurons in the **inferior olivary nuclei** in the rostral medulla. Anatomical and electrophysiological studies have shown that climbing fibers ascend from the inferior olive to the flocculus, carrying visual signals to that area. Fibers that descend to the vestibular nuclei through the inferior cerebellar peduncle, or **restiform body**, carry complex inhibitory signals representing the results of vestibular and visual inputs. This indirect route is one way that visual information enters the vestibular nuclei. The complex connections in this area form a functional triad of the vestibular nuclei, vestibulocerebellum, and part of the in-

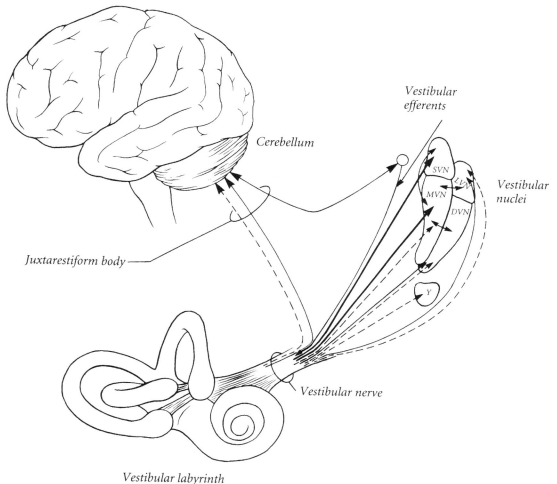

Figure 10–6. Projections of the vestibular nerve to the vestibular nuclei and the cerebellum. Note the somatotopic distribution of some information with the vestibular nuclei. *Broken lines* represent input from the otoliths; *solid lines,* input from the semicircular canals. *Small double arrows* represent local interneurons. The *small unmarked circle* represents other small vestibular nuclei originating vestibular efferent signals. SVN, superior vestibular nuclei; MVN, medial vestibular nucleus, LVN, lateral vestibular nucleus; DVN, descending vestibular nucleus; Y, Y nucleus.

ferior olive. This triad is important for the generation of eye movements,[13] discussed later in this chapter and in Chapter 11.

The visual input to the vestibular nuclei forms the anatomical basis for several phenomena. Vection illusions are illusions of self-motion caused by moving visual stimuli. For example, you might go to the movies or to an amusement park, where the entire visual scene might move, if you were to watch a film of

someone parachuting from an airplane. You might feel as if you had moved. This sensation would be caused by visual signals exciting some, although not all, higher-order neurons in the vestibular nuclei. In this way, the vestibular system responds to motion of the entire visual scene. In real life, rather than an amusement park, apparent motion of the entire visual scene is usually a cue that the individual has moved her head, rather than a cue that the external world has moved. Therefore the nervous system interprets such stimuli to mean self-motion rather than world motion.

Physiological studies illustrate the anatomic underpinning of this sensation. When recording the activity of individual neurons in the vestibular nuclei, vestibular stimulation in one direction (e.g., to the right) elicits the same response as motion of the entire visual surround in the opposite direction (i.e., to the left). Thus, the neuron responds to motion, regardless of the original stimulus.[14]

The internal anatomy of the vestibular nuclear complex is complicated. The nuclei communicate with each other by local projections. Some fibers connect the two sets of vestibular nuclei. Some fibers leave the nuclei, projecting to other small nuclei in the brainstem concerned with control of eye movements, which are too numerous to be detailed here. Suffice to say that these other nuclei are concerned with generation of the various parameters of the several kinds of eye movements. From these oculomotor nuclei, projections return to the vestibular nuclei before their signals are sent further along. The complex anatomy of the vestibular nuclei and oculomotor pathways has been described in detail elsewhere.[12,15]

Descending Projections

The two **vestibulospinal tracts** leave the medial, lateral, and descending nuclei and project to the spinal cord for postural control, as shown in Figure 10–7. The lateral vestibulospinal tract (LVST) descends from primarily the LVN, with a small contribution from the MVN. It descends primarily ipsilaterally, and synapses directly with extensor motoneurons in the cervical and lumbosacral levels of the cord, to influence physiologic extensors of the neck, trunk, and knees. The LVST also makes interconnections within several levels of the spinal cord to influence extensors of the contralateral side.

The medial vestibulospinal tract (MVST) descends bilaterally to cervical and thoracic levels and synapses both directly and by interneurons with extensor motoneurons of the axial musculature. Because the MVST synapses with interneurons, it may take somewhat longer for signals from that tract to influence spinal motoneurons than do signals from the LVST. These pathways form the anatomical basis for the vestibular influence on posture, manifested through the labyrinthine reflexes that are often seen in infants. Older children and adults also demon-

strate these reflexes, which are apparent when the system is stressed, such as when you lose your balance because you slip on an icy sidewalk.[16,17] Posture and balance, however, involve many factors, of which vestibular input is just one. Because the vestibular system includes these pathways, the loss of balance is seen in patients with vestibular impairments, such as bilateral otitis media with effusion in young children or disequilibrium in vestibularly impaired adults.[18,19]

Ascending Projections

Control of Eye Movements

Two kinds of pathways ascend from the vestibular nuclei. Some are concerned with oculomotor control and some are concerned with spatial orientation. Signals concerned with control of eye movements ascend the medial longitudinal fasciculus to the nuclei of CN III, IV, and VI, the oculomotor, trochlear, and abducens nerves, respectively. Both sets of vestibular nuclei send bilateral projections to the cranial nerves, some of which are excitatory and some of which are inhibitory. The effect of this rather complicated arrangement, diagrammed in Figure 10–8, is that the eyes usually move in parallel, in the same direction at the same time, rather than in opposite directions.

The two eyes make five kinds of eye movements, all of which are discussed in Chapter 11. One kind, however, the **vestibuloocular reflex** (VOR), is discussed here in some detail because the VOR represents a major output of the vestibular system. The VOR is a compensatory eye movement, made in response to head movements, to stabilize gaze in space, that is, to enable you to see clearly while moving. You use this reflex as you move through space and try to look at something. For example, as you walk, your head moves up and down and side to side. If your eyes did not counterrotate, you would see only a blur. Try it: have someone else look at your nose and make yaw head rotations left and right. The person's eyes should move right and left as the head moves left and right. You use the VOR during the social gesture of nodding your head during a conversation to indicate understanding, and you use it whenever you sit at the dinner table, lean forward, and pick up a cup. You also use it to compensate for the slight motion of your head that occurs during normal physiologic sway, probably caused by the shift in

(text continues on page 161)

Vestibulospinal Tracts

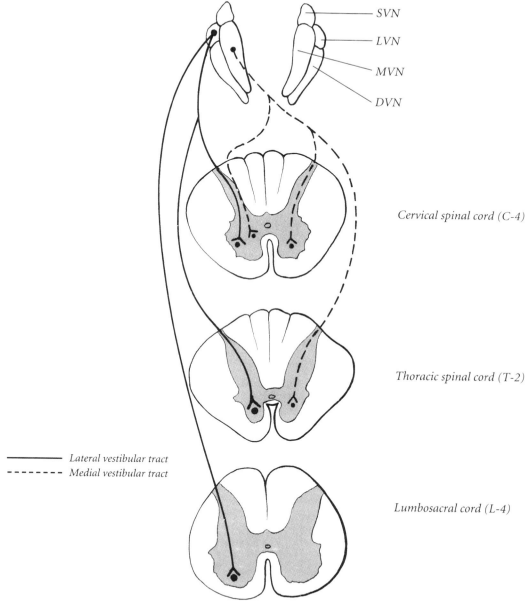

Figure 10–7. The medial and lateral vestibulospinal tracts, descending from the vestibular nuclei to levels in the spinal cord. *Solid lines* represent the lateral vestibulospinal tract; *broken lines* represent the medial vestibulospinal tract.

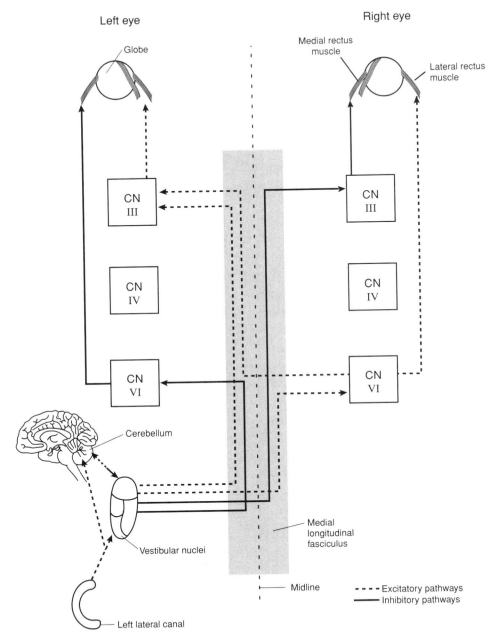

Figure 10–8. The pathways of the horizontal vestibulo-ocular reflex stimulated from excitatory input to the left horizontal semicircular canal when the head turns to the left. The right lateral and left medial recti contract, pulling the eyes to the right, as the left lateral and right medial recti are inhibited so that they relax. Only the pathways that respond to the excitatory input from the left lateral canal side are shown; parallel pathways that respond to the inhibitory input from the right side are not shown. The nuclei of cranial nerves III, IV, and VI are shown; note that the trochlear nerve and nucleus do not participate. Note also that some fibers from the vestibular nuclei decussate and ascend in the medial longitudinal fasciculus, but other fibers do not decussate.

your center of gravity as your heart beats and as you breathe. You see clearly because the VOR compensates for those head motions so you maintain a stable gaze.

Consequently, in the absence of vestibular function caused, for example, by loss of hair cells after having taken ototoxic medications such as streptomycin or gentamicin, people have blurred vision while moving because of loss of the VOR.[20] People with no vestibular function have blurred vision even while standing or sitting still,[20,21] and tend to make few spontaneous head movements during conversation.

In the dark, the pure VOR is approximately 70% accurate. When complemented by optokinetic nystagmus in the light (see Chap. 11), this reflex allows you to compensate completely for head movements. The VOR is stimulated by vestibular signals elicited by rapid head movements, in the range of 0.1 to 7.0 Hz, which is the range of frequencies for normal head movements. When combined with eye movements elicited by movements of the entire visual field about the person, and which are responsive to very low frequencies—below 0.1 Hz—the nervous system can respond to movement of the visual world or the person through a wide range of frequencies.

The ability to maintain gaze stabilization is important for recognizing objects and people while ambulating because your head moves as you walk. Gaze stabilization is also important for normal social interactions. Loss of vestibular function, or loss of visual function in the accessory optic tract or other brainstem visual areas, causes loss of visual acuity. To maintain a clear visual image, you must focus the image on the center of the eye, as you will learn in Chapter 11. As you move your head when you walk, the visual world changes position in reference to your position. Therefore you must constantly update the position of your eye in your head to see clearly.

Pathways

The VOR was once considered the classic three-neuron arc with an input, output, and an interneuron to connect them (see Chap. 13). This concept is now outdated. Even as simple a reflex as the VOR has a much more complex set of underlying pathways. The output of the VOR is directly related to the direction of stimulation to the vestibular labyrinth.[22,23] The VOR output, however, can be adapted to match the size of the visual input as it changes, as when looking through eyeglass lenses.[24,25] We know now that the side loop through the cerebellum,[26] which in-

volves so-called mossy fibers carrying input from the labyrinth and vestibular nuclei and climbing fibers from the inferior olive in the pons, is important for motor learning (e.g., for maintaining an appropriate size of the reflex).[27,28] Mossy fibers and climbing fibers have different physiologic characteristics and carry different kinds of information. For example, mossy fibers fire regularly and carry processed vestibular signals, whereas climbing fibers fire irregularly and carry processed visual signals from the accessory optic tract (see Chap. 11). Because the VOR is easily modified with lenses to change the amplitude of the reflex, and because it is virtually unchanged across many species, it is an ideal behavior to use in studying the neural mechanisms of motor learning.

Mathematical Integration

The VOR compensates for head movements because of a mathematical mechanism in the vestibular system. Because of the fluid mechanics of the labyrinths when they respond to head acceleration, the signal actually ascending the vestibular nerve represents velocity rather than acceleration.[29] Velocity is mathematically related to acceleration, obtained by the mathematical operation of integration. Likewise, position information is obtained by mathematically integrating velocity. So, position can be obtained from acceleration with a few relatively simple calculations. For example, if you walk down the hall, accelerating at 10 feet/second forward, after 10 seconds you will be moving at a velocity of 100 feet/second forward. If you walk at a velocity of 100 feet/second forward for 10 seconds, your new position will be 1000 feet forward of your starting point.

Some of the signals ascending the medial longitudinal fasciculus toward the oculomotor nuclei (CN III, IV, and VI) represent eye position. The velocity signal on the vestibular nerve is mathematically integrated to obtain position.[30] That signal is then given the opposite sign (e.g., from left to right) and sent to oculomotor neurons. So, when your head rotates 10 degrees to the right in the light, when you are watching something, your eyes rotate 10 degrees to the left, maintaining a stable gaze. The **velocity storage integrator**, another mathematical mechanism that operates in the vestibular nuclei, collects and stores velocity information from the vestibular nerve. It releases that information slowly, during the generation of **nystagmus**, a combination eye movement pattern that includes slow phases, from the VOR or optokinetic eye movements, to maintain a stable gaze, and fast phases to reset the position of the eye in the orbit.[31–33] In the VOR, the slow phases are in the opposite direction to the direction of head motion. If, however, the person remains stationary, and the visual surround rotates, such as during some amusement park rides, the optokinetic system generates slow phases in the same direction as the moving stimulus. When a normal person or animal is spun repeatedly, the amount of velocity storage decreases, so that nystagmus occurs for shorter periods of time. Lesions of the cerebellar nodulus interfere with this reduction of velocity storage.[34] Therefore, the inability to shorten the duration of nystagmus is one indicator of a central lesion in the vestibular system.

Adaptive Plasticity

The VOR is a simple, well defined motor behavior that is used in daily life by virtually all vertebrate animals. It is also easily modified with changes in the visual input or with repeated testing, making it an excellent model for the study of motor learning. If you wear eyeglasses that magnify the world, you use this adaptive plasticity daily. The change in the size of the visual image caused by your glasses requires a change in the magnitude of the VOR to maintain a stable gaze during head movement. You learn to increase and decrease the magnitude of the reflex as you view the world with and without your eyeglasses. Similarly, because water magnifies a visual image, divers learn to modify the VOR as they see the world in air and under water. In fact, as you walk toward a visual target (i.e., something that you are watching), you must modify the size of the VOR to maintain a stable gaze. As you near the target, the vertical movement of your head as you walk causes increasingly larger vertical shifts in the image of the target on your eye. To compensate, you must change the vertical component of the VOR. Studies of adaptive plasticity in the VOR and in another simple, habitual motor behavior, the blink reflex, indicate the importance of cerebellar mechanisms in motor learning.[28] Interfering with the vestibular nuclei–vestibulocerebellum–inferior olive triad impairs modification of the amplitude or timing of these reflexes.

In a famous example of ontogenetic modification, flatfish undergo a metamorphosis. The larval fish have eyes on both sides of the head, swimming along in the usual upright position. As the fish develops, the eyes migrate so that both eyes are on one side of the head. The mature fish swims with its eye side up and its blind side down. Remarkably, however, the fish continues to have a normal VOR. To perform this feat, the horizontal canals must respond to vertical rotations and both the LARP and RALP pairs of vertical canals must respond to horizontal rotations. Therefore, this transformation necessitates a 90-degree transformation of the spatial coordinate system of the central vestibular pathways, probably by underlying changes in the anatomical pathways between the vestibular nuclei and the nuclei of the CN III, IV, and VI, the cranial nerves that control eye movements (see Chap. 11).[35,36] This example of plasticity is very unusual, but illustrates another way in which the nervous system modifies itself as needed.

These and other mechanisms of adaptive plasticity are essential to maintaining functional motor behavior over the life span. With age comes loss of peripheral and central neurons and related support structures. People with intact nervous systems compensate for these changes probably by using mechanisms that involve the vestibular nuclei–vestibulocerebellum–inferior olive triad. Therefore, despite some deterioration in balance and the accuracy of the VOR,[37–39] most people continue to function normally. Adaptive changes in neurons use increased calcium uptake and other processes described in Chap. 21. People fail to compensate or to recover when these adaptive mechanisms are inadequate.

Spatial Orientation

Information from the vestibular system also ascends, by a separate set of pathways, to higher centers in the brain (Fig. 10–9). In these areas the neurons responsive to vestibular signals also respond to other sensory stimuli. Therefore, unlike many other sensory systems, above the level of the primary central nuclei the nervous system has no pure vestibular signals. Small groups of fibers terminate in parts of the thalamus, including part of the medial geniculate nucleus, and those neurons respond to auditory as well as vestibular signals. In the ventroposterior inferior nucleus of the thalamus, neurons that respond to electrical stimulation of the vestibular nerve also respond to proprioceptive input. A small projection of fibers from the ventroposterior inferior nucleus ascends to the cerebral cortex, where they disperse in small, diffuse areas also responsive to somatosensory, auditory, or visual stimuli. A small projection has also been found to an area in the caudate nu-

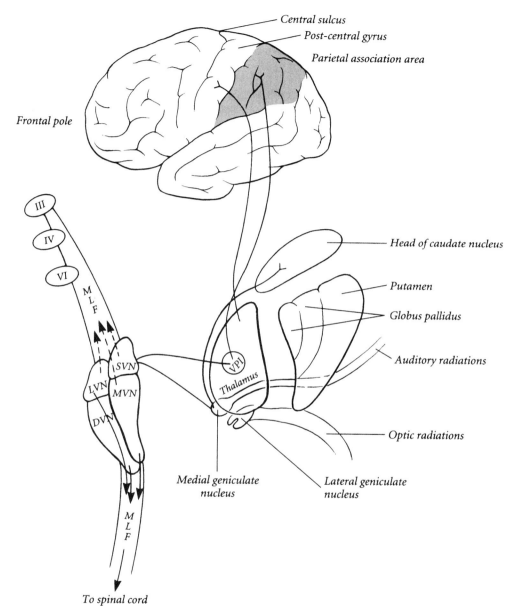

Figure 10–9. Vestibular projections to higher centers. From the vestibular nuclei, some fibers ascend to the medial geniculate nucleus and the ventroposterior inferior nucleus (VPI) in the thalamus. A few fibers go off to the caudate nucleus; others project to association areas in the cerebral cortex. The pathways are smaller and more diffuse than the large projections ascending the medial longitudinal fasciculus (MLF) to CN III, IV, and VI, and descending to the spinal cord.

Vestibulo-autonomic "relay"

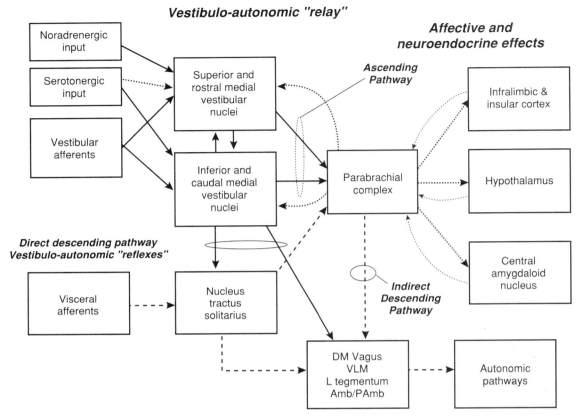

Figure 10–10. The organization of the vestibulo-autonomic connections. (From Balaban CD, Porter JD. Neuroanatomic substrates for vestibulo-autonomic interactions. *J Vestib Res* 1988;8:7–16. Used by permission.)

cleus that also responds to stimulation of the auditory nerve.[40] These findings in rats, cats, and primates suggest that in higher centers pure vestibular information is not represented but, instead, is mixed with signals from other senses.

Behavioral studies with lower animals and humans suggest that these areas, combined with input to the hippocampus, are involved with spatial orientation.[41,42] Information derived from the otoliths is important for knowing about the location of the gravitational vertical. Information from the entire labyrinth is probably important for egocentric (with reference to the self) orientation, as when knowing the direction of rotation,[43] or for short-distance navigation in the absence of visual information.[44–46] These tasks typically move the subject through space, either passively in a moving or rotating vehicle or chair, or actively by walking along some trajectory with vision or visual cues eliminated. Vestibular-deficient people and animals are unable to perform spatial orientation tasks that require this kind of information.[47–49]

One mechanism probably involved in upright spatial orientation is velocity storage. A unique way to study the role of the otoliths is by unloading the otolithic membrane, which occurs during exposure to microgravity (i.e., during space flight). The resulting changes in the VOR that have been observed immediately after space flight in primates suggest that velocity storage undergoes a transformation, probably based on a reinterpretation of otolith gravitational signals as linear translation.[50]

Autonomic Functions

As you will learn in Chapter 15, the **autonomic nervous system** is that part of the central and peripheral nervous systems that controls automatic, involuntary motor functions that are essential for life, including heart rate, respiration, sexual function, urinary control, and digestive control. It also controls some aspects of vision through innervation of intrinsic muscles of the eyes (see Chap. 11). Because these functions are involved in preserving life, it is sometimes called the "fight-or-flight" system. The vestibular system sends some projections to the autonomic nervous system and probably influences postural set and gaze stabilization, which has some practical value as the individual sets his or her or its posture and gaze to do combat with another person or beast or to flee.[51]

The vestibular pathways involved in autonomic regulation include output from the superior, lateral, and descending vestibular nuclei to several areas in the cerebellum, brainstem, caudate nucleus, and related areas involved with various autonomic functions (Fig. 10–10). These pathways probably underlie the neural mechanisms causing the nausea, vomiting, increased heart rate, increased respiration, and other symptoms common to motion sickness, vestibular impairments, and acute responses to initial exposure to microgravity.[52,53] The complex vestibulo-autonomic relationships have been discussed in detail by Yates and Miller.[54]

Clinical Correlations

An important diagnostic test is based on the fact that the labyrinths are filled with fluid. The consistency of a fluid can be affected by changes in temperature. Changing the temperature of the fluids in the inner ear sets up convection currents in the labyrinths, causing the cilia to bend and excite the basal membranes of the hair cells, which release neurotransmitter, eventually exciting the vestibular nerves. This procedure, known as **caloric testing**, is used to evaluate peripheral vestibular function. Warm or cool water is injected into the external ear canal, causing a change in the temperature of the middle ear. The temperature change in that space induces a temperature change in the labyrinths. With this procedure, the two labyrinths can be tested separately, which allows detection of unilateral lesions, such as damage to one nerve.

Because the vestibular and cochlear parts of CN VIII lie close together, tumors of one nerve may cause symptoms in the other system. For example, an **acoustic neuroma** is a benign tumor of the Schwann cells of the vestibular nerve. It is most often manifested, however, by auditory impairments. Because these tumors grow slowly over years, people with otherwise intact nervous systems compensate unknowingly for the vestibular loss. As the tumor grows, it compresses the auditory nerve, causing hearing loss for which patients then seek medical attention. Similarly, because of their close anatomical relationships, other disorders causing hearing impairments may also cause loss of vestibular function.

Causes of bilateral vestibular loss sometimes affect the neighboring auditory labyrinth and sometimes do not. Some medications, such as gentamicin, are primarily toxic to vestibular hair cells, suggesting some differences between auditory and vestibular hair cells. Some metabolic and autoimmune disorders, however, involve both systems. For example, diabetes mellitus and Cogan's syndrome both cause vestibular and hearing impairments.[19,55]

The most common peripheral vestibular disorder is benign paroxysmal positional vertigo, in which otoconial matter from the otoliths becomes displaced into the posterior semicircular canal.[56] Patients experience vertigo when stimulating the involved canal by pitching the head up or by lying down and rolling over onto the involved side. It is easily treated by moving the head in such a way as to move the otoconial matter out of the canal.[57]

Patients have unilateral vestibular loss from viral infections of the vestibular nerve, processes related to aging, or from falls. Many head-injured patients have unilateral vestibular loss and may have positional vertigo, caused by a high-acceleration impact that loosens otoconia from the otoliths. These patients experience **vertigo**, the illusory sensation of motion. Vertigo is caused by unequal signals from the two vestibular nerves projecting to the vestibular nuclei. The vestibular nuclei misinterpret the difference between the signals as indicating movement. These patients may also have impaired postural control, impairments or loss of the VOR and optokinetic nystagmus, and disorientation. Patients can be taught to reduce their vertigo using the intact visual input to the vestibular nuclei. Staring at a stationary object, such as a picture, effectively dumps the vertigo because the visual signals indicate to the vestibular nuclei that the person is not moving, even though disordered vestibular signals may indicate otherwise. Repeatedly experiencing vertigo with rapid visual–vestibular interactions eventually causes it to decrease or dissipate altogether.[58]

Patients with bilateral vestibular loss do not have vertigo, although they may complain of **oscillopsia**, or apparent movement of objects within the visual field, during high-frequency head movements. These patients have no VOR to maintain gaze stabilization, and therefore cannot distinguish details, such as letters on signs and facial expressions, while moving rapidly. At low frequencies of movement, however, visual acuity should be intact.

If you understand the behaviors in which the vestibular system is involved, then you will understand the diverse symptoms of vestibular disorders. Virtually all patients with vestibular disorders complain of blurred vision and poor balance under some circumstances. Sometimes they complain of vertigo and spatial disorientation, such as past-pointing or veering off course when trying to walk in a straight line. Because the autonomic nervous system is involved with control of heart rate, respiration, gut motility, and other basic functions, patients with vestibular disorders may complain of autonomic signs such as increased heart rate, respiration, and stomach awareness.

Acknowledgments

Supported by the Clayton Foundation for Research and NIDCD grant DC02412. Ruth Anne Eatock, PhD, provided invaluable guidance for the section on hair cells.

REFERENCES

1. Cohen B. The roots of vestibular and oculomotor research: introduction. *Hum Neurobiol* 1984;3:121.
2. Wilson VJ, Melvill Jones G. *Adaptive mechanisms of gaze control*. New York: Plenum Press, 1979.
3. Graf W, Spencer R, Baker H, Baker R. Excitatory and inhibitory vestibular pathways to the extraocular motor nuclei in goldfish. *J Neurophysiol* 1997;77:2765–2779.
4. Lysakowski A. Synaptic organization of the crista ampullaris in vertebrates. *Ann NY Acad Sci* 1996;781:164–82.
5. Jones GM, Spells KE. A theoretical and comparative study of the functional dependence of the semicircular canals upon its physical dimensions. *Proc R Soc Med B* 1963;175:403–419.
6. Kevetter GA, Correia MJ, Martinez PR. Morphometric studies of type I and type II hair cells in the Bergil's posterior semicircular canal crista. *J Vestib Res* 1994;4:429–436.
7. Guth PS, Perin P, Norris CH, Valli P. The vestibular hair cells: post-transductional signal processing. *Prog Neurobiol* 1998;54:193–247.
8. Eatock RA. Stimulus processing in vertebrate hair cells. In: Meza Ruiz G, ed. *Neurobiologica de los systemas sensoriales*. Mexico City: Universidad Nacional Autonoma de Mexico, 1995:239–268.
9. Lysakowski A, Goldberg J. A regional ultrastructural analysis of the cellular and synaptic architecture in the chinchilla cristae ampullares. *J Comp Neurol* 1997;389:419–443.
10. Purcell IM, Perachio AA. Three-dimensional analysis of vestibular efferent neurons innervating semicircular canals of the gerbil. *J Neurophysiol* 1997;78:3234–3248.
11. Cheun-Huang C, McCrea RA, Goldberg JM. Contributions of regularly and irregularly discharging vestibular-nerve inputs of the discharge of central vestibular neurons in the alert squirrel monkey. *Exp Brain Res* 1997;114:405–422.
12. Buettner-Ennever JA, ed. *Neuroanatomy of the oculomotor system*. Amsterdam: Elsevier, 1998.
13. Kaufmann GD, Mustari MJ, Miselis RR, Perachio AA. Transneuronal pathways to the vestibulocerebellum. *J Comp Neurol* 1969;370:501–523.
14. Keller EL. Visual–vestibular responses in vestibular nuclear neurons in the intact and cerbellectomized, alert cat. *Neuroscience* 1979;4:1599–1613.
15. Buettner-Ennever JA, Horn AK. Anatomical substrates of oculomotor control. *Curr Opin Neurobiol* 1997;7:872–979.
16. Allum JHJ, Hollinger M, eds. *Afferent control of posture and locomotion*. New York: Elsevier, 1990.
17. Mergner T, Hlavacka F, eds. *Multisensory control of posture*. New York: Plenum, 1995.
18. Cohen H, Friedman EM, Lai D, Duncan N, Pellicer M, Sulek M. Balance in children with otitis media with effusion. *Int J Pediatr Otorhinolaryngol* 1997;42:107–115.
19. Baloh RW, Halmagyi GM, eds. *Disorders of the vestibular system*. New York: Oxford University Press, 1996.
20. JC. Living without a balancing mechanism. *N Engl J Med* 1952;246:452–460.
21. Hillman EJ, Bloomberg JJ, McDonald VP, Cohen HS. Dynamic visual acuity while walking: a measure of oscillopsia. *J Vestib Res* 1998;8 (in press).
22. Cohen B, Suzuki J-I, Bender MB. Eye movements from semicircular canal nerve stimulation in the cat. *Ann Otol Rhinol Laryngol* 1964;73:153–158.
23. Cohen B, Suzuki J-I, Shanzer S, Bender MB. Semicircular canal control of eye movements. In: Bender MB, ed. *The oculomotor system*. New York: Harper and Row, 1964:163–172.
24. Miles FA, Eighmy BB. Long-term adaptive changes in primate vestibuloocular reflex: I. behavioral observations. *J Neurophysiol* 1980;43:1406–1425.

25. Gonshor A, Melvill Jones G. Short-term adaptive changes in the human vestibulo-ocular reflex arc. *J Physiol* 1976;256:361–379.
26. Robinson DA. Adaptive gain control of vestibulooocular reflex by the cerebellum. *J Neurophysiol* 1976;39:954–968.
27. Lisberger SG. The neural basis for learning of simple motor skills. *Science* 1988;242:728–735.
28. Raymond JL, Lisberger SG, Mauk MD. The cerebellum: a neurological learning machine? *Science* 1996;272:1126–1131.
29. Fernandez C, Goldberg JM. Physiology of peripheral neurons innervating semicircular canals of the squirrel monkey: II. response to sinusoidal stimulation and dynamics of peripheral vestibular system. *J Neurophysiol* 1971;34:661–665.
30. Skavenski AA, Robinson DA. Role of abducens neurons in vestibuloocular reflex. *J Neurophysiol* 1973;36:724–736.
31. Cohen B, Matsuo V, Raphan T. Quantative analysis of velocity characteristics of optokinetic nystagmus and optokinetic after-nystagmus. *J Physiol* 1997;270:321–344.
32. Raphan T, Matsuo V, Cohen B. Velocity storage in the vestibulo-ocular reflex arc (VOR). *Exp Brain Res* 1979;35:229–248.
33. Raphan T, Cohen B. Integration and its relation to ocular compensatory movements. *Mt Sinai J Med* 1980;47:410–417.
34. Cohen H, Cohen B, Raphan T, Waespe W. Habituation and adaptation of the vestibulo-ocular reflex: a model of differential control by the vestibulo-cerebellum. *Exp Brain Res* 1992;90:526–538.
35. Graf W, Baker R. Adaptive changes of the vestibulo-ocular reflex in flatfish are achieved by reorganization of central nervous pathways. *Science* 1983;221:777–779.
36. Graf W, Baker R. Neuronal adaptation accompanying metamorphosis in the flatfish. *J Neurobiol* 1990;21:1136–1152.
37. Cohen H, Heaton LG, Congdon SL, Jenkins HA. Changes in sensory organization test scores with age. *Age Aging* 1996;25:39–44.
38. Paige GD. Senescence of human visual-vestibular interactions: 1. vestibulo-ocular reflex and adaptive plasticity with aging. *J Vestib Res* 1992;2:133–151.
39. Peterka RJ, Black FO. Age-related changes in human postural control: motor coordination test. *J Vestib Res* 1990;1:87–96.
40. Fukushima K. Corticovestibular interactions: anatomy, electrophysiology, and functional considerations. *Exp Brain Res* 1997;117:1–16.
41. Blair HT, Sharpe PE. Visual and vestibular influences on head-direction cells in the anterior thalamus of the rat. *Behav Neurosci* 1996;110:643–660.
42. Knierim JJ, Skaggs WE, Kudrimoti HS, McNaughton BL. Vestibular and visual cues in navigation: a tale of two cities. *Ann N Y Acad Sci* 1996;781:399–406.
43. Barry SR, Bloomberg JJ, Huebner WP. The effect of visual context on manual localization of remembered targets. *NeuroReport* 1997;8:469–473.
44. Potegal M. Vestibular and neostriatal contributions to spatial orientation. In: Potegal M, ed. *Spatial abilities: development and physiological foundations*. New York: Academic Press, 1982:361–387.
45. Cohen H, Potegal M. Effects of semicircular canal lesions on spatial ability. *Soc Neurosci Abstr* 1983;9:523.
46. Ivanenko YP, Grasso R, Israel I, Berthoz A. The contribution of otoliths and semicircular canals to the perception of two-dimensional passive whole-body motion in humans. *J Physiol* 1997;502:223–233.
47. Beritoff JS. *Neural mechanisms of higher vertebrate behavior*. Boston: Little, Brown, 1965.
48. Barlow JS. Inertial navigation as a basis for animal navigation. *J Theor Biol* 1964;6:76–117.
49. Bloomberg JJ, Merkle LA, Huebner WP, Barry SR, Cohen HS. Adaptation of vestibularly mediated manual pointing responses. *Soc Neurosci Abstr* 1997;23:775.
50. Young LR, Sinha P. Spaceflight influences on ocular counterrolling and other neurovestibular reactions. *J Vestib Res* 1998;118:S31–S34.
51. Cohen H, Keshner EA. Current concepts of the vestibular system reviewed: 2. visual/vestibular interaction and spatial orientation. *Am J Occup Ther* 1989;43:331–338.
52. Porter JD, Balaban CD. Connections between the vestibular nuclei and brainstem regions that mediate autonomic function in the rat. *J Vestib Res* 1997;77:63–76.
53. Oman CM. Sensory conflict theory and space sickness: our changing perspective. *J Vestib Res* 1998;8:51–56.
54. Yates BJ, Miller AD. *Vestibular autonomic regulation*. Boca Raton, FL: CRC Press, 1996.
55. Baloh RW, Honrubia V. *Clinical neurophysiology of the vestibular system*. 2nd ed. Philadelphia: FA Davis, 1990.
56. Baloh RW, Honrubia V, Jacobson K. Benign positional vertigo: clinical and oculographic features in 240 cases. *Neurology* 1987;37:371–378.
57. Brandt T, Steddin S, Daroff RB. Therapy for benign paroxysmal positioning vertigo, revisited. *Neurology* 1994;37:371–378.
58. Cohen H, Kane-Wineland M, Miller LV, Hatfield CL. Occupation and visual/vestibular interaction in vestibular rehabilitation. *Otolaryngol Head Neck Surg* 1995;112:526–532.
59. Brodel M. *Three unpublished drawings of the anatomy of the human ear*. Philadelphia: WB Saunders, 1946.

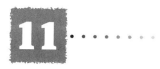

11

Special Senses 3: The Visual System

CHARLES R. FOX, OD, PhD

• • •

Vision, one of the special senses, has receptors in the eyes that detect light and differences in light patterns. Much of what we know about the external world comes through vision. It is particularly impor-

tant for relating to distant objects that cannot be identified and located by the other senses. From an evolutionary point of view, information from vision has three primary uses: 1) watching moving or stationary objects such as potential food, 2) maintaining an appropriate posture, and 3) knowing about your own position in space. These functions may sound similar to those of the vestibular system. If so, you should not be surprised, because these two sensory systems are related physiologically. All of these functions have obvious survival value for lower animals as well as for humans.

Research on visual anatomy and physiology has an important place in neuroscience. Because vision is so important for acquiring knowledge about the external world, structures concerned with vision occupy much of the brain.[1,2] For example, the **visual cortex** is relatively large. It has been studied extensively and the general rules determined for its function have been used as a model to study other areas of the cerebral cortex.

The visual system includes the eye and the related neural structures of the visual pathways (Fig. 11–1). So that you understand the most significant aspects of the anatomy of the peripheral receptor organ, the beginning of this chapter describes the structures of the eye. Then, the visual pathways, subcortical structures, and visual cortex are described. Later, control

Visual Field

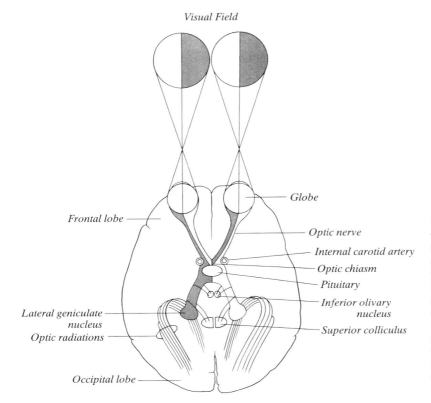

Frontal lobe

Lateral geniculate
nucleus

Optic radiations

Occipital lobe

Globe

Optic nerve

Internal carotid artery

Optic chiasm

Pituitary

Inferior olivary
nucleus

Superior colliculus

Figure 11–1. An overview of the visual system, including the three major projections of the optic nerve: 1) the optic radiations to the occipital lobe; 2) the brachium from the optic tract, along the lateral geniculate nucleus, terminating in the superior colliculus; and 3) the accessory optic tract originating at the posterior chiasm and running through the cerebral peduncles to the inferior olivary nuclei.

of eye movements is discussed. Structures are generally presented from the outside toward the inside and from anterior to posterior in the visual pathway.

Peripheral Visual System

External Structures

The **orbit** is the bony socket containing the eye, orbital fat, fascia (connective tissue sheaths), the levator muscle of the upper lid, the lacrimal gland, extraocular muscles, and the nerves and blood vessels for the orbital contents and some of the face.[3] Seven bones, fused together at **sutures**, form the orbit: the maxilla, frontal, zygomatic, ethmoid, lacrimal, palatine, and sphenoid bones. Eight openings, or foramina, allow arteries, veins, and nerves serving the orbital contents and parts of the face to enter and exit the orbit.

Reinforced folds of skin called the eyelids, or **palpebrae**, protect the eye and the orbit. The eyelids close rapidly and forcefully to protect the eye mechanically from small foreign bodies and excessive light. They also help maintain the quality and quantity of the tear film, the fluid that bathes the eye. The tear film helps maintain the optics and health of the eye. Spontaneous blinking replenishes the tear film, spreads it evenly, and pumps the tears through the drainage system of the eyelids. When the eyelids are open, the upper lid usually covers a small portion of the superior **cornea**, the clear covering in front of the colored part of the eye. The lower lid usually covers the **globe** as far as the inferior aspect of the corneal **limbus**, the junction of the clear cornea and the white **sclera**. The space between the lids, the palpebral aperture, measures approximately 10 mm wide at its widest point. In general, if the palpebral fissures of the two eyes are not equal, the patient may have some pathologic condition, such as Horner's syndrome.

The eyelids contain several muscles that act synergistically. The **orbicularis oculi muscle** occupies the entire length of the eyelid and is responsible for eye closure. It is controlled by the facial nerve (cranial nerve [CN] VII). The **levator palpebrae superioris muscle** occupies the entire width of the lid; it is the prime effector for eyelid retraction (i.e., eye opening) and is under control of the superior branch of the oculomotor nerve (CN III). **Ptosis**, or drooping of the eyelids, may result from disease of CN III or dysfunction of the levator; normal aging, however, may cause drooping eyelids, a nonneurologic ptosis based on tissue elasticity changes. If ptosis is bilateral, the patient may adopt an abnormal head posture, typically tilted back, to look out from under the drooping lids. Abnormalities of eye opening or closing may indicate dysfunction of CN III or CN VII and may result in "dry eye syndrome" through decreased tear film secondary to evaporation. Dry eye syndrome can result in damage to the cornea and subsequent vision problems.

The **conjunctiva**, a clear mucous membrane, forms the deepest layer of the eyelids. It is loosely connected to the lids and is folded back onto the globe, covering the eyeball as far as the cornea. Blood vessels lie in and just below the conjunctiva; irritation, infection, or injury of the eye may cause an inflammatory engorgement of these vessels (conjunctivitis) and edema.

The Lacrimal System

The lacrimal system produces and maintains the tear film. Tears provide a smooth, optically clear surface for the cornea; they wash away debris and cellular waste products produced by the conjunctival and corneal epithelia; they nourish and protect the eye from disease as part of the body's immune system. Tearing is controlled by the autonomic nervous system, discussed in Chapter 15. Basic tearing is indirectly controlled by nerves from the cervical spinal cord that regulate blood flow. The lacrimal gland is innervated by parasympathetic fibers from the greater, or superficial, petrosal nerve, a branch of CN VII that travels with the maxillary branch of CN V. The lacrimal gland also receives innervation from sympathetic fibers of the lesser, or deep, petrosal nerve of CN VII that travels with the ophthalmic branch of CN V. The ophthalmic branch passes through but does not directly influence the lacrimal gland. Reflex or **psychogenic tearing**,

known to most people as weeping, is influenced directly by both parasympathetic (increased tears) and sympathetic (decreased tears) influences on the lacrimal gland. Some disorders of the lacrimal system that lead to dry eye syndrome (see earlier discussion) can be related to neurologic disease.

The Globe

The eyeball itself, also called the **globe**, includes three concentric spheres, or tunics, and is filled with fluids. The spheres are, from outside to inside: 1) the fibrous tunic, including the cornea and sclera; 2) the vascular tunic, including the **iris**, **ciliary body**, and choroid; and 3) the nervous tunic, including the **retina** and **retinal pigment epithelium**. Figure 11–2 illustrates the major structures of the globe.

Fibrous Tunic

Cornea. The cornea is the major light-focusing surface of the eye. It is unique because it is transparent. The cornea is innervated by the sensory branches of the trigeminal nerve (ophthalmic branch, CN V) that are responsible for pain, temperature, and touch. The nerves reach the front of the eye by running through the choroid as the long ciliary nerves, and then run toward the outside of the eye. The nerves of the cornea terminate as free nerve endings between the cells of the central layer of this five-layered structure, so that the cornea is sensitive to even slight stimulation. This arrangement allows for a simple, standard test for the integrity of CN V—lightly touching the cornea with a wisp of cotton. In response to a light touch, the blink reflex causes the eyelids to close rapidly. Normally, the response in each eye is equal. Decreased or unequal responses of the two eyes may suggest a lesion of the ophthalmic branch of CN V.

Sclera. The sclera, or the white of the eye, begins at the cornea and comprises the posterior five sixths of the fibrous tunic. The sclera and the cornea are both made of similar collagen fibers. The cornea's fibers are regularly arranged and are transparent; the sclera's fibers, however, are randomly arranged and opaque. The sclera provides a rigid protective shell for the inner contents of the globe while allowing for variations in intraocular pressure. It also provides a relatively elastic insertion point for the extraocular muscles.

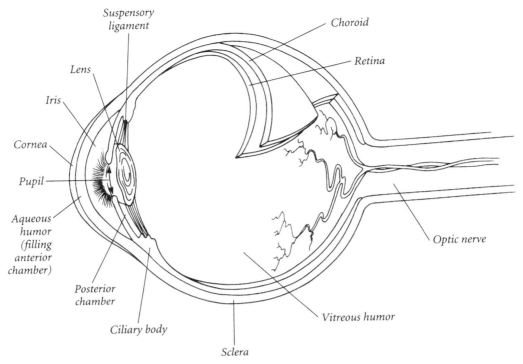

Figure 11-2. The contents of the globe, including the three tunics described in the text. The figure is shown in sagittal section.

Vascular Tunic

Iris. The iris is the colored part of the eye. It divides the eye's internal space into the anterior chamber, in front of the iris, and the posterior chamber, between the iris and the lens (see Fig. 11-2). Its three main layers are perforated in the center, creating the **pupil**, which is an opening, not an actual structure. The front of the iris is made of loosely structured collagen fibers. It contains **melanocytes**, or pigment cells, the **sphincter muscle** that reduces the size of the pupil in bright light, and the blood vessels of the iris. The central layer of the iris is nonpigmented epithelium, and includes the **dilator muscle** that opens the pupil in the dark.

The dilator and sphincter muscles are involuntary and have opposite functions. Therefore, the control of these two muscles must be accurately coordinated. These muscles are not under voluntary control but are both innervated by nerves from the autonomic nervous system. The sphincter is controlled by parasympathetic autonomic fibers traveling with

the inferior division of CN III that synapse in the ciliary ganglion and project to the pupillary sphincter as several short ciliary nerves. The dilator is controlled by sympathetic autonomic fibers traveling with the nasociliary division of the ophthalmic branch of CN V that segregate inside the orbit into two long ciliary nerves. Remember that the innervation for these muscles is different; changes in pupil size or reactivity to light reflect disturbances in the autonomic nervous system. Therefore, testing the pupillary light responses is a sensitive method for examining the integrity of the nervous system.

The deepest layer of the iris includes the pigmented epithelium, and the tangential structure, the lens. These structures have no significant neurologic function and are not discussed further.

Ciliary Body. Immediately behind the iris and just inside the sclera, the ciliary body is composed of several layers that are similar to the iris. The most external layer, the **ciliary muscle**, contains the stromal blood vessels and ciliary processes. The ciliary muscle is innervated by the same short ciliary nerves that innervate the lacrimal gland (CN VII). The blood vessels of this area produce a fluid called the **aqueous humor** that fills the anterior chamber. The aqueous enters the posterior chamber in front of the lens, flows through the pupil into the anterior chamber, filters through a membranous mesh, and eventually empties into veins in the sclera, to be removed from the eye. Aqueous humor provides metabolic support for the lens and posterior cornea and is largely responsible for the intraocular pressure. If too much aqueous is produced, or not enough drains, the pressure in the eye increases. Extremely high pressure can damage the **optic nerve**, resulting in the most common form of glaucoma (intraocular dependent form), the end stage of which is tunnel vision or blindness.

The ciliary body serves several other functions. Contracting and relaxing the ciliary muscle adjusts the tension on the capsule of the lens, allowing the lens to adopt different shapes that result in different refractive powers. This process, called **accommodation**,[4] helps focus light entering the eye. Owing to the deterioration of accommodation, many of us who have passed our 40th birthdays must hold reading material at arm's length. The ciliary body also secretes one component of the **vitreous humor**, a gel-like material that fills the main cavity of the eye behind the iris and in front of the retina (see Fig. 11–2). The vitreous helps to maintain the shape of the globe. With age it coagulates and condenses, causing tension on the retina that, if severe enough, can result in localized retinal detachments.

Choroid. Posterior to the ciliary body, the vascular tunic is called the choroid. It forms a network of blood vessels providing metabolic support for the outer layers of the retina as well as the inner layers of the sclera. Damage to this network interferes with vision.

Nervous Tunic

Retina. The retina[5,6] has 10 layers, divided into 2 general sections: the retinal pigment epithelium (outer layer) and the sensory or neural retina (layers 2 through 10), shown in Figure 11–3. The retina converts light energy falling on it into electrical impulses that can be analyzed by the brain. Interconnections among retinal elements provide extensive processing of the information extracted from the light patterns.

Nonneural Structures of the Retina. The retinal pigment epithelium (RPE) is the outermost retinal layer. It is in contact with the choroid. The RPE helps to nourish and support the **photoreceptors**, those retinal elements that actually convert light to bioelectrical impulses. It helps maintain proper retinal physiology by providing vitamin A and other nutrients to the photoreceptors. Vitamin A is a major component of the chemicals that capture the light energy for conversion. The RPE actively transports nutrients into the retina and removes waste from the photoreceptor cells. When this metabolic support system breaks down, various forms of retinal degeneration occur, such as macular degeneration or retinitis pigmentosa. In addition, processes from the RPE envelop each individual photoreceptor, improving the efficiency of the retina by holding the photoreceptors in the proper alignment for maximal absorption of light. This supporting function also absorbs stray light and prevents intraocular reflection and scatter. Layer 10, discussed later, is also a nonneural layer. Thus, the innermost and outermost layers of the retina are nonneural structures that enclose the neural structures in layers 2 to 9.

Neural Structures of the Retina. The neural retina begins at layer 2. It is a unique sense organ because it is actually part of the central nervous system (CNS). It is a unique neural structure because most neurons in the retina do not generate action potentials; instead, they simply hyperpolarize or depolarize.

Layer 2 is the photoreceptor layer. The human eye has two classes of photoreceptors, **rods** and **cones**. These two types differ in their anatomy, physiology, and distribution throughout the retina. Regardless of their differences, rods and cones all convert light energy into neural impulses through a series of biochemical and electrochemical reactions involving the photopigments present in the outer segments. Receptors are partly depolarized in the dark; their axon terminals continuously leak neurotransmitter substance in the dark. When light impinges on the retina, several events occur. Individual small packets of energy, **quanta**, are absorbed by individual photopigment molecules in the outer segments, leading to a series of molecular changes over a few milliseconds. The molecular changes generate a weak biphasic electrical response called the **early receptor potential** (ERP). The ERP is the first electrical response to light. It occurs immediately and is highly resistant to drugs, hypoxia, or even death because it involves only biochemical mechanisms without

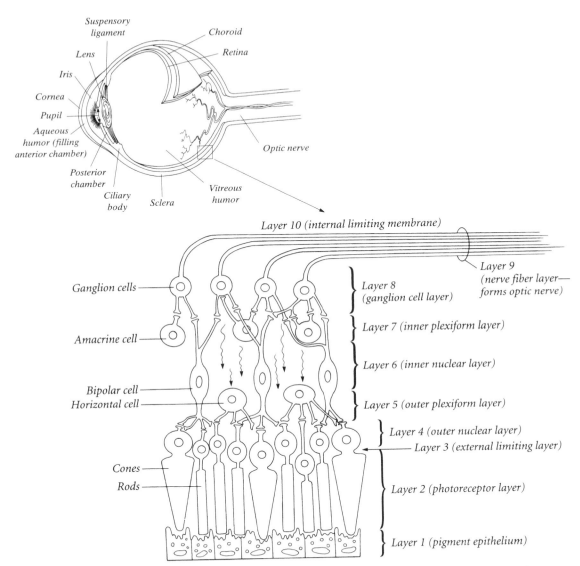

Figure 11–3. Nervous tunic showing the 10 layers detailed in the text. Downward arrows represent light.

membrane potential changes. The ERP is followed by a hyperpolarization of the receptor membrane. Therefore, absorption of light actually reduces the release of neurotransmitter.

Functionally, the responses of the rods and cones are based on the presence or absence of light; in addition, cones are responsible for color discrimination. Rods can be stimulated in dim illumination, but cones require more light. Therefore, when light is minimal, the rods do the "seeing," and the cones are relatively inactive. Because of that difference, you cannot see color in dim illumination. The differential responses of the rods and cones to color and darkness form the basis of clinical testing to investigate this layer of the retina.

Rods and cones have different distributions in the retina. The retina is divided into concentric circular zones based on anatomic and physiologic characteristics. In the central 1-cm–diameter area of the retina, called the **macula lutea** or just **macula**, the photoreceptors—mainly cones—are the most dense. The central 1.5-mm–diameter area of the macula has a concave area, the **fovea**, that contains an even smaller region with only cones, the **foveola**. These anatomic distinctions are not used by clinicians. The rest of this chapter uses clinical terms, but you should be aware of the different uses of these terms. Clinicians refer to the macula and fovea as the macula, and the foveola as the fovea. This central macular/foveal area is responsible for the fine discriminations and high visual acuity in humans. Insult to this area, as in age-related macular degeneration, causes decreased visual acuity. Insults that leave the macula intact, such as diabetic retinopathy without macular edema, do not affect acuity. Outside of the macula, rod density increases and cone density decreases toward the periphery, along with a corresponding decrease in acuity and an increase in light sensitivity. By testing the peripheral retina as opposed to the central retina, rods can be preferentially tested without the cones involved, and vice versa.

Layer 3, just interior to the photoreceptors, is the **external limiting membrane** of the retina. This structure is not really a membrane, but is the point at which the photoreceptors are joined together by a specific type of cellular junction called the **zonula adherens**. It marks the midpoint of the length of the rods and cones. The cell bodies of the photoreceptors are inside the external limiting membrane, in the fourth layer, known as the **outer nuclear layer**. These cell bodies perform the typical metabolic support functions and transmit the electrical responses started in the outer segments of the photoreceptors.

Layer 5, the **outer plexiform layer**, contains the first synapses in the visual pathway; "plexiform" refers to layers without cell bodies that contain synaptic sites. In this layer, the terminal ends of photoreceptors synapse with dendrites of bipolar cells and **horizontal cells**. The cones have synaptic ends that are flat, called **pedicles**, and rods have round ends called **spherules**. The bipolar cells transmit visual signals toward the brain in "vertical" transmission of information. Some bipolar cells relay information from single foveal cones, so that each cell represents a single point in space. In addition to the higher density of cones in the fovea, this direct transmission of information through the bipolar cells accounts for the high spatial resolution and better visual acuity of the fovea. Other bipolar cells receive

and integrate inputs from several peripheral cones or rods. This early many-to-one mapping of information from multiple receptors to a single bipolar connection represents very early processing of information in the visual system.

Layer 5 also contains horizontal cells that connect receptors to other receptors and other horizontal cells. This horizontal processing integrates the input from groups of cells into **receptive fields**. Integration reduces the spatial specificity of each photoreceptor, resulting in poor resolution but high spatial integration in the peripheral retina. To demonstrate this functional differentiation between the central and peripheral areas of the retina, try to read the text on this page while looking off to the side; it will not be as clear as when you looked at it directly because of the higher spatial resolution in central vision. Although this arrangement might appear to be disadvantageous, in fact it is adaptive. This organization increases sensitivity for luminance detection across the retina and underlies **edge enhancement**. To demonstrate enhanced luminance detection, look at a small, dim light in a dark room. You will not be able to see it by looking at it directly, with your fovea, but you will see it clearly when you look to the side. You may have had the experience of being out in the woods on a dark night and noticing a light off to the side that disappears when you look directly at it. Enhanced luminance detection is also useful to law enforcement agents, who are trained to use this peripheral sensitivity when entering a dark environment.

Layer 6, the **inner nuclear layer**, contains the cell bodies of bipolar cells, horizontal cells, **Müller cells**, and **amacrine cells**. Müller cells, which are glia rather than neurons, provide nutritional and mechanical support. They are actually scattered throughout all the layers internal to the outer nuclear layer (i.e., layers 5 through 9). This layer is the most external layer that is completely supplied by the retinal circulation instead of the choroidal circulation. Blood vessels are located in all the layers internal to layer 6, as well. This dual blood supply is clinically important in vascular accidents and disease.

Amacrine cells have no axons. For this reason, unlike typical unidirectional neurons, they behave in an unusual manner: they conduct impulses bidirectionally. Amacrine cells integrate information from **ganglion cells**, providing further enhancement of border detection. They may also be involved in processing temporal information such as movement of the visual image across the retina. The amacrine cell's processes and the axons of the bipolar cells synapse on the dendrites of ganglion cells in layer 7, the **inner plexiform layer**. Ganglion cells are the next step in vertical processing and are the first neurons in the visual pathway to demonstrate the true action potentials found in the CNS. The nearly one-to-one relationship of receptor to bipolar cells is preserved for information from the foveal receptors, resulting in a three-to-one relationship between cones and ganglion cells. Information from the peripheral retina is integrated again because several bipolar cells may synapse on one ganglion cell.

Layer 8, the ganglion cell layer, contains the cell bodies of the ganglion cells, axons of which carry visual information out of the eye. The axons run across the inside of the retina, constituting layer 9, the **nerve fiber layer**, and then form a bundle called the optic nerve (CN II). Layer 10 is the **internal limiting membrane**, which separates the ganglion cell layer from the face of the vitreous that fills the posterior chamber. This membrane is composed of collagen fibers connecting the Müller cells.

To summarize, the retina is divided into 2 sections with a total of 10 layers that are numbered from the outer to the inner. Layers 1 to 5 are supported by the circulation of the choroid, and layers 6 to 10 by the circulation of the retina. The RPE is the outer retina; the inner layers make up layers 2 through 10. In general, the input from 126 million photoreceptors is contained in, and transmitted through, 1 million optic nerve fibers, which are the ganglion cell axons. Most convergence of information occurs in the peripheral retina; the foveal cones in the central retina have a 1:1 relationship with their ganglion cells and thus with the optic nerve fibers that carry their information. This organization results in maximum visual acuity in the fovea.

The Visual Pathway

The Visual Field

The amount of the world you can see at any one time, without eye or head movements, is your **visual field**.[7,8] The organization of the visual field is a direct result of the anatomy of the visual pathway. Visual **field defects** can help localize lesions of the visual pathway and serve as a primary tool for traditional neuroophthalmology.[8] To trace the visual pathway systematically and correlate it to the visual field, the retina is usually considered in quarters (Fig. 11–4). These quarters, called quadrants, are created by imagining a vertical line through the fovea separating the nasal (toward the nose) from the temporal (toward the temple), retinal halves, and a horizontal line through the fovea dividing these hemiretinal fields into superior and inferior quarters. The retinal elements in any quadrant actually represent the visual field that is opposite to it in the physical world. For example, the superior nasal quadrant is stimulated by light from the inferior temporal field. Thus, visual information about the area below and lateral to your eye is gathered by receptors in the superior nasal retina. This inverted representation of the visual field is continued in higher centers in the brain, as shown in Figure 11–4.

Central Visual Pathways

Subcortical Centers

Optic Nerve and Tract. Axons of retinal ganglion cells collect to form a tract known as the optic nerve (CN II). At a point called the **optic chiasm**, some fibers from each side of the visual field decussate, so that some fibers from the nasal retina of each eye join the temporal fibers of the other eye. In this way, each **optic tract** carries signals from one half of the visual field, rather than from an eye. For example, the left optic tract carries visual information from the right visual field of both eyes, rather than information from both the left and right visual fields from the left eye (see Fig. 11–4). Inside the brain these visual afferents continue as the optic tract. Both the optic tract and the optic nerve also contain efferent fibers innervating the sphincter and dilator muscles described previously.

Lateral Geniculate Nucleus. The optic tract projects to three known areas.[9] The largest projection goes to the **lateral geniculate nucleus** (LGN), caudal and lateral to the thalamus. The LGN has six layers, each of which receives input from only one eye, so that each eye is represented in three layers. The ipsilateral eye projects to layers 2, 3, and 5; the contralateral eye projects to layers 1, 4, and 6. The layers of the LGN are arranged so that the same point in space is represented in similar points in adjacent layers. The optic tract carries information from both eyes, from one side of the visual field. Neurons in the LGN project to the primary visual cortex, also known

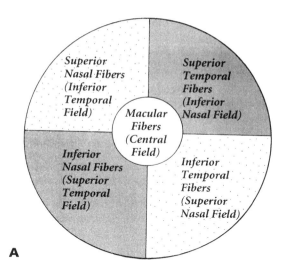

A

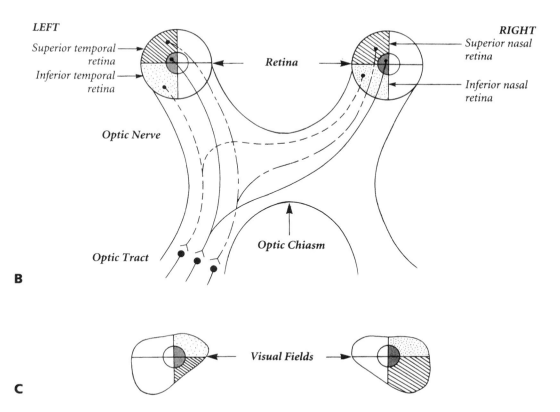

B

C

Figure 11–4. Relationships among visual field structure and visual pathway anatomy. **A:** The visual fields and their corresponding neural substrate. The inferior temporal neural fibers receive information from light originating in the superior nasal field. **B:** The organization of optic nerve fibers as they leave the retina and form the left optic nerve. Note the decussation of fibers from the right eye at the optic chiasm. Solid lines represent information flow from macula; uneven, broken lines represent flow from the left superior quadrant; even, broken lines represent flow from the left inferior quadrant. **C:** The visual fields corresponding to the neural organization described in **B.**

as Brodmann's area 17, in the **occipital lobe**. The LGN is the first brain center where information from the retina is represented.

Superior Colliculus. The optic tract sends a smaller projection to the **superior colliculus** (SC), known as the tectum in lower animals. These fibers from the optic tract run alongside the LGN as part of the **brachium of the superior colliculus**. The macula, however, does not project directly to the SC. Instead, the visual cortex sends processed signals back to the colliculus. Within the SC, the visual field is represented in a distorted manner; the central 30 degrees is represented in the rostral three fourths, whereas the remainder of the visual field is represented in the caudal quarter. SC neurons have large receptive fields and respond to unidirectional horizontal movement from the central to the peripheral visual field. Thus, this structure is a mechanism for detecting specific movements in the field, such as those resulting from body movement.

The SC receives and integrates information from three main sources: the optic tract, the occipital cortex—which projects to the brachium and thus to the SC—and the **spinotectal tract**, which carries somatosensory input from the spinal cord and the medulla. Some SC fibers project to the contralateral nucleus so that signals from both visual fields can be processed together. Other fibers form the **tectothalamic tract** and project to the pulvinar in the thalamus, the LGN, and perhaps the **pretectum**, which is an area caudal to the SC with many small nuclei involved in controlling eye movements. Still others project to the accessory oculomotor nuclei as part of the tectoreticular tract. The vast numbers of nuclei involved in generating eye movements are beyond the scope of this chapter, but the most significant centers are discussed later. For now, you should appreciate that many fibers from these pathways are involved in generating eye movements. Tectopontine fibers convey visual information to the cerebellum. Other projections form the **tectospinal tract**, which sends descending input down the **medial longitudinal fasciculus** (MLF) to the spinal cord. Tectospinal signals are probably involved in the visual control of posture. The ascending MLF is a larger fiber bundle that also carries efferent signals to the oculomotor nuclei (CN III, IV, and VI) for control of eye movements, discussed later in this chapter. The MLF is so large that it can be seen in unstained longitudinal sections of the brainstem. MLF lesions cause impairments in oculomotor control and gaze stabilization, sometimes indicated by complaints of blurred vision.

The functional distinction between the tectopontine and tectospinal tracts has been demonstrated by several experiments on animals in which one of the tracts has been cut. If the brachium of the SC is lesioned, animals that have been trained to make spatial judgments are no longer able to do so. For example, after a lesion of the SC, an animal that was previously trained to run a maze making left turns when a light is on, but right turns when it is off, is no longer able to perform this spatial task. However, the animal retains the ability to make fine, nonspatial discriminations, such as acuity tasks. The reverse is true for lesions of the pathway from the optic chiasm to the LGN. If the LGN is intact, people with lesions of the visual cortex continue to have postural and oculomotor responses to visual stimuli, even though they cannot "see" in a traditional sense. This phenomenon is known as cortical blindness. In short, the geniculocortical tract is involved in identifying objects (the "what" system), whereas the geniculocolliculus tract is involved in spatial localization (the "where" system).

Accessory Optic Tract. The third, and probably smallest, projection from the optic tract is the **accessory optic tract** (see Fig. 11–1). In this phylogenetically old pathway, some fibers separate from the optic tract and project to the nucleus of the optic tract and then to several sites, including the small, accessory optic nuclei around the nucleus of CN III, the medial vestibular nucleus, the LGN, and some nuclei in the thalamus. The major projection is to the inferior olivary nucleus, a large nuclear group that gives the lateral pons its characteristic bulge.[10,11] From the pons, projections ascend by climbing fibers and mossy fibers to the cerebellar flocculus, a phylogenetically old area related to the vestibular system, which is involved in control of eye movements. Climbing fibers have a characteristic slow, intermittent firing pattern. Mossy fibers fire more regularly. This pathway is involved in oculomotor adaptation.

Cortical Projections

Pathways from the LGN to the visual cortex project as the **optic radiations** to the **calcarine sulcus** of area 17 in the occipital lobe. The optic radiations run posteriorly, through Wernicke's area in the temporal lobe (see Chap. 18), just lateral to the lateral ventricles. At the lateral ventricles, the fibers fan out in a broad band as they sweep posteriorly to the visual cortex. The most ventral portions of the radiations actually turn anteriorly for a short distance before turning posteriorly toward the occipital lobes (see Fig. 11–1). A lesion in this anterior section of the radiations causes a characteristic loss of vision in one quarter of the visual field (see later discussion on lesion effects). After turning posteriorly, the optic radiations course through the center of the middle temporal gyrus. Therefore, a lesion in this part of the temporal lobe, which is usually considered a language area, can cause a visual field deficit.

Visual Cortex

The visual cortex[8,12,13] occupies the visual lobe and is anatomically defined as Brodmann's areas 17, 18, and 19 based on the cytoarchitecture (Fig. 11–5). The anatomical boundaries of the occipital lobe are difficult to define; it is generally demarcated by a theoretic line from the parietooccipital fissure to the temporooccipital incisure (see Fig. 11–5). Most of the visual cortex is located on the medial aspect of the occipital lobe in and around the calcarine sulcus, but some of the area extends onto the lateral aspect of the **occipital pole**, to the cuneate and lingual gyri. The gross anatomy of this area varies considerably among individuals.

Area 17, where the optic radiations synapse, contains distinctive white and gray "stripes" or lines known as the striae of Gennari. Because of these stripes, area 17 is also known as the **striate cortex.** It receives input from the LGN and is considered the major gateway for visual information into the cortex. The striae are actually the fibers of the optic radia-

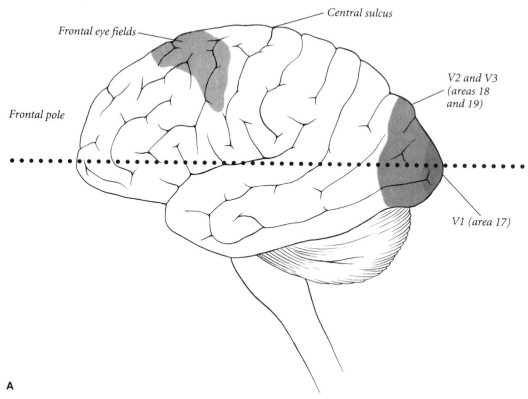

A

Figure 11–5. A: Lateral surface view of the cerebral cortex showing the main visual areas in the occipital lobe (V1–V3) as well as the frontal eye fields for oculomotor control. *Dotted line* shows level of scan in Fig. 11–5B. (continued)

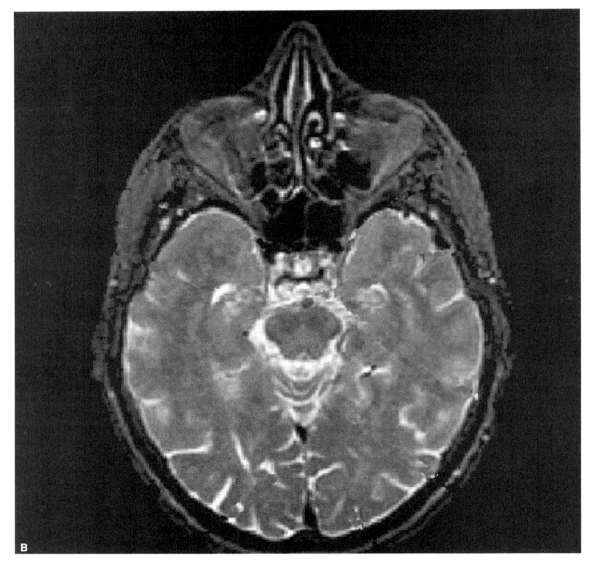

B

Figure 11–5 (continued). B: Radiologic view of a horizontal slice of the cortex at the level indicated by the dotted line in **A.**

tions mixed with intracortical fibers that connect the striate cortex with other areas of the cerebral cortex. These myelinated neurons send their processes past darker local neurons, causing the striped pattern. Areas 18 and 19, visual association areas to which area 17 projects, are difficult to identify histologically and probably do not correspond as directly to functional specialization as other areas such as motor and sensory cortex.

These anatomically defined areas contain five physiologically defined visual processing areas. These areas, V1 to V5, perform different visual tasks. Some other visual areas are also located outside of the visual cortex, such as the frontal or **motor eye fields**, but most visual information processing takes place in areas V1 to V5. Sub-areas such as V3A and V5A have been found in lower species, but they have not been described in detail for humans. Areas V1 through V5 have been relatively well described anatomically, physiologically, by microelectrode studies, by functional magnetic resonance imaging, and by positron emission tomography studies.

Visual Cortical Anatomy

Under the microscope, the visual cortex has a well defined organization. Hubel and Wiesel[14] and other investigators have studied the physiologic properties of cells in area V1 (area 17) using implanted electrodes. Because of the extensive body of research on the visual cortex, the structure of this area is better understood than that of the rest of the cerebral cortex. Most parts of the cortex have six distinct layers. Visual cortex, however, has eight layers. The optic radiations project to granular cells in layer IV. Granular cells project to other neurons within the striate cortex, and also to oculomotor neurons in the brainstem along the **corticomesencephalic tract**. This tract is involved in generating rapid eye movements to objects in the visual field.

Area 17, also known as primary visual cortex, contains a topographic map of the retina. All submodalities of vision are represented there. V1 responds to motion, color, and position (orientation and disparity) in the visual field. V1 receives topographically organized projections from the LGN and projects either topographically or functionally, or both, to all the other visual areas. Area 18 (V2) surrounds V1, primarily dorsally and ventrally, in a horseshoe shape. Adjacent retinal points in V1 connect with adjacent points in V2. Therefore, V2 has a second detailed topographic map of the retina. V2 is also maximally responsive to orientation, direction, and color. Neurons in V2 are color selective, broad band oriented, and disparity selective. Area V2 primarily projects information about the peripheral retina to V4.

Area V3 lies next to V2 in area 18 and receives direct projections from V1, creating a mirror of V2 that primarily represents peripheral retinal orientation information. V3 responds to orientation information but not to color information. V4, lateral to V3 along the occipitotemporal region, primarily receives input from V2, with a smaller input from V1. Thus, the entire retina is represented, although not topographically. V4 responds to large fields and color. It shows

some orientation-specific response, but color is also important. V5 is anterior to V4 along the lateral posterior temporal lobe and receives projections from V1. V5 responds primarily to unidirectional motion and does not respond to color. Area V6 has been described in monkeys; it probably is equivalent to the medial superior temporal area (area MST) in humans. Area MST is anterior to V3 and receives complex projections from V2. Area MST responds to complex, multidirectional movement. All of the visual areas have multiple cortical outputs and are extensively interconnected, projecting to at least two other cortical areas and to subcortical structures.

Visual Cortical Function

Historically, neuroscientists thought that all attributes of a visual image are analyzed in a single cortical area. This concept arose from the integrated and unitary nature of the visual perceptual image, that is, the visual image displays attributes of form, color, motion, and distance seen in precise spatiotemporal registration in the external world. We now know, however, that the experience of a unitary visual image does not imply a unitary visual process. Instead, it represents the integration of many processes. Consider the following clinical example. Cerebral dyschromatopsia is the loss of color vision while maintaining form vision. Dyschromatopsia is probably due to an ischemic lesion of color-specific neurons in the fusiform and lingual gyri. This separation of color and form vision suggests that different aspects of the same visual image are processed in anatomically separate areas and are "bound" into a unified perception of visual objects. This perceptual binding probably occurs through attention-mediated mechanisms.

Classically, the definition of a cortical area has been based on a single topographic representation within that area. In effect, topographic organization delineates cortical areas. Discontinuities are taken as evidence of boundaries between separate cortical areas. This concept is true of area V1 as well as motor areas and most other sensory areas. V1 shows a mapping of the visual field that is continuous in receptor field location. Even in V1, however, multiple functional domains are represented in single cortical areas. Specifically, ocular dominance and orientation columns are evidence of anatomic grouping of cells with common function rather than common retinal loci. Functional grouping is also evident in the directional columns in V5 and the color and disparity organization of V2.

The striate cortex (V1) contains a cortical map of the retina, representing the retinal image. Envision half of the retina spread over the striate area; the macula is represented most posteriorly and the peripheral retina is represented most anteriorly. The upper retina is represented above the calcarine sulcus and the lower retina below it. The macula, responsible for maximal visual acuity, is represented by a huge portion of the striate cortex occupying the caudal one third of the calcarine area. The paracentral and peripheral retina occupy more rostral areas. The relative dimensions of this map indicate the survival value of accurate, foveal vision.

Neuroscientists once believed that each macula was represented bilaterally in the visual cortices. This notion was based on clinical observations of **macular sparing**, a phenomenon in which the central 2 to 5 degrees of vision is intact after a cerebral vascular accident (CVA) involving area 17. Anatomic research, however, demonstrates complete unilateral representation of the macula in the contralateral visual cortex. The apparent discrepancy can be resolved if you understand the vascular supply to the occipital lobe. The occipital pole, where most macular information is represented, is located at the border of the areas supplied by the middle and posterior cerebral arteries. CVAs that affect this area usually involve the posterior cerebral artery. Most of the time, a CVA of that artery causes damage to areas representing one half of the peripheral visual field. The macula is affected minimally because the collateral circulation provided by the middle cerebral artery continues metabolic support to the posterior pole.

Anatomically and functionally, V1 is the first site of integration of information from the two retinas. Up to this point, all areas have been biocular. For example, the LGN receives projections from both eyes, but those inputs are segregated in different layers. VI is also the first site for perception of color, contour, form, and relative localization of objects. Lesions in V1 can impair these functions. For example, a lesion of V1 can cause letter agnosia, the inability to recognize letters, because this skill requires perception of contour and relative location.

In the visual cortex, V1, and perhaps V2, can be considered a neural segregator that receives direct projections from the LGN and parcels out different signals by functional domain, sending them to specialized visual processing areas. For example, consider V2, which is a major projection region for V1. V2 has a striped architecture that anatomically separates color and disparity function. That is, color information from a particular location in the visual field is processed in the thin stripes, disparity from the same physical location is processed by the thick stripes, and orientation from that location is represented by interstripe neurons. In effect, V2 contains multiple, interleaved visual maps for color, disparity, and orientation. The same region in space is represented by each anatomically distinct stripe. Adjacent stripe cycles represent adjacent locations in space so the visual maps are continuous across like stripes. Overall, V2 shows multiple and discontinuous representations of visual space across three types of functional stripes. Each locus in the visual field is represented three times: in the color domain, and in the orientation domain. Domains are continuous within the stripes and from one stripe to the next like stripe, but are discontinuous at stripe borders. Similarly, area V5 has multiple representations with two interdigitated organizations, one representing local motion sensitivity and the other representing global motion sensitivity.

These multiple representations within a single cortical area suggest multiple functional maps of visual space. These maps serve a practical, easily understood function. Think back to the clinical example of dyschromatopsia and consider visual function as a simple paint program on your computer. You would first create a region defined by a disparity contour, such as a black-lined circle on a white field. Defining this region would be done in the disparity domain. Next you would ask your computer to fill the region with red, so you now have a red circle on a white field. Filling in the region would be done in the color domain. By having multiple domains in a single anatomic area, we can easily understand how coherent perceptions, such as the red circle, arise. This organization is a relatively simple one-to-many mapping of the three-dimensional spatial domain to the visual functional domains. A key concept here is that visual input goes through successive physiologic areas in the visual cortex, making successive transformation from visuotopic to functional maps, ascending through the cortical hierarchy.

Receptive Fields

In the same way that individual tactile receptors are sensitive to stimulation in specific locations on the skin, individual retinal cells and the related pathways are sensitive to light stimuli in specific spatial locations known as receptive fields. A visual receptive field is the region of the visual field where the activity of a ganglion cell or higher pathways can be influenced.[15,16] Experiments in receptive fields are typically performed with single-unit recordings in which the activity of individual neurons, or units, are recorded with electrodes while the animal is presented with well defined visual stimuli in different regions in visual space.

In the retina, the receptive field is determined by the photoreceptors and other cells that influence the activity of a single ganglion cell. Retinal ganglion cells have receptive fields that can be represented as two concentric circles with opposite effects (Fig. 11–6). These fields can be of two types: 1) "on" center with "off" surround, and 2) "off" center with "on" surround. When describing receptive fields, "on" means excitatory, and "off" means inhibitory. A diffuse light that stimulates both the center and the surrounding area has little effect on ganglion cell activity. The maximum response occurs when a spot of light corresponds exactly to the excitatory region: a small spot that precisely fills the central area for the

"on center" cells and a doughnut shape that precisely fills the peripheral area for the "on surround" cells. In the LGN, neurons are similar to, but more specific than, retinal ganglion cells. LGN neurons respond to changes in retinal illumination and not just to the presence or absence of illumination.

In the visual cortex, receptive fields are more complex than in the LGN (see Fig. 11–6). For example, neurons that respond to orientation are not concentric. Instead, they respond maximally to either of two kinds of stimuli: dark or light narrow rectangles on a contrasting background—bars—or straight-line borders separating two areas of different brightness—edges. Cortical neurons respond vigorously to retinal stimuli of specific sizes in specific orientations. This specificity of orientation, called the **receptive field axis of orientation**, is critical and constant for a particular cell but differs among cells. Any deviation results in a less than maximal response.

Consider the theoretic receptive field represented in Figure 11–6B. It has a maximum response of 10 magnitude units to a stimulus 10 width units wide at a 90-degree angle. (The units of measurement here are undefined and are not relevant to the example.) A light bar of precisely these parameters will cause a +10 response. A bar 5 units wide will not fully excite all of the "on" cells represented in this field, so the output of the cortical cell will be less than 10. If the bar is 15 units wide, it will excite all of the on cells and some of the off cells, so, again, the response of the cortical neuron will be less than 10. If the bar is exactly 10 units wide but at an angle of 45 degrees rather than 90 degrees, some but not all of the retinal on cells and some but not all of the off cells will be stimulated. Again, the response of the cortical cell will be less than 10. In the extreme case, if the stimulus axis is at 90 degrees to the receptive field axis of orientation, the cortical neuron will not respond.

Primary visual cortex (V1) is organized in discrete columns running from the cortical surface to the white matter. All cells in each column have the same receptive field axis of orientation. These columns are fundamental functional units of the cortex. Each region of the visual field is anatomically represented in V1 many times in columns with different receptive field orientations. The cells in these columns can be divided into two functional categories: 1) **simple cells**, and 2) complex cells (see Fig. 11–6B, C).

Simple cells have a proper receptive field axis of orientation with on/off areas. The on areas are rectangular with specific sizes and widths, surrounded

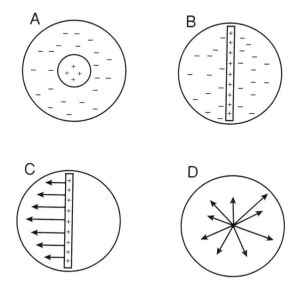

Figure 11–6. Receptive fields of cells in the visual pathway. **A:** Receptive field of a retinal ganglion cell. **B:** Receptive field of a simple type cortical cell. **C:** Receptive field of a complex cortical cell. **D:** Receptive field of a hypercomplex cortical cell. Retinal ganglion cells and simple cells respond to static stimuli; complex and hypercomplex cells respond to dynamic stimuli.

by large off regions. These properties are determined by anatomic connections and probably are hardwired (i.e., they do not change). A given **cortical column** has cells of a single receptive field axis of orientation, but the axis varies from column to column. Remember, neurons in layer 4 receive input directly from the LGN. Each simple cell probably receives inputs from many LGN neurons with their on-centers arranged in a straight line. The response properties of these cells are described in the example given previously. From the example, you can see that a large spot of light that covers the entire retina does not evoke a response in the simple cortical cells that respond to contrasts.

V1 has primarily simple cells. V2 and V3 have mostly complex cells. Complex cells also respond to bars and edges of the appropriate orientations, but they have another unique feature. They respond maximally to unidirectional movement of the stimulus, provided the stimulus orientation remains unchanged. Stimulus movement in one direction increases the cells' response, but stimulus movement in the opposite direction diminishes the response. These cells do not have an on/off organization. Instead, the specific change in position of the stimulus causes these cells to respond. Each complex cell probably receives inputs from many simple cells with the same axis of orientation. Thus, the striate cortex includes vast networks of highly specific intracortical connections between simple and complex cells. Some investigators have also speculated on the existence of **hypercomplex cells** in higher cortical areas that have more elaborate response properties, such as responses to multidirectional movements. These hypercomplex cells might receive inputs from multiple **complex type cells** that are either excitatory or inhibitory to unidirectional movements of retinal stimuli of specific sizes and orientations. These inputs could combine to produce the sensitivity to bidirectional motion seen in these hypercomplex cells. Even higher-order neurons have more complex response properties. Neurons in area MST show large receptive fields that respond to large-pattern motion such as expansion patterns. Expansion patterns are optically similar to patterns generated by observer movements in three-dimensional space. For example, when you walk toward a visual array, the scene appears to expand in size, and the change in size across the array has particular geometric properties. These changes provide visual cues that help to guide the motion. Neurons in area MST probably carry out

sophisticated, higher-order analyses of visual motion that may be the underlying neural mechanism for complex spatial behavior such as locomotion, driving, and wayfinding (spatial orientation).

Binocularity

As mentioned previously, V1 receives projections from both eyes and is the first opportunity for true binocular information representation.[17] More than three fourths of cortical neurons are influenced independently by the two eyes. **Binocular cells**, however, have receptive fields with point-by-point correspondence of organization and axes of orientation on the retina. Binocularity occurs when these corresponding points are stimulated simultaneously. The evidence indicates overwhelmingly that early visual experience can alter the distribution of the axis of orientation of striate cortical neurons, especially in binocular cells. Controlled visual deprivation experiments in animals have demonstrated that early visual experience, within the first 1 to 3 months of life, with binocular stimuli, not merely biocular stimuli, is critical to normal development of binocular cortical cells. Furthermore, binocular visual experience has a continuing and lasting effect on the functional organization of the striate cortex. From this work has come the concept of critical periods in development, and our understanding of the effects of sensory deprivation. These concepts are relevant to patients who are born with cataracts, and to those who lose binocularity and have double vision as the result of severely constricted visual fields or oculomotor paralysis.

Functional Organization

The first functional processing of visual input results from synchronous firing of retinal ganglion cells,[18] which fire in a time locked fashion when near one another but asynchronously when far from one another. Processing mechanisms, such as lateral inhibition and temporal adaptation, help maintain a high fidelity of visual representation while minimizing the amount of information transmitted, a feat that is accomplished by decreasing redundancy in the neural code. Therefore, multineuronal firing patterns provide important information to higher centers.

One result of this visual information processing is found in the dorsal aspect of the area MST of the monkey cerebral cortex, an area similar to area V5 in humans. Cells in this area have been shown to respond to expanding radial motion even though no receptors for radial motion have been found.[19] Optically, such a radial flow field occurs naturally as a result of self-motion through a static environment. These cells are sensitive to the direction, speed, and location of the center of motion.[20,21] Thus, they may be a class of hypercomplex cells the responses of which may be related to naturally occurring optical flow patterns that result from self-motion through a static environment, specifying important global parameters of self-motion.[22] More localized spatial parameters have been found in the supplementary eye fields of the monkey, an area responsible for higher-order oculomotor control.[23] These neurons do not encode visual or retinal space in any general sense. Rather, they include sensory or motor information defined in reference to the current object of interest. This information allows purposeful, visually guided behavior in reference to objects in the visual field. This ability is impaired in hemifield neglect, a clinical phenomenon in which the patient does not respond to object features on the side contralateral to the lesion, even though he or she sees the entire object with the intact visual field.

The phenomenon of subjective contours is also based on the functional organization of cortical cells. An example is a luminance border, which has no spatial discontinuity but is perceived as an edge. You may have been fooled by a shadow on a flat, two-dimensional wall that creates the impression of a three-dimensional surface. Neurons in V1 and V2 respond to subjective edges; these neurons are organized into discrete columns and spatial maps. Some cells respond to a combination of subjective and objective edges. These perceptual phenomena suggest an intricate level of network organization that begins in V1, continues in V2, and perhaps continues to higher centers.

Visual Spatial Orientation

The visual system provides information about spatial localization. To localize an object visually in space, such as that snack I so desperately want but can't have until I finish writing this section, the CNS needs information about the position of the retinal image and the orientation of the eye in the head. The problem can be simplified as follows: given a movable eye and movable objects, how are changes in the retinal image pattern evaluated? The receptive field of any given cell moves with the retina, so after an eye movement that cell covers a different point in vi-

sual space. If an object enters a receptive field, how does the CNS distinguish between an object that has moved while the eye is stationary and eye movement that brings a stationary object into the field? To experience the problem, look quickly from the left to the right margin of this page. Now look straight ahead at the page while you move the page from right to left. Although your eye receives the same stimulation in both situations, you have no doubt that your eye, not the page, moved. Models of various types of comparator mechanisms suggest that retinal image slip is evaluated against independent kinesthetic information about eye position.[24–28]

One possible set of comparator neurons may be located in the parietal lobe. These neurons have receptive fields that change in anticipation of eye movements and predict the retinal consequences of such a movement. In addition, neurons in area MST are maximally responsive to expansion patterns with centers of motion that are off center in the receptor field. This finding indicates that more complex spatial behavior such as obstacle avoidance and nonlinear approach have their neural underpinnings in this area, and the results indicate the dynamic nature of visual information processing even on a single-cell level.

Vision also influences posture, presumably through the visual input to the vestibular nuclei (see Chap. 10). Neurons carrying eye movement signals to the oculomotor centers have also been found to project downward as far as the cervical levels of the spinal cord. Presumably these visual/vestibular eye movement signals are involved in control of neck reflexes, such as the vestibulocollic reflex.

Control of Eye Movements

Vision is a distance sense that is largely dedicated to localizing objects in space. Detailed visual information can be obtained only through the fovea, a very small area in the central retina. To obtain detailed information about a large object of interest, the eyes must scan the object by moving the fovea over the area. Therefore the visual system must be involved in controlling eye movements.

The Extraocular Muscles

One of the major pathways of association fibers in the cortex is from the visual cortex to the motor eye fields, which is part of Brodmann's area 8. The motor eye fields seem to be responsible for planning voluntary eye movements not dependent on visual stimuli. Area 8 is located in the frontal lobe, principally on the caudal part of the middle frontal gyrus (see Fig. 11–5), and extends into contiguous portions of the inferior frontal gyrus. Electrical stimulation of the eye fields results in **conjugate** deviations of the eyes to the side contralateral to the stimulation. Data from electrical stimulation and lesion studies in monkeys suggest the presence of an occipital eye center responsible for conjugate eye movements to the opposite side. This occipital center is not localized to any one visual area, although V1 seems to be the most sensitive. These centers control eye movements in response to visual stimuli. Both the frontal and occipital eye fields probably control eye movements indirectly through projections to the SC, which, in turn, projects to nuclei in the pontine and medullary reticular formations and the accessory oculomotor nuclei.

Accurate eye movements, regardless of the original stimuli for them, require coordination between the two eyes. Coordination is accomplished through the coordinated manipulation of six distinct extraocular muscles attached to the globe: the medial, lateral, superior, and **inferior rectus muscles** and superior and **inferior oblique muscles**. These muscles have few muscle fibers, each of which is controlled by an individual nerve fiber, which allows for highly accurate control of eye movements. All of the extraocular muscles are striated muscles, although some aspects of their structures differ from skeletal muscles, as discussed in Chapter 13. The recti and the **superior oblique muscles** originate from a tendon that surrounds the optic foramen at the back of the orbit, "the common tendinous ring" or "the annulus of Zinn." This tendon inserts into the sphenoid bone. The recti insert into the sclera in front of the equator and the obliques insert into the sclera behind the equator. The "equator" refers to the area that is roughly halfway from the cornea to the macula along the sclera or retina (i.e., the midpoint of the eye). The location, actions, and innervation of each muscle are discussed in the following paragraphs and summarized in Table 11–1.

The medial and lateral recti move the eye in yaw rotation. The **medial rectus** runs from its origin at the optic foramen, along the medial wall of the orbit to its insertion onto the sclera 5.5 mm behind the limbus. It is the most powerful of the extraocular muscles, and has only one action, **adduction**, that is, turning the eye toward the nose. It is controlled by the inferior division of the oculomotor nerve (CN III). The **lateral rectus** runs along the lateral wall of the orbit to its insertion onto the sclera 7 mm behind the limbus. Like the medial rectus, the lateral rectus has only one action. It abducts the eye, moving the eye away from the midline, to look away from the nose. The lateral rectus is controlled by the abducens nerve (CN VI).

The inferior rectus runs along the floor of the orbit from the orbital apex to its insertion 6.5 mm behind the limbus. It makes a 23-degree angle with the medial wall of the orbit. Because of this angle, contraction of the inferior rectus makes the eye move in more than one direction. The primary action of this muscle is depression of the globe, that is, rotating the eye down toward the maxillary bone. The inferior rectus also assists in adducting the eye, and weakly assists in extorting it. **Extorsion** is a motion in which the top of the eye rotates out, toward the temple, and the bottom of the eye rotates in, toward the nose. This muscle is also controlled by the inferior division of the oculomotor nerve (CN III).

The **superior rectus** runs along the roof of the orbit from the orbital apex to its insertion 7.7 mm behind the limbus. Like the inferior rectus, it also makes a 23-degree angle with the medial wall. Therefore, it also has several actions, which are directly opposite those of the inferior rectus. The primary action of the superior rectus is elevation. It rotates the eyeball upward toward the frontal bone. The secondary action of the superior rectus is **abduction**, and the tertiary action is **intorsion**, rolling the top of the eye toward the nose and the bottom of the eye toward the temple. This muscle is controlled by the superior division of the oculomotor nerve (CN III).

The superior oblique muscle originates on the annulus of Zinn, or very near it on the sphenoid bone. It runs along the superior medial wall to a small bony loop at the front of the orbit, called the **trochlea**, which acts as its functional origin. The ligament of the muscle passes through the trochlea and is reflected back onto the globe to its insertion just behind the equator of the globe. This ligament makes an angle of 51 to 53 degrees with the medial wall. Therefore, this muscle also has several actions. The primary action is depression, turning the eye down toward the maxillary bone. Its secondary action is abduction, turning the eye away from the nose. The tertiary action of the superior oblique is intorsion. The superior oblique is controlled by the trochlear nerve (CN IV).

TABLE 11-1

Individual Extraocular Muscles and Their Actions

Muscle	Innervation	Primary Action	Secondary Action	Tertiary Action
Medical rectus	CN III	Adduction	—	—
Lateral rectus	CN VI	Abduction	—	—
Superior rectus	CN III	Elevation	Intorsion	Adduction
Inferior rectus	CN III	Depression	Extorsion	Adduction
Superior oblique	CN IV	Intorsion	Depression	Abduction
Inferior oblique	CN III	Extorsion	Elevation	Abduction

The inferior oblique is the only extraocular muscle that originates at the front of the orbit. It begins at a fossa (depression) in the maxillary bone near the lacrimal sac, and runs between the eye and the inferior rectus. It, too, makes an angle of 51 to 53 degrees—the same angle as the superior oblique tendon—to its insertion just below the lateral rectus. The actions of the inferior oblique are opposite those of the superior oblique. Its primary action is elevation, with adduction and extorsion being the secondary and tertiary actions. It is also innervated by the inferior division of the oculomotor nerve (CN III).

The six extraocular muscles of each eye are arranged as three opponent pairs, so the action of one muscle of each pair is directly opposed by the action of the other muscle. These pairs, called antagonists or yoked muscle pairs, are listed in Table 11–2. The pairing of muscles of the two eyes that move the eyes in the same direction (i.e., to the left, or up) is an im-

portant association. These pairs are called agonists, and their action relative to eye movements are illustrated in Figure 11–7. The muscle pairs must respond properly to the neural signal to move the eyes if proper binocular alignment is to be maintained. If one muscle is paretic or paralytic, **strabismus** results. Strabismus is the inability to direct both eyes to an object of regard at the same time. It can indicate an underlying neurologic deficit or muscular damage.

Neural Control of Eye Movements

Gaze is eye movement that brings an object of interest onto the fovea. The two eyes make five kinds of eye movements: four conjugate, (i.e., in the same direction) and one **disconjugate** (i.e., in the opposite direction). The four conjugate eye movements are the **vestibuloocular reflex** (VOR), **optokinetic nystagmus** (OKN), pursuit, and **saccadic** eye movements or **saccades**. The disconjugate eye movements are **vergence** eye movements. Except for some saccades and vergence movements, all eye movements are reflexes, and are not considered to be under voluntary control. The VOR is, as its name implies, a vestibularly driven, conjugate, compensatory movement of the eyes in response to head movement (see Chap. 10). OKN can be considered a special case of **smooth pursuit** eye movements elicited by whole-field moving visual stimuli combined with refixation saccades.

Smooth pursuit eye movements are stimulated by "slip" of visual images across the retina. This retinal

TABLE 11-2

Yoked Extraocular Muscle Pairs

Ipsilateral Eye	Contralateral Eye
Medical rectus	Lateral rectus
Superior rectus	Inferior oblique
Inferior rectus	Superior oblique

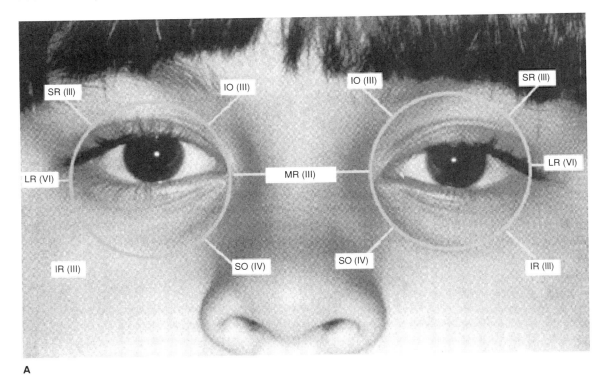

A

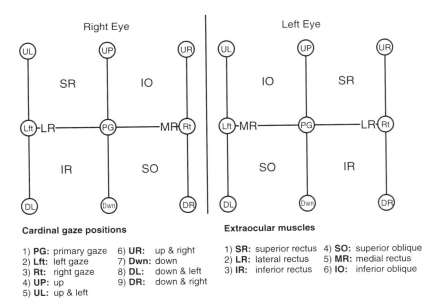

B

Figure 11-7. A: Muscle action planes. The lines normal to the circle indicate direction of eye movement. The primary extraocular muscle involved is indicated by initials and the cranial nerve innervating this muscle is indicated in parentheses. See **B** for abbreviations. **B:** The nine clinical standard positions of gaze and their relation to the action planes of the extraocular muscles.

image slip generates an error signal that stimulates the oculomotor pathways to move the eyes at the same rate as the moving image, to keep the visual image on the fovea. If you have ever watched a sail drift slowly on the horizon or watched someone walk across your visual field from one side to the other, you have used your smooth pursuit system. Last year I watched my nephew taking his first few steps: I pointed my fovea on the proud face of this new walker and as he moved forward his image moved off my fovea. I, the proud but cautious uncle, moved my eye to keep his face fixed on my fovea. This smooth, slow visual following is accomplished by the pursuit system.

When the entire visual field moves, rather than a discrete stimulus, OKN is elicited. If you have ever gone to the movies and watched a scene in which the camera looked out the window of an airplane so that the entire visual scene moved, you used OKN to watch the scene. Likewise, if you have ever sat in a stationary train and looked out the window as an adjacent train moved past in the opposite direction (with the confusing sensation that you were moving), you used OKN to watch the train as the visual input fooled your vestibular system momentarily. OKN is a slow system, most accurate at low frequencies, below 0.1 Hz. It probably shares many parts of the pathway with smooth pursuit, but also may involve some projections from the nucleus of the optic tract to accessory oculomotor nuclei.[29]

Saccades are rapid eye movements that occur so quickly that you do not see during them. They can be as fast 1,000 degrees per second. Saccades are stimulated by changes in the position of the image on the retina, such as the rapid changes that occur when watching a quickly moving stimulus such as a tennis ball. Perhaps while watching a tennis game one day you fixated on the server, but, with the explosive speed of the serve, you were unable to watch the ball with the slow eye movements of pursuit. To catch up with the image, you generated saccades reflexively. Saccades are also generated voluntarily, as when scanning a stationary visual field. You are using saccades to read this page.

Figure 11–8 illustrates the neural mechanisms for generation and control of some eye movements. Many tiny nuclei in the medial pons and medulla are involved. The final signals, however, ascend from higher-order neurons in the vestibular nuclei, carrying complex signals that have been processed many times, to the nuclei of CN III, IV, and VI through the

MLF. The MLF is, in effect, the final common pathway for eye movements. The term, **final common pathway**, refers to the last point at which information is collected before being sent to the motor efferents for control of movement.

More specifically, signals for a saccade to the right (i.e., activation of the right lateral rectus and the left medial rectus) begin in the left frontal eye field of the premotor cortex, travel down through the anterior limb of the internal capsule, and reach the medial cerebral peduncle. At the level of the trochlear nucleus, the fibers decussate and synapse in the paramedian pontine reticular formation. Here neurons project to the abducens nucleus, and interneurons decussate to the opposite MLF and ascend the brainstem to the medial rectus subnucleus. In addition, the paramedian pontine reticular formation contains an inhibitory system for the right medial rectus and left lateral rectus. A parallel pathway originates in the SC. The pursuit gaze center is in the deep parietooccipital junction near the occipital trigone of the lateral ventricle. It receives its driving commands from the ipsilateral V1. The pursuit system is still poorly delineated, but seems to include visual areas of the temporal and parietal lobes, the pontine nuclei, and the cerebellar flocculus.[8] Lesions in these areas impair conjugate eye movements.

Vergence movements include both **convergence** and **divergence**. Convergence, where both eyes turn toward the nose, helps maintain clear vision as objects approach from optical infinity (more than 3 m) to near the eye. Accommodation, a focusing mechanism, and pupil constriction, which increases the depth of focus, are also involved in maintaining a clear visual image. The neural circuitry controlling convergence is poorly understood, but animal experiments have suggested that the nucleus perlia in the midbrain might be an important control center. Divergence, where both eyes turn away from the nose, is not a unique control system but rather a relaxation of the convergence response to a neutral distance point.

The VOR is a compensatory eye movement, made in response to head movements, to stabilize gaze in space while the head is moving. In the dark, the pure VOR is inaccurate, but when complemented by OKN in the light, the reflex compensates completely for head movements. The VOR is stimulated by vestibular signals, and is responsive at the high frequencies that usually encompass the range of normal head movements. OKN is stimulated by slow slip of the vi-

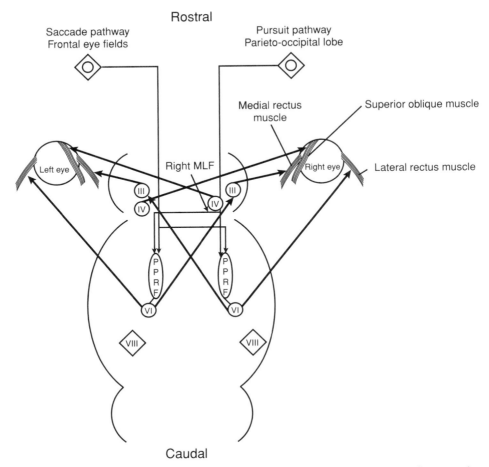

Rostral

Saccade pathway
Frontal eye fields

Pursuit pathway
Parieto-occipital lobe

Medial rectus
muscle

Superior oblique muscle

Left eye

Right MLF

Right eye

Lateral rectus muscle

III

IV

III

IV

P
P
R
F

P
P
R
F

VI

VI

VIII

VIII

Caudal

Figure 11–8. Pathways for control of the three major conjugate eye movements: saccades, smooth pursuit, and vestibulo-ocular reflex. VIII: Vestibular nuclei. VI: Abducens nucleus. III: Oculomotor nucleus. IV: Trochlear nucleus. MLF: Medial longitudinal fasciculus. PPRF: Paramedian pontine reticular formation.

sual image across the peripheral retina and is responsive at very low frequencies, below 0.1 Hz. The combination of these eye movements makes the system able to respond to movement of the visual world or the person through a wide range of frequencies. This ability to maintain gaze stabilization is important for recognizing objects and people while moving, because your head moves as you walk and even during conversation as you nod to indicate comprehension. Loss of vestibular function or loss of visual function in the accessory optic tract or other brainstem visual areas causes loss of visual acuity, charac-

terized by complaints of blurred vision. Remember that to maintain a clear visual image, you must focus the image on the retinal fovea. As you move your head when you walk, the visual world changes position in reference to your position. Therefore you must constantly update the position of your eye in your head to maintain a stable, clear gaze.

As you learned in Chapter 10, the pathways for the VOR are well known. They involve input from the vestibular portion of CN VIII, neurons in the vestibular nuclei, secondary pathways in the vestibulocerebellum, and signals ascending the MLF to the nuclei of the oculomotor cranial nerves. Damage to the vestibular labyrinth or to any of the central pathways impairs this reflex.

Clinical Correlations

Loss of visual information, or the ability to use vision, is extremely disabling. Most people rely heavily on vision to orient to and interact with the world. Loss of the information or impairment in visual function is disorientating. Perhaps 90% of our spatial information is visual in origin. Epidemiologically, decreased vision is the third-ranking reason for limiting activities of daily living (heart disease and arthritis are the top two), and half of all people with decreased vision report difficulty performing activities of daily living.

Oculomotor Abnormalities

Deviation of the visual axes relative to each other is the most common sign in all neuromuscular anomalies of the eyes, except for supranuclear lesions. Strabismus causes either **diplopia** or suppression of vision from one eye. These symptoms are potentially problematic to adults, but may critically interfere with the developing visual system in children and may prevent the development of normal visual acuity. The visual system is organized to receive inputs from corresponding loci on the retina and process these signals into a single visual percept. Strabismus creates a situation in which yoked retinal loci receive different retinal images because of the misalignment of the eyes (as in a "wall-eyed" person), so the brain cannot resolve the two disparate images into a single percept. This situation is not tolerable to the visual system, so the system ignores the input from one eye. If suppression occurs while the visual system is still developing (in children younger than 8 years of age), the system will not develop normally.

The underlying causes of strabismus are varied and include mechanical abnormalities, accommodative dysfunction, muscle paresis, brainstem lesions, and vestibular abnormalities.[30] In adults, sudden onset of strabismus and diplopia often indicates CNS lesions. Also, any lesion in the cortex or brainstem above the level of the ocular motor nuclei may cause a gaze palsy. Hemispheric lesions produce tonic deviation of both eyes toward the side of the lesion and away from the side of hemiparesis, which can last for several days. Seizure activity in the frontal eye fields and motor cortex also causes gaze deviations. Lesions of the dorsal midbrain may cause upward gaze paralysis and downgaze nystagmus. Brainstem lesions at the level of the pons cause eye deviation toward the side of the hemiparesis because ascending gaze control fibers have decussated but descending motor fibers have not.

Diplopia is a main symptom of patients with any type of ocular motility dysfunction. Intermittent diplopia occurs either because ocular alignment occurs only some of the time or because vision from one eye is suppressed intermittently. Lesions of the MLF between the pons and the oculomotor nucleus cause a characteristic pattern of disconjugate gaze with impaired adduction and nystagmus of the adducting eye. Usually, although not always, young patients have multiple sclerosis and old patients have cerebral vascular disease.

Lesions of CN IV (trochlear nerve) cause paresis of the superior oblique muscle, resulting in a failure of the eye to depress in adduction with consequent vertical diplopia. The eye is extorted and hypertorted, sometimes with a compensatory head posture in which the head is tilted, the chin depressed and the face turned toward the unaffected side. These lesions are typically caused by head trauma, although vascular disease may also be involved. Lesions of CN VI (abducens nerve) cause paresis of the lateral rectus muscle. Because the medial rectus retains normal tone, the eye is pulled inward, causing esotropia accompanied by horizontal diplopia and sometimes a compensatory head posture with the face turned to the affected side. These lesions are typically idiopathic or caused by vascular disease, including diabetes.

Lesions of CN III can effect all of the remaining extraocular muscles. These lesions therefore present in many ways that often involve other symptoms such as impaired pupillary light responses. In the case of a complete third nerve palsy, the affected eye is exotropic, intorted, and somewhat hypotropic. Usually patients do not have diplopia because the ptosis makes binocularity impossible. For the same reason, compensatory head postures are not present.

Nystagmus is a combination of slow and fast eye movements that can be normal in some circumstances and abnormal in others. Specific types of nystagmus can arise from lesions at various sites. For example, periodic alternating nystagmus can be due to lesions of the cervicomedullary junction or lesions in the vestibulocerebellum. It can also be caused by CVA, tumors, multiple sclerosis, drug intoxication, degenerative diseases, or dense cataracts. If the lesion is central, nystagmus has a fast phase that changes with the direction of gaze, cannot be suppressed by visual fixation, and may even be enhanced by fixation.

Insults to the Visual Pathway

Because of its peculiar anatomy, an insult to the visual pathway causes characteristic losses of visual sensitivity known as field defects, or **scotomas**. In classic neurology and in areas where advanced brain imaging techniques are not available, the ability to determine the lesion location based on visual field defects is important for diagnosis. A field defect that affects approximately one fourth of the visual field in either eye is called a **quadrantanopsia** or **quadrantanopia**. A loss of half of the visual field of either eye is called a **hemianopsia** or hemianopia. If a field defect such as a hemianopsia exists in both eyes, and if it affects the same field in each eye, it is called **homonymous**. For example, a scotoma involving the right half of the visual field in both eyes is homonymous. A field loss that involves the right half of the visual field in the right eye and the left half of the visual field of the left eye is not homonymous.

Lesions of the retina or the optic nerve cause unilateral field defects. Bilateral, often homonymous, losses occur with chiasmal and postchiasmal lesions (see Fig. 11–4). If the lesion is at the chiasm, the visual field defect is usually bilateral. Combining this knowledge with the area of the field affected helps locate the lesion. For example, a pituitary adenoma, a cancer of the pituitary gland, destroys the crossing nasal fibers because of its location directly above the chiasm, resulting in a characteristic loss of the temporal field in both eyes, a bitemporal hemianopsia. The temporal fibers can be damaged by compressing the chiasm from the sides, which can occur in the case of an internal carotid artery aneurysm. Because the internal carotid arteries run vertically up the sides of the chiasm, a bulge in the wall of the internal carotid artery may push against the side of the chiasm where the fibers representing the temporal field are located. The field defect that results from damage to the temporal fibers is a binasal hemianopsia because the temporal fibers convey the information from the nasal field. Binasal and bitemporal scotomas are not homonymous because they do not affect the same side of the visual field in each eye. Lesions of the optic tract produce homonymous hemianopsias that affect the field on the opposite side. For example, an injury to the left optic tract produces a right homonymous hemianopsia; that is, the vision in the right half of the visual field of both eyes is lost.

Because of the close alignment of neurons representing the same spatial locations in the LGN, lesions of the LGN or deeper in the CNS create identical defects in each eye. All such defects are homonymous and identical. This information helps to localize lesions in the postchiasmal part of the pathway because lesions between the chiasm and the LGN produce similar, but usually not identical defects in the two eyes. The long path of the inferior fibers in the optic radiations makes them susceptible to insults to the temporal lobe, resulting in a homonymous superior quadrantanopsia. This field defect is often wedge shaped and stops at the midline, causing a "pie-in-the-sky" defect. Because of the anatomy of the parietal lobe pathways, a lesion in the parietal lobe can cause complete homonymous hemianopsia with macular splitting. Information from one half of the visual field, including the ipsilateral half of the retinal macula, never reaches V1. Also common are abnormal eye movements due to damage to the corticomesencephalic tract between areas 18 and 19 and a nucleus in the pons concerned with eye movements.

Specific lesions in the visual areas demonstrate the functional processing distinctions based on the site of the lesion. For example, a CVA of area 17 can lead to a hemianopsia. A left hemianopsia creates a reading problem because the patient gets to the end of the line, on the right of the page, and cannot find the beginning, on the left. A right hemianopsia creates a related problem because the patient is not aware of the end of the line and so never finishes. A CVA of area 17 can also cause cortical blindness,[31] in which light patterns are detected by the lower centers such as the retina and the lower visual pathway, but cannot be interpreted by the cortex, so the person appears to be functionally blind. For example, the patient can, on instruction, reach to the right and pick up some keys, but cannot identify them visually. These patients, however, retain OKN and show almost normal VORs in the light. They can also use visual information to modify their posture, but they cannot see in the ordinary sense. Another example is cerebral dyschromatopsia (mentioned previously), a condition in which the person is unable to see the world in color after a cortical lesion despite normal retinal color mechanisms. In this condition, form vision can be essentially normal. Another condition, cerebral **akinetopsia**, may follow lesions to V5. In this syndrome, the patient is unable to perceive an object in motion but perceives the object normally when stationary. Again, retinal mechanisms are not involved. Experimental lesions in V4 and V5 support these clinical observations. Similarly, a selective inability to see objects in depth (i.e., disparity) has been described clinically and may be caused by lesions of V1, V2, or V3 but not V4 or V5. Animal models of these impairments have not yet been developed.

Conclusions

Vision is one of the ultimate achievements of human evolution. The extent of neurologic complexity in the visual system is slowly being revealed as increasingly sophisticated techniques are used to investigate visual cortical areas. For example, functional magnetic resonance imaging has revealed visual areas that are probably related to reading ability, contrast sensitivity, and visually guided behavior.[32,33] These modern techniques have established that over half of the nonhuman primate neocortex is concerned with visual information processing. Over 25 separately identifiable visual areas beyond V1 have been mapped by modern techniques. These findings suggest that much of the human neocortex, far beyond the currently identified five visual areas, may also be involved in visual information processing. In addition, experiments on human visual perception have demonstrated the critical importance of visual memory and visual attention. The neural mechanisms underlying these processes remain unclear, but imaging studies in humans and lesion studies in lower animals are beginning to reveal the underlying neural mechanisms.

Acknowledgment

Preparation of this manuscript was partially supported by an unrestricted grant to the Department of Ophthalmology, University of Maryland, Baltimore, from Research to Prevent Blindness, Inc.

REFERENCES

1. Zeki S. The visual image in mind and brain. *Sci Am* 1992;267:68–76.
2. Stoerig P, Cowey A. Visual perception and phenomenal consciousness. *Behav Brain Res* 1995;71:147–156.
3. Warwick R, ed. *Eugene Wolff's anatomy of the eye and orbit*. 7th ed. Philadelphia: WB Saunders, 1976.
4. Koretz J, Handelman G. How the human eye focuses. *Sci Am* 1988;259:92–99.
5. Dowling J. *The retina: an approachable part of the brain*. Cambridge, MA: Harvard University Press, 1987.
6. Kuffler S, Nicholls J, Martin A. *From neuron to brain*. Sunderland, MA: Sinauer Associates, 1984.
7. Towsend J, et al. *Visual fields: clinical case presentations*. Boston: Butterworth, 1991.
8. Walsh T. *Neuro-opthalmology: clinical signs and symptoms*. Philadelphia: Lea & Febiger, 1992.
9. Celesia G, DeMarco P. Anatomy and physiology of the visual system. *J Clin Neurophysiol* 1994;11:482–492.
10. Mustari MJ, Fuchs AF, Kaneko CR, Robinson FR. Anatomical connections of the primate pretectal nucleus of the optic tract. *J Comp Neurol* 1994;349:111–128.
11. Büttner-Enever JA, Cohen B, Horn AKE, Reisine H. Efferent pathways of the nucleus of the optic tract in monkey and their role in eye movements. *J Comp Neurol* 1996;373:90–107.
12. Netter F. Nervous system, part 1: anatomy and physiology. In: Brass A, ed. *The CIBA collection of medical illustrations*. Vol. 1. Summit, NJ: CIBA Medical Education, 1986.
13. Zeki S. *A vision of the brain*. Oxford: Blackwell Scientific, 1993.
14. Hubel D, Wiesel T. Brain mechanisms of vision. *Sci Am* 1979;241:150–162.
15. Hartline H. The response of single optic nerve fibers of the vertebrate eye to illumination of the retina. *Am J Physiol* 1938;121:400–415.
16. Riggs L. Electrophysiology of vision. In: Graham C, et al, eds. *Vision and visual perception*. New York: John Wiley & Sons, 1965:81–131.
17. Hubel D. Exploration of the primary visual cortex, 1955–78. *Nature* 1982;299:515–524.
18. Meister M, Lagnado L, Baylor D. Concerted signaling by retinal ganglion cells. *Science* 1995;270:1207–1210.
19. Duffy C, Wurtz R. Response of monkey MST neurons to optic flow stimuli with shifted centers of motion. *J Neurosci* 1995;15:5192–5208.
20. Duffy C, Wurtz R. Planar directional contributions to optic flow responses in MST neurons. *J Neurophysiol* 1997;77:782–796.
21. Duffy C, Wurtz R. Medial superior temporal area neurons respond to speed patterns in optic flow. *J Neurosci* 1997;17:2839–2851.
22. Gibson J. *The ecological approach to visual perception*. Boston: Houghton Mifflin, 1979.

23. Olson C, Gettner S. Object-centered direction selectivity in the macaque supplementary eye field. *Science* 1995;269:985–988.

24. Fox C. Some visual influences on postural equilibrium in humans: binocular and monocular fixation. *Perception and Psychophysics* 1990;47:409–422.

25. Leigh RJ, Zee DS. *The neurology of eye movements.* Philadelphia: FA Davis, 1991.

26. Buettner-Ennever JA, ed. *Neuroanatomy of the oculomotor system.* Amsterdam: Elsevier, 1988.

27. Wurtz RH, Goldberg ME, eds. *The neurobiology of saccadic eye movements.* Amsterdam: Elsevier, 1989.

28. Matin L, Li W. Multimodal basis for egocentric spatial localization and orientation. *J Vestib Res* 1995;5:499–518.

29. Büttner-Ennever JA, Cohen B, Horn AKE, Reisine H. Pretectal projections to the oculomotor complex of the monkey and their role in eye movements. *J Comp Neurol* 1996;366:348–359.

30. von Noorden G. *Burian-von Noorden's binocular vision and ocular motility: theory and management of strabismus.* St. Louis: CV Mosby, 1980:150–165.

31. Gazzaniga M, Fendrich R, Wessinger M. Blindsight reconsidered. *Current Directions in Psychological Sciences* 1994;3(3):93–96.

32. Sereno M, et al. Borders of medical visual areas in humans revealed by functional magnetic resonance imaging. *Science* 1995;268:889–893.

33. Tootell R, et al. Functional analysis of human MT and related visual cortical areas using magnetic resonance imaging. *J Neurosci* 1995;15:3215–3230.

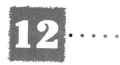

Special Senses 4: The Chemical Senses

MARION E. FRANK, PhD
JANNEANE F. GENT, PhD

• • •

The three external chemical senses are taste (gustation), smell (olfaction), and the **common chemical sense** (irritation). These three senses are anatomically and physiologically separate, but are often confused.[1] For example, before we even put pieces of our mother's famous enchiladas into our mouths, our sense of smell has already told us if it has too much oregano in it. Once in our mouths, our sense of taste tells us that it is not too salty, as our sense of smell continues to report that the amount of cumin is just right, and our common chemical sense begins to beg us to take a drink of water soon because the habañero chili pepper really has a bite to it. In fact, it is nearly impossible for people to identify reliably which system is telling us what. It is no wonder that patients with head trauma, for example, which can result in damage to the olfactory nerve, often report losing their sense of *taste* after their accident. The loss of the sense of smell, which is what these patients have actually experienced, has a tremendous impact on the perception of flavor, which includes the sensations of smell as well as taste and irritation.

Each of these three specialized chemical senses has a role to play in maintaining a healthy human being: the taste system evaluates the nutritional value or harmful nature of chemicals taken into the mouth and contributes to the pleasure of eating; the olfactory system is highly developed for the detection and analysis of environmental chemicals, and contributes to social, reproductive, and nutritional

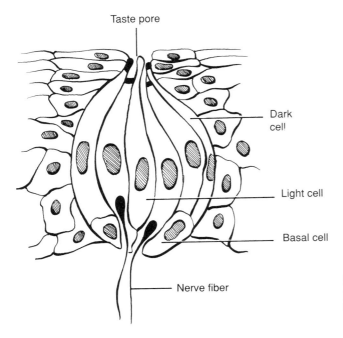

Taste pore

Dark cell

Light cell

Basal cell

Nerve fiber

Figure 12–1. A taste bud. (Adapted and used with permission from Frank ME, Rabin MD. Chemosensory neuroanatomy and physiology. *Ear Nose Throat J* 1989;68: 292–296.)

choices, as well as choices of habitat; and the common chemical sense detects chemicals that injure contacted tissue and is responsible for reflex responses (such as gagging, coughing, sneezing) to irritating chemicals in the oral/nasal cavity.

The Gustatory System

Taste Receptors

Taste **receptor** cells are modified epithelial cells that are found in spherical clusters called taste buds (Fig. 12–1) within the lingual **epithelium** and elsewhere in the oropharyngeal **mucosa**. Cells in taste buds are constantly regenerating, having an average life span of about 10 days.[2] The interaction between gustatory nerve endings and taste buds is an example of **neurotrophism**: if denervated, taste buds degenerate but do not disappear.[3]

Lingual taste buds are dispersed over the **dorsal** surface of the **anterior** two thirds of the tongue (Fig. 12–2) in hundreds of **fungiform papillae**, as well as on the **lateral** edges of the **posterior** tongue, in a few **foliate papillae**, and on the dorsum of the posterior tongue in a few **circumvallate papillae**. Each

fungiform papilla contains a few taste buds. Each foliate or circumvallate papilla contains hundreds of taste buds.[4] Taste buds are also located in places other than on the tongue, namely on the soft palate and oral pharynx, including the epiglottis.

Taste Stimulus Transduction

Oral solutions enter taste pores and interact with membranes of taste receptor cells that project into taste pores (see Fig. 12–1) as **microvilli**. The type of chemical present determines how the taste system translates, or transduces information about that chemical.[5,6] In general, all chemicals can be classified as ionic or nonionic. Some ions, such as Na^+, are basic to sustaining physiologic function. Specific pathways (ion channels) permit passage of ions into cells. Initial **transduction** of ionic taste stimuli uses membrane ion channels directly. For example, Na^+Cl^- (the positive sodium ions and negative chloride ions that make up salt) is transduced by influx of Na^+ through amiloride-sensitive ion channels, which results in a **depolarization** of the receptor cell. The fact that the ion channels are "amiloride sensitive" puts them into a class of channels, such as

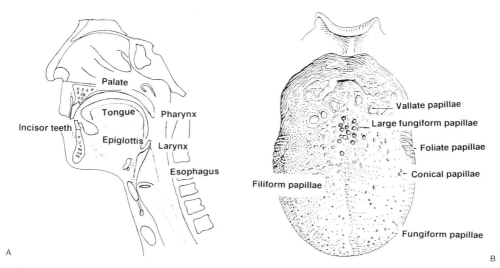

Figure 12–2. A: Human oropharyngeal cavity. **B:** Human tongue. (Adapted and used with permission from Miller IJ Jr, Bartoshuk LM. Taste perception, taste bud distribution, and spatial relationships. In: Getchell TV, Doty RL, Bartoshuk LM, Snow JB Jr, eds. *Smell and taste in health and disease.* New York: Raven Press, 1991:216.)

those in the gut, that are blocked by the diuretic, amiloride. Nonionic taste stimuli (such as sugars) are transduced by binding to proteinaceous receptor molecules in the membrane, which are coupled to second-messenger systems (see Chapter 4 on neurotransmitters). A G-protein **(gustducin),** with a subunit very similar to **transducin** in the retina, is expressed specifically in taste bud tissue. For nonionic stimuli, initial transduction is followed by cascades of intracellular biochemical events, which may use **cyclic adenosine monophosphate (cAMP).** Resulting changes in receptor cell potential opens voltage-dependent Ca++ (positive calcium ions) channels. Finally, increase in intracellular Ca++ leads to transmitter release at synapses located at the base of taste receptor cells, activating gustatory nerve endings.

Chemicals that are usually considered to elicit the primary taste sensations (e.g., sweet, bitter, salty, sour) fall into different chemical groups.[7] For example, sweet-tasting chemicals are typically caloric sources with a limited number of **hydrophilic** molecular structures such as sugars, certain amino acids, and artificial sweeteners (e.g., saccharin, aspartame). Bitter-tasting chemicals are typically poisons with diverse **lipophilic** chemical structures, such as **alkaloids,** thioureas, bile acids, and glycosides. Certain amino acids and salts (e.g., potassium

chloride [KCl]) are also bitter. Interestingly, genetically altered animals that do not express gustducin demonstrate profound deficits in sweet and bitter taste.[8] Only sodium and lithium salts have a pure salty taste—hence the difficulty in designing a substitute for the salt craving. Acids are sour tasting, but are also irritants.

Taste Nerves

One reason that a true, total, and complete loss of the sense of taste is so rare[9] is that the taste system is served by six nerves: branches of three cranial nerves, bilaterally (Fig. 12–3). The primary **afferent** relay neurons for taste are **pseudounipolar** neurons with **somata** in three **peripheral nervous system** ganglia (plural of **ganglion**) and small **myelin**ated and unmyelinated **axons.** Taste buds in the fungiform papillae are innervated by the **chorda tympani nerve** and taste buds on the palate are innervated by the greater superficial petrosal nerve. These nerves are both sensory branches of the facial nerve (cranial nerve VII), with cell bodies in the geniculate ganglion and central axonal processes in the intermediate nerve. The taste buds that they innervate are well located for a role in food selection. Taste buds in the foliate and circumvallate papillae are inner-

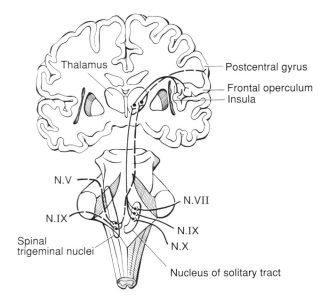

Figure 12–3. Neural pathways for taste (solid lines) and the common chemical sense (dotted lines) on the dorsal surface of the brainstem and a coronal section through the forebrain. (Adapted and used with permission from Frank ME, Rabin MD. Chemosensory neuroanatomy and physiology, *Ear Nose Throat J* 1989:68:292–296.)

vated by the lingual branch of the **glossopharyngeal nerve** (cranial nerve IX), with cell bodies in the petrosal ganglion. The taste buds that they innervate are well located to play a role in reflexes and swallowing. Extralingual taste buds of the pharynx are innervated by the superior laryngeal branch of the **vagus nerve** (cranial nerve X), with cell bodies in the nodose ganglion. These taste buds are well located to initiate reflexes that protect the airway.

Coding in Primary Taste Afferent Neurons

The activity of the taste nerves codes the information about the taste of a particular chemical that is present in the mouth. Different chemicals produce different levels of activity in the various single nerve fibers that make up each nerve. The pattern of activity is the code that is sent to the brain; different types of chemicals produce different patterns. Many single taste nerve fibers in the chorda tympani and glossopharyngeal nerves of rodents are selectively sensitive to compounds of one taste quality[10] (Fig. 12–4). For example, fibers that are sensitive to sucrose respond to fructose and D-phenylalanine, which are also sweet. They typically do not respond to NaCl, HCl, or quinine, which are not sweet. Similarly, nerve fibers that are sensitive to NaCl respond to other so-

dium salts and lithium salts, which are all salty. In contrast, other taste nerve fibers respond nonselectively. For example, chorda tympani and glossopharyngeal nerve fibers that are sensitive to HCl and that respond to other acids that are sour, also respond to many salty and bitter salts. These neural units have been termed *generalists*, in contrast to the *specialists* that respond to taste stimuli of one quality.[7] Different parts of the oral cavity are innervated by nerve fibers that respond selectively to different chemicals. For example, receptive fields of specialist nerve fibers that respond most strongly to quinine are located on the posterior tongue and receptive fields of specialist fibers that respond most strongly to NaCl are located on the anterior tongue. Thus, in rodents, all taste bud regions do not show the same taste receptor sensitivity. Regional differences in sensitivities to taste stimuli are also seen in humans.[11]

Central Pathways for Taste

The messages from the periphery of the taste system follow specific pathways on their way to the cerebral **cortex**. Along the way, the inputs from the different fibers converge and become part of feedback loops, with some fibers exciting and others inhibiting neural activity. Information from taste neurons is integrated with input from the **somatosensory** system

A. Pathways

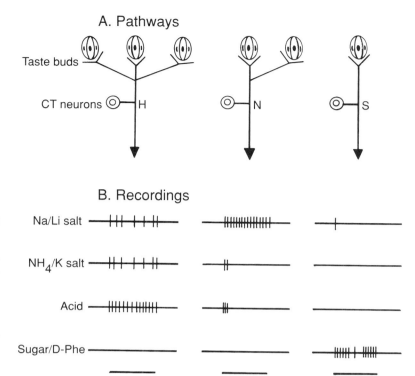

Taste buds

CT neurons   H   N   S

B. Recordings

Na/Li salt

NH$_4$/K salt

Acid

Sugar/D-Phe

Figure 12–4. Response spectra of chorda tympani (CT) generalist (H) and specialist (N, S) neurons in the hamster. The bars beneath the recordings indicate a 3-second stimulation period, and the short vertical lines in the recordings mark occurrences of nerve impulses. (Adapted and used with permission from Frank ME, Hettinger TP, Mott AE. The sense of taste: neurobiology, aging and medication effects. *Crit Rev Oral Biol Med* 1992;3:38L)

and eventually sent to the areas of the brain responsible for appetite, behavior, motivation, and emotion. Taste is crucial to the survival of the organism: we must eat.

Central axonal processes of primary taste afferent neurons enter the **brainstem** and join the **solitary tract**, ending in the surrounding cells of the **nucleus** of the solitary tract (nucleus tractus solitarius), which spans the length of the **medulla oblongata**. Facial taste afferents of the intermediate nerve enter the brainstem most **rostrally**, followed by glossopharyngeal and vagal taste afferents; finally, vagal **visceral** afferents enter most **caudally** (see Fig. 12–3). Taste-responsive neurons are concentrated in the rostral pole of the solitary nucleus. Some of these secondary taste neurons are less specifically tuned to taste quality than are primary afferent neurons. For example, secondary neurons that respond best to sucrose may also respond to NaCl, which is not sweet. Other solitary nucleus neurons that are excited by sucrose, however, are inhibited by stimuli that are not sweet[12]; the inhibition is a consequence of inhibitory circuits of the solitary nucleus.[13] Recep-

tive fields of some secondary taste neurons include receptive fields served by different nerves. For example, one solitary nucleus cell may respond to sucrose applied to the palate and NaCl applied to the anterior tongue.[14] The convergence of diverse inputs on single neurons results in a loss of the quality-specific or place-specific information that is present in the separate primary neural inputs.

Taste-responsive neurons in the nucleus of the solitary tract project to a **medial parvocellular** (small-celled) portion of the ventral posteromedial nucleus of the **thalamus** in primates (see Fig. 12–3). The thalamic taste area is just medial to the somatosensory representation of the tongue in the ventral posteromedial nucleus. Visceral afferents project to a **parabrachial nucleus** of the **pons** and, from there, to parts of the **ventral forebrain (limbic system).** In nonprimate species such as rats, the parabrachial nucleus is an obligatory relay in the taste afferent pathway and projects bilaterally to the thalamus and **ipsilaterally** to the ventral forebrain. Thalamic taste neurons appear to have more complex response properties than brainstem taste neurons.[7]

Thalamic taste neurons project to primary taste cortex, which in primates is found in the **insula** and adjacent **frontal opercular** cerebral cortex[15] (see Fig. 12–3). The cortical taste area is close to, but separate from, the cortical somatosensory representation of the tongue. Taste and somatosensory pathways are bilateral in primates. Taste pathways are primarily uncrossed, but lingual somatosensory pathways are primarily crossed. Cortical taste neurons can have more specific response properties than lower-order taste neurons. For example, one cell may respond best to a "natural" sweet stimulus mixture (e.g., fruit juice), whereas another cell may respond best to glucose. Other cortical cells appear to be less quality specific, responding to preferred stimuli of different taste quality (e.g., NaCl and sucrose). A secondary cortical taste area is found in the **orbitofrontal cortex** in primates. Taste-responsive cells in this secondary cortical taste area can become less responsive to a taste stimulus as it is repeatedly sampled, showing a "stimulus-specific satiety."[15]

Behaviors Mediated by the Gustatory System

The conscious experience of taste sensation, presumably a cortically mediated phenomenon, is composed of four very different qualities in people. Early in the century, Henning[16] proposed that all taste sensations could be represented by the surface of a tetrahedron. "Sweet," "salty," "sour," and "bitter" (taste primaries) were located at the four corners, and intermediate tastes, such as salty-sweet, were located appropriately elsewhere on the surface of the tetrahedron. Investigators still debate whether there are primary taste sensations.[17,18]

The learning of taste aversions also depends on the cerebral cortex. After one experience, the taste of a food item that is followed by gastrointestinal upset becomes aversive.[19] Other behaviors elicited by taste do not require the forebrain. For example, decerebrates, including **anencephalic** human infants,[20] still make the facial expressions of acceptance and rejection associated with sweet and sour stimuli.

Clinical Correlations

The complaints of taste dysfunction among patients presenting to special taste and smell clinics far exceed the number of patients with clinically measurable taste loss.[9] This phenomenon primarily reflects the nature of "flavor" perception and the difficulty we all have in separating olfaction (which is more vulnerable to damage due to trauma and disease) from gustation. As mentioned previously, complete loss of the sense of taste **(ageusia)** is very rare. Partial losses of taste sensitivity **(hypogeusia),** however, do occur. Age takes its toll on the taste system.[21,22] Taste loss in one taste bud field can also occur as a result of damage to peripheral taste nerves[23] (e.g., lingual nerve injury during oral surgery) or damage to the chorda tympani during ear surgery. Usually, other taste fields can compensate for these losses and patients may not notice the damage.[24] Damage to the taste areas of the brain, such as might occur from head trauma, can also result in hypogeusia; patients with head trauma may show losses in their ability to detect tastes.[25] **Dysgeusia**, a persistent, unpleasant taste, has a number of possible causes, such as exudates of oral disease or taste nerve injury.[9] Taste perception can also be altered as a side effect of certain medications. For example, the perception of the saltiness of NaCl is enhanced by systemic use of the diuretic amiloride (for the treatment of hypertension).[26] Alternatively, the perceived intensity of NaCl is profoundly reduced by topical treatment of gingivitis with the mouthwash chlorhexidine.[27] These effects are reversed with the cessation of medication.

The Olfactory System

The Olfactory Receptor Mucosa

Olfactory receptor cells occur in large numbers (5×10^6) in small, bilateral patches (2–5 cm^2) of olfactory mucosa (Fig. 12–5) that line parts of the upper nasal cavity (the superior and middle turbinates), as well as the upper part of the nasal septum[28] (Fig. 12–6). During normal breathing, the structure of the nasal cavity causes air to be deflected upward, giving odorous molecules access to the receptors.

The olfactory mucosa includes olfactory receptor cells, supporting cells (see Fig. 12–5), and glands, which secrete mucus. Supporting cells contain secretory granules and project microvilli into the mucus layer. An olfactory receptor cell is a **bipolar neuron**, possessing one dendritic (from a **dendrite**) and one axonal process. The dendritic process is topped by a knob, from which **cilia** project about 0.1 mm into the mucus.

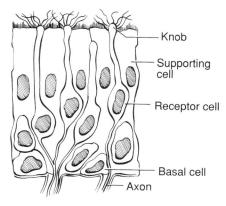

Figure 12–5. Olfactory receptor cells in the olfactory mucosa. (Adapted and used with permission from Frank ME, Rabin MD. Chemosensory neuroanatomy and physiology. *Ear Nose Throat J* 1989;68:292–296.)

Olfactory receptor neurons turn over in adult mammals, having a life span of approximately 50 days.[28] The basal cells of the olfactory epithelium (see Fig. 12–5) comprise the generative cell population. If the axons in olfactory receptor neurons are cut and the olfactory epithelium degenerates, a new olfactory epithelium can regenerate.[29] The reconstitution of the olfactory epithelium begins with increased mi-

totic activity of basal cells. Thereafter, differentiated olfactory receptor neurons appear, dendritic processes grow toward the epithelial surface, and axonal processes grow toward the **olfactory bulb**. Eventually, olfactory knobs are covered with cilia, the olfactory bulb is innervated, and the system appears to function again. This ability of the olfactory epithelium to respond to injury may account for the return of the olfactory function months after it has been lost as a result of head trauma.[30] With age, however, the receptor population is not strictly maintained and the sense of smell deteriorates.[31]

Olfactory Stimulus Transduction

The membranes of olfactory cilia contain proteins (comparable to **opsin**) with seven **hydrophobic** transmembrane segments,[32] which suggests they are coupled to G-proteins. The hundreds of such "receptor proteins," which are restricted to the olfactory mucosa, are thought to bind specific olfactory stimuli. A tissue-specific G-protein alpha-subunit (G_{olf}) and adenylyl cyclase provide the basis for one second-messenger pathway for olfactory signaling, which results in stimulus-evoked increases in cAMP.[33] With the opening of a specific cyclic-nucleotide–

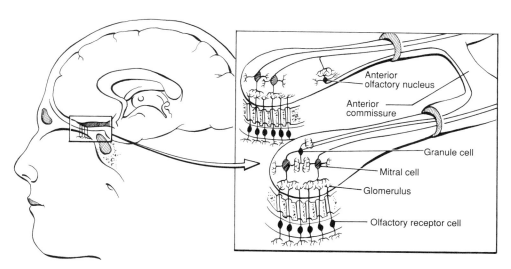

Figure 12–6. Projections of olfactory receptor neurons to the olfactory bulbs that connect through the anterior commissure. (Adapted and used with permission from Dodd J, Castellucci VF. Smell and taste: the chemical senses. In: Kandel ER, Schwartz JH, Jessell TM, eds. *Principles of neural science.* 3rd ed. New York: Elsevier, 1991:514.)

gated Na$^+$ channel, the olfactory receptor cell is depolarized and **action potentials** generated in the receptor neuron's axon. The olfactory cation (positively charged ion) channel is homologous to the channel involved in visual transduction.

Classification of perceptual odor qualities for humans has been attempted a number of times, but investigators have no general agreement on a single, valid, and complete set of perceptions. Early in this century, Henning proposed a "smell prism," the corners representing six primary odor qualities: flowery, foul, fruity, burnt, spicy, and resinous[34] (odors of such compounds as phenethyl alcohol, ethanethiol, geranial, acrolein, cinnamaldehyde, and pinene, respectively). Many other odor qualities, however, such as sweaty (isovaleric acid), fecal (methylindole), camphorous (cineole), and sweet (vanillin) have been proposed. Names of odors are often associated with environmental processes, objects, and events. They are not abstractions of perceptions, as are the names for tastes.

The Olfactory Nerve

The fine axons (0.1–0.3 mm in diameter) of olfactory receptors comprise the *fila olfactoria*, or **olfactory nerve** (cranial nerve I), in which several small bundles of axons are surrounded by a single Schwann cell. Maintaining some of the topography of the mucosa, the olfactory nerve fibers project to the olfactory bulb through the **cribriform plate** of the ethmoid bone (see Fig. 12–6).

Slow potentials (surface negative voltages) can be recorded with an electrode placed on the olfactory mucosal surface and action potentials can be recorded with a microelectrode inserted to the base of the epithelium.[35] The electroolfactogram reflects the generator potentials (voltages) of receptor cells, and the action potentials are recorded from olfactory nerve axons. Different regions of the mucosal surface show different chemical sensitivities. For example, n-butanol, which has an unpleasant odor, is more effective when the electroolfactogram electrode is placed anteriorly, but d-limonene, which has a pleasant odor, is more effective when the electrode is placed on the posterior mucosal surface.[36] Furthermore, one of four subfamilies of receptor proteins is exclusively expressed in olfactory receptor neurons located in one of four separate regions of the olfactory mucosa.[37] Individual olfactory receptor axons typically show excitatory responses to a number of odor chemicals. Some stimuli elicit a short-latency response that is maintained until the stimulus is removed, but other stimuli are not effective (Fig. 12–7).

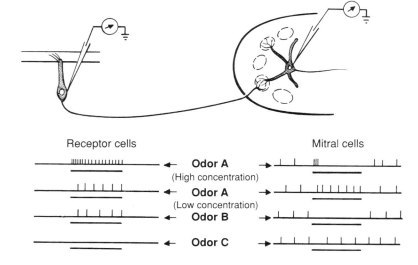

Receptor cells   Mitral cells

Odor A
(High concentration)

Odor A
(Low concentration)

Odor B

Odor C

Figure 12–7. Responses of olfactory receptor cells (left) and mitral cells (right) in the salamander. (Adapted and used with permission from Shepherd GM. *Neurobiology.* 2nd ed. New York: Oxford University Press, 1988:241.)

The Olfactory Bulb

Axons of olfactory receptor neurons enter the olfactory bulb (see Fig. 12–6)—a complex, layered central neural structure (Fig. 12–8) in the olfactory nerve layer. In spherical **neuropil** in the glomerular layer, axonal endings of the receptor neurons form excitatory synapses with primary dendrites of **mitral** and tufted cells, output neurons of the olfactory bulb.[28] An individual **glomerulus** may receive input exclusively from receptor neurons using a single receptor protein.[38] Periglomerular cells, which are **intrinsic** to the bulb, form inhibitory synapses with primary dendrites of output cells in the glomerular layer. In the external **plexiform** layer, secondary dendrites of the output neurons receive inhibitory synapses from granule cells, which are also intrinsic to the olfactory bulb. Reciprocal excitatory–inhibitory synapses are seen between dendrites of output and intrinsic cells of the olfactory bulb. Reciprocal synapses between mitral cells and granule cells are common.[28]

Mitral cells of the olfactory bulb respond selectively to odor quality and odor intensity. Some odor stimuli affect an individual mitral cell; other stimuli do not.[39] In fact, mitral cells are tuned to stereochemical features of odor stimuli. Mitral cells can also show excitatory–inhibitory responses to odor stimuli. A low-level stimulus elicits a response in the mitral cell that is simply excitatory. A higher-level stimulus, however, elicits a short excitatory response that is followed by inhibition (see Fig. 12–7). This inhibition lengthens with increasing intensity, may be

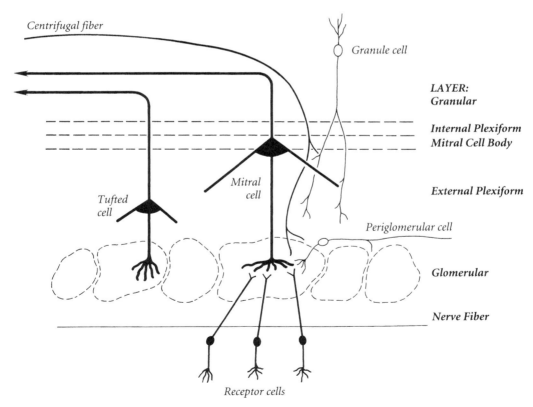

Figure 12–8. Neurons and layers of the olfactory bulb. Axons of the receptor cells project upward from the olfactory epithelium to reach the bulb. Deepest bulbar layers are in the upper part of the figure.

a self-inhibition of the excited mitral cell by a granule cell by way of a reciprocal synapse,[40] and may explain the profound **adaptation** of smells.

Receptive fields for excitatory responses are small areas of the olfactory mucosa. In contrast, receptive fields for inhibitory responses are large. The inhibition may be a lateral inhibition mediated by periglomerular cells, which span several glomeruli in the glomerular layer. All response types are seen in individual mitral cells, but the chemicals that elicit them differ across mitral cells.[41] Response to a particular chemical is typically greater in some regions of the bulb than in others, and different chemicals elicit different patterns of activity across the bulb. The patterns are sharpened by inhibitory bulbar circuits.[42] The intensity and quality of an odor is represented in a spatiotemporal pattern of neural activity in the olfactory bulb.[41]

Higher Olfactory Pathways

Axons of mitral and tufted cells leave the olfactory bulbs in **olfactory tracts**, which project to five sites, including the anterior olfactory nucleus; **piriform cortex** (a three-layered **paleocortex**); **olfactory tubercle**; as well as the **amygdala** and **entorhinal cortex** (Fig. 12–9).

The anterior olfactory nucleus, which is caudal to the olfactory bulb, projects to the **contralateral** bulb through the **anterior commissure**. The piriform cortex and olfactory tubercle project to the medial dorsal thalamus, and from there to the orbitofrontal cerebral cortex, structures that are thought to be involved in conscious odor perception. The topography of the olfactory mucosa is not clearly preserved in the projections to the piriform cortex.[43] The olfactory projection goes to the corticomedial nucleus of the amygdala and the lateral entorhinal cortex, limbic system structures that have roles in reproductive behavior and memory. Olfactory projections from these structures go to the **hypothalamus** and **hippocampus**. Thus, the output neurons of the olfactory bulb project directly, or by a few synapses, to the **diencephalon** and limbic system. Such diverse projections may help explain why an odor can elicit complex, specific situational and emotional memories.[44] Based on such nonperceptual effects of odors, therapies have been devised to alleviate psychological stress with presentation of pleasant, familiar odors.[45] Most of the sites of olfactory projec-

tions send **centrifugal** input back to the olfactory bulb, and projections to the bulb also ascend from the brainstem. These feedback and brainstem projections can control effects of olfactory inputs.

Clinical Correlations

The regenerative capabilities of the olfactory system diminish as we age, and **hyposmia** (partial loss of smell) is not uncommon among the elderly.[46] One nontrivial public health consequence of this fact is the diminished ability to detect natural gas warning agents among our aging population.[47] The olfactory system is also vulnerable to trauma and disease. **Anosmia** (complete loss of smell) is a frequent consequence of head trauma.[30] Recovery from trauma to the olfactory receptor neurons, whose axons have the ability to regenerate, is possible. Chronic nasal and sinus disease, characterized by abnormal thickening of the mucosal walls of the sinuses, can also result in hyposmia or anosmia by impairing airflow to the tiny patch of olfactory mucosa. Often, treatment of severe forms of this disease with topical **corticosteroids** results in recovery of olfactory function.[48] Hyposmia after viral upper respiratory infections is also not uncommon.[49] Unfortunately, the mechanism for damage to the olfactory system is unknown, and there is no known treatment. **Parosmia** (smelling odors, usually foul or unpleasant, that others do not) or dysosmia (distortions in odor perceptions) are symptoms of nasal and sinus disease that are eliminated with treatment of the disease.[50]

Common Chemical Sense

The "common chemical sense," a term in use since 1912,[51] is separate from gustation and olfaction. In the context of the oral and nasal cavities, it is the sense of irritation caused by chemical stimulation of the free nerve endings buried deep in nasal and oral mucous membranes.[52,53] These finely myelinated or unmyelinated fibers that respond to chemicals are part of the trigeminal system. Figure 12–10 illustrates the sensory innervation to the epithelia of the head, including nasal and oral surfaces, provided by the **trigeminal nerve** (cranial nerve V). This nerve gets its name from its three branches, the ophthalmic, maxillary, and mandibular nerves. The mucosa of the nasal cavity is innervated by the ethmoid (a divi-

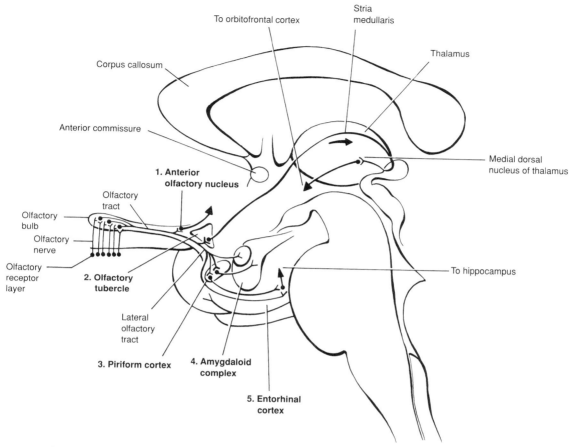

Figure 12–9. The central projections of the olfactory system. (Adapted and used with permission from Dodd J, Castellucci VF. Smell and taste: the chemcial senses. In: Kandel ER, Schwartz JH, Jessell TM, eds. *Principles of Neural Science.* 3rd ed. New York: Elsevier, 1991:517.)

sion of the ophthalmic) and the nasopalatine (a division of the maxillary) branches of the trigeminal nerve. The mucosa of the oral cavity is innervated by the maxillary and mandibular divisions. Central projections of the trigeminal nerve are shown by the dotted line in Figure 12–3.

Many of the chemicals that we can smell and taste are also perceived as irritating or painful if presented in high enough concentrations. Some odorless or tasteless chemicals have only irritating properties, such as CO_2 and capsaicin (the active ingredient in chili peppers). Stimulation of the trigeminal receptors elicits reflexes that are designed to protect the organism from prolonged exposure to noxious chemicals. For example, a whiff of CO_2 in the nose can cause reflex **apnea**, an involuntary interruption of respiration,[53] sneezing, tearing, and increased mucous production. Stimulation of the **nociceptors** in the mouth with capsaicin can produce a reflexive increase in salivation, facial sweating, tearing, and coughing.[54]

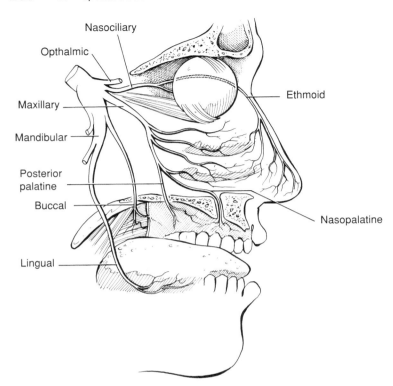

Nasociliary

Opthalmic

Maxillary

Mandibular

Posterior palatine

Buccal

Lingual

Ethmoid

Nasopalatine

Figure 12–10. Branches of the trigeminal nerve that innervate the nasal and oral cavities. (Adapted and used with permission from Silver WL. The common chemical sense. In: Finger TE, Silver WL, eds. *Neurobiology of taste and smell.* New York: John Wiley & Sons, 1987:67.)

Conclusions

All three of our chemical senses are involved in the evaluation of food, yet all three are anatomically and physiologically distinct systems. The receptors for taste, smell, and irritation are located physically near each other in the nasal and oral cavities, and all have projections into the limbic system, the area of the brain involved with motivation and emotion. The common activation of these three systems by the same stimuli makes it very difficult for patients with chemosensory problems to identify which system is involved.

Acknowledgment
This work was supported in part by research grant 2P50 DC00168 from the National Institute on Deafness and Other Communication Disorders, National Institutes of Health, Bethesda, Maryland.

REFERENCES

1. Gent JF, Goodspeed RB, Zagraniski RT, Catalanotto, FA. Taste and smell problems: validation of questions for the clinical history. *Yale J Biol Med* 1987;60:27–35.
2. Kinnamon JC. Organization and innervation of taste buds. In: Finger TE, Silver WL, eds. *Neurobiology of taste and smell.* New York: John Wiley & Sons, 1987:277–297.
3. Whitehead MC, Frank ME, Hettinger TP, Hou L-T, Nah H-D. Persistence of taste buds in denervated fungiform papillae. *Brain Res* 1987;405:192–195.
4. Miller IJ Jr. Anatomy of the peripheral taste system. In: Doty RL, ed. *Handbook of olfaction and gustation.* New York: Marcel Dekker, 1995:521–547.
5. Margolskee RF. Receptor mechanisms in gustation. In: Doty RL, ed. *Handbook of olfaction and gustation.* New York: Marcel Dekker, 1995:575–595.
6. Kinnamon SC. Taste transduction: a diversity of mechanisms. *Trends Neurosci* 1988;11:491–496.
7. Frank ME, Hettinger TP, Mott AE. The sense of taste: neurobiology, aging and medication effects. *Crit Rev Oral Biol Med* 1992;3:371–393.

8. Wong GT, Gannon KS, Margolskee RF. Transduction of bitter and sweet taste by gustducin. *Nature* 1996;381: 796–800.

9. Doty RL, Bartoshuk LM, Snow JB Jr. Causes of olfactory and gustatory disorders. In: Getchell TV, Doty RL, Bartoshuk LM, Snow JB Jr, eds. *Smell and taste in health and disease.* New York: Raven Press, 1991:449–462.

10. Smith DV, Frank ME. Sensory coding by peripheral taste fibers. In: Simon SA, Roper SD, eds. *Mechanisms of taste transduction.* Boca Raton, FL: CRC Press, 1993: 295–338.

11. Sandick B, Cardello AV. Taste profiles from single circumvallate papillae: comparison with fungiform profiles. *Chem Senses* 1981;6:197–214.

12. McPheeters M, Hettinger TP, Nuding SC, Savoy LD, Whitehead MC, Frank ME. Taste-responsive neurons and their locations in the solitary nucleus of the hamster. *Neuroscience* 1990;34:745–758.

13. Smith DV, Liu H, Vogt MB. Neural coding of aversive and appetitive gustatory stimuli: interactions in the hamster brain stem. *Physiol Behav* 1994;56:1189–1196.

14. Travers SP, Pfaffmann C, Norgren R. Convergence of lingual and palatal gustatory neural activity in the nucleus of the solitary tract. *Brain Res* 1986;365:305–320.

15. Rolls ET. Central taste anatomy and neurophysiology. In: Doty RL, ed. *Handbook of olfaction and gustation.* New York: Marcel Dekker, 1995:549–573.

16. Henning H. Psychologische Studien am Geschmackssinn. In: Abderhalden E, ed. *Handbuch der biologischen Arbeitsmethoden.* Berlin: Urban & Schwarzenberg, 1927.

17. Erickson RP. The role of "primaries" in taste research. In: LeMagnen J, MacLeod P, eds. *Olfaction and taste VI (proceedings of the Sixth International Symposium).* London: IRL Press, 1977:369–376.

18. McBurney DH, Gent JF. On the nature of taste qualities. *Psychol Bull* 1979;86:151–167.

19. Nowlis GH, Frank ME, Pfaffmann C. Specificity of acquired aversions to taste qualities in hamsters and rats. *Journal of Comparative and Physiological Psychology* 1980;94:932–942.

20. Steiner JE. Oral and facial innate motor responses to gustatory and to some olfactory stimuli. In: Kroeze JHA, ed. *Preference behavior and chemoreception (ECRO proceedings).* London: IRL Press, 1979:247–261.

21. Stevens JC, Cruz LA, Hoffman JM, Patterson MQ. Taste sensitivity and aging: high incidence of decline revealed by repeated threshold measures. *Chem Senses* 1995;20:451–459.

22. Stevens JC. Detection of tastes in mixture with other tastes: issues of masking and aging. *Chem Senses* 1996; 21:211–221.

23. Barry MA, Frank ME. Response of the gustatory system to peripheral nerve injury. *Exp Neurol* 1992;115:60–64.

24. Miller IJ Jr, Bartoshuk LM. Taste perception, taste bud distribution, and spatial relationships. In: Getchell TV,

Doty RL, Bartoshuk LM, Snow JB Jr, eds. *Smell and taste in health and disease.* New York: Raven Press, 1991: 205–233.

25. Costanzo RM, DiNardo LJ, Zasler ND. Head injury and taste. In: Doty RL, ed. *Handbook of olfaction and gustation.* New York: Marcel Dekker, 1995:775–783.

26. Mattes RD, Christensen CM, Engelman K. Effects of therapeutic doses of amiloride and hydrochlorothiazide on taste, saliva and salt intake in normotensive adults. *Chem Senses* 1988;13:33–44.

27. Helms JA, Della-Fera MA, Mott AE, Frank ME. Effects of chlorhexidine on human taste perception. *Arch Oral Biol* 1995;40:913–920.

28. Greer CA. Structural organization of the olfactory system. In: Getchell TV, Doty RL, Bartoshuk LM, Snow JB Jr, eds. *Smell and taste in health and disease.* New York: Raven Press, 1991:65–81.

29. Graziadei PP, Karlen MS, Monti Graziadei GA, Bernstein JJ. Neurogenesis of sensory neurons in the primate olfactory system after section of the fila olfactoria. *Brain Res* 1980;186:289–300.

30. Costanzo RM, DiNardo LJ, Zasler ND. Head injury and olfaction. In: Doty RL, ed. *Handbook of olfaction and gustation.* New York: Marcel Dekker, 1995:493–502.

31. Stevens JC, Cain WS. Age-related deficiency in the perceived strength of six odorants. *Chem Senses* 1985;10: 517–529.

32. Buck L, Axel R. A novel multigene family may encode odorant receptors: a molecular basis for odor recognition. *Cell* 1991;65:175–187.

33. Reed RR. Signaling pathways in odorant detection. *Neuron* 1992;8:205–209.

34. Henning H. *Der Geruch.* Leipzig: Barth, 1916.

35. Shepherd GM, Getchell TV, Kauer JS. Analysis of structure and function in the olfactory pathway. In: Tower DB, ed. *The nervous system. Vol 1: The basic neurosciences.* New York: Raven Press, 1975:207–220.

36. Mackay-Sim A, Shaman P, Moulton DG. Topographic coding of olfactory quality: odorant-specific patterns of epithelial responsivity in the salamander. *J Neurophysiol* 1982;48:584–596.

37. Ressler KJ, Sullivan SL, Buck LB. A zonal organization of odorant receptor gene expression in the olfactory epithelium. *Cell* 1993;73:597–609.

38. Vassar R, Chao SK, Sitcheran R, et al. Topographic organization of sensory projections to the olfactory bulb. *Cell* 1994;79:981–991.

39. Mori K, Mataga N, Imamura K. Differential specificities of single mitral cells in rabbit olfactory bulb for a homologous series of fatty acid odor molecules. *J Neurophysiol* 1992;67:786–789.

40. Scott JW, Harrison TA. The olfactory bulb: anatomy and physiology. In: Finger TE, Silver WL, eds. *Neurobiology of taste and smell.* New York: John Wiley & Sons, 1987: 151–178.

41. Kauer JS. Coding in the olfactory system. In: Finger TE, Silver WL, eds. *Neurobiology of taste and smell*. New York: John Wiley & Sons, 1987:205–231.

42. Yokoi M, Mori K, Nakanishi S. Refinement of odor molecule tuning by dendrodendritic synaptic inhibition in the olfactory bulb. *Proc Natl Acac Sci U S A* 1995;92: 3371–3375.

43. Price JL. The central olfactory and accessory olfactory systems. In: Finger TE, Silver WL, eds. *Neurobiology of taste and smell*. New York: John Wiley & Sons, 1987: 179–203.

44. Ackerman D. *A natural history of the senses*. New York: Random House, 1990.

45. King JR. Scientific status of aromatherapy. *Perspect Biol Med* 1994;37:409–415.

46. Murphy C. Taste and smell in the elderly. In: Meiselman HL, Rivlin RS, eds. *Clinical measurement of taste and smell*. New York: Macmillan, 1986:343–371.

47. Stevens JC, Cain WS, Weinstein DE. Aging impairs the ability to detect gas odor. *Fire Technology*, 1987:23:198–204.

48. Mott AE, Cain WS, Lafreniere D, et al. Topical corticosteroid treatment of anosmia associated with nasal and sinus disease. *Arch Otolaryngol Head Neck Surg* 1997;123: 367–372.

49. Leopold DA, Hornung DE, Youngentob SL. Olfactory loss after upper respiratory infection. In: Getchell TV, Doty RL, Bartoshuk LM, Snow JB Jr, eds. *Smell and taste in health and disease*. New York: Raven Press, 1991: 731–734.

50. Mott AE, Leopold DA. Disorders in taste and smell. *Med Clin North Am* 1991;75:1321–1353.

51. Silver WL. The common chemical sense. In: Finger TE, Silver WL, eds. *Neurobiology of taste and smell*. New York: John Wiley & Sons, 1987:65–87.

52. Dodd J, Kelly JP. Trigeminal system. In: Kandel ER, Schwartz JH, Jessell TM, eds. *Principles of neural science*. 3rd ed. New York: Elsevier, 1991:701–710.

53. Dunn JD, Cometto-Muniz JE, Cain WS. Nasal reflexes: reduced sensitivity to CO_2 irritation in cigarette smokers. *J Appl Toxicol* 1982;2:176–178.

54. Green BG, Lawless HT. The psychophysics of somatosensory chemoreception in the nose and mouth. In: Getchell TV, Doty RL, Bartoshuk LM, Snow JB Jr, eds. *Smell and taste in health and disease*. New York: Raven Press, 1991:235–253.

section three

MOTOR SYSTEMS

Motor I: Lower Centers

MEENAKSHI B. IYER, PhD, OTR/L
ANDREW R. MITZ, PhD
CAROLEE WINSTEIN, PT, PhD

• • •

Every movement, whether voluntary or reflexive, is achieved by contraction of skeletal muscles. An elaborate nervous system provides fine control of muscular contractions, from the simple act of standing to the acrobatics of a gymnast. To perform a movement effectively, the adjacent body parts and the body as a whole must assume a stable and appropriate posture. The process of **motor control** is complicated;

209

any therapist treating neurologically impaired patients must understand the major neural interactions associated with the performance of movement.

In this chapter, you will study muscles and their connections to the spinal cord, the spinal cord itself, and the brainstem. Because the motor neurons in the spinal cord and the motor nuclei of the cranial nerves located in the brainstem constitute the **final common pathway**[1] for determining muscle action, they are collectively known as the **lower motor neurons**. These "lower" motor centers provide many of the automatic functions of movement. They receive inputs from **segmental** and suprasegmental (spinal, medullary, midbrain, and cortical) areas. The integrated activity of these converging inputs is responsible for posture and movement. In the next chapter, you will study "higher" motor centers: the cerebral cortex, cerebellum, and basal ganglia, which are crucial for coordinated, goal-directed movement.

Organization of the Neural Substrates Responsible for Movement

The four general processes involved in the performance of voluntary movement are motivation, ideation, programming, and execution.[2] Figure 13–1 depicts these four aspects and the general scheme of neuronal connectivities associated with the performance of movement. According to this scheme, the neuronal substrates contributing to motor control subserve two distinct but interactive systems: the limbic system and the sensorimotor system. The limbic system includes cortical structures that connect with areas of the midbrain and brainstem that control vital functions such as hunger, thirst, heart rate, body temperature, and blood pressure. The sensorimotor system deals with sensations, perceptions, and motor actions. Although the motor centers are chiefly responsible for the motor action, keep in mind that motor performance relies heavily on sensory feedback and stored perceptions of the movement. For this reason, the term "sensorimotor system" denotes the combination of all the processes involved in the production of coordinated movement.

The limbic system is involved in the control and regulation of emotional behavior and basic biological drives.[3] More important, it is involved in the process of learning. Its connections with the sensorimotor system are critical for the execution of goal-directed movement.[4,5] *Motivations* (needs or drives) arising through the limbic system are analyzed and transformed into *ideas* through cortical processing carried out in the association cortex (frontal, parietal, temporal, occipital lobes). *Ideas* are formatted into **motor programs** through processes *(programming)* carried out in the sensorimotor cortex, cerebellum, basal ganglia, and related subcortical nuclei. A motor program is an algorithm of neuronal activities that encodes the movement strategy for execution of a desired motor behavior. *Programming* encodes all aspects of the movement, from the general to the specific. At the general level, the temporal order or goal may be specified; at the specific level, the muscles to be activated are selected and parameters such as how and when to activate them are determined.

In the process of *programming* a voluntary movement, the precentral gyrus or motor cortex is the last center to be activated before the **central command** is relayed down to the brainstem and spinal cord for *execution*. The descending central command is also transmitted back to the higher centers involved in programming the movement. This internal loop relaying descending motor signals back to the higher centers is known as **corollary discharge**. It provides a reference by which the system can distinguish incoming sensory stimuli resulting from externally imposed events (exafference) from those that are a consequence of self-motion (corollary copy or reafference). The descending central command acts on the lower motor neurons of the brainstem and spinal cord to *execute* the desired movement. Movement is produced by precise, well coordinated muscular contractions that, in turn, are activated by the lower motor neurons that send nerve fibers to innervate them. The muscles that are activated generally subserve two semidistinct functions: they are directly responsible for the skilled voluntary activity, and they coordinate postural adjustments to provide a stable background for the movement.

Movement alters the sensory input from muscles, tendons, joints, and skin. During and after the movement, feedback about the motor action ascends to spinal and supraspinal centers. During a movement, the system uses this continuous sensory feedback to

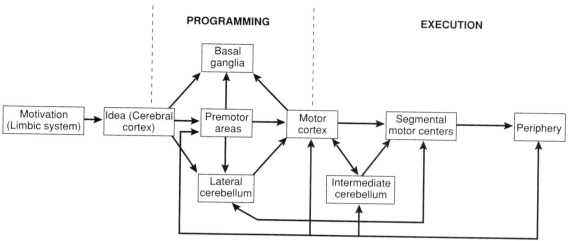

Figure 13–1. General scheme of neuronal connectivities associated with the performance of movement. (From Cheney PD. Role of cerebral cortex in voluntary movements: a review. *Phys Ther* 1985;65:624–635, with permission.)

adjust and smooth the movement. Sensory feedback plays a pivotal role in the acquisition of new motor skills. In fact, feedback is so important in controlling movement that some theoretic models of motor control have been based on its presence or absence. Movement performed in the presence of sensory feedback is said to be performed "closed loop"; movement performed in the absence of sensory feedback is said to be performed "open loop."

Models of Neural Control: Open-Loop and Closed-Loop Control

Closed-loop processes are based on the feedback "loop" between sensory information and motor actions. The feedback helps to monitor discrepancies in motor performance; these discrepancies can be used to refine motor programs leading to actions. In contrast, *open-loop* movements are performed without the benefit of feedback, or in a **feedforward** mode. For example, during the performance of very fast or "ballistic" movements, the desired action is completed before sensory loops can provide information that would be used to modify the action.

A simple example of motor control illustrates the value of mechanical feedback. Figure 13–2A shows the key components of a simple cruise control for a car. The driver sets the desired speed. The desired speed feeds into the accelerator and, as we all know, the accelerator affects the car speed. Wind resistance reduces the car's speed (we will ignore all other factors for the moment), as indicated by the minus sign ($-$). If the effects of wind resistance were entirely predictable, the feedforward *open-loop* control system shown in Figure 13–2A would work well. Some desired speed value would always balance the wind resistance perfectly, and would give the correct car speed. In other words the "plus" ($+$) of the accelerator and the "minus" of the wind resistance would be exactly equal at this speed. Thus, feedforward anticipates the relation between the system (in this case, the accelerator value) and the environment (wind resistance) to determine a course of action (car speed).[6]

Of course, this system fails on windy days. Wind resistance can be less because of a tail wind or much greater because of a head wind. One improvement is to measure the car speed and use that information to

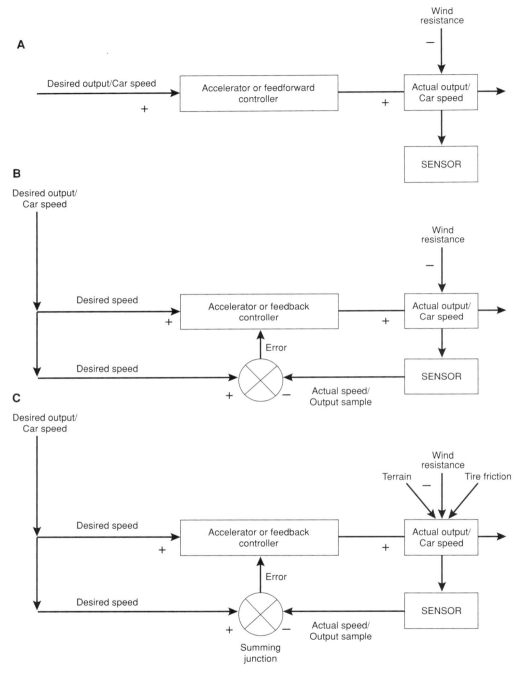

Figure 13–2. Example of simplified control problem: automobile cruise control. **A:** Open-loop control of car speed. Car speed will vary on a windy day. **B:** Closed-loop control using negative feedback. Feedback compensates for any shift in the wind pushing on the car. **C:** The closed-loop system automatically compensates for other environmental factors.

adjust the accelerator (see Fig. 13–2B). If the car is going too fast because of a tail wind, then the accelerator signal is reduced; if the car is going too slow because of a head wind, then the accelerator signal is increased. In other words, the accelerator signal is always adjusted in the opposite direction of the car speed. This adjustment is called **negative feedback**. The circle in the figure, called a "summing junction," shows that the desired speed signal, which still has a "plus" sign, and the actual car speed signal, which has a "minus" sign, combine to have a net effect on the accelerator. Note that the signal going to the accelerator is the difference between the desired speed and the car speed. This difference is called the "error signal." A closed loop is formed by the accelerator, car speed sensor, and summing junction; thus, this arrangement is called *closed-loop* control.[7] In Figure 13–2C, we have added other factors that directly affect car speed. These other factors, however, do not affect the basic performance of the system. Whatever the disturbances to car speed, as long as the accelerator can supply sufficient power, the closed control loop will compensate.

The delay in time is a disadvantage of the closed-loop system. Although not shown in the drawing, the control loop requires time for the feedback to come around the loop and modify the error signal before it influences the output (car speed). In some circumstances, such as a speed bump or a pothole, insufficient time is available to improve the outcome with feedback. If closed-loop control is used in such a case, the feedback can actually lead to instability, because any modification it introduces to the movement is too late, and inappropriate.

The open-loop controller (see Fig. 13–2A) monitors the environment directly; it must know the state of the system before generating its control signal, but it does not monitor that output. In contrast, the closed-loop controller relies on feedback. It continuously monitors the relation between the actual and desired state of the system or the error signal, while generating its control signal.

Problems of Moving

The problem of motor control is load compensation, or moving against varying weights and loads. Sometimes the loads are minimal, as when lifting a pencil, but sometimes the load is substantial, as when carrying a knapsack full of books. Sometimes loads are predictable, such as writing with a pen or offsetting the effects of gravity on a limb, but often loads are unpredictable. The load is uncertain if someone hands you a sealed package, or when you begin a handshake with a stranger. In some situations you know to expect uncertainty. What about completely unexpected events? Have you ever tried to open a door without knowing it was locked? Through judicious use of sensory feedback, the central nervous system averts disaster in extreme situations and provides smooth and accurate movements during more favorable circumstances. Motor control requires more than just planning specific muscle activities. It requires planning contingencies in case unexpected "perturbations" arise.[7]

Although feedforward and feedback are two different models of neural control, a third scheme that more effectively describes the neural control of skeletal muscle is shown in Figure 13–3. In this scheme, the discharge of the hypothetical motor neuron maintains a specific desired level of muscle length and tension. It receives input from both the open-loop feedforward and the closed-loop feedback controllers. The two controllers, in turn, are *coactivated;* that is, the hypothetical descending central command conveys the desired output signal to both the feedforward and feedback systems. The feedforward system sets the output—the specific level of muscle length and tension; the feedback system acts to make the finer adjustments by compensating for any inaccuracy from the desired value.[8,9] Receptors in the muscles, themselves, are important for the moment-to-moment control of limb position and force generation.

When first learning a new motor skill, movements may be slow, vacillating, and poorly coordinated. However shaky the performance, each trial is an attempt to achieve a target or other goal. At this early stage, learning relies heavily on feedback to control each action. The unskilled performer pauses between movements as visual information is evaluated and the movement is attempted again with a revised plan. Eventually, the sequencing and timing of the movements becomes automated, shifting from direct visual control to a more internalized form of control.[10] The learned movement becomes smooth and coordinated, and requires little attention. The goal can be achieved without conscious intervention. The ease of the learned skill can make us take it for granted. Sometimes we forget the degree of work that went into learning how to open a door.

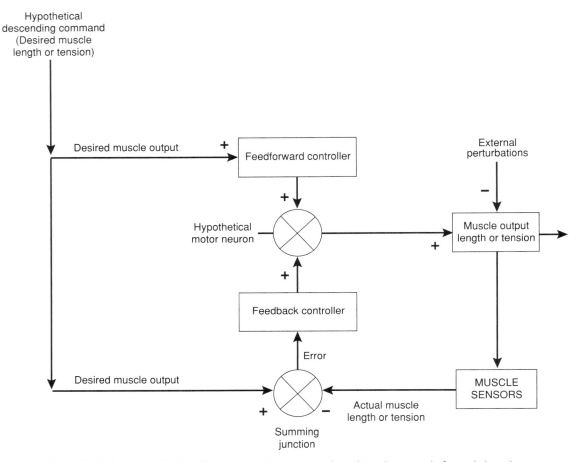

Figure 13–3. Example of a simplified coactivation strategy describing the control of muscle length or tension. The feedforward system sets the output of the muscle and the feedback system compensates for any discrepancies from the desired output.

Peripheral Motor System and Motor Control

Skeletal Muscle: Structure and Function of the Contractile Unit

The primary constituent of skeletal muscle is a collection of long, thin **muscle fibers**. The contractile properties of a muscle reside in the muscle fibers. Each muscle fiber is an unusually large cell formed by the fusion of many separate cells. Like other cells in the body, the muscle fiber is composed of cytoplasm, in this case called **sarcoplasm**, enclosed in a cell membrane called the **sarcolemma** or plasma membrane. Muscle fibers produce force when activated by the central nervous system through axons in the muscle nerve. Impulses traveling in the muscle nerve generate contractions in muscle fibers. This process is described later in some detail. Let us first look at the muscle structure and mechanism of contraction.[11,12]

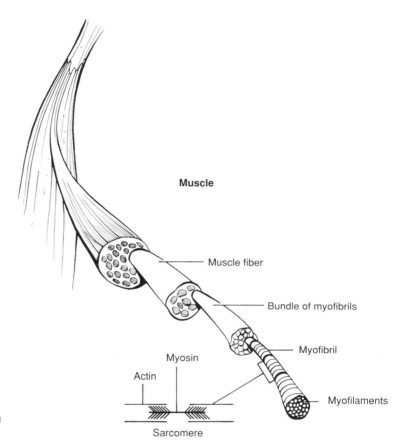

Figure 13–4. Perspective drawing of muscle fiber. A single muscle fiber has many bundles of myofibrils. The myofibrils contain long series of sarcomeres, each with interdigitating actin and myosin molecular filaments.

Muscle fibers in the muscle contain bundles of substructures, called **myofibrils**, that run the length of the cell (Fig. 13–4). A microscopic pattern of stripes runs the entire length of the myofibril. Skeletal muscle is called striated muscle because of this pattern. The pattern is absent from the smooth muscle of the viscera. Each repeat of the pattern is called a **sarcomere**, and is only a few micrometers (2.5 μm) long. The striping effect is due to the alternation of thin protein filaments, called actin, and thick protein filaments, called myosin. Actin and myosin are the protein moieties responsible for muscle contraction.

Fine extensions of the myosin filaments, **crossbridges**, contact the actin filaments, forming attachments at specific binding sites on the actin molecule. During contraction, energy is expended to make and break cross-bridges, pulling the two actin filaments toward the center of the sarcomere (Fig. 13–5). The actin filaments from the opposite ends of the sarcomere slide over the myosin filaments and approach each other, and the muscle shortens. Tension is generated in a muscle whenever cross-bridges are formed. The active shortening of a muscle due to sliding of the actin filaments is called a **shortening** or **concentric** contraction. If the filaments are not free to move because of external forces, the repeated making and breaking of cross-bridges exerts a steady tension that is proportional to the degree of overlap. In this case, a contraction occurs without an appreciable decrease in the length of the whole muscle, and an *isometric* force is generated. When a muscle is relaxed, however, and an external force is applied to

A

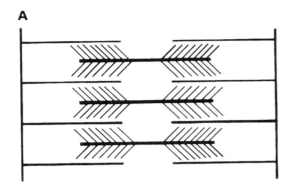

B

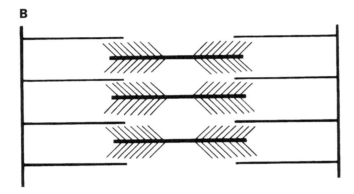

C

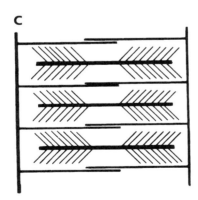

Figure 13–5. Schematic drawing of the sarcomere. Thin horizontal lines represent actin filaments. Thick horizontal lines represent myosin filaments. Short diagonal lines show cross-bridges emanating from the myosin. **A:** With the muscle at its rest length, most of the cross-bridges are able to contact binding sites on the actin filaments. **B:** When the muscle is stretched, fewer cross-bridges can form, so less active force can be produced. **C:** At very short muscle lengths, the overlapping actin molecules interfere with each other and reduce the number of available cross-bridge sites. Again, fewer cross-bridges can form compared with the resting muscle length.

stretch it, the filaments slide past each other without cross-bridge formation, allowing an easy stretch of the muscle fibers.

This model, in which the actin filaments slide over the myosin filaments by cross-bridge formation, is known as the **sliding filament model** of muscle contraction.[12,13] The energy expended during muscular contraction is in the form of adenosine triphosphate (ATP), which is degraded to adenosine diphosphate (ADP). ATP is synthesized in the mitochondria of the muscle fiber from the oxidation of food. Each cross-bridge is formed in the presence of calcium ions, then ATP is expended to generate force and release the cross-bridge. The cycle is repeated as long as calcium ions are present. In normal muscle at rest, ATP is freely available but sarcoplasmic calcium ion concentrations are low. More important, the actin binding sites are covered by a protein called tropomyosin that, in turn, is linked to a smaller protein called troponin. An increase in calcium ion concentration in the sarcoplasm (to about 10^{-6} molar) initiates a contraction. When calcium ions are available, troponin binds to the calcium ions. This action permits movement of the tropomyosin molecule, thereby uncovering the actin binding sites. The next section discusses how the sarcoplasmic concentration of calcium ions is controlled.

Skeletal Muscle: Excitation of Muscle Fibers

The Neuromuscular Junction

Skeletal muscle is entirely controlled by the central nervous system. Muscles contract only when nerve impulses propagate down the motor axon from the spinal cord to the muscle. Earlier in this book, you learned about synapses between neurons. A similar junction is formed between the spinal motor nerve, to which executive instructions for contractions are passed, and its target muscle. This synapse is aptly called a **neuromuscular junction** (NMJ).

The **prejunctional terminal** of the NMJ, analogous to the presynaptic terminal, is widespread and highly folded, forming a large area of interaction between the nerve and the muscle fiber.[12,14] Just as with a synapse, a transmitter substance, in this case **acetylcholine** (ACh), is released by the nerve terminal when an action potential travels along the axon and invades the prejunctional terminal. The ACh diffuses across the space between the nerve and the muscle to act at specific **acetylcholine receptor sites** in the postsynaptic muscle membrane. The transmitter–receptor interaction leads to depolarization of the muscle membrane, producing an **end-plate potential** analogous to the postsynaptic potential. The action of ACh is terminated by an enzyme that is imbedded in the membrane of the muscle fiber, **acetylcholinesterase** (AChE). AChE is essential for proper operation of the NMJ. If the action of AChE is inhibited, as is the case with rat poison and certain chemical warfare agents, ACh acts too long at the receptor sites and produces uncontrolled muscle contractions. Sustained contractions interfere with the cyclic activity of respiration, and can lead to asphyxiation.

Unlike the synapse, the amount of transmitter released at the NMJ always produces a large enough end-plate potential to evoke an action potential in the muscle. Synapses between neurons are usually not strong enough to make the postsynaptic neuron reach threshold every time the presynaptic neuron fires. Synapses rely on spatial and temporal summation. At the NMJ, however, every impulse from the nerve fiber produces an impulse in the muscle fiber. In certain disorders, such as **myasthenia gravis**, the number of ACh receptors in the postsynaptic muscle membrane is reduced.[15-17] Too little ACh is released from the prejunctional terminal to activate the muscle cells effectively, causing muscle weakness. Therefore, one treatment to improve muscular performance in patients with myasthenia gravis is to administer AChE inhibitors. The inhibitors increase the concentration of ACh in the synaptic cleft, allowing a greater activation of the ACh receptors that remain intact.

Muscle Action Potentials and Calcium Ions

Muscle action potentials propagate along the muscle fiber, just as action potentials travel along nerve axons. Because the NMJ is usually somewhere near the middle of the muscle fiber, the muscle action potential propagates outward in both directions—toward both tendons of the muscle. The electrochemistry of the muscle action potential is essentially the same as for a neuron. Sodium, potassium, and, to some degree, calcium channels on the membrane surface react to changes in membrane potential and produce the all-or-none phenomenon discussed earlier in this book. A series of membranous folds, the **transverse tubules** or **T tubules**, run through the muscle cell, increasing its surface area within the interstitial space. The T tubules extend inward to surround each myofibril. The muscle action potential signal, initiated at the NMJ, is passed through the T tubules to all of the myofibrils in the cell, so that the entire muscle contracts synchronously.

Whenever an action potential propagates along the muscle cell, the resulting changes in membrane voltage lead to sharp increases in the intracellular concentration of calcium ions. The primary mechanism for this increase in intracellular calcium is a special structure inside the cell, the **sarcoplasmic reticulum**. The sarcoplasmic reticulum is a sheath of anastomosing, flattened vesicles derived from the endoplasmic reticulum that acts as as a calcium ion reservoir. It surrounds each myofibril and lies adjacent to the T tubules. The electrical activity carried by the T tubules is somehow transferred to the sarcoplasmic reticulum, which then releases its calcium ions into the sarcoplasm.

The consequence of increasing sarcoplasmic calcium is to trigger the formation of actin–myosin bonds or the contraction mechanism. Thus, the electrical activity of the cell is coupled to the contractile activity of the cell by the sarcoplasmic calcium ion concentration. This relationship is called **excitation–contraction coupling**.[11,12] Excitation–contraction coupling implies that an appropriate ionic environment is essential for muscle contraction.

Once the action potential ends, special transport molecules in the membrane of the sarcoplasmic reticulum rapidly "pump" the calcium out of the sarcoplasm and back into the sarcoplasmic reticulum. Because the calcium ions must move in the direction of greater concentration, the process requires energy in the form of ATP. Once the calcium ion concentration falls below a critical level (approximately 10^{-6} molar), contraction ceases. Thus, both contraction and relaxation of muscle require ATP.

The muscle membrane is very sensitive to external stimulation. Although the muscle action potential normally begins at the NMJ, the action potential can be started artificially from elsewhere in the muscle cell. Experiments with tiny electrodes show that excitation–contraction coupling is a very localized phenomenon. If the voltage of the muscle is changed over only a tiny region of the cell, that tiny region shows contraction.

Skeletal Muscle: Mechanical Properties

Skeletal muscle is composed of two types of tissues: muscle tissue (contractile element) and connective tissue (noncontractile element). The interaction of the properties of these two tissues gives muscles their unique set of mechanical characteristics.[12,18] Let us first look at the properties of the whole muscle when excited by electrical stimulation of its nerve (Fig. 13–6A). A single shock to the nerve causes the muscle fibers to exhibit a single **twitch**, a brief contraction followed by a relaxation (see Fig. 13–6B). The force of a twitch rises rapidly and decays more slowly. The twitch starts approximately 2 millisec-

onds after the application of the electrical stimulus. Every fiber in the muscle contributes to this twitch. (The twitch of a single fiber in a muscle would be difficult to detect, because the force it produces is very small.) Repeated action potentials to the muscle produce repeated twitches unless the time between each stimulus is too short to allow the muscle fully to relax. **Summation of contractions**, or additional activation of the contractile element, is brought about when stimulation occurs before relaxation. When stimulation is faster, the individual twitches fuse into one continuous contraction. The muscle maintains its force throughout the period of stimulation; this maintained force is called **tetanus** (see Fig. 13–6B). The force produced during a tetanic contraction is larger than the twitch force.

If we string up a muscle (usually from a frog) and mount it on a frame and attach the other end to an electronic force gauge (see Fig. 13–6A), we can measure a few of its properties. First, we can stretch it a little and see how much resistance is in the connective tissue. The resistance to stretch, or **passive tension**, is due to the noncontractile elements that behave like a stiff elastic band[19,20] (see Fig. 13–6C). We can then place the muscle at different lengths and measure the passive tension or electrically stimulate its nerve, and measure the force the muscle can produce at each length. Because we fix the length, each time we stimulate the measurement is isometric. The total force of the muscle minus the passive tension gives us the **active tension**, or the tension produced by the contractile elements in the muscle (see Fig. 13–6C). The length of the muscle at which the active tension is maximal is called the **rest length**. Thus, the force-generating mechanism in the muscle works optimally at the muscle's rest length. Note that at shorter muscle lengths, total muscle force is primarily due to the contractile elements; at longer muscle lengths, muscle tension is primarily due to the noncontractile elements.

The sliding–filament model explains why the force-generating capacity of a muscle depends on muscle length.[21] Each cross-bridge contributes to force. The number of cross-bridges that can form per unit area of the muscle determines the total force a muscle can develop. At longer muscle lengths, actin and myosin overlap less. Fewer cross-bridges form between the myosin molecule and the actin binding sites. With fewer cross-bridges pulling, less force can be generated. At short muscle lengths, the two adja-

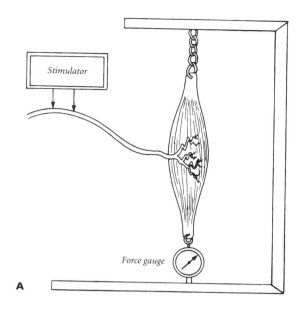

A

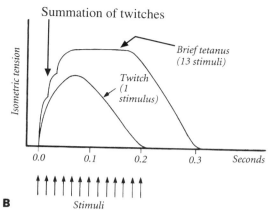

Summation of twitches

Brief tetanus (13 stimuli)

Twitch (1 stimulus)

B

Stimuli

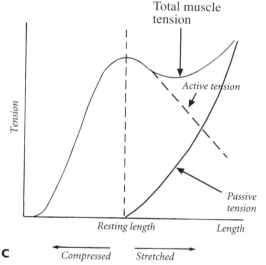

Total muscle tension

Active tension

Passive tension

Resting length

Length

C

Compressed   *Stretched*

Figure 13–6. Isometric properties of muscle. **A:** Experimental arrangement suitable for measuring whole-muscle properties. Stimulator is set to excite entire muscle through its nerve. The chain is adjusted to set the muscle length. **B:** Time course of muscle tension during a twitch and a brief tetanus. Arrows on the bottom show timing of stimuli during tetanus. **C:** Maximum tension of a muscle at different lengths. Passive tension is measured without stimulation. Active tension is measured during a brief tetanus. The dashed line on the curve is at the muscle's resting length.

cent actin fibers overlap and interfere with each other, again reducing the number of cross-bridges formed. Thus, at very short and very long lengths, the muscle generates force but less efficiently than at intermediate lengths.

Because muscles may be needed for various types of work, the contractile properties of the muscle fibers vary. Muscle fibers are divided into three major groups.[22–24] **Slow muscle fibers** cannot generate force very quickly, but they can operate for long periods of time without fatiguing. This type of muscle fiber is very important for postural muscles where

the force of gravity must be opposed constantly. Slow fibers tend to be smaller in diameter than fast muscle fibers. They also tend to be innervated by smaller-diameter nerve fibers. **Fast muscle fibers**, as the name suggests, can produce large forces quite rapidly, and may take several minutes to recover after a maximal effort. Axons leading to fast fibers are usually large-diameter axons that conduct action potentials more quickly than smaller-diameter axons. Finally, an intermediate type, **fast fatigue-resistant muscle fiber**, has properties, including fiber size, that are intermediate between the slow and fast muscle fibers. Axons to these fibers tend to be intermediate in size.

Muscles require energy to operate, and a muscle's fiber type is related to the way it uses energy. Fast muscle fibers derive their energy from burning glycogen, using **anaerobic metabolism**, a process that does not require a constant source of oxygen. The amount of energy that can be extracted from glycogen during anaerobic metabolism is relatively small compared with the amount of glycogen that can be stored in a muscle. Therefore, fast fibers fatigue readily. These fibers are fast because the energy from glycogen can be released quickly. Slow fibers metabolize fats with the aid of oxygen, which is a slower process. Because fast muscle fibers use glycogen, they are often called fast-glycolytic (FG) fibers. Likewise, slow fibers that use oxidative metabolism are called slow-oxidative, or SO fibers. The process of burning fats with oxygen is called **aerobic metabolism**. Aerobic metabolism can be sustained for longer periods of time, as long as oxygen is present, thanks to the greater energy capacity of fats. To help with oxygen storage, slow fibers have molecules similar to those found in red blood cells. In the muscle, **myoglobin** stores oxygen in the same way hemoglobin does in the blood. The reddish tint of myoglobin is the pigmentation in red meat. Birds, for example, have dark leg muscles for brief, energetic activity, and light breast muscles for sustained flight, whereas all human muscles are a mixture of muscle types.

The process that determines which muscle fibers are fast and which are slow is complex and still not fully understood. In experimental studies, muscles that are continuously electrically stimulated at low frequencies tend to develop a higher percentage of slow fibers.[25,26] Other experiments, however, show that the nerve leading to the muscle can influence the muscle fiber type. When a nerve that is removed from a muscle containing mostly slow fibers is allowed to grow into a muscle that normally has mostly fast fibers, the fast fibers are transformed into slower fibers.[27-29] This finding indicates that the motor neurons in the spinal cord somehow signal the muscle fibers to change their type.

Skeletal Muscle: The Functional Unit

The nerve entering a muscle is mixed; it is composed of both sensory **(afferent)** and motor **(efferent)** axons. Thus, it is the pathway by which descending motor commands reach the muscle, and by which sensory signals from the muscle, regarding tension, stretch, and external loads, are passed on to the central nervous system. Except for the cranial nerves, the sensory axons arise from cell bodies in the dorsal root ganglia, just outside the spinal cord. The axons split (bifurcate), sending one branch into the dorsal horn of the spinal cord as the dorsal spinal root. The other branch joins with the peripheral nerves until the appropriate axons reach the muscle. The motor axons of the muscle arise from **motor neurons** in the ventral horn of the spinal cord and exit as the ventral root.

Like muscle fibers, nerve fibers, or axons, have different sizes. Nerve fiber size affects conduction velocity: larger axons conduct action potentials more quickly than do smaller axons. For the purpose of classification, the fastest sensory nerve fibers are called *Type I*, the next fastest *Type II*, then *Type III*, and so on. Greek letters are used to indicate motor axon fiber sizes. The fastest are alpha (α), the next fastest (β), the next gamma (γ), and so on. Motor neurons in the spinal cord are of two sizes: α and γ. The larger, α motor neurons innervate the **extrafusal** muscle fibers, the force producing fibers of the muscle, and are referred to as the *skeletomotor system*. The smaller γ motor neurons innervate the **intrafusal** muscle fibers in the sensory (spindle) apparatus of the muscle, and are known as the *fusimotor system*. The intrafusal muscle fibers are part of a length-sensing apparatus; they generate no detectable tension in the muscle, but their contraction increases the frequency of firing of the sensory inflow to the spinal cord. Studies have identified a group of α motor neurons that innervate both extrafusal and intrafusal fibers, referred to as the *skeletofusimotor system*.[30]

Spinal motor neurons are multipolar cells with vast dendritic arborizations. Each neuron receives thousands of synapses from such diverse sources as the cerebral cortex, brainstem, distant spinal afferent neurons, nearby interneurons, and primary muscle afferents. By convention, cells that are contained wholly within the spinal cord, that is, not motor neurons and not dorsal root ganglia neurons, are called **interneurons**. All the different inputs converge on the motor neuron, and together they regulate how close the neuron is to threshold, called **motor neuron excitability**, and when it fires an action potential.

Because a single axon branches to innervate many muscle fibers distributed over a wide area within the same muscle, an action potential in the neuron leads to the more-or-less synchronized twitch of a group of fibers in that muscle. In other words, the motor neuron and the fibers it innervates work together as a unit, and are therefore known as a **motor unit**. The central nervous system plans movements in terms of motor units rather than individual muscle fibers. For this reason, it is more valuable to discuss the properties of a motor unit in a muscle rather than the properties of a single nerve or single muscle fiber. All the muscle fibers of a motor unit are of the same type (e.g., fast, slow, fatigue-resistant) and are of the same general size. Thus, based on the type of muscle fibers they innervate, three types of motor units can be identified: **fast fatigable** motor units, **slow** motor units, and **fatigue-resistant** motor units.[22–24] All human muscles are a mixture of all three motor unit types. The number of muscle fibers in a motor unit, however, varies according to the muscle. Small muscles, such as extraocular muscles or hand muscles, have three to six muscle fibers per motor unit. These muscles are capable of producing fine, graded, precise movement. In contrast, muscles involved in more forceful, less precise movements, such as large muscles of the leg and back, have 200 to 2,000 fibers per unit.[31]

The motor neurons associated with a muscle are mixed with other neurons of the spinal cord, but still tend to be relatively near each other; they form a vertical column in the ventral horn of the spinal cord. The motor neurons to a muscle live together and work together. They operate in a coordinated manner, like a pool of laborers at a construction site. Like the laborers, the motor neurons innervating a muscle are called a **motor neuron pool**.[32] Also like a pool of laborers, at any given moment some percentage of the total population is active. Sometimes, 10% are active; on rare occasions, 100% are active. The force requirement of a task determines how many motor units are active during that task. If more force is needed, more motor units are **recruited**, which means a greater percentage of the motor neuron pool is active. Thus, the strength of contraction is graded by the number or motor units recruited.

Animal studies have shown a general relationship among the motor neuron soma size, the size of its axon, and the size of the muscle fibers it innervates.[33,34] Large motor neurons give rise to large-diameter axons that innervate fast muscle units, and slow muscle units are innervated by small, slowly conducting motor neurons. When relatively low forces are required for a task, the body automatically uses the motor units with smaller muscle fibers. This observation makes sense, because these motor units are the least likely to fatigue (see earlier discussion). If more force is needed, fast units are recruited, until the force requirement is met. Stated another way, motor neurons in a pool are recruited according to their size, from small to large. This principle is called the **size principle**.[34,35]

In addition to recruitment, a muscle's force output depends on how rapidly it is being excited by its nerve. The amount of force a muscle produces (up to the fusion frequency) depends on how often it is excited; the more frequently the muscle is activated, the larger the force it produces (see Fig. 13–6B). This increase in force is brought about by changing the discharge rates of the recruited motor neurons, and is known as **rate coding**. Several studies have shown that the firing rate of the recruited motor neurons increases proportionately with increasing force output.[34,36–38]

We now have touched on two ways muscle force can be regulated at any given moment: 1) recruitment, and 2) rate coding. Both variables are used to control force during normal muscle operation. The twitch, or tetanus, of any one motor unit is hardly detectable. So, for any submaximal pulling force exerted by the muscle, the two mechanisms work together to adjust force up or down in steps so tiny that muscle action appears totally smooth.

A skeletal muscle is a rather unintelligent organ. Muscles follow the dictates of the motor neuron pools. The motor neuron pool is smarter. It is wired for the size principle. Ultimately, however, the motor neuron pool follows the dictates of the rest of the nervous system. The motor neuron pool collects information from sensory neurons within the muscle, and less directly from a wide variety of sources, including skin, joint receptors, the inner ear, and eventually from whatever parts of the brain are responsible for conscious thought. In fact, for any part of the nervous system to contribute to the control of a muscle, it must ultimately do so through the muscle's motor neuron pool. For this reason, the motor neuron pool is called the final common pathway to the muscles. Understanding how the central nervous system controls movement depends largely on understanding the various ways different parts of the nervous system affect muscles through the final common pathway.

Sensory Organs of the Muscle

The sensory organs play important roles in the reflex regulation of motor unit activity. They convey information about mechanical forces arising from the muscle and include **Golgi tendon organs (GTO)** and **muscle spindles**. The sensory axons that innervate GTO are about as large as any other sensory fiber in the body. Thus, they are classified as Type I. Because two different Type I sensory fibers are found in the muscle nerve, they are designated Type Ia and Type Ib. Type Ia fibers come from spindles, Type Ib come from GTO.

Golgi Tendon Organ

The GTO are distributed among the collagenous fascicles of the muscle's tendon. They lie in series with the extrafusal muscle fibers, 3 to 25 muscle fibers per tendon organ. The GTO detects tension generated by both passive stretch and active contraction of the muscle. The amount of stretch at the tendon is proportional to the force on the muscle during contraction.[39] Passive stretch of the muscle is not very effective at activating the tendon organs, because the more elastic muscle fibers take up much of the stretch. Thus, to generate nervous activity from the sensory fiber (Type Ib) innervating the tendon organ, the muscle must contract. Activation of the Type Ib fibers leads to inhibition of the motor neurons that supply the muscle from which they arise. The inhibition is mediated by inhibitory interneurons. The Type Ib fibers discharge whenever the muscle contracts. Thus, the GTO functions as a sensor in a feedback system that regulates muscle force by bringing about changes in muscle tension by increasing or decreasing the inhibition on the α motor neurons.[40]

Muscle Spindle

The muscle spindle is a complex sense organ located in the muscle itself. The spindle has a fusiform shape, composed of tiny, *intrafusal* muscle fibers (approximately four to eight) that are bundled together, and sit astride or parallel to the more massive extrafusal fibers. Because of their position in the muscle, changes in the length of the whole muscle are reflected as changes in the length of the muscle spindle.[39] The spindle fibers are innervated by both motor and sensory axons, and together they supply detailed information about muscle length and movement to the central nervous system.[40,41] The number of spindles in skeletal muscle varies. Small muscles that produce precise movements have many spindles, reflecting the need for sensory information for accurate performance of these movements. Large muscles producing less precise movements have few spindles; muscles of the ear have no spindles at all.

The spindle has two types of intrafusal muscle fibers: **nuclear bag fibers** and **nuclear chain fibers** (Fig. 13–7A,B). The nuclear bag fibers contain many nuclei in an enlarged central area called the bag, whereas the nuclei are lined up in a single file in the nuclear chain fibers. The ends of the nuclear chain fibers connect to the sides of the nuclear bag fibers. The intrafusal muscle fibers can contract and, like all other skeletal muscle fibers, they receive motor neuron innervations. The innervating axons are very thin and come from small γ motor neurons in the spinal cord. For reasons discussed later, the nuclear chain fibers receive γ static motor axons and the nuclear bag fibers receive γ dynamic axons. Like the motor innervations, spindles have two different types (sizes) of sensory axons: *Type Ia* and *Type II*. Type Ia or primary endings wrap around the center of the nuclear bag fibers and nuclear chain fibers. Type II or secondary endings innervate only the nuclear chain fibers. The arrangement of the afferent and efferent elements of the muscle spindle allows the central nervous system to control the information coming from the spindle sensory organ. The nuclear bag fiber and the nuclear chain fiber have different mechanical properties. Their efferent innervations regulate these properties. Type Ia endings are affected by both kinds of intrafusal fibers, and therefore affected by both types of γ innervation; Type II endings are affected only by the nuclear chain fibers, and are therefore influenced only by the γ static innervations.

The operation of the muscle spindle is easiest to describe, beginning with the Type II sensory ending. (We will ignore, for the moment, Type Ia afferent endings.) Action potentials recorded from Type II spindle afferents show that their firing rate depends on the length of the muscle. If the muscle is lengthened passively by an external force, the firing rate increases linearly with the change in whole muscle length. If the muscle is held at this length, the Type II afferent continues to fire at the new (higher) rate (see Fig. 13–7C). The Type II afferent reacts to the stretch of the nuclear chain fiber, which tugs on its wrapped ending (see Fig. 13–7A). This mechanism suggests an alternate way to affect the Type II ending. Activation of the γ static innervation causes the end

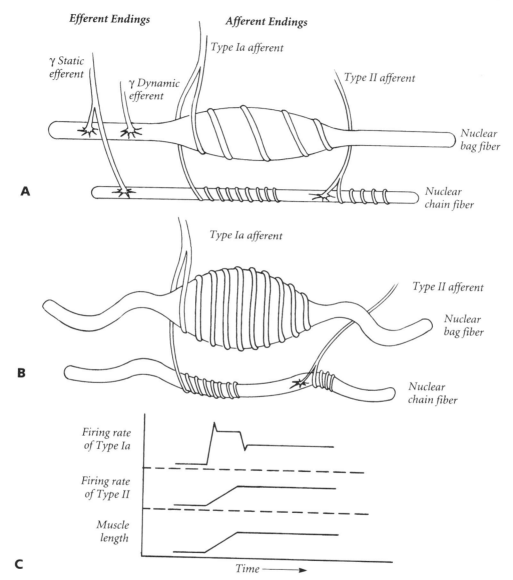

Figure 13–7. Muscle spindle fiber and its properties. **A:** The muscle spindle has two types of intrafusal muscle fibers: nuclear bag and nuclear chain, each with its own γ motor innervation: γ dynamic and γ static, respectively. It also has two types of afferent (sensory) fibers: Type Ia and Type II. Type Ia endings always span both types of intrafusal fibers. Stretching the whole muscle stretches the intrafusal fibers. This stretches the afferent endings, setting up action potentials in the afferents. **B:** Without efferent endings, shortening the muscle causes the spindle to lose all its tension and the afferent ending ceases to generate action potentials. With γ activity, the slack spindle in **(B)** straightens up, as in **(A)**. **C:** Type Ia and Type II endings have different responses to stretch. The bottom trace shows the length of a muscle during a smooth stretch. The middle trace shows that the firing rate of Type II afferent endings faithfully reproduces the muscle length. (We are assuming that the spindle is not slack.) The top trace shows the effect of dynamic sensitivity. The Type Ia and II afferents in this example have similar static sensitivities. The difference occurs only when the muscle length changes.

of the nuclear chain fiber to contract. This action, in turn, stretches the Type II sensory ending, just as if the muscle had been stretched. This arrangement serves a useful function. Instead of lengthening the muscle, what happens when the muscle is shortened? During a typical movement, a muscle shortens as it contracts. As the muscle length is reduced, so is the firing rate of the Type II ending. At some muscle lengths, the Type II afferents turns off completely. At this point, the nuclear chain fiber is limp (see Fig. 13–7B). Further muscle shortening does not affect the Type II endings on the nuclear chain fiber. This circumstance poses a problem for the central nervous system because, until the spindle is stretched again, it no longer supplies information about muscle length. (Remember, we are ignoring Type Ia afferents right now.) The central nervous system does not know if the muscle shortens further, because Type II afferents cannot fire at a rate less than zero. The solution is the γ static innervation. The γ static activity shortens the nuclear chain fiber, so it is no longer limp, and brings the Type II afferent firing rate above zero. The central nervous system controls the intrafusal fiber length with the γ innervation, so the Type II afferents are always providing information about muscle length.

Type Ia afferents have more complex responses to muscle stretch because their activity is determined by stretch of both the nuclear chain fiber and the nuclear bag fiber. If the muscle lengthens very slowly, then the Type Ia afferent behaves much like a Type II axon. If the same stretch happens rapidly, the Type Ia afferent shows a great burst of activity and then settles down to its normal value sometime after the end-point is reached. So, although Type Ia activity depends somewhat on static muscle length, much of its discharge rate depends on the rate (i.e., velocity) of muscle stretch. The Type Ia axon is said to have both **static** and **dynamic sensitivity**, whereas the Type II axon has only static sensitivity.[40,42]

It is easy to understand why static sensitivity is a valuable commodity. It supplies the central nervous system with a faithful description of moment-to-moment muscle length. The utility of dynamic sensitivity may be less obvious and is worth reviewing here. The main assets that dynamic sensitivity provides are sensitivity and speed. Many of the sensory organs of the human body are acutely tuned to detect changes in the environment. The pacinian corpuscle, for example, does not detect skin pressure per se, but rather detects *changes* in pressure on the skin. This fact explains why a hand lying still on a surface does not activate these receptors, but if the hand should suddenly slip or the surface should start to move, the pacinian corpuscles in the hand signal the environmental change. Similarly, if the same motion leads to a change in the length of some muscle in the hand, which it almost certainly will, the Type Ia axon of the muscle spindles responds vigorously to the rapid change in muscle length. As the muscle begins to change length, the Type II axons begin to change their firing rate. Even before a significant change in length occurs, however, the Type Ia axons may send a strong signal telling the central nervous system that a rapid change is underway. The central nervous system receives advance warning that a significant length change will take place. The speed advantage imparted by the dynamic sensitivity is crucial because muscle is an inherently sluggish device. Action potentials can move from the spinal cord to the hand within 20 milliseconds, but it takes 50 to 100 milliseconds for a muscle to produce significant force once the signal reaches the NMJ. Our ability to respond quickly and accurately to unexpected perturbations depends on a sensory system with dynamic sensitivity. This dynamic sensitivity helps to make up in part for the time delay inherent to this feedback system.

The amount of dynamic sensitivity, measured as the **dynamic index**, and the amount of static sensitivity must be adjusted constantly by the central nervous system to ensure that no unexpected perturbation goes undetected. Too much dynamic sensitivity can create a problem. If the muscle is rapidly shortened, Type Ia axons go completely silent as soon as the shortening begins. During this silent period, the central nervous system stops receiving information from the Type Ia axons, so details about the rest of the movement are lost. The solution is the γ dynamic innervation. The effect of γ static axons was discussed earlier; the γ dynamic axons work in a similar manner. Activation of the γ dynamic efferents causes the contractile ends of the intrafusal fibers to shorten, which, in turn, stretches the nuclear bag portion of the spindles and initiates impulses in the Type Ia fibers. Thus, activation of γ motor neurons ensures that spindle afferents continue to transmit information when the extrafusal muscle shorten during voluntary contraction. Thus, α-γ **coactivation** is essential to keep the Type Ia sensory fibers from falling silent as the muscle is shortened. It also helps to adjust the sensitivity of the Type II fibers. The α-γ

coactivation appears to be common, both during conscious, goal-directed movements, as well as during more automatic movements, such as respiration and walking.

The primary or Type Ia endings make direct excitatory connections with α motor neurons supplying the same muscle; therefore, stretch of the extrafusal fibers produces a rapid increase in muscle tension and opposes the stretch. It can also be viewed as a feedback loop that tends to maintain the length of the extrafusal fibers at a constant value. The desired muscle length is specified by the descending pathways that bring about α-γ coactivation. Deviations from the desired length are reflected in the activity of the muscle spindle, which in turn influences the activity of the α motor neurons. If the muscle is stretched more than the desired length, spindle activity is increased and shortening is produced. If, however, the muscle shortens more than the desired length, spindle discharge decreases and the muscle relaxes. Several studies have shown that γ efferents discharge along with α motor neurons.[39,40,43–45] The pervasiveness of α-γ coactivation, however, does not mean that γ activity strictly mimics α activity *all* the time. The evidence suggests that α and γ motor neurons can be differentially controlled by separate control centers in the brain.[40,46–48] Furthermore, modulation of γ motor neurons activity during walking, for example, does not appear to match changes in α motor neuron activity exactly.

Clinical Correlations

Primary Muscle Disease

Two types of disorders affect muscle directly: those that affect the motor neurons—either the cell body or axon—and those that affect the muscle cell itself. Diseases that affect the motor neuron are known as **neurogenic** disorders, and those that affect the muscle cell directly are termed **myogenic** disorders. *Neurogenic* diseases have been divided into those that affect the motor neuron cell body (i.e., motor neuron disease) and those that affect the peripheral axon (i.e., peripheral neuropathies).

A well known neurogenic disease is amyotrophic lateral sclerosis (ALS), also called Lou Gehrig's disease. The cause of ALS is unknown, although about 10% of the cases are familial (autosomal dominant), exhibiting a mutation in the long arm of chromosome 21.[49,50] The disease attacks the cell bodies of motor neurons in the spinal cord and brainstem,

and neurons in the cerebral cortex that synapse on motor neurons (see Chapter 14). The affected neurons degenerate, leading to muscle weakness beginning first in the hands and feet. Degeneration is associated with fasciculations or spontaneous twitches of the denervated motor units. The spontaneous muscle activity can be recorded on an electromyogram. Damage to the motor neurons leads to muscle wasting or atrophy; damage to the cortical neurons causes hyperreflexia. Remarkably, all sensory innervation is unaffected by the disease process. When the disease progresses to the muscles of respiration, it is usually fatal.

In contrast to ALS, Guillain-Barré syndrome is an acute polyneuropathy causing diffuse lesions of the mixed peripheral nerves, not the motor neuron cell bodies.[51] It causes both sensory and motor disturbances. On the sensory side, disturbances are commonly in the distal part of the extremities, leading to a stocking-and-glove pattern of numbness, often with a tingling sensation. On the motor side, muscular weakness and reduced reflexes are observed.

Myogenic diseases of skeletal muscle can be either inherited or acquired. The most common inherited myopathy is Duchenne muscular dystrophy. The Duchenne myopathy is inherited as an X-linked recessive trait and thus affects males only.[52] It manifests as a relatively rapid progression of muscle weakness, beginning before the age of 5 years. These patients are usually wheelchair bound by the age of 14 years, and usually die by the third decade of life because of weakness of the respiratory muscles. Other forms of inherited muscular dystrophy include the fascioscapulohumeral, myotonic, and limb-girdle types, each with its own age of onset, pattern of weakness, and progression. All three are carried by an autosomal dominant trait. Alterations in ion channel (Cl^-, Ca^{++}, or Na^+) genes also have been shown to produce myotonia (muscle stiffness) or paralysis.[53,54]

Dermatomyositis is an example of an acquired myopathy. In this disease, muscle weakness primarily affects proximal limb muscles. It is accompanied by a skin rash of the face, chest, and extensor surfaces of the joints. The cause is unknown, but an autoimmune origin is suspected.

Peripheral Nerve Injury

Peripheral nerve injury usually involves both sensory and motor axons. Because each nerve supplies a particular part of the body, the location of the injury can often be inferred from the symptoms. Large nerve trunks, closer to the spinal cord, involve a more widespread territory. The effects of small nerve branch lesions are more localized. The sensory and motor losses may not exactly coincide if the sensory and motor axons in the nerve have slightly different target areas of the body. The motor loss is called paralysis or paresis and its severity depends on the extent of the injury. Injuries of the motor neurons and peripheral nerves also result in areflexia (loss of reflexes) and loss of muscle tone (decreased resistance to passive stretch). Reflexes and muscle tone are discussed in the next section.

Large and small axons react to injury differently. Compression selectively inactivates larger nerve fibers first. The sensation of your leg "falling asleep" is a reversible compression injury. The smaller pain fibers are still operational, but the larger sensory fibers (i.e., Types Ia and Ib) and motor fibers (i.e., α motor neurons) are dysfunctional. Therefore, do not try to walk! Lesions that cut off blood flow—ischemic lesions—affect smaller axons first, which has the reverse effect. Dull pain is absent, although sharp pain can still persist; the smaller sensory fibers are af-

fected (i.e., spindle Type II fibers), as are the γ motor fibers. Because partial ischemic lesions are rare, this constellation of symptoms is also rare.

Spinal Mechanisms and Motor Control

General Anatomy

The spinal cord, like other areas of the central nervous system, contains both gray and white matter, arranged in a systematic manner. The human spinal cord consists of approximately 18 inches of gray matter, surrounded by an outer layer of white matter. While sheathed in dura, it has the consistency of rope; with the dura removed, the spinal cord is no firmer than Jell-O. If the spinal cord is sliced perpendicular to its long axis, it can be viewed in cross-section, which reveals a tiny central canal filled with cerebrospinal fluid, and the gray matter core (Fig. 13–8). The core is shaped like the wings of a butterfly. Focusing on one side (wing), the central gray that bulges

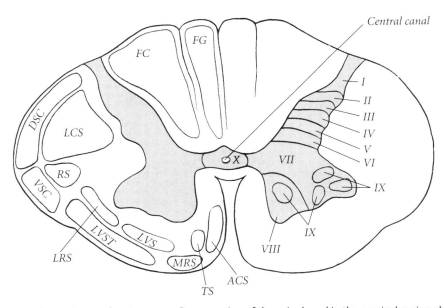

Figure 13–8. Laminae and major tracts. Cross-section of the spinal cord in the cervical region showing gray matter divided according to Rexed's laminar organization on the right, and selected white matter tracts on the left. LCS, lateral corticospinal tract; MRS, medial reticulospinal tract; LRS, lateral reticulospinal tract; LVST, lateral vestibulospinal tract; ACS, anterior corticospinal tract; RS, rubrospinal tract; VSC, ventral spinocerebellar tract; DSC, dorsal spinocerebellar tract; TS, tectospinal tract; FG, fasciculus gracilis; FC, fasciculus cuneatus.

anteriorly is called the ventral horn, where motor neuron cell bodies, also called ventral horn cells, are located. The efferent fibers leave through the ventral roots. The posterior horn is invaded by sensory fibers (dorsal roots) from the dorsal root ganglia. These ganglia reside outside the spinal cord proper, but are covered by the same dural sheath. The supposition that in the spinal cord dorsal roots are sensory and the ventral roots are motor is known as the **Bell-Magendie's law**.

Remember from Chapter 2 that each level of the spinal cord is identified by the same system used to identify bony vertebrae in the vertebral column (C-1 through C-8, T-1 through T-12, and so forth). Because of the different rates of growth of the spine and the spinal cord, the correspondence is not exact. Spinal nerves exit the vertebral column caudal to where they exit the spinal cord. Therefore, a compression lesion that affects one level of the spinal cord usually also affects the spinal nerve from a higher level of the spinal cord.

The relative proportions of gray and white matter vary along the spinal cord, as does the cord size. The cord is largest rostrally to accommodate axons that must pass the upper segments to reach either the brain (ascending fibers) or the lower segments (descending fibers). The gray matter thickens dramatically where motor and sensory neurons and their fibers must be included to communicate and process information for the upper and lower limbs.

Based on a cross-sectional view of the spinal cord, the gray matter can be divided into 10 distinct regions, or laminae, based on the careful cytoarchitectonic studies of Rexed.[55] These laminae are numbered I through X (see Fig. 13–8). Motor neurons are usually arranged in Rexed lamina IX of the ventral horn. Motor neurons associated with the extremities are located more laterally in lamina IX, whereas those associated with the trunk (i.e., axial musculature) are located more medially. Along the anteroposterior axis, motor neurons innervating extensor muscles (i.e., antigravity muscles) are found more anteriorly than those innervating flexor muscles.

Surrounding the central gray area are ascending and descending pathways arranged in each of the major funiculi or regions of white matter. Ascending sensory information from the periphery is carried in the posterior funiculus (fasciculus cuneatus, fasciculus gracilis), and these fibers together constitute the posterior columns. Descending motor pathways are found in the lateral and anterior funiculi. In gen-

eral, the descending pathways in the lateral funiculus, such as the lateral corticospinal tract (see Chapter 14), influence all muscles. In contrast, those descending pathways found in the anterior funiculus, such as the anterior corticospinal tract, primarily influence axial and trunk musculature involved in postural stabilization and equilibrium responses.[56]

Understanding the general anatomy of the gray and white matter is important for understanding the clinical manifestations of localized tumors, spinal cord injuries, infections, or vascular disturbances. Lesions of the gray matter cause problems localized to the particular spinal segments involved, whereas lesions of the white matter usually produce more widespread dysfunctions. For example, damage to the ventral horn of the spinal cord at C-5 affects the lower motor neuron innervation to the muscles at that specific level (e.g., deltoid, supraspinatus). Such an impairment would manifest itself as difficulty with shoulder movements ipsilateral to the lesioned side. Clinically, this pattern is known as a lower motor neuron lesion, and is discussed in more detail later.

Spinal Reflex Mechanisms

Maintenance of Upright Posture

The muscles of the legs, back, and neck constantly wrestle with gravity to maintain an upright posture. Even during quiet stance, many small corrective muscle actions are needed to prevent toppling over. A simple series of actions—shaking the hand of a stranger, for instance—shifts the center of gravity, generates unexpected perturbations, and requires constant postural support to make the primary actions fluid.

When upright, the body rests on a tiny surface area circumscribed by the two feet, and is levered by a 1.5- to 2-m moment arm. The complex central nervous system network that controls upright stance can operate without conscious intervention, and is imbued with precision, speed, flexibility, and adaptability.

Spinal cord circuitry plays a major role in posture. Many postural reflexes can be elicited after complete transection of the spinal cord, although without the brainstem, the surviving reactions to stimulation cannot support standing posture even in quadrupeds. For example, experimental animals with spinal transections have stretch and withdrawal reflexes. They show compensatory activity in the opposite limb during a withdrawal reflex (crossed extensor reflex), which ensures that when one leg is lifted during withdrawal, the other is prepared to bear more weight.[5,57] In general, a vast spinal network supports interlimb coordination in response to stimulation from receptors in the skin, muscles, joints, and special senses.

Those muscles that oppose the force of gravity are grouped together as physiologic extensors. Physiologic extensors have reflexes in common with each other and are characteristically different from their antagonists, the physiologic flexors. For example, the withdrawal reflex is a reflex that activates flexors and inhibits extensors.

Simple Reflexes

Reflexes are a form of sensorimotor integration because they involve connections between the afferent and efferent neurons. Spinal reflexes are mediated at the spinal level, in contrast to others mediated at the brainstem and higher centers (see Chapter 14). Spinal reflexes serve three important functions in motor control: 1) to adjust for unexpected perturbations; 2) to organize patterns of coordination, such as **reciprocal inhibition**; and 3) to allow for rapid protection from painful or damaging stimuli. Spinal reflexes that are nonpathologic provide efficiency in motor planning and effectiveness of movement without the need for conscious thought or continuous supraspinal modulation. For example, higher centers may provide a goal-directed plan for skipping rope, but the details of this plan, such as the reciprocal activation of flexors and extensors, is enabled by the spinal cord reflex circuitry rather than by direct supraspinal control.

I hand you a box that is small, but unexpectedly heavy for its size. Without too much effort, you are able to compensate for this unexpected weight automatically. The adequate stimulus for load compensation is muscle stretch; thus, the reflex is called the **stretch reflex**, also known as the **myotatic reflex**. The stretch reflex is present even after total destruction of the cerebral cortex. Even though the cortex is involved in the myotatic reflex, the remainder of the central nervous system makes its own contribution. Several different neural circuits are responsible for increasing muscle activation in response to an increased load. Much of the circuitry for the stretch reflex appears to be wired into the spinal cord.

Returning to the example, when you received the box, the very first change in your muscle activity occurred quickly. Type Ia spindle afferents were excited by the stretch on the muscle due to the weight of the box. These afferents enter the spinal cord through the dorsal root and synapse directly on motor neu-

rons of the same muscle. If enough Type Ia afferents release enough transmitter on the motor neurons, the motor neurons generate action potentials that travel back out the ventral root of the cord and activate the muscle. We can measure the **reaction time** or time for action potentials to travel from the muscle spindles to the spinal cord, plus the time for action potentials induced in the motor neurons to travel back to the muscle.[57] In humans, the stretch reflex has a reaction time of 19 to 24 milliseconds. Based on the very first action potentials in the muscles, action potentials from the stretch reflex spend approximately 0.5 millisecond in the spinal cord. This time period is called the **central delay**. You may remember from Chapter 3 that this period of time is just long enough to send transmitter across one synapse. We conclude that the fastest component of the stretch reflex required only one synapse. That synapse must be formed by a Type Ia afferent connected directly to an α motor neuron. The pathway for the earliest component of the stretch reflex, as opposed to other components that take many milliseconds longer to begin, is called the **monosynaptic** pathway. It consists of the shortest possible neuronal circuit—one synapse.

The traditional definition of a spinal reflex is one in which an adequate stimulus leads to a stereotypic motor response that is graded with the stimulus. A reflex has 1) a sensor, 2) a processor, and 3) an effector. The sensor, or "afferent limb," consists of the receptor and its primary sensory afferent. For example, the muscle spindle and the Type Ia afferent are considered the sensor in the stretch reflex. The processor is the integration center in the spinal cord, such as the synapse in the ventral horn in the case of the monosynaptic stretch reflex. Finally, the effector is the "efferent limb," including the α motor neuron and muscle fibers it innervates (i.e., motor unit) in the muscle.

Spinal reflexes can be localized in the spinal cord so that the sensor, processor, and effector are all associated with the same spinal segment. Alternatively, intersegmental spinal reflexes that involve several spinal segments use interneurons to transmit afferent limb signals to higher or lower spinal segments. Intersegmental reflexes underlie synergistic effector responses, such as the **flexor withdrawal reflex**, discussed later.

Stretch Reflex

The stretch reflex is mediated by the muscle spindle with its intrafusal fibers and Type Ia and II afferents.[58]

When a muscle is stretched, axons from Type Ia afferents from that muscle enter the spinal cord through the dorsal root. Branches of these axons cross through the gray matter of the spinal cord to the ventral horn and synapse directly on motor neurons projecting to the same muscle. Therefore, any external force stretching the muscle excites the Type Ia axons, which excite the motor neuron pool, which oppose the external force by activating the muscle. This process is termed **autogenic facilitation**; the stretch stimulus originated in the same muscles that were activated by the reflex. In addition, through an inhibitory interneuron (Type Ia interneuron, or Ia-IN), the antagonistic muscle is inhibited.

Each Type Ia afferent projects to nearly all of the motor neurons in the homonymous motor neuron pool.[33] The recruitment of motor neurons by the stretch reflex follows the size principle: small, slow motor units are recruited first, and only rarely are large, fast units recruited during a stretch reflex. The size principle also applies to the inhibitory action of Type Ia-INs: the antagonist muscle slow motor units are *inhibited* more easily than the antagonist fast motor units.

In contrast to the monosynaptic pathway of the Type Ia afferent, the Type II afferents make polysynaptic connections with the same motor neuron pool. In addition, the average excitatory effect from a Type II afferent on the postsynaptic cell is about one half the size of that from a Type Ia afferent. Thus, the recruitment capability of the Type II afferent is less effective than that of the Type Ia. Because the monosynaptic pathway is driven by Type Ia sensory fibers, a very rapid stretch should be more effective at activating this pathway than a slow stretch. Remember, the monosynaptic pathway is only one part of the stretch reflex; other pathways are better suited to deal with slow stretches.

The easiest way to demonstrate a rapid stretch is with the knee-jerk response, elicited by striking the tendon distal to the patella. The muscle is stretched very rapidly, but only a short distance. The characteristic kick of the knee results from maximal stimulation of the monosynaptic pathway. Remember, Type Ia fibers are exquisitely sensitive to rapid stretch, owing to their dynamic sensitivity. Thus, the knee-jerk reflex, or more generally the deep tendon reflex (DTR), is simply a special case of the stretch reflex. The signal is almost a pure velocity signal (its rate of change is very high), and the response is dominated by the Type Ia synapse on motor neurons of the same muscle.

This description of a DTR does not address an important problem. When the knee kicks because of the reflex activation of the knee extensor muscles, a rapid stretch of the knee flexors is produced. What prevents the knee flexors from responding with their own jerk reflex? This action, of course, would cause another jerk in the extensors, which in turn would lead to another flexor jerk, and so on. When the sensory axons from the extensors excite the extensor α motor neurons, they simultaneously inhibit the flexor motor neurons through the Type Ia-IN described earlier. This two-synapse path ensures that the antagonist muscles do not interfere with the DTR or, more generally, with the stretch reflex. Whenever antagonist muscles are inhibited during the activation of agonist muscles, the process is called **reciprocal inhibition**.[59,60] Reciprocal inhibition helps coordinate action at a joint. This coordination is hard-wired at the spinal cord level. Higher centers can use the hard-wired spinal circuits, such as reciprocal inhibition, in the coordination of more complex actions like locomotion.

Before leaving the stretch reflex, we should examine how it is controlled by other neural circuits. Although this reflex has only one synapse to homonymous motor neurons and only two synapses to antagonist motor neurons, it is actually under considerable "external" influence.[61] The central nervous system can reduce spindle sensitivity to regulate the stretch reflex in three ways: 1) in presynaptic inhibition (see Chapter 3), a tiny synapse at the presynaptic terminal of the Type Ia axon, as it makes contact with the α motor neuron, can inhibit the monosynaptic pathway and render it ineffective; 2) inhibitory synapses onto the Type Ia-IN can prevent reciprocal inhibition; and 3) γ motor neuron control can affect muscle spindle sensitivity.

The sensitivity of the muscle spindle to stretch can be regulated by the γ motor neurons by way of the intrafusal fibers—that is, the γ motor neurons help to set the gain of the stretch reflex. If the γ dynamic motor neurons are highly activated, the reflex is even more responsive to rapid stretch. In other words, if the gain is high, a small stretch can produce a large increase in muscle tension. Less γ dynamic activity means less velocity sensitivity of the Type Ia axons and greater difficulty in producing a reflex response. Therefore, if the gain is low, a greater stretch is required to produce a similar change in muscle force.

Research has shown how this process might work to improve motor control.[40,62] The level of activation of γ motor neurons varies in accordance with the motor task and context; the sensitivity of the muscle spindle is adjusted appropriately for the specific requirements of a task. For example, in the cat, during slow walking on a level surface in a predictable environment, where muscle length changes slowly, only static γ motor neurons are active. In contrast, during unpredictable conditions, as when the animal is lifted off the ground, dynamic γ motor neurons are highly active, reflecting an increased spindle responsiveness. These examples show how external conditions modulate muscle spindle sensitivity to provide the most appropriate information during any given motor task. Thus, even the simplest reflex mechanism has all the properties of any reflex, including mechanisms to modulate the reflex action from outside the reflex loop.

Therapeutic Considerations. You have just learned why most stretching exercises should be performed slowly. A slow stretch is less likely to elicit a stretch reflex—a counterproductive contraction in the stretched muscle—than a fast stretch.

To facilitate a muscle that is already contracting, a quick stretch to that muscle increases the contraction through autogenic facilitation. Muscles of the face and the digastric (a jaw-opening muscle), however, do not have muscle spindles, so this facilitation technique applied to the facial muscles cannot be mediated by the stretch reflex. Instead, it may be mediated by certain cutaneous reflexes discussed later in this section.

Tendon Organ Reflex

Recall that the GTO is most sensitive to force when the muscle is contracting. The tendon organ reflex provides negative feedback to regulate the excessive development of muscle force. The Type Ib afferent carries signals from the tendon organs located at the musculotendinous junction. The Type Ib afferent influences the homonymous motor neuron pool through an inhibitory Type Ib-IN that inhibits the α motor neuron of the muscle that is generating the force. This process is termed **autogenic inhibition**. In addition, the antagonist motor neurons are facilitated disynaptically by an excitatory Type Ib-IN. This process is termed **reciprocal excitation**.[57]

This reflex arrangement suggests a kind of protective function for the tendon organ. It can keep the discharge frequency of the α motor neuron at a safe level to avoid spontaneous microruptures of musculotendinous tissues. Not surprisingly, the Type Ib-IN has the most influence on large motor neurons associated with FG type motor units. The FG motor units are also the largest force producers of the three motor unit types. The Type Ib-IN has the least influence on α motor neurons of slow motor units, which produce the lowest levels of force. The tendon organ and muscle spindle have opposing influences. Thus, investigators sometimes refer to the **tendon organ reflex** as the **inverse myotatic reflex** or **inverse stretch reflex**.

Functionally, the tendon organ serves more than a protective role. Because of its exquisite sensitivity to muscle force and its anatomic location, which allows it to sample a large number of motor units, the GTO probably acts with the muscle spindle to regulate muscle tone and compliance of the muscle. Similar to the muscle spindle, the influence of the GTO on the α motor neuron pool can be regulated centrally by convergent input onto the Type Ib-IN.[61,63] Input converges on the Type Ib-IN from multiple sources, including muscle spindle Type Ia afferents, joint capsule afferents, cutaneous afferents, and excitatory and inhibitory descending input from higher centers. The functional importance of this convergence for motor control may be considered in the context of fine control of grip force during the physical manipulation of objects. Suppose I am holding a videotape between my index finger and thumb. I am counteracting its weight with the force of my fingers. If this force is a little too low, the object may begin to slip between my fingers. Cutaneous receptors would then be excited, and through their input to the Type Ib-IN, the tendon organ inhibitory effect could be reduced, allowing an increase in muscle tension to increase my grip force and to stop the slippage. Because the Type Ib-IN also receives descending input, the strength of the inverse myotatic reflex can be tuned up, for example, with a more fragile object, or tuned down when more force is needed.

Therapeutic Considerations. Therapeutic intervention relies on the GTO for a stretching technique called "contract–relax." A forceful contraction of a muscle to be stretched invokes autogenic inhibition through the tendon organ reflex. After this contraction, the muscle is more likely to undergo a larger passive stretch before invoking a stretch reflex than if the stretch had not been preceded by the contraction. The suppression of the stretch reflex is most likely due to some form of persistent inhibition (i.e., posttetanic potentiation; see Chapter 3) of the agonist motor neuron pool created by autogenic inhibition mediated by the GTO.

Cutaneous Reflexes

Of all the spinal reflexes, cutaneous reflexes are probably the least understood.[61,64] These reflexes are polysynaptic and involve at least two or more interneurons in the reflex arc. The flexor reflex is a protective reflex that can be initiated by a painful stimulus (nociceptive stimuli), such as a hot or sharp object touched by the hand. Here, the cutaneous receptors are free nerve endings innervating the skin on the fingertips. The afferent fibers from these free nerve endings, sometimes called **flexor reflex afferents**, synapse onto interneurons in the dorsal horn. These interneurons excite α motor neurons of flexor muscles and inhibit α motor neurons of extensor muscles. This response occurs along several spinal segments to produce a synergistic flexion response, and the limb is withdrawn from the painful stimulus. This flexor withdrawal can occur within 50 milliseconds of touching the object. In fact, this spinal-mediated response occurs well before higher centers of the brain process the information that a hot object was touched. Conscious realization occurs well after the limb has been withdrawn. This intersegmental spinal reflex mechanism allows the rapid speed of this protective response.

A more complicated but equally useful cutaneous reflex specific to the lower extremities is the combined flexor withdrawal and **crossed extensor reflexes**. Here again, the adequate stimulus is pain mediated by free nerve endings in the foot—for example, as one steps on a sharp object. Through a series of polysynaptic connections, the flexor motor neurons of the ipsilateral limb are excited and the extensor motor neurons are inhibited. Through commissural spinal interneurons, the opposite response is elicited in the contralateral limb; the flexor motor neurons are inhibited and the extensor motor neurons are excited. These reflexes allow the ipsilateral limb to be withdrawn from the sharp object and the contralateral limb to support the body weight. Thus, these two complementary reflexes have functional utility for both protection and the maintenance of balance.

Some therapeutic techniques have been developed that involve the application of heat, cold, ice, light stroking, brushing, and deep pressure to invoke cutaneous reflexes leading to muscle contraction (facilitation) or relaxation (inhibition), especially in cases where voluntary control is diminished or absent. Light tactile stimulation of the skin facilitates a contraction in the muscle underlying the stimulated area.[65] Similarly, applications of ice also facilitate contraction, and heat may inhibit or relax the underlying muscle.[66] In general, the neurophysiologic reflex mechanisms underlying such techniques are poorly understood. The more synapses in the reflex arc, the more points for potential modification of the output from multiple sources, both centrally and peripherally. Therefore, the response to any specific stimulus cannot be predicted reliably.

In summary, spinal reflexes are not learned. They are innate neural circuits that serve to improve the efficiency of motor control by allowing for rapid protective responses (i.e., flexor withdrawal), rapid adjustments to perturbations (i.e., myotatic reflex), and regulation of muscle tension (i.e., the tendon organ reflex).

Central Pattern Generators

Central pattern generators (CPGs) have been identified across the phylogenetic spectrum, from worms to mammals. These neuronal circuits can generate stereotypic, rhythmic neural activity that is responsible for patterned movements such as locomotion, respiration, chewing, scratching, and paw shaking. Walking and other forms of locomotion were once assumed to be controlled by various combinations of spinal reflexes. Now, however, the evidence suggests that these neural circuits, or CPGs, are capable of generating the coordinated activity patterns of agonists and antagonists for reciprocal locomotion, and other stereotypic, rhythmic activities in animals.[67–69]

If the spinal cord of a cat is transected at the lower thoracic level, all segments below this level are disconnected from the brain. When placed on a specially constructed treadmill, and after some initial training, these cats are able to "walk" with their hind limbs moving in a coordinated, reciprocal manner. The lower limb muscle activity pattern resembles that of the intact cat. If the dorsal roots are also sectioned, the cat continues to exhibit locomotive movements.[67,69] This finding suggests that the spinal cord circuitry is sophisticated enough to produce relatively complex patterns of motor behavior without requiring sensory input from the periphery and input from supraspinal centers for coordination. Thus, the CPG may be defined as a neural network that is capable of generating coordinated activity patterns (e.g., alternate flexion and extension of the limbs) in the absence of sensory input. Each limb may have a CPG that is coupled with that of the other limb to generate the rhythmic movement of walking. Supraspinal centers are important for "turning on" the CPG and controlling its rate, but the actual stepping pattern seems to be part of the spinal cord circuitry. In humans with transected spinal cords, some locomotive movements can be elicited, but these movements are, by far, less robust than that seen in a cat, because in humans the CPGs are critically dependent on descending pathways.[70,71] In addition, the postural control requirements in humans are far more demanding than can be accommodated by spinal circuitry alone. Some studies, however, suggest that the treadmill training with body weight support that is routinely used with the spinal cats could also be appropriate as a retraining strategy for patients with certain neurologic disorders.[70,72,73]

Locomotor CPGs regulate reflexes as well as the basic stepping pattern. For example, when a cat with a transected spinal cord is not walking but standing, a contact-reaction reflex, similar to the flexor withdrawal in humans, can still be elicited with a light touch on the top of the paw. This reflex is mediated by cutaneous receptors and causes the cat to flex its ipsilateral limb. If the cat is walking, and the top of the paw is touched when it is in the swing phase of locomotion, the ipsilateral limb flexes as expected and the contralateral limb extends, like the crossed extensor reflex. If the limb is in the stance phase of locomotion, however, and the top of the paw is touched, the ipsilateral limb extends. The usual flexion response would be inappropriate, given that the stimulated paw is supporting body weight. Thus, during locomotion the response evoked by the same stimulus (i.e., tactile input to the top of the paw) depends on the phase of the step cycle. This state-dependent reflex action is known as a **reflex-reversal**.[67,68] The locomotor CPG appears to regulate spinal reflexes and thereby allows for more functional motor control.

Clinical Correlations

The clinical test of the intactness of the monosynaptic stretch reflex is the DTR test mentioned earlier. Typically, DTR testing with a reflex hammer is part of a routine neurologic examination. Unusually brisk responses are associated with states of **hyperreflexia**, whereas absent or weak responses are associated with states of **hyporeflexia**. Hyperreflexia can result from damage to the lateral columns of the spinal cord. Hyporeflexia is seen locally during nerve compression. These situations are just examples; the constellation of symptoms and test results permits a diagnosis.

In normal cases, if a tendon jerk in the legs is weak or difficult to elicit, **Jendrassik's maneuver** is used. As the subject forcefully attempts to pull her interlocked hands apart, a tendon tap on the Achilles or patellar tendon may result in a markedly increased response because the excitatory signal to the α motor neurons of the arms and hands is distributed to a larger segment of the cord, perhaps for postural needs. Therapists can use this effect. For example, when assisting a patient with weak leg muscles to arise from a chair, resistance to voluntary activation of neck and arm muscles would elicit a Jendrassik effect in the leg muscles, providing the patient with the additional force necessary for standing up.

In general, spinal reflexes improve the effectiveness of motor control, but sometimes a spinal reflex can interfere with action. Descending input from supraspinal centers can suppress or inhibit reflex activity as needed. In pathologic conditions, the loss of this descending regulation can lead to disorders of muscle tone, such as spasticity and rigidity.

Disorders of Muscle Tone. Muscle tone refers to the resistance that an examiner perceives when moving someone's limb in a passive manner. It is the resting level of tension that keeps the muscle primed for reflexive or voluntary movement. When the limb of someone with a normal nervous system is passively moved at a particular joint, a certain amount of resistance is felt by the examiner. This resistance is not related to any conscious, voluntary effort on the part of the subject but reflects the normal state of neuromuscular tone. In the abnormal state, muscle tone is either hypotonic, with decreased resistance to passive manipulation, or hypertonic, with increased resistance to passive manipulation.

Hypotonia can be produced immediately if either the ventral roots containing the motor nerves innervating the limb are cut (ventral rhizotomy), or the dorsal roots containing the sensory nerves from the limb are cut (dorsal rhizotomy). Hypotonia also results from diseases of certain supraspinal centers, such as the cerebellum (see Chapter 14). Reflex activity, therefore, appears to contribute to muscle tone.

In contrast to hypotonia, hypertonia characterizes two abnormal states of muscle tone—**spasticity** and **rigidity**.[74] Spasticity is usually accompanied by the **clasp-knife** form of resistance and the DTRs are exaggerated; that is, there is an increased responsiveness of the α motor neurons to Type Ia sensory input. The clasp-knife phenomenon refers to the relatively greater resistance to passive manipulation during the initial range of motion (either flexion or extension) and the rapid decline in resistance as the limb is manipulated further through the range of motion. The initial resistance of the clasp-knife response is due to hyperactivity of the stretch reflex, whereas the GTO is probably involved in the sudden give of the stretch reflex. **Clonus**, the regular, oscillatory movement of a limb segment due to the alternating pattern of stretch reflex and inverse stretch reflex of a spastic muscle, is also associated with spasticity. Ankle clonus may be elicited by a brisk, maintained dorsiflexion of the ankle. Rigidity, unlike spasticity, is not associated with the clasp-knife form of resistance or with increased DTRs. It has two forms: 1) a plastic or lead-pipe rigidity, which is uniform throughout the range of motion; or 2) a series of jerks called **cogwheel rigidity**, seen most commonly in Parkinson's disease.

Severe hypertonia can result in disability related to the associated motor control problems and also to secondary problems involved with difficulty in delivering proper skin care, the development of muscle contractures, and difficulty positioning the patient in bed or in a chair. Many therapeutic intervention techniques claim to reduce spasticity, although the efficacy and long-term effectiveness of these procedures have not been established. Pharmacologic and surgical advances, including antispastic medications (e.g., baclofen) and selective dorsal rhizotomies, respectively, have shown promising results.[74] The improved function in patients treated with these procedures has been attributed to changes in the spinal cord rather than to any supraspinal reorganization of motor commands. To assess their effectiveness, continued research is needed to examine the relative permanence of these improvements and the precise criteria for use.

Specific Lesions of the Spinal Cord. Lesions to the spinal cord result from trauma, tumors, degenerative and demyelinating diseases, infections, and disorders of blood supply. Various clinical tests of cutaneous sensation, voluntary muscle force, and reflex contraction of muscles through stretch or tendon tap reflexes are used to evaluate the precise location of the lesion.

The impairment that results depends to a large extent on the location of the spinal cord lesion. As noted earlier, lesions to the gray matter manifest locally, but lesions to the white matter tracts manifest at distant sites. For example, the poliovirus selectively attacks motor neurons in the spinal cord and brainstem. In general, this kind of lower motor neuron lesion results in 1) hypotonia or absent muscle tone, 2) weak or absent DTRs, 3) progressive muscle atrophy restricted to those muscles innervated by the affected nerve, and 4) fibrillation potentials, seen with electromyography, due to the loss of muscle innervation.

By contrast, a traumatic spinal cord injury almost invariably damages both gray and white matter at the level of the lesion and causes both upper and lower motor neuron symptoms. The clinical term, "upper motor neuron lesion," is nonspecific but refers to a lesion anywhere in the central nervous system that affects any descending pathway controlling the activity of ventral horn cells. Upper motor neuron symptoms include varying degrees of paresis of voluntary movement, **Babinski's sign** (i.e., extension of the great toe and abduction of the toes in response to stroking of the sole of the foot), hypertonicity, and increased DTRs.

A partial transection of the spinal cord or hemisection results in the **Brown-Séquard syndrome** caudal to the level of the lesion.[75] Although it is unusual in nature, a discussion of this syndrome has heuristic value. First, damage to the lateral descending tracts results in paresis of muscles *ipsilateral* to the lesion, with spasticity, increased DTRs, loss of superficial reflexes, and a positive Babinski's sign. Damage to the dorsal columns results in loss of position sense, vibratory sense, and tactile discrimination *ipsilateral* to the lesion. Damage to the anterolateral system results in loss of pain and temperature sensation *contralateral* to the lesion beginning one or two dermatomes below the level of the lesion.

In addition to these effects related to disruption of the long ascending and descending tracts, symptoms are possible from damage to the ventral and dorsal spinal roots at the level of the lesion. These symptoms occur ipsilateral to the lesion. They can include flaccid paralysis of the muscles innervated by the destroyed ventral roots, a band of anesthesia over the dermatome innervated by the destroyed dorsal root, paresthesias, and radicular pain over the affected dorsal root zone from irritation of the dorsal root fibers.[75]

Subacute combined degeneration results from a lesion involving the posterior and lateral funiculi. It is associated most commonly with pernicious anemia related to vitamin B_{12} deficiency. Although the dorsal and lateral tracts degenerate, the gray matter is not usually affected. This disorder is associated with both sensory and motor impairments, including lower extremity paresis, spasticity, increased DTRs, a positive Babinski's sign, loss of position and vibration sense in the legs, and a positive **Romberg's sign**, indicated by a loss of balance while standing with the feet close together and the eyes closed.[75]

Finally, thrombosis of the anterior spinal artery affects the ventral and lateral funiculi as well as most of the gray matter of the spinal cord. If the thrombosis occurs in the cervical region, the lesion results in flaccid paralysis at the level of the lesion, spastic paresis, and a loss of pain and temperature sensation below the level of the lesion.

Brainstem and Motor Control

Inside the skull, the brainstem is the continuation of the spinal cord through the foramen magnum. The brainstem connects the cerebral hemispheres with the spinal cord and consists of the medulla oblongata, pons, and midbrain. Although each region has special features, together they serve as a common conduit for certain fiber tracts, and each region includes nuclei of cranial nerves. Descending central commands control the primary brainstem and spinal cord neurons critical for producing voluntary, goal-directed movements. The brainstem is particularly concerned with postural control. It receives and integrates inputs from the vestibular apparatus, cerebral cortex, and cerebellum. Its major efferent projections are from the vestibular nuclei, reticular formation (RF), and red nucleus.

Relationship to Spinal Motor Control

Even after complete removal of the cortex in experimental animals, these animals can right themselves from lying down, stand up, react to shifts of a standing platform, and walk.[69,76] This eerie picture of behavior from totally unconscious animals attests to the complex automatic circuitry of the brainstem working in conjunction with the spinal cord. Much of the circuitry for simple behaviors resides in the spinal cord, but the brainstem coordinates these circuits by mixing in information from the special senses and commands from the cerebellum and cerebrum. Our ability to stand, walk, and chew gum without conscious intervention shows the degree of automation the subcortical motor system possesses. We can move smoothly from standing to sitting, and chewing to talking, because the brainstem nuclei coordinate with the cerebellum and cerebrum, using many complex connections among these structures. For example, in addition to its direct line to spinal motor neuron pools through the corticospinal pathway, the primary motor cortex has parallel neuronal projections to brainstem nuclei. Brainstem nuclei act reflexively to stimuli and in response to commands issued by other motor centers. The vestibular nuclei are a good example. They coordinate body adjustments in response to head tilt as reflex responses to changes of head position and velocity, detected by the vestibular labyrinth. The vestibular nuclei also produce body adjustments in response to descending input from higher centers.

The brainstem nuclei influence motor neuron pools both directly and through spinal reflex pathways. These two classes of projections regulate muscle tone by the constant activation of the motor neurons, either by synapsing directly on the motor neurons, or by way of interneurons, or by adjusting reflex thresholds. The motor neuron pool contribution may be in the form of detectable muscle tone, or may be **subliminal excitation**. Lowering the threshold of a reflex can also affect muscle tone. In the standing posture, for instance, as gravity pulls on the body and stretches the physiologic extensors, tone increases depending on the threshold of the stretch reflex. Thus, static posture is an active state. Descending signals from the brainstem establish a sensitive balance between flexor and extensor muscle groups and their reflex pathways. The "quiet" nature of posture should not lull us into treating posture as a neurologically quiet state. The extreme postures manifested clinically (e.g., various forms of rigidity) are not due to new signals to the spinal cord after an injury. They result from the loss of one side of a balanced system, because descending motor control signals from the brainstem are carefully balanced. Like a teeter-totter, if one rider jumps off, the other person falls to the ground. This loss of descending control is called a **release phenomenon**, or release from inhibition, whenever a balanced neural system loses one input, and the other input suddenly dominates.[77]

Studying the effects of brain lesions in experimental animals has been extremely useful for understanding brainstem organization and its relationship to other central nervous system structures.[78,79] A complete transection of the spinal cord just caudal to the medulla produces spasticity, affecting primarily the extensors. Spasticity is not seen until a few days after a lesion, owing to the phenomenon of **spinal shock**, a period when the spinal reflexes are greatly depressed. In humans, spinal shock lasts at least 2 weeks. A brainstem transection made more rostrally, leaving the medulla and spinal cord intact, is called a low **decerebration**. Here, the extensor muscles develop a hypertonus that leads to the extension of all four limbs. **Decerebrate rigidity**, a form of spasticity, is, in a sense, an antigravity posture, but it does not change if the animal is laying down or held so that its weight is on its limbs. An experimental lesion of the mesencephalon makes a high decerebrate animal. In this preparation, decerebrate rigidity ensues but changes after approximately 10 days. The unconscious animal can still spontaneously right itself, stand, and walk. Decerebrate rigidity is evident when the animal is quietly standing, but "melts" away as the animal starts to move. In a high decerebrate animal, rigidity is a more passive state that is overridden when one of the automatic functions of the brainstem takes over. In disease states decerebrate rigidity occurs rarely, and the defects that produce it are inevitably fatal.

When only the cortex of the animal is sectioned, the intact brainstem is operational immediately.[80,81] This state is called the **decorticate** preparation. It also produces a rigidity, but one that quickly disappears as the animal rights itself, walks, runs, and so forth. The behaviors are smooth and often appropriate for the environment (e.g., faster walking when a treadmill is run faster), but without goals or clear purpose. In humans and arboreal primates, such as many monkeys and apes, the static decorticate posture is slightly different from the decerebrate posture. Humans have arboreal nervous system features because we evolved from arboreal ancestors. Arboreal animals flex their arms and extend their legs to counter gravity while in trees, and the flexed arm posture of decorticate humans is an antigravity pos-

ture. In contrast, the decorticate posture in quadrupeds, such as cats and dogs, is with all four limbs extended.

Reticular Formation

The RF is not a unitary structure and it has no single role. Because its many nuclei were too small for the early anatomists to see with primitive microscopes, they thought it was a simple netlike or reticular structure; hence its name. The RF is involved with a broad range of automatic, or unconscious, neural functions. Various parts of the RF regulate oculomotor reflexes, postural tone, conscious state (e.g., waking/sleeping), and autonomic activity, described in a later chapter. Other parts relay somatic and special sensory information to the cerebellum and are involved in emotional behavior.

The RF is a collection of small nuclei and fiber tracts that run through the core of the brainstem, extending from the caudal medulla, where it is continuous with the spinal cord reticular formation, to the diencephalon, where it invades the intralaminar parts of the thalamus. The RF can be divided into a lateral and a medial group. The medial group gives rise to long ascending and descending fiber pathways, many of which project both rostrally into the thalamus and caudally as far as the sacral levels of the spinal cord, influencing the axial and proximal limb muscles. The lateral group has primarily local connections, including many projections into the medial group.[82]

Reticular Nuclei Related to the Cerebellum

Inputs to the Cerebellum. The lateral reticular nucleus has two main divisions, parvicellular and magnocellular, and other, smaller divisions. Both main divisions supply inputs to the cerebellum, each to a different part. The parvicellular division relays somatosensory information from the spinal cord to mossy fibers of the cerebellar vermis. The magnocellular division receives primarily cerebral cortical input, which influences the cerebellar hemispheres. Other parts of the lateral reticular nucleus provide a means for the red nucleus, and for the cerebellar fastigial nucleus, to influence the vermis.

In addition to the lateral reticular nucleus, the paramedian reticular nucleus and the nucleus reticularis tegmenti pontis provide pathways by which cerebellar nuclei can influence the cerebellar cortex. Like the parvicellular lateral reticular nucleus, the paramedian reticular nucleus receives inputs from the fastigial nucleus and projects back to the vermis. This pathway is also influenced by inputs from the cerebral cortex. The nucleus reticularis tegmenti pontis receives projections from both the dentate and interpositus cerebellar nuclei and projects to all parts of the cerebellar cortex. It, too, is influenced by descending cerebral cortical inputs.

Outputs From the Cerebellum. The cerebellum has no direct pathway to the spinal cord. It influences the activity of other systems, such as the reticulospinal system, that project to the cord.[83] The RF gives rise to the lateral and medial reticulospinal tracts. Projections from the ipsilateral dentate nucleus of the cerebellum have an excitatory influence on medial reticulospinal tract cells. These neurons modulate sensory pathways in the spinal cord, produce Type Ia presynaptic inhibition, and affect various aspects of autonomic control. Signals from the contralateral fastigial nucleus are relayed to the spinal cord directly through the medial reticulospinal tract, and indirectly from the medial bulbar RF to the lateral bulbar RF to the spinal cord by way of the lateral reticulospinal system. The dentate nucleus receives signals from the motor and primary sensory areas of the cerebral cortex, and may be involved in movement planning. The fastigial nucleus is more involved with reflexes of vestibular and somatosensory origin, and modulation of ongoing voluntary movements.

Reticular Activating System
Reticular formation fibers that ascend into the intralaminar nuclei of the thalamus are essential for the conscious state of wakefulness.[82] Electrical stimulation of certain parts of the RF awakens a sleeping or lightly anesthetized animal. Lesions of the **reticular activating system** in the lower brainstem can induce coma, and are associated with respiratory and cardiovascular complications. Lesions higher in the brainstem can produce a variety of states. Slowly progressing lesions, like the growth of a tumor, may have only subtle effects on wakefulness until the disease state is advanced. Rapid lesions, like vascular accidents, can cause deep coma. Small lesions of the rostral brainstem lead to **hypersomnia**, including akinetic mutism, a sleep state but with the eye movements typical of wakefulness. The locus ceru-

leus of the mesencephalon and the raphe nuclei of the pons may play roles in states of wakefulness.

Reticular Contributions to Postural Tone
Posture depends on the effects of gravity and the influence of flexors and extensors at each joint. The muscle tone of the flexors and extensors is regulated by spinal reflexes and tonic supraspinal descending activity to the motor neuron pools.[84,85] Tonic input comes from two different parts of the RF. The medial group at the medullary level provides a tonic inhibition of physiologic extensors and a tonic excitation of flexors. The lateral group in the pons, which is closely tied to the vestibular nuclei, provides the opposite influence on motor neuron pools. It tonically excites physiologic extensors, and inhibits flexors. Both sources of tonic activation also influence the γ motor neurons of these motor neuron pools, which contributes to the control of the stretch and other spindle afferent reflexes.

These two competing, descending reticulospinal systems receive different inputs. The lateral pontine RF receives input from the major vestibular nuclei. The vestibulospinal tracts also excite extensors in parallel with this part of the RF. Muscle spindle and other somatic input are also involved in controlling the excitation to physiologic extensors. These sensors send ascending projections to the same RF region. The medial medullary input to the spinal cord inhibits extensors based on inputs from a variety of structures, including the cerebral cortex. The cerebral cortex uses the medullary RF to counteract the antigravity effects of the vestibulospinal and pontine reticulospinal systems. Presumably, the medial medullary RF tones down the antigravity system at the appropriate moments to allow voluntary flexion of the joints.

The two opposing RF systems are carefully balanced for normal motor behavior. The effects of imbalance are apparent in disease and serve to explain the results of decerebrate rigidity.[84] If a serious injury destroys all descending pathways above the pons (decerebration), the descending cerebral cortex excitation of the medial medullary RF can no longer supply adequate extensor inhibition, which produces the release from inhibition described earlier. The cortex and cerebellum both supply continuous excitatory influences on the medullary RF. So, disrupting either of these areas produces rigidity. Less excitatory synaptic drive to this part of the RF causes the same release of inhibition, albeit not as strong, as in the case of damage to the reticulospinal tract.

The effects of cerebellar lesions in quadrupeds and primates show one important difference.[86,87] If the cerebellum, or just the anterior lobe of the cerebellum, is removed in a decerebrate cat that already has increased tonic activity in the physiologic extensors, the extensor tone increases even more. The anterior lobe of the cerebellum exerts a strong inhibitory effect on the lateral vestibular nucleus. When this inhibition is removed, the descending pathway from the lateral vestibular nucleus, the lateral vestibular tract, exerts a strong excitatory effect primarily on extensor motor neurons. Because this effect is primarily due to excitation of the α motor neurons, it is said to be "alpha rigidity." If the cerebellum is removed in primates, it produces hypotonia, tremor, difficulty controlling the force and rate of muscle contractions, and a general decrease in γ motor neuron activity. This difference in cerebellar lesions in cats and primates is probably due to species differences in the output of the anterior lobe of the cerebellum and in the relatively enlarged cerebellar hemispheres in primates. In humans and other primates, if the direct projection from the anterior cerebellum to the lateral vestibular nucleus is removed, the effect is less robust. Instead, the major output of the primate cerebellum is from the lateral hemispheres, which is responsible for regulating the rate and force of muscle contractions.[88]

Induced Locomotion

As explained earlier, decerebrated experimental animals can perform smooth stepping when placed on a moving treadmill. Experimental recordings show that many reticulospinal tract neurons are modulated in synchrony with the step cycle of walking.[89] The exact role these neurons play in walking is not yet known, but they lose their synchrony with the step cycle if the cerebellum is removed.

Human locomotion differs dramatically from that of other animals. Humans are erect bipeds; we rarely hop. We must, therefore, interpret the study of locomotion in other animals carefully. If the brainstem is surgically severed in exactly the right place in an experimental animal, and an electrode is placed in a particular part of the RF, then electrical stimulation at this site induces "walking" on a treadmill.[69] If the stimulus speed is increased, the walking speed increases. With enough stimulation, the animal breaks into a trot or gallop. If the treadmill is tilted on a

steep incline, the gallop returns to a walk. Not only do the brainstem and spinal cord have the necessary circuitry for walking, trotting and galloping, but these areas can determine which gait is appropriate, based on the drive (stimulation) and work load (incline).

Cranial Motor Nerves

The characteristics of spinal motor neurons hold true for the cranial motor neurons. The unique structure of the brainstem changes the location, but not the function, of the motor neuron pools that reside there. The motor nerves of the eye (III, IV, and VI) are discussed earlier in this book. The trigeminal (V), facial (VII), glossopharyngeal (IX), vagus (X) cranial nerves are **mixed nerves**; they carry both sensory and motor information. Only their skeletomotor contributions are discussed here. The motor nuclei of the cranial nerves receive inputs from the brainstem as well as from the cerebral cortex. In some cases, the cortical projection is primarily to the contralateral motor nucleus, whereas in other cases, each side of the cerebral cortex projects bilaterally to both left and right cranial motor nuclei. In the cases of bilateral cortical projections, a unilateral motor deficit can usually be traced to cranial nerve nucleus damage. In cases of primarily contralateral cortical projections, a unilateral deficit can result from a nerve, brainstem, or cortical lesion. Except in those cases indicated later, the cranial nerve nuclei receive primarily contralateral cortical projections, like the spinal motor nuclei.[90]

The trigeminal nerve controls muscles of the jaw and inner ear and the mylohyoid muscle. Its motor neurons are located at the mid-level of the pons. Many of these motor neurons are involved in jaw reflexes and contribute to control of mastication. The forces involved in chewing and biting are massive, with great potential to damage teeth and bones. The reflex regulation of force production in the presence of unexpected loads (e.g., an unpopped kernel of popcorn) is as demanding as in the skeletal motor system. Therefore, the trigeminal nerve is part of an important brainstem network for automatic jaw control.

The motor neurons of the facial nerve are located in the pons, caudal to those of the trigeminal nerve. The facial nerve innervates the superficial muscles of the face and the middle ear, and the platysma and stylohyoid muscles. Cerebral cortical control of motor neurons innervating the forehead differs from control of the motor neurons innervating muscles below the forehead. Both cortical hemispheres project to the frontalis motor neurons on either side of the pons, so that motor cortex lesions or lesions affecting their fibers (e.g., upper motor neuron lesions) do not dramatically affect the frontalis muscles, whereas lesions of the cranial nuclei (lower motor neuron lesions) can cause paralysis. Below the forehead, an upper motor neuron lesion appears as a contralateral facial palsy because the cortical projection is only to that side.

Like the trigeminal and facial nerves, the glossopharyngeal and vagus nerves are mixed nerves, but they have significantly smaller motor components. The glossopharyngeal nerve supplies primarily a sensory innervation of the tongue, soft palate, and viscera, and the vagus nerve provides a sensory innervation of the soft palate and pharynx. The motor components originate from the nucleus ambiguus and are discussed in the chapter on the autonomic nervous system.

The internal ramus of the accessory nerve also originates from the nucleus ambiguus. The internal ramus of this purely motor nerve innervates the intrinsic muscles of the larynx. The external ramus of the accessory nerve innervates the upper shoulder girdle and the sternocleidomastoid and trapezius muscles. Although the accessory nerve is a cranial nerve, the external ramus originates from the cervical segments of the spinal cord. The cerebral cortex projection to the accessory nerve, as well as to the other cranial motor nerves for controlling speech, is primarily contralateral. In the event of damage to the accessory nerve, however, speech may not be spared, even with paralysis of only one side.

The hypoglossal nerve is a motor nerve originating from the hypoglossal nucleus of the medulla. These fibers control movements of the tongue. Cortical projections to the hypoglossal nucleus are contralateral and come from the pyramidal tract. Lesions of the medulla can affect the pyramidal tract before fibers cross the midline, and at the same time impinge on the adjacent hypoglossal nerve. This scenario can produce a contralateral upper motor neuron hemiplegia with additional ipsilateral lower motor neuron symptoms involving the hypoglossal nucleus.

Red Nucleus

The red nucleus, a pink structure in the midbrain tegmentum surrounded by the midbrain RF, has a

rostral, parvicellular division and a caudal, magnocellular division. The magnocellular division has direct projections to the spinal cord, with a terminal distribution similar to the corticospinal tract. In apes and humans, the magnocellular division is proportionally small compared with the parvicellular division. In carnivores, the magnocellular division is proportionally large. The significance of evolutionary changes in the red nucleus is unknown, but the magnocellular division may be less important in humans than in other animals.[91,92]

Electrical stimulation of the red nucleus shows that it is somatotopically organized. The magnocellular division supplies the cerebellum with a fairly direct crossed pathway to the spinal cord. Contralateral inputs from the interpositus nucleus (in monkeys) or emboliform nucleus (in humans) of the cerebellum form powerful synapses on cells that descend to the spinal cord along the rubrospinal tract. Projections from the ipsilateral primary motor cortex synapse on the same neurons, providing a background modulation of rubrospinal tract cell activity. Thus, the primary motor cortex gradually sets the background level, and the cerebellum imposes moment-by-moment changes on the tract cells. In parallel with this cerebellorubrospinal pathway is a cerebellothalamocortical pathway, which seems to provide similar information. If the corticospinal pathway is damaged, the rubrospinal pathway helps compensate, and vice versa. One explanation for this redundancy is that the rubrospinal pathway is used for motor behaviors that are very well learned and almost completely automatic, assigning the motor areas of the cortex to more complex tasks, such as motor learning.

The parvicellular division of the red nucleus also receives cerebral cortical and cerebellar nuclei inputs. The role of the parvicellular division, however, is quite different. The cortical inputs are bilateral and come primarily from premotor cortical areas. Moreover, the output of the parvicellular division is aimed at the ipsilateral inferior olivary complex and is presumably important for influencing the climbing fiber projection from the olivary complex back to the cerebellum.

Thalamus

The thalamus is rostral to the brainstem, surrounded by the cerebral cortex. The thalamus handles all ascending signals to the cortex.[56] All sensory information, except olfactory, all signals from the cerebellum, basal ganglia, and RF—virtually everything destined for the cerebral cortex—must pass through the thalamic "office administrator," which then relays information to the cortex. Each part of the thalamus projects to a specific cortical area. Each cortical area that receives thalamic input also sends its signals back to the same part of the thalamus. Apparently, the thalamus is under the direct control of the cortex.

The thalamus has four main nuclear groups (lateral, dorsomedial, centromedian, and ventral), plus laminae that separate the main groups. The exact location of each nucleus is difficult to imagine in three dimensions, and the nomenclature for thalamic nuclei is confusing, at best. The main thalamic nucleus that handles ascending information to the motor areas of the cerebral cortex is the ventrolateral nucleus (VL). The VL can be divided into the oral (VLo), medial (VLm), and caudal (VLc) parts. The oral part of another nucleus, the ventroposterolateral nucleus (VPLo), also serves motor areas of the cortex, as does the intralaminar zone called area X. The VL, VPLo, and area X receive contralateral inputs from the dentate and interposed nuclei of the cerebellum, and bilateral inputs from the fastigial nucleus. Anterior parts of each cerebellar nucleus project to lateral parts of the VL, which, in turn, project to medial parts of the primary motor cortex. A similar relationship exists between the posterior parts of the cerebellar nuclei, medial VL, and lateral primary motor cortex. Because the primary motor cortex is somatotopically organized along the lateral-to-medial axis, both the VL and the cerebellar nuclei are probably somatotopically organized. Thus, each part of the body has its own relay system from the cerebellum to the cortex.

Separate from the cerebellar inputs are projections to the anterior part of the VL (VLo) from the internal segment of the globus pallidus. These projections are relayed not to the primary motor cortex, but to the premotor areas. Also separate from the cerebellar inputs, in the medial part of the VL (VLm), are projections from the pars reticulata of the substantia nigra (see Chapter 14). These projections are relayed to the limbic cortex on the medial surface of the frontal lobe.

You might expect that damage to the thalamus mimics damage to the subcortical systems that project to the motor areas of the cortex. Clinically, however, discrete lesions of the motor parts of the thalamus are rare. Thalamic involvement usually manifests itself as sensory symptoms, typically diffuse pain.

Clinical Correlations

A common lesion of the brainstem is stroke. Depending on which brainstem artery is involved, different portions of the brainstem can be damaged.[75] For example, a unilateral lesion of the anterior spinal artery and its paramedian branches can affect the medial zone of the medulla at the level of cranial nerve XII (hypoglossal nerve). Because this lesion affects the ipsilateral lower motor neuron of cranial nerve XII and upper motor neurons of descending motor fiber tracts (pyramidal tract fibers), it is known as an alternating hemiplegia. The disorder is manifested as an ipsilateral paralysis of the tongue, contralateral somatosensory loss due to medial lemniscus involvement, and a contralateral spastic paresis. The spastic paresis is contralateral because the pyramidal tract crosses the midline well below the level of the lesion, at the medulla, before these fibers descend in the spinal cord as the lateral corticospinal tract. Other brainstem syndromes include 1) Wallenberg's syndrome, or lateral medullary syndrome due to a posterior inferior cerebellar artery lesion; 2) Weber's syndrome, affecting the basal region of the midbrain due to occlusion of the branches of the basilar and posterior cerebral arteries; and 3) Benedikt's syndrome, affecting the upper midbrain core, also called the tegmentum.

REFERENCES

1. Sherrington C. *The integrative action of the nervous system*. 2nd ed. New Haven: Yale University Press, 1947.
2. Cheney PD. Role of cerebral cortex in voluntary movements: a review. *Phys Ther* 1985;65:624–635.
3. Holstege G. The emotional motor system. *Eur J Morphol* 1992;30:67–79.
4. Brooks VB. *The neural basis of motor control*. New York: Oxford University Press, 1986.
5. Rothwell JC. *Control of human voluntary movement*. 2nd ed. London: Chapman and Hall, 1994.
6. Minsky ML. Steps towards artificial intelligence. *Proc Inst Radio Eng* 1961;49:9–30.
7. Arbib MA. Perceptual structures and distributed motor control. In: Brookhard JM, Mountcastle VB, Brooks VB, Geiger SR, eds. *Handbook of physiology*. Section 1, Vol II. Bethesda, MD: American Physiological Society, 1979: 1440–1480.
8. Feldman AG. Functional tuning of the nervous system with control of movement or maintenance of a steady posture: II. controllable parameters of the muscles. *Biophysics* 1966;11:565–578.

9. Houk JC. Motor control processes: New data concerning motor servo mechanism and tentative model for stimulus–response processing. In: Talbott RE, Humphrey DR, eds. *Posture and movement*. New York: Raven Press, 1979:231–241.

10. Schmidt RA. *Motor control and learning: a behavioral emphasis*. 2nd ed. Champaign, Illinois: Human Kinetics, 1988.

11. Almers W. Excitation–contraction coupling in skeletal muscle. In: Patton HD, Fuchs AF, Hille B, Scher AM, Steiner R, eds. *Textbook of physiology: excitable cells and neurophysiology: I*. Philadelphia: WB Saunders, 1982: 156–170.

12. McComas AJ. *Skeletal muscle form and function*. Champaign, Illinois: Human Kinetics, 1996.

13. Gordon AM. Molecular basis of contraction. In: Patton HD, Fuchs AF, Hille B, Scher AM, Steiner R, eds. *Textbook of physiology: excitable cells and neurophysiology: I*. Philadelphia: WB Saunders, 1982:171–195.

14. Hille B. Neuromuscular transmission. In: Patton HD, Fuchs AF, Hille B, Scher AM, Steiner R, eds. *Textbook of physiology: excitable cells and neurophysiology: I*. Philadelphia: WB Saunders Co, 1982:130–155.

15. Drachman DB. Myasthenia gravis. *N Engl J Med* 1994; 330:1797–1810.

16. Elmqvist D, Hofmann WW, Kugelberg J, Quastel DM. An electrophysiological investigation of neuromuscular transmission in myasthenia gravis. *J Physiol (Lond)* 1964; 174:417–434.

17. Patrick J, Lindstrom J. Autoimmune response to acetylcholine receptor. *Science* 1973;180:871–872.

18. Gordon AM. Contraction of skeletal muscle. In: Patton HD, Fuchs AF, Hille B, Scher AM, Steiner R, eds. *Textbook of physiology: excitable cells and neurophysiology: I*. Philadelphia: WB Saunders, 1982:196–213.

19. Ralston HJ, Inman VT, Strait LA, Shaffrath MD. Mechanics of human isolated voluntary muscle. *Am J Physiol* 1947;151:612–620.

20. Rack PMH, Westbury DR. The effects of length and stimulus rate on tension in the isometric cat soleus muscle. *J Physiol (Lond)* 1969;204:443–460.

21. Gordon AM, Huxley AF, Julian FJ. The variation in isometric tension with sarcomere length in vertebrate muscle fibers. *J Physiol (Lond)* 1966;184:170–192.

22. Burke RE. Motor units: anatomy, physiology and functional organization. In: Brooks VB, ed. *Handbook of physiology*. Section 1, Vol II. Bethesda, MD: American Physiological Society, 1981:345–411.

23. Lewis DM. The physiology of motor units in mammalian skeletal muscle. In: Towe AL, Luschei ES, eds. *Handbook of behavioral neurobiology: V*. New York: Plenum Press, 1981:1–67.

24. Burke RE, Edgerton VR. Motor unit properties and selective involvement in movement. *Exerc Sport Sci Rev* 1975;3:31–81.

25. Salmons S, Vrbová G. The influence of activity on some contractile characteristics of mammalian fast and slow muscles. *J Physiol* 1969;201:535–549.

26. Gorza L, Gundersen K, Lømo T, Schiaffino S, Westgaard RH. Slow-to-fast transformation of denervated soleus muscles by chronic high-frequency stimulation in the rat. *J Physiol* 1988;402:627–649.

27. Edgerton VR, Bodine-Fowler S, Roy RR, Ishihara A, Hodgson JA. Neuromuscular adaptation. In: Rowell LB, Shepherd JT, eds. *Handbook of physiology*. Section 12. Bethesda, MD: American Physiological Society, 1996: 54–88.

28. Dubowitz V. Cross-innervated mammalian skeletal muscle: histochemical, physiological and biochemical observations. *J Physiol (Lond)* 1967;193:481–496.

29. Romanul FCA, Van Der Meulen JP. Slow and fast muscles after cross innervation: enzymatic and physiological changes. *Arch Neurol* 1967;17:387–402.

30. Windhorst U. *How brain-like is the spinal cord?* Berlin: Springer-Verlag, 1988.

31. Feinstein B, Lindegård B, Nyman E, Wohlfart G. Morphologic studies of motor units in normal human muscles. *Acta Anat* 1955;23:127–142.

32. Burke RE, Strick PL, Kanda K, Kim CC, Walmsley B. Anatomy of medial gastrocnemius and soleus motor nuclei in cat spinal cord. *J Neurophysiol* 1977;40:667–680.

33. Henneman E, Mendell LM. Functional organization of the motoneuron pool and its inputs. In: Brooks VB, ed. *Handbook of physiology*. Section 1, Vol I. Bethesda, MD: American Physiological Society, 1981:423–507.

34. Binder MD, Heckman CJ, Powers RK. The physiological control of motoneuron activity. In: Rowell LB, Shepherd JT, eds. *Handbook of physiology*. Section 12. Bethesda, MD: American Physiological Society, 1996:3–53.

35. Henneman E. Relation between size of neurons and their susceptibility to discharge. *Science* 1957;126: 1345–1347.

36. Milner-Brown HS, Stein RB, Yemm R. Changes in firing rates of human motor units during linearly changing voluntary contractions. *J Physiol (Lond)* 1973;230:371– 390.

37. Monster AW, Chan H. Isometric force production by motor units of extensor digitorum communis muscle in man. *J Neurophysiol* 1977;40:1432–1443.

38. De Luca CJ, LeFever RS, McCue MP, Xenakis AP. Behavior of human motor units in different muscles during linearly varying contractions. *J Physiol (Lond)* 1982; 329:113–128.

39. Al-Falahe NA, Nagaoka M, Vallbo ÅB. Response profiles of human muscle afferents during active finger movements. *Brain* 1990;113:325–346.

40. Prochazka A. Proprioceptive feedback and movement regulation. In: Rowell LB, Shepherd JT, eds. *Handbook of physiology*. Section 12. Bethesda, MD: American Physiological Society, 1996:89–127.

41. Matthews PBC. *Mammalian muscle receptors and their central actions*. Baltimore: Williams & Wilkins, 1972.

42. Houk JC, Rymer WZ. Neural control of muscle length and tension. In: Brooks VB, ed. *Handbook of physiology*. Section 1, Vol II. Bethesda, MD: American Physiological Society, 1981:257–323.

43. Vallbo ÅB. Discharge patterns in human muscle spindle afferents during isometric voluntary contractions. *Acta Physiol Scand* 1970;80:552–566.

44. Vallbo ÅB. Basic patterns of muscle spindle discharge in man. In: Taylor A, Prochazka A, eds. *Muscle receptors and movement*. London: Macmillan, 1981:219–228, 263–275.

45. Vallbo ÅB, Hagbarth KE, Torebjörk HE, Wallin BG. Somatosensory, proprioceptive, and sympathetic activity in human peripheral nerves. *Physiol Rev* 1979;59: 919–957.

46. Prochazka A, Hullinger M, Zangger P, Appenteng K. "Fusimotor set": new evidence for α-independent control of γ-motoneurons during movement in the awake cat. *Brain Res* 1985;339:136–140.

47. Prochazka A, Wand P. Independence of fusimotor and skeletomotor systems during voluntary movement. In: Taylor A, Prochazka A, eds. *Muscle receptors and movement*. London: Macmillan, 1981:229–243.

48. Prochazka A, Hullinger M, Trend P, Durmuller N. Dynamic and static fusimotor set in various behavioral contexts. In: Hnik P, Soukup T, Vejsada R, Zelena J, eds. *Mechanoreceptors: development, structure, and function*. New York: Plenum Press, 1988:417–430.

49. Siddique T, et al. Linkage of a gene causing familial amyotrophic lateral sclerosis to chromosome 21 and evidence of a genetic locus heterogeneity. *N Engl J Med* 1991;324:1382–1384.

50. Brown RH Jr. Amyotrophic lateral sclerosis: recent insights from genetics and transgenic mice. *Cell* 1995; 80:687–692.

51. Walton JN. *Disorders of voluntary muscle*. 5th ed. Edinburgh: Churchill Livingstone, 1988.

52. Hoffman EP, Wang J. Duchenne-Becker muscular dystrophy and the nondystrophic myotonias: paradigms of loss of function and change of function of gene products. *Arch Neurol* 1993;50:1227–1237.

53. Barchi RL. Molecular pathology of the skeletal muscle sodium channel. *Annu Rev Physiol* 1995;57:355–385.

54. Hoffman EP, Lehmann-Horn F, Rudel R. Overexcited or inactive: ion channels in muscle disease. *Cell* 1995;80: 681–686.

55. Rexed B. The cytoarchitectonic organization of the spinal cord in the cat. *J Comp Neurol* 1952;96:415–495.

56. Martin JH. *Neuroanatomy: text and atlas*. 2nd ed. Stamford, CT: Appleton and Lange, 1996.

57. Patton H. Spinal reflexes and synaptic transmission. In: Ruch T, Patton HT, eds. *Physiology and biophysics: IV*. Philadelphia: WB Saunders, 1982:261–302.

58. Matthews PBC. The human stretch reflex and the motor cortex. *Trends Neurosci* 1991;14:87–91.

59. Day BL, Marsden CD, Obeso JA, Rothwell JC. Reciprocal inhibition between the muscles of the human forearm. *J Physiol (Lond)* 1984;349:519–534.

60. Katz R, Penicaud A, Rossi A. Reciprocal Ia inhibition between the elbow flexors and extensors in the human. *J Physiol (Lond)* 1991;437:269–286.

61. Baldiserra F, Hultborn H, Illert M. Integration in spinal neuronal systems. In: Brooks VB, ed. *Handbook of physiology*. Section 1, Vol II. Bethesda, MD: American Physiological Society, 1981:509–597.

62. Prochazka A, Hullinger M. Muscle afferent function and its significance for motor control mechanisms during voluntary movements in cat, monkey, and man. *Adv Neurol* 1983;39:93–132.

63. Rudomin P. Presynaptic inhibition of muscle spindle and tendon organ afferents in the mammalian spinal cord. *Trends Neurosci* 1990;13:499–505.

64. Lundberg A, Malmgren K, Schonberg EB. Reflex pathways from group II muscle afferents: papers 1, 2, and 3. *Exp Brain Res* 1987;65:271–306.

65. Hagbarth KE. Excitatory and inhibitory skin areas for flexor and extensor motoneurons. *Acta Physiol Scand* 1952;26(Suppl 94):1–58.

66. Davies CTM, Young K. Effects of temperature on the contractile properties and muscle power of triceps surae in humans. *J Appl Physiol* 1983;55:191–195.

67. Grillner S, Wallen P. Central pattern generators for locomotion, with special reference to vertebrates. *Annu Rev Neurosci* 1985;8:233– 261.

68. Grillner S, Wallen P, di Prisco V. Cellular network underlying locomotion as revealed in a lower vertebrate model: transmitters, membrane properties, circuitry, and simulation. *Cold Spring Harb Symp Quant Biol* 1990;55:779–789.

69. Rossignol S. Neural control of stereotypic limb movements. In: Rowell LB, Shepherd JT, eds. *Handbook of physiology*. Section 12. Bethesda, MD: American Physiological Society, 1996:173–216.

70. Muir GD, Steeves JD. Sensorimotor stimulation to improve locomotor recovery after spinal cord injury. *Trends Neurosci* 1997;20:72–77.

71. Calancie B, Needham-Shropshire B, Jacobs P, Willer K, Zych G, Green BA. Involuntary stepping after chronic spinal cord injury: evidence for a central rhythm generator for locomotion in man. *Brain* 1994;117:1143–1159.

72. Wernig A, Muller S, Nanassy A, Cagol E. Laufband therapy based on "rules of spinal locomotion" is effective in spinal cord injured persons. *Eur J Neurosci* 1995;7: 823–829.

73. Wernig A, Muller S. Laufband locomotion with body weight support improved walking in persons with severe spinal cord injuries. *Paraplegia* 1992;30:229–238.

74. Young RR. Spasticity: a review. *Neurology* 1994;44: S12–S20.

75. Rowland LP. Clinical syndromes of the spinal cord and brainstem. In: Kandel ER, Schwartz JH, Jessell TM, eds.

Principles of neuroscience. New York: Elsevier, 1991: 711–731.

76. Sherrington CS. Decerebrate rigidity and reflex coordination of movements. *J Physiol (Lond)* 1898;22:319–332.

77. Roberts TDM. *Neurophysiology of postural mechanisms*. London: Butterworths, 1979.

78. Luccarini P, Gahery Y, Pompeiano O. Cholinoceptive pontine reticular structures modify the postural adjustments during the limb movements induced by cortical stimulation. *Arch Ital Biol* 1990;128:19–45.

79. Mori S. Contribution of postural muscle tone to full expression of posture and locomotor movements: multifaceted analyses of its setting brainstem–spinal cord mechanisms in the cat. *Jpn J Physiol* 1989;39:785–809.

80. Dufosse M, Macpherson J, Massion J, Sybirska E. The postural reaction to the drop of a hindlimb support in the standing cat remains following sensorimotor cortical ablation. *Neurosci Lett* 1985;55:297–303.

81. Ioffe ME, Ivanova NG, Frolov AA, Birjukova EV. On the role of motor cortex in the learned rearrangement of postural coordinations. In: Gurfinkel VS, Ioffe ME, Massion J, Roll JP, eds. *Stance and motion, facts and concepts*. New York: Plenum Press, 1988:213–226.

82. Wilson VJ, Peterson BW. Vestibulospinal and reticulospinal systems. In: Brooks VB, ed. *Handbook of physiology*. Section 1, Vol II. Bethesda, MD: American Physiological Society, 1981:667–702.

83. Diener HC, Dichgans J. Postural ataxia in late atrophy of the cerebellar anterior lobe and its differential diagnosis. In: Black FO, Igarshi M, eds. *Vestibular and visual control on posture and locomotor equilibrium*. Houston: Karger, 1985:282–289.

84. Mori S. Integration of posture and locomotion in acute decerebrate cats and in awake, freely moving cats. *Prog Neurobiol* 1987;28:161–195.

85. Mori S, Matsuyama K, Kohyama J, Kobayashi Y, Takakusaki K. Neuronal constituents of postural and locomotor control systems and their interactions in cats. *Brain Dev* 1992;14:S109–S120.

86. Mori S, Sakamoto T, Takakusaki K. Interaction of posture and locomotion in cats: its automatic and volitional control aspects. In: Shimamura M, Grillner S, Edgerton VR, eds. *Neurological basis of human locomotion*. Tokyo: Japan Scientific Societies Press, 1991:21–32.

87. Ito M. *Cerebellum and neural control*. New York: Raven Press, 1984.

88. Dichgans J, Diener HC. Different forms of postural ataxia in patients with cerebellar diseases. In: Bles W, Brandt T, eds. *Disorders of posture and gait*. Amsterdam: Elsevier, 1986:207–215.

89. Gelfand IM, Orlovsky GN, Shik ML. Locomotion and scratching in tetrapods. In: Cohen AH, Rossignol S, Grillner S, eds. *Neural control of rhythmic movements in vertebrates*. New York: John Wiley & Sons, 1988:167–199.

90. Role LW, Kelly JP. The brainstem: cranial nerve nuclei and the monoaminergic systems. In: Kandel ER, Schwartz JH, Jessell TM, eds. *Principles of neuroscience*. New York: Elsevier, 1991:683–700.

91. Nathan PW, Smith MC. The rubrospinal and central tegmental tracts in man. *Brain* 1982;105:223–269.

92. Kuypers HGJM. Motor units: anatomy of the descending pathways. In: Brooks VB, ed. *Handbook of physiology*. Section 1, Vol II. Bethesda, MD: American Physiological Society, 1981:597–666.

14

Motor 2: Higher Centers

LINDA L. PORTER, PT, PhD

• • •

Voluntary movement is a complex behavior that requires the coordination of many brain regions. This chapter discusses the higher motor centers, including the motor areas of the cerebral cortex, the basal ganglia, and the cerebellum. The motor cortex is a complex structure comprising several functionally different regions. Extensive incoming and outgoing pathways keep it well informed of activity occurring in other regions of the brain. An enormous bundle of axons arising from the motor cortex and traveling the great distance to the spinal cord tightly links the motor cortex to the spinal cord, giving the motor cortex potent control over voluntary movement. Its control over highly skilled movements, particularly that of hand movement in humans, makes it a fascinating focus of study. Its ability to adapt to internal structural changes or external manipulations makes it of great clinical interest as well.

The **basal ganglia** are a set of subcortical nuclei, and their related pathways link several motor centers through a complex system of internal motor control loops. They have no direct output to the spinal cord, and therefore their role in modulating voluntary movement is mediated through the internal loops. The severity of motor symptoms in diseases affecting the basal ganglia (e.g., Parkinson's and Huntington's diseases) indicates the importance of the basal ganglia in motor control. The cerebellum is also interesting from many points of view. Its highly stereotyped structure would appear to preclude any functional heterogeneity, but the cerebellum has some clever means to provide different and relevant information to its target structures. The cerebellum is a great integrator of information. It receives constant updates on the state of spinal cord activity and ongoing movements, descending commands from the motor cortex, and peripheral perturbations to movement. It coordinates these vast incoming signals and alerts the appropriate motor centers to make any necessary corrections to achieve smooth, purposeful movements.

Although this chapter discusses these higher motor centers separately, they are intimately related through a complex network of connections. Therefore, their functions are difficult to isolate from one another. Their concerted efforts result in an amazing ability to learn and control posture and balance, muscle tone and reflex strength, and highly skilled motor tasks.

The Motor Cortex

Historical Perspectives

In 1870, Hughlings Jackson,[1] a British neurologist, published his observations of patients with epilepsy. He concluded that focal motor seizures beginning in the hand were caused by localized changes in blood flow to the cerebral cortex. This idea led to his proposal that higher brain centers, including the cerebral cortex, controlled movement. He perceived a "motor" cortex that contained multiple locations to control different movement patterns. Jackson's insightful hypothesis that movements are controlled by multiple sites in the cortex took a century to confirm. These ideas were revolutionary for his time. The contemporary thinking was that the cerebral cortex was devoted to intellectual and perceptual functions, whereas lower brain centers controlled motor functions. Two German scientists shared the belief that the cortex controlled movement and provided timely evidence to support this theory. In 1870, Fritz and Hitzig[2] applied galvanic current directly to the exposed cortical surface of dogs. Electrical stimulation activates neurons and, because of the connections from the motor cortex to the spinal cord, the outcome of activation of this brain region is movement. The crude methods that they used produced movements on the side of the body opposite to the cerebral hemisphere that they stimulated. Their conclusion that a large area of the cortex was "excitable," and therefore was involved in the control of purposeful movement, led to a flurry of activity. As techniques of electrical brain stimulation were refined, more discrete cortical functions were determined. Ferrier,[3] in 1875, described a more precisely delineated region of the primate cortex that responded to small amounts of electrical current. To support his physiologic data, he removed the entire "motor cortex" **unilaterally** and noted a resultant persistent paralysis of the opposite side of the body.

At the turn of the century, Sherrington[4] attempted to localize motor cortex function accurately in primates. In doing so, he made several notable observations: localized electrical stimulation produced isolated and **synergistic** movements (involving a few to several muscles), rather than contraction of individual muscles. Localized **ablation** of the region of the cortex controlling hand movements led to immediate **paresis** of the hand, followed by a delayed and partial recovery of function. Thus, the idea of cortical control of movements rather than muscles gained support, and the ability of the cortex to adapt to change was noted. In 1930, Penfield,[5] a noted neurosurgeon, stimulated the human motor cortex during surgery for intractable epilepsy (uncontrolled seizures) and found that it was arranged like that of nonhuman primates. When he stimulated discrete regions of the precentral cortex, movements of discrete body parts were produced. He described a complete cortical representation or map of the body, with the feet located medially and the head laterally. A notable feature of his **homunculus** was that body parts that participate in fine motor skills are represented over disproportionately large areas of the motor cortex. The map is shown in Figure 14–1. He also described a second motor area. When he applied high levels of electrical current to an area medial to that considered the "motor area," complex orienting movements of the head and arms were produced. He proposed that different parts of the excitable cortex controlled different aspects of movement, and termed his newly found region the supplementary motor area (SMA).

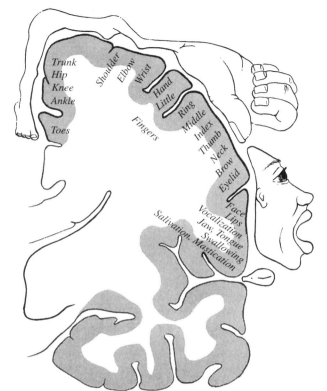

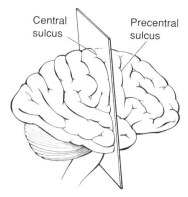

Figure 14–1. The motor homunculus. A slice through the precentral gyrus in the motor cortex shows Penfield's vision of the organization of the motor cortex map. The body parts are represented in a medial to lateral manner, with the feet on the medial wall and the face on the lateral surface of the cerebral hemisphere. The hand and mouth are proportionally larger than the body part to which they are connected. The inset shows the location from which the slice was taken in the brain.

Much has been learned from research using electrical stimulation techniques and from studies correlating brain lesions with motor dysfunctions. Other techniques have been added to researchers' repertoires. Animal studies in which neuronal activity is recorded during specific aspects of motor tasks have added tremendously to our current knowledge. More recently, human studies using noninvasive techniques for imaging localized brain activity, such as positron emission tomography (PET) and functional magnetic resonance imaging, or techniques for evoking localized moments, such as transcutaneous magnetic stimulation, have also been valuable.

Structural Organization of the Motor Cortex

We now know that the motor cortex comprises several distinct regions. These regions can be defined structurally according to their distinctive **cytoarchitecture** and to their connections with other areas of the brain. They can also be defined functionally, according to how neuronal activity is correlated with specific motor tasks or components of a task. Different terminology has evolved, but the most widely accepted defines a primary motor area (M1), a premotor area (PM), and an SMA. Two other, more recently defined motor areas are based on anatomic connections and lie in the cingulate cortex.[6] These areas are called the rostral cingulate motor area (rCMA) and the caudal cingulate motor area (cCMA). M1 lies along the anterior bank of the precentral sulcus and in the precentral gyrus. Rostral and medial to it is the PM and its SMA subdivision. The cingulate motor areas lie in the medial wall of the hemisphere. The locations of the motor regions are shown in Figure 14–2. All of these areas possess the basic characteristics that define them as motor areas: electrical

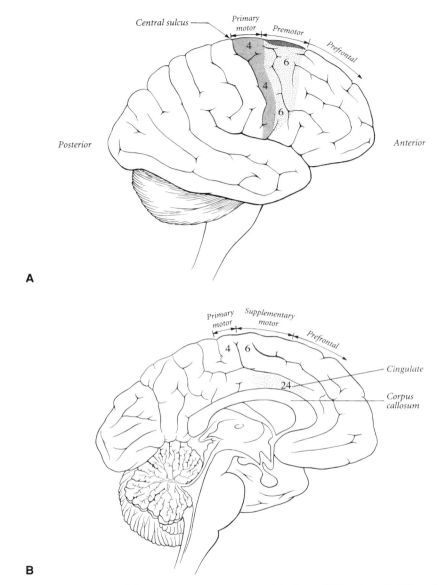

Figure 14–2. The location of the motor cortex. Drawings of the lateral **(A)** and medial **(B)** surfaces of the cerebral hemispheres show the extent of the motor areas. Area 4 corresponds to the primary motor area (MI), and is just in front of the central sulcus. Area 6 corresponds to the premotor (PM) and supplementary motor (SMA) areas, which are both in front of the MI. Most of the SMA and the cingulate motor areas (24) are on the medial wall of the hemisphere.

stimulation produces movement, neurons in the area project directly to the spinal cord (corticospinal neurons), and connections are formed with other motor centers. Underlying differences in these characteristics delineate functional differences of the motor areas. For example, the amount of electrical current needed to produce a movement and the resultant movements are unique to each area. Each area preferentially controls movement of different body parts. The density and destination of corticospinal cells varies for each area. Finally, the pathways that carry afferent signals in and efferent signals out are unique to each area.

The Motor Cortex: Cytoarchitecture

The motor areas have different cytoarchitectonic features. In fact, differences in cell and fiber patterns exist across the cortex. Distinct cytoarchitectonic regions were first delineated according to cell and fiber size, density, and laminar organization by Brodmann in 1909.[7] He assigned numerical designations such that M1 is in area 4, PM and SMA are in area 6, and rCMA and cCMA are in areas 24 and 25, respectively. Overall, the motor areas share certain cytoarchitectonic features. They are distinguished by unusually large pyramidal cells in layer V and the absence of a granular layer IV. In most neocortical regions, layer IV is the target of signals from the thalamus. In the "agranular" motor areas, thalamic signals still reach the cortex, but spread diffusely throughout all other cortical layers. The individual motor areas have subtle cytoarchitectonic distinctions. Area 4 is particularly distinct, because it has the largest layer V pyramidal cells, called Betz cells after their discoverer. Except for the absence of layer IV, the laminar arrangement of cell types according to their projection targets is similar to that in other neocortical areas. Layer I contains mainly axons and dendrites. Layers II and III contain the cell bodies of small to medium-sized pyramidal cells whose axons project to other parts of the cortex (corticocortical projections), including the opposite cerebral hemisphere. Layer V contains mainly medium and large pyramidal neurons, whose primary axons project subcortically. These neurons include cells that project to the thalamus and spinal cord. Layer VI contains medium pyramidal cells that also send axons to the thalamus, as well as to the striatum and claustrum. Some pyramidal cells in layers V and VI also

have axonal branches or collaterals that remain within the cortex, and all have branches that end in the vicinity of the cell body. Pyramidal cells use the neurotransmitter glutamate and have excitatory effects on their target cells. Nonpyramidal cells account for about one third of all motor cortex neurons. They are distributed across layers II to VI. These cells use gamma-aminobutyric acid (GABA) as their neurotransmitter and have inhibitory effects on the cells that they contact. Their axons are **intrinsic** to the cortical region from which they arise. The dense network of intrinsic connections in the motor cortex is functionally very important. Incoming axons from other areas are distributed in a laminar organization as well. Unlike projection neurons, however, they usually terminate in more than one layer.

Corticocortical Connections

Pathways leading in and out of the motor cortex to other cortical regions are numerous, and only the most relevant ones are discussed. The connections of the individual motor areas with other parts of the brain are different from one another and form the basis for their functional roles. The M1 receives proprioceptive information from joint and tendon receptors from area 3a of the somatosensory cortex.[8] These signals tell the M1 about body position and the amplitude, speed, and direction of ongoing movements. The M1 also receives **exteroceptive** information from areas 1 and 2 of the somatosensory cortex. This sensory feedback pathway reports to the M1 on peripheral events detected by the skin, such as object texture, shape, and borders. The PM, SMA, and the opposite motor cortex all project to the M1. The PM and, in turn, SMA receive complex integrated visual, auditory, and somatosensory signals from the sensory association areas as well as from the M1. Most connections between cortical areas are reciprocal. The functional relevance of these connections will be clearer as the roles of the individual motor areas are discussed.

Afferent Subcortical Connections: The Thalamic Relay

The motor cortex is well informed. It receives information from many subcortical structures, but primarily from two important motor centers, the basal ganglia and the cerebellum. These structures work with the motor cortex to control voluntary movement. The thalamus acts as the relay station for input arriving from these, as well as other brain regions, to inform the motor cortex of exteroceptive and proprioceptive events. The thalamus is a collection of nuclei in the rostral diencephalon that directs virtually all the subcortical traffic entering the cerebral cortex. The thalamus has four main nuclei that relay information back and forth to different cortical areas. Groups of cells within the thalamus called the ventrolateral (VL) nuclei are connected to the motor cortex. Subdivisions of the VL relay signals through three somewhat separate systems to specific regions of the motor cortex.[9,10] The cerebellum uses two of the three paths. Cerebellar output travels to the cortex through paired deep cerebellar nuclei. The rostral parts of these nuclei send signals primarily through the ventroposterolateral pars oralis portion of the VL to the M1, but also through a caudal subdivision of the VL to the M1 and cCMA.[11] The caudal parts of these same nuclei send signals by way of nucleus X, a medial subdivision of the VL, to the PM and SMA. The basal ganglia use the third path. Their primary

output travels through the globus pallidus to the ventrolateral pars oralis nucleus of the thalamus mostly to the SMA, but also to the cCMA, the M1 hand representation, and other parts of the frontal cortex. These pathways are summarized in Figure 14–3.

Efferent Subcortical Connections

The Corticospinal Tract. Information received and processed by the motor cortex must eventually reach the musculature to produce movement, the most direct route for which is the corticospinal tract (CST). This important outflow path has origins common to all of the motor cortex and to the parietal cortex. It consists of a huge bundle of axons arising from large pyramidal cells in layer V, including the Betz cells. Most CST cells are in the M1, but also in the SMA, PM, and the somatosensory cortex. The cortical distribution of the cells of origin of this pathway is shown in Figure 14–4. The axon bundle or tract travels through the internal capsule to the medulla,

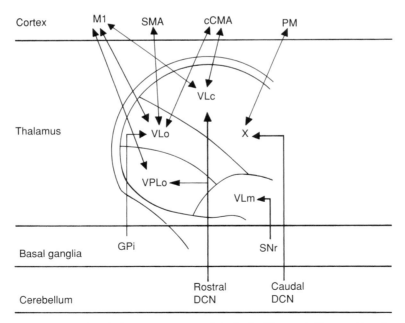

Figure 14–3. Thalamic relays linking motor areas of the brain. The cerebellum and basal ganglia inputs to the ventral-tier thalamic nuclei are summarized. These signals are relayed preferentially to specific areas of the motor cortex as shown, which in turn are reciprocally connected with the thalamus. DCN, deep cerebellar nuclei; cCMA, caudal cingulate motor area; GPi, globus pallidus internal segment; M1, primary motor area; PM, premotor area; SMA, supplementary motor area; SNr, substantia nigra reticulata; VLc, m, o, ventrolateral thalamic nucleus; caudal, medial, oral portions; VPLo, ventroposterolateral thalamic nucleus, oral portion; X, thalamic nucleus X.

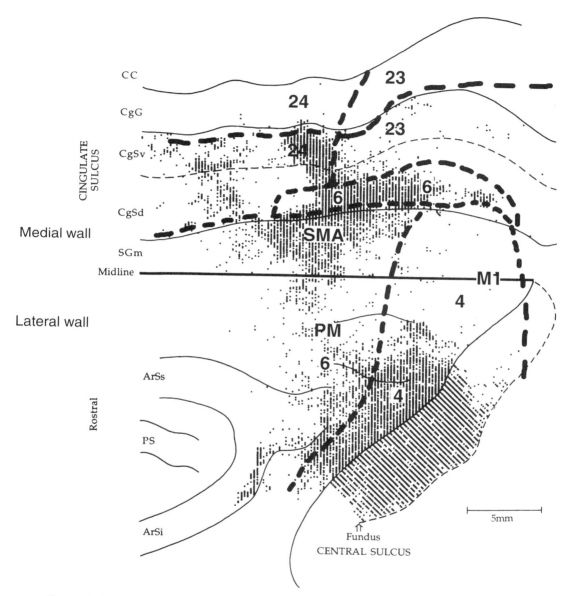

Figure 14–4. Surface map of the motor areas of the primate cortex showing the origin of corticospinal tract (CST) neurons. The three-dimensional cortex has been unfolded and flattened along the midline and along its sulci into a two-dimensional diagram. Each dot represents the location of a CST neuron whose axon descends to the cervical or thoracic levels of the spinal cord. The dashed lines represent the approximate locations of boundaries between the motor areas of the primate cortex. MI, primary motor area; PM, premotor area; SMA, supplementary motor area. CST neurons in the somatosensory cortex are not shown. (Modified from Dum RP, Strick PL. The origin of corticospinal projections from the premotor areas in the frontal lobe. *J Neurosci* 1991;11:667–689.

where it forms a bulge on the medullary surface. This pyramid-shaped bulge earned the CST a second name, the pyramidal tract. At the junction of the medulla with the spinal cord, nearly all CST fibers (90%) cross the midline and descend along the lateral aspect of the spinal cord in the lateral CST. This crossing accounts for the fact that one hemisphere controls movements primarily on the opposite side of the body. A smaller bundle of uncrossed fibers also descends in the spinal cord as the anterior CST. Many of these cross within the spinal cord. Most CST axons end by contacting **interneurons** in the spinal cord. Some, however, end directly on motor neurons, forming a tight link between the cortex and the muscles (one synaptic relay). Such CST cells are given a special name, corticomotoneurons, and are restricted to area 4. Corticomotoneurons project only to muscles that innervate the distal upper extremities. Gradual myelination of these fibers after birth corresponds to the development of skilled hand movements.[12]

The CST is likely to subserve more than one function because it has multiple origins from different cortical regions that have distinct patterns of termination in the spinal cord. The tract acts as a conduit for the movement parameters controlled by each cortical region. For example, signals for force of muscle contraction, motor learning, or preparation for internally generated movements originate in the M1 or SMA. Sensory signals needed for tactile exploration originate in the parietal cortex. These signals are directed to appropriate spinal targets by the CST. In other words, the higher-level processing of the cortex is enabled through the CST. It is involved with the fine tuning of volitional movements, with particular focus on skilled, independent finger control. Some evidence suggests that fine precision grip is controlled by the CST. The amounts of force exerted by the index finger and thumb muscles during precision grip are under separate control by CST neurons, allowing for a high level of independent function and fine motor control to the fingers. The continuous sensory input to CST neurons during movement aids in fine control by providing these cells with the means to adjust their output rapidly in response to changes in peripheral conditions. In animal models of CST lesions, distal movements deteriorate behaviorally and can no longer be produced by electrical stimulation.

Nonpyramidal Descending Pathways. The motor cortex indirectly affects spinal cord activity through other descending pathways. Its neuronal projections go to the basal ganglia, pons, reticular formation, and the red nucleus. These projections are discussed in the following sections.

Functional Organization of the Motor Cortex

Now that we know how the motor cortex is structurally divided, it is easier to understand its functional delineations. Much of our current knowledge of the division of labor in the motor cortex comes from the electrophysiologic techniques developed by Evarts[13] in the 1960s. He devised experiments in which the activity of single neurons was recorded during carefully designed behavioral tasks. Activity that was correlated to a certain aspect of the movement indicated neuronal control over that part of the movement.

Primary Motor Cortex

Neuronal Activity, Electrophysiology. Primary motor area neurons are involved in control of several aspects of voluntary movements, as determined by their activity during motor tasks. The close correlation between M1 neuronal firing and the beginning of muscle contractions indicates that the M1 is responsible for the actual execution of movements. Most M1 cells fire just before movement begins and their activity is temporally linked to electromyographic (EMG) activity in target muscles. M1 cells also control the pattern and time course of activation of synergistic muscles, but the extent of their effectiveness is limited to restricted regions of the body. M1 neurons discharge primarily during movement of synergistic muscles around only one or at most two joints of the contralateral side.[14] Some M1 neurons, however, can control reciprocal effects on agonist and antagonist muscles at the same time. In other words, they can activate one muscle group and inhibit the opposing group. M1 neurons also control specific parameters of muscle contraction, including force, speed, and direction. Some M1 neurons fire when the limb is in a particular static or dynamic joint position. These neurons are likely to control the force of isometric and dynamic muscle contractions (torque), respectively. Other M1 neurons fire in relation to the velocity of a movement, and these neurons control the speed of muscle contraction. Other cells are selectively active when movement is in a particular direction, regardless of the level of force or velocity. These cells control the direction of a movement. Direction-selective cells have preferred directions in that they fire through a wide range of directions, but fire most strongly in a limited range. Many of these cells work together to control the direction in which the body part is moved.[15]

Sensory Influences on Neuronal Activity. Remember that the M1 receives rapid tactile and proprioceptive input through corticocortical connections. This sensory input is continuous throughout the movement, even while the motor cortex neurons are active.[16] Most cells in the M1 (60%) respond to proprioceptive, and some (30%) respond to cutaneous input.[17] The proprioceptive information comes primarily from the muscles that the neuron controls and the joint that is affected by those muscles.[18] Tactile information comes mostly from the skin that is in the field of action of the relevant muscles. Thus, the sensory feedback is current, relevant, and rapid, allowing for quick and continuous adjustments in the movement. M1 cells that respond to tactile cues are more active during exploratory movements when force adjustments are needed to probe or grasp an object. Those cells that respond to proprioceptive cues are activated during velocity and force changes in antagonist muscles. Ultimately, changes in M1 neuronal activity in response to sensory cues are translated into signals that are sent to the spinal cord interneurons or motor neurons to alter the movement.

The Motor Map, Electrical Stimulation. The M1 is able to control movement of all body parts. In fact, the M1 motor map contains the most detailed and complete body representation of all the motor cortex areas. The M1 has the most dense population of CST neurons and is the only region thought to contain corticomotor neurons. The high density of CST cells accounts for the fact that very small amounts of electrical current applied to this area are capable of producing movement.

The M1 is especially well designed to control skilled hand movements, and the mechanisms by which it does this have been studied extensively. Remember the disproportionately large hand representation in the homunculus. From this area, CST neurons travel to the spinal cord. Even for the intrinsic muscles of the hand, which are densely innervated, a single CST neuron projects to several spinal cord motor neuron pools. Therefore, one cell innervates more than one muscle. This relationship is difficult to reconcile with

cortical representation based on control of muscles rather than of movements. Direct stimulation of the CST cell layer in the cortex has shown that small groups of M1 neurons are clustered into "efferent or movement zones" that elicit discrete movements of the digits.[19] Multiple noncontiguous efferent zones in the M1 control movements that involve the same muscles in different tasks. For example, flexion of the index finger in a task that requires grasping a small object between the finger and the thumb can be produced by stimulating one efferent zone. Flexion of the index finger to tap a piano key can be produced by stimulation of a different, nonadjacent zone. Thus, the index finger flexors may be represented multiple times in the motor map. Related studies in which single-neuron activity in the M1 hand region is recorded during different tasks show that the same neuron is active during movements of several digits.[20] Usually, however, the neuron fires most robustly during one preferred movement. In other words, during control of a specific finger movement, widespread and noncontiguous regions of the cortical hand representation are active. This pattern is not inherent in the classic homunculus, which shows adjacent digits occupying somatotopically organized adjacent sites in the cortex. Thus, the motor map has been redrawn for the M1, with the forelimb region organized as a motor "mosaic" with multiple, non-overlapping movement representations, as depicted in Figure 14–5.

Supplementary Motor Cortex

Neuronal Activity, Electrophysiology, and Imaging. Unlike M1 cells, SMA cells are not tightly coupled to the actual movement. They are active at long and variable time periods before muscle activity and show a poor correlation with EMG activity. Furthermore, their activity does not correlate well with physiologic parameters of muscle contractions such as force, velocity, or direction.[21]

The SMA does, however, have an important role in motor control. It is involved with preparation for movement, especially self-initiated (internally generated) movement. Electrophysiologic studies show that SMA neurons become active well in advance of an intended movement. Their activity is correlated with differences in instructional cues given to begin a movement. Memorized cues, rather than sensory cues (e.g., a bell or a light) are the most effective in triggering SMA activity, but both work. Cells in this re-

Map 1

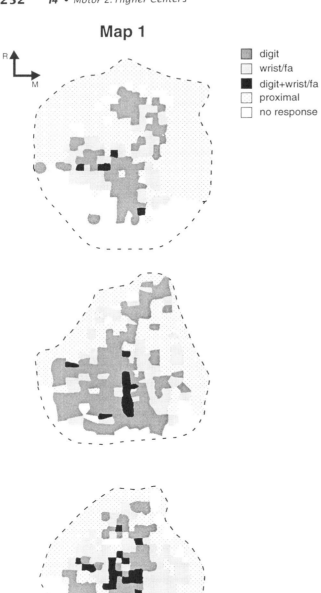

digit
wrist/fa
digit+wrist/fa
proximal
no response

Figure 14–5. The motor map of the hand in the primary motor area (MI) of the left primate cortex. Small amounts of electrical current were passed through a microelectrode that was moved in a gridlike pattern across the hand representation of the MI. Movements of the hand and wrist that occurred in response to the stimuli were marked on this surface map of the cortex. The movements are coded as shown by the key. Note that the body parts are organized in a noncontiguous manner. fa, forearm. (From Nudo RJ, et al. Use-dependent alterations of movement representations in primary motor cortex of adult squirrel monkeys. *J Neurosci* 1996;16: 785–807.

gion respond more robustly to visual and auditory cues than to proprioceptive and tactile cues. (Remember that the M1 receives the latter through dense projections from the somatosensory cortex, whereas the SMA receives auditory and visual signals from the association cortices.) It is interesting that SMA cells respond to visual and auditory cues only if they are relevant to an intended movement.[22] For example, if a bell rings, the SMA neurons do not respond. If the subject has been trained to perform a movement in response to the bell, however, then its sound activates SMA cells, but SMA cells are not particularly excited by the ensuing movement and, as mentioned, their activity is not tightly coupled to the movement. In other words, they are goal oriented. All in all, the SMA cells are not concerned with how the goal is accomplished but with the anticipated goal itself.

Imaging studies such as PET scans can show changes in localized brain activity in awake subjects asked to perform a specific task. One technique is to measure cerebral blood flow by imaging radioactive dyes in the blood. Localized increases in blood flow during the task are interpreted as indications of increased neuronal activity. During such a test, blood flow to the SMA is increased during the preparatory phase of movement, such as at the time of the sensory cue to move, but not once the movement has been initiated. A clever study by Roland et al.[23] used PET to study SMA. Subjects were instructed to imagine that they were performing a movement without actually moving. Under these conditions, blood flow to the SMA increases, indicating its role in movement preparation.

The Motor Map, Electrical Stimulation. The SMA is smaller in extent than the M1 and less somatotopically organized. The SMA contains only 15% to 20% of all CST cells, and so the anatomic linkage to actual movement, like the physiologic linkage, is not as strong as that in the motor cortex. Results of electrical stimulation to the SMA are difficult to interpret. Large amounts of electrical current are needed to elicit movements, reflecting the low density of CST cells. Stimulation results in complex orienting movements of predominantly proximal and axial musculature both bilaterally and contralaterally. Some distal extremity movements are observed, but SMA control over distal limb movements is much less extensive than that of the M1.

Premotor Cortex

Neuronal Activity, Electrophysiology. Far less is known about PM function. PM neurons are variably active during different aspects of movement, but some trends have emerged from the data and suggest a role for the PM in the preparation phase of sensory-triggered movements and for sequencing series of movements. Many PM cells are active during the planning phase of movement, whereas few are active during the actual movement.[24,25] In this respect, they are similar to cells in the SMA. Most PM cells respond to sensory cues, but only if they are triggers for ensuing movement. Auditory, visual, and somatic cues are all effective. An interesting observation is that many PM cells are active during a series of related movements, but not during the individual movements if they are performed separately. These findings led to the suggestion that the PM guides entire behavioral acts such as reaching for food, grasping it, and bringing it to the mouth.[26] This idea is supported by PET studies that show bilateral increases in blood flow to the PM while patients are learning a complex sequence of finger movements.

The Motor Map, Electrical Stimulation. The PM also has a somatotopic representation of the body but, again, it is far less organized than in the M1. Not all body parts are clearly represented, and the somatotopy is not discretely arranged. Electrical stimulation of the PM produces movement only if high current intensity is applied, probably because only 5% to 10% of CST cells are in the PM.[27] Stimulation produces complex bilateral movements of axial, proximal, and, to some extent, distal extremities, and facial musculature.

Clinical Correlations

Lesions of Primary Motor Cortex

Localized brain lesions supply pieces to the puzzle of regional cortical function. Lesions in the M1 lead to contralateral weakness or paresis with little or no initial **spasticity**, but some spasticity develops over time. Postural reactions and stretch reflexes are reduced in the acute phase, but show gradual recovery, and eventually an overshoot, such that stretch reflexes become hyperactive. Damage of this sort has been classically defined as "upper motor neuron" dysfunction, the upper motor neurons being those that arise from the cortex and the lower motor neurons those that arise from the spinal cord and brainstem. After the acute phase of the lesion, recovery is typically gradual, but incomplete. Proximal movements usually show the greatest recovery, whereas distal movements remain weak and fractionated. Fine finger movements are the most drastically and permanently affected because they rely heavily on M1 control. Proximal movements show greater recovery because the undamaged PM and SMA may assume some lost function. Both areas have some bilateral control of proximal musculature.

Lesions of Supplementary Motor Cortex

A lesion to the SMA results in complex motor dysfunctions. The symptoms include severe **akinesia** on the side opposite the lesion, **mutism**, loss of facial expression, and difficulty with tasks requiring cooperative movements of both hands. In addition, patients have trouble performing self-initiated tasks. For example, if you hand a tool to such a patient, he is likely to do nothing with it even though he knew how to use the tool before the lesion. He cannot initiate the task himself, but he can learn to use the tool in response to an auditory, visual, or tactile cue. Thus, when the SMA is missing, the ability to self-initiate tasks is disrupted and the brain must depend on other cortical areas to help out. It may be that the intact PM can initiate the same task, but needs the sensory cue to get started.

Lesions of Premotor Cortex

Lesions in the PM result in nonspecific motor disturbances or **apraxia**. The patient's movements are clumsy and slow, with mild proximal joint weakness and loss of coordination of movements around the proximal joints. Rhythmic movements such as typing are disrupted, and **perseveration** may occur. For example, patients with PM lesions would have a difficult time pedaling a bicycle, but could manage to tie their shoes, a task that requires coordination of distal extremity movements. The ability to learn and produce complex or sequential motor tasks is impaired. Previously acquired sequential tasks deteriorate, even though individual movements within the sequence are performed easily. Unlike patients with SMA lesions, they are able to do self-initiated tasks, but have difficulty with sensory-triggered tasks. In this case, the patient would have difficulty learning to use his tool in response to a bell, but could use it unprompted when the need arose.

Lesions of the Sensory Cortex

The importance of sensory information for smooth voluntary movements is exemplified by parietooccipital lobe lesions. Postcentral lesions of the somatosensory cortex lead to **ataxia**, **dysmetria**, and a reluctance to move. Fine finger movements during tactile exploration are disrupted, and visual guidance is needed to increase the accuracy of movements. Parietooccipital lesions result in visuomotor ataxia in that patients cannot guide the arm or eye to a target. In these examples, both the movement and its guidance system are disrupted, even though motor centers are intact.

Plasticity of the Motor Cortex

The motor cortex is able to reorganize and adapt in response to numerous perturbations. This capability is known as plasticity, and is reflected in reorganization of the motor map and in recovery of lost function. It may occur by one or a number of mechanisms, including sprouting of new axon terminals, changes in dendritic organization,[28] altering the effectiveness of synapses, and uncovering or unmasking existing synapses whose functions are blocked by inhibitory influences. Repetitive electrical stimulation of a particular body part representation rapidly and reversibly expands the cortical representation of that body part.[29] Motor representations can also be altered by peripheral manipulations such as forelimb amputation or peripheral nerve damage.[30] Most exciting, because of the potential therapeutic benefits after localized **ischemic** damage, is the ability of the motor cortex rapidly to reorganize the cortical map in response to retraining of skilled motor tasks. After a stroke, patients are left with weakness or paralysis of the contralateral limb. Some gradual recovery in motor function occurs, but skilled digit use rarely recovers. The partial recovery is thought to be a result of undamaged cortical regions taking over the lost function of the damaged area. The hands are represented primarily in the M1 and have little bilateral cortical control. Therefore, other cortical areas or the opposite hemisphere are unlikely to have the ability to take over hand function, and so it shows poor recovery. With intense training of hand skill after a localized stroke, reorganization of the cortical map occurs, such that the hand is now represented in adjacent undamaged cortex that previously contained representations of adjacent body parts.[31] Better yet, this reorganization is accompanied by partial functional recovery in hand skill.[32]

The Basal Ganglia

Historical Perspectives

Our understanding of basal ganglia function began with studies of neurodegenerative disorders involving specific subsets of neurons in the basal ganglia. Early clinical reports of a motor disorder, originally called the "shaking palsy" by James Parkinson in 1817, would later be tied to degeneration of neurons in a region of the basal ganglia called the substantia nigra. Pathologic changes in this nucleus are associated with complex motor symptoms, characterized in general by a slowness or paucity of movement. Cellular changes in other regions of the basal ganglia result in very different motor symptoms, such as the uncontrolled movements of Huntington's disease. These varied symptoms reflect the complex circuitry of this part of the brain.

Structural Organization of the Basal Ganglia

The basal ganglia consist of five subcortical nuclei that span the telencephalon, diencephalon, and midbrain. Different terminology has been used for the group of nuclei that comprise the basal ganglia, but most commonly they are described as the caudate, putamen, globus pallidus (GP), subthalamic nucleus (STN), and substantia nigra (SN). Their general orientation is shown in Figure 14–6. The caudate (medially) and putamen (laterally) share many similarities and together are called the neostriatum, or often just the striatum. They develop from a common origin in the basal telencephalon and therefore have similar cell types. Because they migrate differently, however, they are separated from one another by the internal capsule, a fiber bundle that carries axons away from the cortex. The caudate and putamen together are the primary termination site of incoming

axons to the basal ganglia; they are the main entrance to the basal ganglia. The GP, sometimes called the pallidum and sometimes the paleostriatum because it is phylogenetically older than the rest of the striatum, develops from the diencephalon. The GP is also separated into two parts by a fiber bundle. These parts are the internal and external segments (GPi and GPe). The cells in both parts are similar and both receive input from the neostriatum, but project to different targets. The internal segment is one of two primary routes of information flow out of the basal ganglia—part of the main exit.[33] The GP and putamen, together, are sometimes called the lentiform nucleus because of the bean-shaped structure these adjacent nuclei form. The STN is small and lies on the inner surface of the internal capsule. The SN is a large sheet of cells situated dorsal to the cerebral peduncle. It is also composed of two cell groups. The pars compacta (SNc) portion is the more dorsal of the two, and it has most of the cells that produce the neurotransmitter dopamine. A pigmented substance called melanin that is derived from dopamine makes the tissue appear dark, and is responsible for the name "substantia nigra" ("black substance"). The SN pars reticulata (SNr) is pale and has cells and connections like that of the internal segment of the GP. It forms the other portion, along with the GPi, of the primary output route from the basal ganglia. Functionally these two subnuclei—the SNr and Gpi—may be considered as one structure and will be referred to as the **exit nuclei**.

Afferent Connections

Nearly all incoming information enters the basal ganglia through the striatum. A primary source of afferent input is the ipsilateral cerebral cortex. Virtually all of the neocortex contributes to this vast, topographically organized projection. The sensorimotor cortical areas, including the M1, PM, SMA, and the primary somatosensory cortex, send dense topographic projections to the putamen, the region of the striatum involved mostly with motor function. Caudate projections arise from remaining cortical areas, and this region is functionally related to visuomotor and limbic functions. The cortical neurons from which the corticostriate projection originates are pyramidal cells primarily in layers V and VI. A secondary projection comes from layer VI.[34] Another source of afferents to the striatum comes from the in-

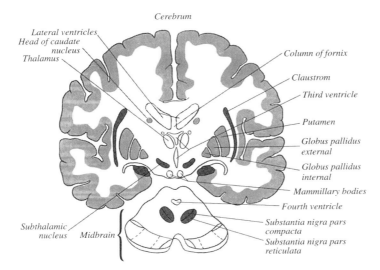

A

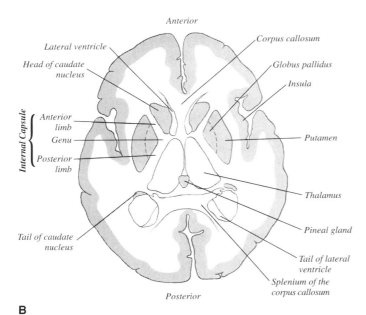

B

Figure 14-6. Anatomy of the basal ganglia. **A:** Frontal section of the brain shows the locations of the basal ganglia nuclei. **B:** Horizontal section of the telencephalon shows the relationship of the basal ganglia nuclei with the internal capsules.

tralaminar thalamic nuclei, the amygdala, and the dorsal raphe. Less extensive projections also go to other areas of the basal ganglia. One of these projections originates from the M1 and PM and projects directly to the STN.

Efferent Connections

The basal ganglia are unique among the motor systems in that they have no direct connections with the spinal cord. Thus, their influence over movement is mediated primarily by their projections to the motor areas of the cerebral cortex (M1, PM, and SMA), which are the major targets of basal ganglia outflow.

Nearly all outgoing signals leave the basal ganglia by way of the GPi and the SNr. These two exit nuclei send inhibitory signals to several motor regions: the VL, ventroanterior, centromedian, and mediodorsal thalamic nuclei, and the pedunculopontine nucleus. The SNr also projects to the superior colliculus.[35] The cortical-basal ganglia loop is one of two important motor loops formed with the motor cortex. The other is the corticocerebellar loop. Cortical signals that enter the striatum from the sensorimotor cortex are processed through the basal ganglia circuitry. The integrated signals leave the basal ganglia through the main exit path and return to the motor cortex by way of the ventral-tier thalamic nuclei. (The mediodorsal nucleus relays to the prefrontal cortex.) The SMA is the primary recipient of basal ganglia output, but the PM and M1 receive some as well. Through this motor loop, the basal ganglia indirectly influence spinal and brainstem motor areas.

Some axons leave the basal ganglia through other exits. These projections may be smaller, but are very important to brain function. For example, dopamine-producing cells in the SNc send axons to many brain regions, including limbic centers and cortical motor centers. Although dopamine input to the cortex is widespread, the motor areas of the cortex, in particular the SMA, receive very dense dopaminergic input.[36,37] It is now easier to see how intimately connected the motor cortex is with the basal ganglia.

Intrinsic Connections

The basal ganglia have three separate internal circuits:

1 The direct path through the basal ganglia goes from the striatum to the two exit nuclei, the GPi and the SNr.

2 The indirect path through the basal ganglia goes from the striatum, to the GPe, to the STN, and then to the exit nuclei. Both the direct and the indirect path are topographic.

3 The SNc sends dopaminergic axons to the striatum, which sends a reciprocal projection back.

The circuitry in these connections may seem too complex to emit any decipherable signals, so let us add the appropriate neurotransmitters and look at it piece by piece.

Neurotransmitter Systems. The complex network of input, output, and internal circuits of the basal ganglia uses many neurotransmitters. The output of this system cannot be predicted by any one input or neurotransmitter system, but results from the effects of all influences. We focus first on the motor cortex–basal ganglia loops. If the direct basal ganglia path is used, axons travel from the cortex, to the striatum, to the exit nuclei, to the thalamus, and back to the cortex. The cortical cells use glutamate and are excitatory. Neurons in the striatum use the neurotransmitter GABA and are inhibitory. Cells in both GPi and SNr also use GABA, and therefore are inhibitory. Stimulation of this pathway is thought to facilitate movement. If we retrace the pathway we can see how this happens; the corticostriate cells excite striatal target cells, increasing their activity, and these cells in turn increase their inhibitory effect on the output cells of the exit nuclei. Neuronal activity in GPi and SNr is reduced, and therefore their inhibitory effects on the thalamus are reduced. Finally, the thalamus is **disinhibited** and excitatory thalamic input to the cortex is increased. This elevated input leads to increased cortical activity and output to the spinal cord and brainstem motor centers.

The indirect motor pathway involves more of the internal circuitry of the basal ganglia. Let us begin with the cortex again. Axons from the cortex go to the striatum. Striatal cells project to the GPe, which projects to the STN. These cells project to the exit nuclei, which take their usual route to the thalamus and then the cortex. The new additions here are the STN, which uses glutamate and is therefore excitatory, and the GPe, which uses GABA and is inhibitory. Activation of this pathway appears to have the opposite effect of the direct path in that it leads to suppression of movement. To see how, let us retrace the steps. Corticostriate axons excite their striatal target cells. Striatal activity increases, causing increased inhibition of target cells in the GP. In this instance, a different subset of striatal cells is activated, as described later. These cells inhibit the GPe. Next, reduced pallidal activity leads to decreased inhibition of the STN. This change results in increased STN activity and thus in increased excitation of the exit nuclei. The resultant increase in inhibitory input to the thalamus leads to a subsequent decrease in excitatory thalamic activation of the motor cortex. Reduced activity in the cortex translates to reduced spinal cord and brainstem motor output and sup-

pression of movement. These two circuits are summarized in Figure 14–7.

To further complicate the picture, remember that other circuits are involved. The SNc sends dopaminergic fibers to the striatum. Dopamine excites the GABAergic cells that project directly to the exit nuclei and thus activates the direct pathway. On the other hand, dopamine inhibits the GABAergic cells that project to the GPe and thus inhibits the indirect pathway. The opposing effects of dopamine are mediated by different subsets of dopamine receptors. Therefore, dopamine can facilitate movement by

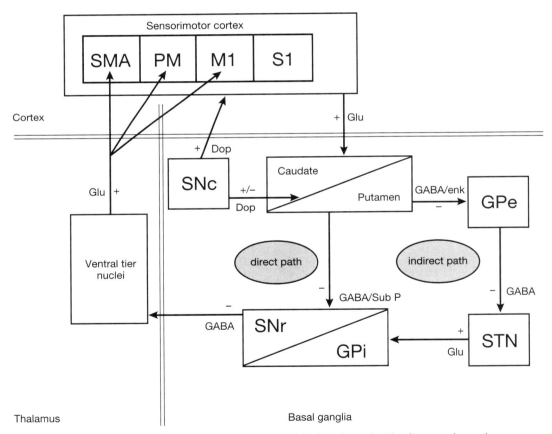

Figure 14–7. The indirect and direct motor loops of the basal ganglia. The diagram shows the connections between the basal ganglia and the motor cortex through the thalamic relay. The projections are depicted by the arrows and the neurotransmitters (+ is excitatory and − is inhibitory) used for the pathways are marked on the arrows. Dop, dopamine; Enk, enkephalin; GABA, gamma-aminobutyric acid; Glu, glutamate; Gpe, i: globus pallidus external, internal segment; Ml, primary motor area; PM, premotor area; Sl, primary somatosensory cortex; SMA, supplementary motor area; Sub P, substance P; SNc, r, substantia nigra compacta, reticulata; STN, subthalamic nucleus.

modulating both the direct and indirect basal ganglia pathways. The striatum sends signals back to the SNc, by way of cells that produce substance P (excitatory). Dopaminergic cells in the SNc also project directly to the motor cortex, but the inhibitory or excitatory nature of this projection is not so clear. Given the idea that different routes through the basal ganglia can either enhance or suppress movement, you should now understand why dysfunction in different areas of the basal ganglia causes such vast differences in motor symptoms.

Compartmental Organization of the Striatum

The striatum has a unique compartmental organization based on neurotransmitter receptors, neuropeptides, and patterns of input and output projections.[38] We examine this complex organization in this section.

Connectional Organization. Let us begin by looking at the arrangement of striatal output cells. Most striatal cells are medium-sized, spiny cells that produce GABA. Two subsets of these cells exist. One group participates in the direct path: striatonigral and striatopallidal (GPi) cells. In addition to GABA, these cells produce the neuropeptides dynorphin and substance P, and they have the D_1 type of dopamine receptor. The other subset, the striatopallidal (GPe) neurons, participates in the indirect path. These cells produce GABA and the neuropeptide enkephalin, and they contain the D_2 type of dopamine receptor. Differential cortical input and dopaminergic modulation of these two groups of cells determine which pathway is activated. Dopamine binding to D_1 or D_2 receptors produces different effects in target cells. Activation of D_2 receptors causes downregulation of enkephalin expression and decreases physiologic activity in the target cell. Activation of D_1 receptors, however, upregulates dynorphin and substance P expression and increases physiologic activity in target cells. Thus, dopamine can alter the balance of the two pathways and affect motor behavior through both the basal ganglia pathways.

Patch–Matrix Organization. Afferents to the striatum are topographically organized, and like the cell bodies of output neurons, are distributed to either patch or matrix compartments. A patch–matrix arrangement was first described in the striatum on the basis of mu (μ) opioid receptor distribution. Gray-

biel[39] first identified patches of tissue that stained for the presence of these receptors. Later studies showed that the same patches also stained for acetylcholinesterase. The matrix contains cells that stain for calbindin (a calcium-binding protein) and fibers that contain somatostatin (a neuropeptide). The massive input from the sensorimotor cortex comes mostly from layer V cells and goes to the large striatal matrix compartment. A smaller projection from deep layer V and layer VI cells goes to patch structures that are embedded within the matrix. Two separate populations of both thalamostriatal and nigrostriatal (dopaminergic) cells also exist; one projects to the matrix and one to the patches. The output of the matrix compartment goes preferentially to the exit nuclei, and that of the patch compartment goes preferentially to the SNc. These pathways are summarized in Figure 14–8. It is interesting that the organizational schemes described here do not completely coincide, in that neurons producing enkephalin, substance P, and dynorphin immunoreactivity are spread across the patches and matrix.

Neuronal Activity of Basal Ganglia Neurons, Electrophysiology

Physiologic studies of the basal ganglia have targeted specific aspects of some subsets of cells, so we must look at them set by set. GP cell activity is strongly correlated with remembered tasks rather than with visually cued tasks, linking them to initiation of internally cued movement.[40] Some pallidal and putamen cell activity is correlated temporally to certain phases of movement. Many of these cells are active only during one part of sequential movement, but not during the entire movement. Other cells are activated by particular sequences of movement. Therefore, they may be involved in programming complex sequential movements. Striatal cells are tonically quiescent; they fire infrequently unless stimulated. Some striatal cells fire similarly to cortical cells. They are active during the same phase of a movement and at the same time as neurons in the M1. This pattern of activity suggests that parallel systems in the cortex and basal ganglia work together to control the same aspects of movement.[41]

Functions of the Basal Ganglia

Our ideas of basal ganglia function have been inferred from lesion studies that need to be carefully

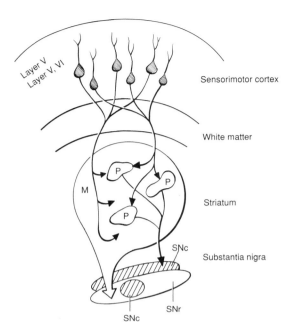

Figure 14-8. The input and output connections of the striatal patches and matrix. Pyramidal neurons in layer V and those in layers V and VI of the sensorimotor cortex are shown projecting to the matrix compartment and patches of the striatum, respectively. Arrows show the output of the striatal matrix and patches projecting primarily to the exit nuclei and SNc, respectively. M, matrix; P, patch; SNc, r, substantia nigra compacta, reticulata.

interpreted. Coupled with information on connectivity and neuronal activity, however, a reasonable definition of their role in motor control can be put forth. Note, first, that their function is not exclusively motor. They are involved in cognitive aspects of movement and in limbic function. Their role in motor control is probably one of programming the initiation of internally generated (but not sensory-triggered) movements and execution of complex motor strategies.[42] They may also be involved in sensorimotor integration and sensory gating. In other words, they help to compare motor commands from the cortex with proprioceptive input. Subsequently, they evaluate the sensory data to determine which stimuli are relevant.

Specific subsets of cells may influence different aspects of movement. For example, pallidal cells may help to set the appropriate sequence of movement components involved in complex motor strategies. Remember that the basal ganglia, like other motor centers, do not function alone. The vast system of interconnections between the motor centers highlights this idea. Furthermore, the basal ganglia depend on the motor loops through the cortex to mediate their effects. The basal ganglia have been described as the major players in the extrapyramidal system, along with the other descending cortical pathways. Their functions and the disorders associated with their

loss were described as somewhat separate and distinct from the pyramidal system (CST). The interconnections and interactions between these two systems, however, make it difficult to define them functionally or structurally as two distinct motor systems with disorders leading to distinctly different syndromes. This differentiation between the extrapyramidal tract system and the pyramidal system is used less frequently today.

Clinical Correlations

Basal ganglia disorders are clinically heterogeneous. As discussed earlier, the vast differences seen in motor symptoms may be due to the effects on different subpopulations of cells that lead to imbalances in basal ganglia output. Damage to the basal ganglia can result from trauma, infection, biochemical processes, tumors, and vascular insufficiency. Disorders of the basal ganglia are often associated with disruption of specific neurotransmitter systems. All of these factors are likely to affect other systems as well. Therefore, the resultant motor deficits must be carefully interpreted to determine functional specificity. Depending on the basal ganglia area involved, paucity of movements or phasic involuntary movements occur. The reduced rate and amount of movement associated with Parkinson's disease are related to loss of nigrostriatal dopamine-producing cells. Athetosis describes slow and continuous writhing movements that are uncontrolled. The hands, lips, and tongue are most affected. Chorea describes rapid and jerky movements that are involuntary and also often involve the hands and face. Both athetosis and chorea are associated with cell loss in the striatum. Ballisimus describes violent, flinging movements, mostly of the proximal musculature. This disorder is usually one sided (hemiballisimus) and is associated with contralateral lesions of the STN.

Biochemical Disorders of the Basal Ganglia

Parkinson's Disease. Parkinsonism is a neurologic disease that affects many elderly people (mean age of onset is 58 years). The hallmark of the disorder is a gradual loss of dopamine-producing neurons in the SNc.[43] In addition, a secondary and less severe reduction in serotonin and norepinephrine occurs. The disease is characterized by **hypokinesia**, **rigidity**, and resting tremor. The progression of symptoms is gradual, but eventually movements become slow **(bradykinesia)** and difficult to initiate. The slowed movements are accurate, however, unlike the movements seen with cerebellar lesions. Furthermore, unlike with cortical lesions, paralysis does not occur. The overall level of movement is reduced and patients may maintain a fixed posture for unusually long periods of time. Even facial expressions are reduced and arm swing is lost from gait. Often, patients freeze midway through a movement (akinesia). These patients have no reflex responses to perturbations in their intended movements. A muscle rigidity develops that is present even during relaxation, but is more severe during passive stretch. Hyperactivity of both alpha and gamma motor neurons leads to the rigidity. A rhythmic resting tremor develops. It usually begins in the thumb and fingers and has been described as a pill-rolling motion. Continuous alterations in agonist and antagonist contractions lead to the tremor, which may be dampened during spontaneous movements.[44] As described previously, dopamine facilitates movement; therefore, its loss leads to decreased movement. Motor symptoms can be alleviated temporarily by treatment with L-dopa, a precursor to dopamine that crosses the blood–brain barrier. Promising therapy now comes

from transplantation of dopaminergic cells or factors to protect these cells from degenerating.

Huntington's Disease.
Huntington's disease is a genetically transmitted disease associated with dementia, chorea, and early death. Cognitive and motor symptoms first appear as clumsiness and slurred speech, but gradually progress to a level at which cognitive decline is severe and uncontrolled movement confines the patient to a wheelchair. The motor symptoms probably result from loss of cholinergic and GABAergic cells in the striatum. The GABAergic neurons are lost first, and this diminishes the inhibitory input to the external pallidum. Thus, activation of the indirect basal ganglia pathway is decreased and basal ganglia inhibition of the thalamus is removed. The thalamus sends more excitatory input to the cortex and upregulates motor cortex activity. Involuntary movements are expressed.

Lesions of the Basal Ganglia
Tardive dyskinesia is a motor disorder that results from prolonged drug therapy for treatment of psychosis. It may or may not be reversed by cessation of drug therapy. The drugs affect dopamine transmission and ultimately lead to hypersensitivity of dopamine receptors, making dopamine more effective in facilitation of movement. The primary symptom is involuntary facial movement. Vascular accidents can cause restricted lesions with symptoms characteristic to the lesion location. Such lesions that affect the STN are usually unilateral and lead to hemiballisimus.[45] Some gradual recovery may occur after the acute episode. Restricted nigral lesions lead to hypokinesia and flexed postures. GP lesions lead to hypokinesia, flexed posture, and loss of ability to perform alternating movements. Striatal lesions lead to hyperactivity and rotation to the side of the lesion.

The Cerebellum

Historical Perspectives

Studies of patients with head injuries suffered during the first World War provided early ideas on cerebellar function. Detailed descriptions of motor deficits after gunshot wounds to the cerebellum were made by Holmes[46] in 1917. Although cerebellar lesions do not cause paralysis or loss of sensation, they do cause devastating changes in the ability to produce smooth, sequenced, complex movements. Supporting postures and balance deteriorate, eye–hand coordination is disrupted, and motor programs degrade into their constituent parts. Holmes described a set of symptoms that included hypotonia to passive stretch, loss of muscle synergy resulting in tremor, and ataxia. These symptoms reflect errors in generating movement parameters of direction, force, velocity, amplitude, and timing.

Structural Organization of the Cerebellum

The cerebellum is unique in that its cellular components and their connections are arranged in a very stereotyped pattern. This structural homogeneity means that neuronal signals are processed in a similar and characteristic way throughout. The heterogeneity of cerebellar function, in that it influences various aspects of movement and different body parts, may lie in the arrangement of its afferent and efferent systems.

Gross Structure

The cerebellar cortex is a large, folded structure tucked under the posterior aspect of the cerebral hemispheres. It consists of an outer gray matter called the cerebellar cortex and an inner core of white matter (medullary substance) containing three paired nuclei. Two deep fissures, primary and posterolateral, divide the cortex into anterior, posterior, and flocculonodular lobes, as seen in Figure 14–9. More superficial fissures subdivide the 3 lobes into 10 lobules, each of which is further subdivided into narrow folia (folds). No clear median division is apparent, but shallow longitudinal furrows delineate a midline vermis from the right and left hemispheres, each of which has an intermediate and a lateral cortical region. Three large tracts, the superior, middle, and inferior cerebellar peduncles, carry axons to and from the cerebellum to other brain structures.

The major lobes can be classified according to their phylogenetic origins. The archicerebellum is phylogenetically the oldest portion and consists of the flocculonodular lobe. The paleocerebellum evolved more recently, and consists of the anterior lobe. The neocerebellum is phylogenetically the newest and consists of the posterior lobe.

Although investigators disagree somewhat on discrete functional localization, the longitudinally oriented structural subdivisions correspond to three functionally different areas. Each subdivision has somewhat different afferent and efferent connections. The vestibulocerebellum corresponds to the archicerebellum in that it consists of the flocculonodular lobe. Its input and output travel through the vestibular nuclei, which act like deep cerebellar nuclei, but are located outside the cerebellum. The vestibulocerebellum controls balance during gait and stance and coordinates eye and body movements. The spinocerebellum comprises the midline vermis and the intermediate cortical region that spans the anterior and posterior lobes. It receives most of its afferents from the spinal cord and sends efferents out by way of the fastigial (from the vermis) and interpositus (from the intermediate cortical region). The spinocerebellum controls coordination of ongoing limb movements. The cerebrocerebellum is composed of the lateral portions of the cortical regions and spans the anterior and posterior lobes. Its afferents come from the sensorimotor regions, by way of the pontine nuclei. It sends efferents out through the dentate, which travel back to the motor cortex by way of the thalamus. The cerebrocerebellum helps in the planning or preparation for intended movements. We will return to these subdivisions later.

Microscopic Structure of the Cortex

The cerebellar cortex is a laminar structure. It is folded into sequential, thin layers, the folia, that run parallel to one another. Within the folia, the cortex consists of an outer molecular layer, a Purkinje cell layer, and a granule cell layer. The molecular layer contains two cell types, both of which are inhibitory. These are the basket cells and stellate cells. Basket cell axons descend deeper into the cortex to contact the cell bodies of Purkinje cells. These axons are distinct in that they wrap around the cell body and axon hillock of Purkinje cells, emulating a "basket." On the other hand, stellate cell axons contact the dendrites of Purkinje cells. The Purkinje cell layer is named for its constituent cells. These cells are large with flattened, fan-shaped dendritic trees that are striking in size and regularity. The distal dendrites have numerous spines. Purkinje cells provide the only route for signals to leave the cortex. Their axons send inhibitory signals out to the deep cerebellar nu-

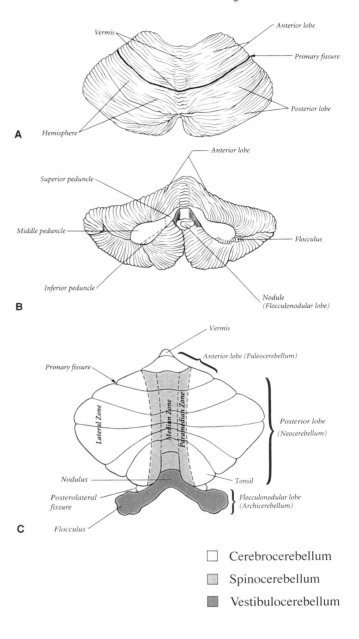

Figure 14-9. Anatomy of the cerebellum.
A: Superior view of the cerebellar surface.
B: View of the cerebellum as it has been
cut away from the rest of the brain. **C:** The
functional subdivisions of the cerebellum
as described in the text.

☐ Cerebrocerebellum

▨ Spinocerebellum

▧ Vestibulocerebellum

clei and the vestibular nuclei. The granule cell layer
is packed with small granule cells. Each one has an
axon that extends out to the molecular layer, where
it divides into a "T." Branches of the "T" run parallel
to the long axis of the folia, and are called parallel
fibers. The parallel fibers uniformly distribute excita-

tory signals to Purkinje cell dendrites over great distances (up to 6 mm). Golgi cells are also found in
the granular layer. They are less common, but exert a
powerful inhibitory influence on granule cells. The
arrangement of cortical neurons is shown in Figure
14-10.

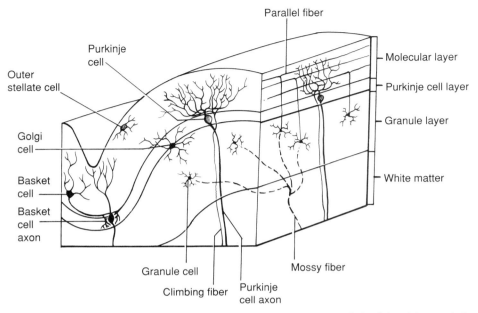

Figure 14–10. Cytoarchitecture of the cerebellum. A cross-section through the folia of the cerebellum shows the cortical layers, the locations of the different types of neurons, and the locations of the afferents.

Cellular Profiles and Circuits Are Stereotyped. A closer look at the cortical circuitry reveals that axons and dendrites of nearly all cell types are organized in a planar fashion. Basket and stellate cell dendrites and axons travel near the surface, perpendicular to the long axis of the folia. The flat Purkinje cell dendrites are organized in stacks, that are also oriented perpendicular to the long axis of the folia. Their primary input from the parallel fibers runs perpendicular to their dendrites. Even this brief description highlights the stereotyped structural organization of the cortex. Further homogeneities, however, are associated with the circuitry. For example, each basket cell axon diverges to contact between 6 and 10 Purkinje cells, whereas axons from many basket cells converge onto one Purkinje cell. Individual parallel fibers synapse at only two sites on a Purkinje cell's dendrites, but approximately 40,000 different parallel fibers contact the dendritic tree of one Purkinje cell. In other words, the anatomy is characterized by tremendous convergence from many parallel fibers onto a single target cell and tremendous

divergence of parallel fibers from one granule cell onto many Purkinje cells. These fibers provide a powerful excitatory input to Purkinje cells.

Organization of Cerebellar Projections

The three pairs of deep cerebellar nuclei communicate with other structures in the brain. The fastigial (medial), the interpositus (middle), and the dentate (lateral) nuclei are groups of cells embedded in the white matter deep to the cerebellar cortex. Axons from the Purkinje cells terminate in these nuclei and in the vestibular nuclei. Together, these nuclei provide the exit route for processed signals to leave the cerebellum. They also receive copies of incoming information destined for the cortex.

Afferent Connections

The cerebellum is well informed on current events. Input to the cerebellum comes primarily from the sensorimotor and visual cortices, the spinal cord, and the vestibular system. It is carried through two systems, the climbing fibers and the mossy fibers, which represent separate modes of activation. Climbing fibers carry input from various sources and synapse directly onto the Purkinje cells, whereas mossy fibers bring diverse input to the Purkinje cells by way of granule cells.

The Climbing Fiber System. Climbing fibers arise from cells in the inferior olive. They cross the midline, travel to the cortex through the inferior cerebellar peduncle, and terminate on Purkinje cell dendrites and interneurons. They send axon collaterals to the deep nuclei. This system is topographically organized along longitudinal zones in the cortex. Their input pattern is stereotyped throughout the cortex. One olivary cell axon divides to as many as 10 climbing fibers, each of which synapses with one Purkinje cell. The climbing fiber wraps around the proximal dendritic tree, forming 200 to 300 synapses. This arrangement establishes a highly specific and powerful excitatory input onto the Purkinje cell such that when a climbing fiber fires, its target cell fires.[47] In fact, synchronous climbing fiber activation simultaneously depolarizes nearly the entire Purkinje cell dendritic tree, leading to a burst of stereotyped action potentials. The resulting distinctive action potentials are called complex spikes. They are large-amplitude action potentials, followed by a burst of small spikes. Complex spikes occur at low frequency (1 Hz). Climbing fibers not only elicit action potentials, but increase Purkinje cell excitability to parallel and mossy fiber input by changing the level of depolarization.

The olivocerebellar projection receives signals from many areas of the brain, including the cerebral cortex, red nucleus, brainstem nuclei, spinal cord, reticular formation, and cerebellar nuclei. Its most important input is from the spinal cord, which sends information on reflex activity in response to unexpected perturbations in movement, and on descending commands obtained by sampling interneuronal activity in the spinal cord. The inferior olive compares, processes, and forwards this information to the cerebellum. It makes sense, then, that olivary neurons respond to interruption of an intended posture or movement caused by an unexpected event such as displacement of the standing surface. They are not, however, interested in uninterrupted movements. The perturbations

are detected as changes in joint position, movement, velocity, and acceleration.[48]

The Mossy Fiber System. Mossy fibers are the largest afferent system to the cerebellar cortex. They comprise a diverse conglomeration of inputs originating in the spinocerebellar, corticopontocerebellar, and reticulocerebellar paths, as well as from the vestibular and deep cerebellar nuclei.[49,50] They discharge at high frequency, which maintains the high level of tonic activity in the cerebellum and ensures that changes in mossy fiber activity are detected rapidly. Mossy fibers continuously update the cerebellum on the status of ongoing and intended movement by eliciting simple spikes in Purkinje cells. These signals are small-amplitude, high-frequency (50–100 Hz) action potentials. Mossy fibers send collaterals to the deep nuclei, enter the cortex, and branch repeatedly before contacting granule cells. They excite the granule cells, which, in turn, influence the Purkinje cells. Climbing and mossy fibers that carry information about the same body part project to overlapping areas of the cortex.

Spinocerebellar Input. The main input to the spinocerebellum is somatosensory information from the spinal cord by way of the dorsospinocerebellar (lower extremity) and the cuneocerebellar tracts (upper extremity). These tracts carry precise (**modality** and spatially specific) proprioceptive information from muscle and joint receptors, and exteroreceptive information from skin mechanoreceptors.[51,52] They report to the cerebellum on position, velocity, and force of muscle contractions,[53] and peripheral events. The ventrospinocerebellar tract and its forelimb equivalent, the rostrospinocerebellar tract, carry more complex signals to the spinocerebellum. Their cells of origin receive multimodal signals from widespread regions of the body, along with copies of descending cortical and subcortical signals. They have little modality and spatial specificity. They report to the cerebellum on the state of ongoing spinal cord activity. As mentioned, the input to the three functional cerebellar regions overlaps. The motor cortex sends some afferents to the spinocerebellum. Furthermore, the vermis receives visual, auditory, and vestibular signals.

Corticopontocerebellar Input. Although the entire cerebral cortex contributes input to the cerebrocerebellum, most input comes from primary sensorimotor, association, and visual areas. The pontine nuclei serve as an integration center and relay for this input. Cortical afferents to the pons are topographically organized. Although pontine efferents converge extensively to nearly all of the cerebellar cortex (except the nodulus), some specific cortical information is relayed to the cerebrocerebellar region. These axons travel through the middle peduncle. This pathway reports to the cerebellum on the programming and execution of intended movements.

Reticulocerebellar Input. Certain reticular nuclei, such as the lateral reticular nucleus and the reticulotegmental nucleus, send input to the cerebellar cortex through the inferior peduncle. They relay updated motor information from the sensorimotor cortex, red nucleus, spinal cord, and fastigial nucleus. This convergent and varied input is reflected in the large, complex receptive fields exhibited by these cells. These reticulocerebellar nuclei have been implicated in regulation of tonic firing levels in the cerebellar cortex,[54] in facilitation of rapid corrections during movement, and in coordination of central corollary discharges from visual and vestibular circuits to control eye movement.

Vestibulocerebellar Input. Vestibular information reaches the cerebellum by way of the vestibular nerve and vestibular nuclear complex. Signals reporting head position are conveyed to the flocculonodular lobe (vestibulocerebellum), along with visual information from the cortex, superior colliculus, and lateral geniculate. Integration of these signals allows the vestibulocerebellum to control balance and equilibrium and to influence head and eye movements relative to gaze.

Efferent Connections

The cerebellum processes the combined mossy and climbing fiber input and sends the information out to higher and lower motor centers, where adjustments to ongoing or intended movements are made. Purkinje cell axons send inhibitory signals (GABA) to the ipsilateral deep cerebellar nuclei and the vestibular nuclei (from the flocculonodular lobe). The projections to the deep nuclei are topographic and follow the functional classification described previously. The vermis portion of the spinocerebellum projects to the fastigial and the intermediate cortical area projects to the interpositus. The lateral hemispheres, or cerebrocerebellum, project to the dentate nucleus. A more discrete topography based on longitu-dinal zones within the cortex to nuclear regions has been described. Purkinje cell signals converge temporally with excitatory signals from mossy and climbing fiber collaterals onto the deep nuclei.[55] The signals resulting from this convergence are excitatory and leave the nuclei through the superior peduncle. The nuclei send copies back to the cerebellar cortex. The fastigial nucleus projects to the reticular formation and vestibular nuclei, both of which send descending signals to the spinal cord. Some axons also ascend to the motor cortex by way of the thalamus. Through these routes, spinal control of axial and proximal musculature is achieved. Projections from the interpositus to the inferior olive,[56,57] red nucleus, and the limb representations of the motor cortex by way of the thalamus influence descending paths that control distal limb musculature. The dentate nucleus is the main link to the motor areas of the cerebral cortex by way of the thalamic nuclei. The afferent and efferent pathways are summarized in Figure 14–11.

Cerebellar Function

The role of the cerebellum lies between the sensory and motor realms. Its unique construction and connections allow it to upgrade and integrate information about the outside world continuously with information about body position, movement, and signaling along central motor pathways. This information is shared with other central sensorimotor systems, which use it to produce smooth volitional movements. The cerebellum functions as a regulator of postural control and coordinated movement. It guides postures and ongoing movements of the eyes, head, body, and limbs, and it plays a role in learning motor skills.

The cerebellum contributes an intermediate step in the production of coordinated movements. It can be considered as an integrator of signals from the periphery and the body, and of feedback on current movement and ongoing activity in central nervous system pathways. The substrate for the integration of signals necessary for postural control and coordinated limb movements is the unique circuitry that supports parallel subsystems modulated by climbing fibers and linked by parallel fibers. Remember, however, that brain regions work in concert. Other brain areas determine how and if to use the signals to adjust central motor commands for the production of smooth purposeful movements.

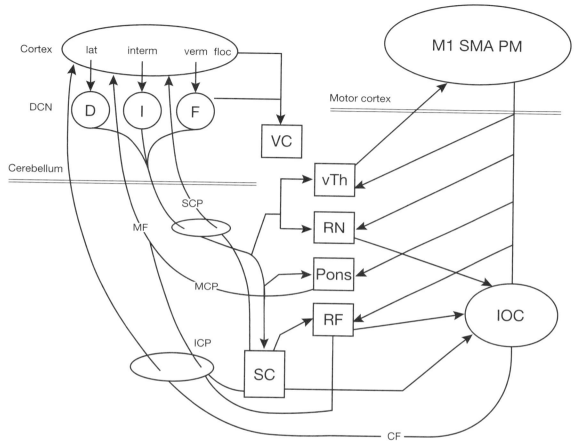

Figure 14–11. Summary of the pathways linking the cerebellum with subcortical and cortical motor areas. The motor cortex (primary motor cortex [MI], supplementary motor area [SMA], and premotor cortex [PM]) sends descending projections to the ventral-tier thalamic nuclei (vTh), the red nucleus (RN), the pons, the inferior olivary complex (IOC), and the reticular formation (RF). Signals are sent from these structures by way of certain relay nuclei, as either mossy fibers (MF) or climbing fibers (CF) through the cerebellar peduncles (SCP, MCP, ICP; superior, middle, and inferior) to the cerebellum. The cerebellum, in turn, sends information from the lateral (lat), intermediate (interm), vermal (verm), and floccular (floc) regions of its cortex to the dentate (D), intermediate (I), and fastigial (F) deep cerebellar nuclei (DCN) and to the vestibular complex (VC). From these structures, signals are passed to various cortical and subcortical structures and the spinal cord (SC).

Regionalized Function

Now you should understand the difficulty in delineating localized functional regions of the cerebellum. The uniform structure and the widespread convergence of afferent input make this task difficult. A large-scale assessment of patients in whom localized cerebellar lesions[58–60] correspond to distinct motor deficits, however, supports the notion of regional specificity, probably through the inhibitory circuitry. Interneurons may sustain inhibition of patches of Purkinje cells, thus isolating the effective circuitry. The topography of input and output connections, which is more defined in the efferent system, is likely to contribute. Based on the latter, the functions of the sagittal subdivisions[61] described earlier can be summarized. The spinocerebellum uses its cortical input on intended movement and its spinal input on peripheral activity to correct for perturbations encountered during movement. It adjusts muscle tone and synergy to compensate for changes in load and to smooth movement oscillations. The cerebrocerebellum is involved in initiation of movement, timing of coactivation of muscles (especially during rapid movements), and timing of sequential movements, all elements that contribute to precise control of skilled movements.

Neuronal Activity of the Deep Nuclei. Differences in neuronal activity among the deep nuclei are consistent with the notion of heterogeneous output. For example, dentate cells are active during preparatory phases of movements that are triggered by sensory cues, but not during the actual movement. They signal joint position, direction of intended movements, and patterns of compound movements. The dentate relays information to the motor cortex to adjust timing, intensity, velocity, and the start–stop of intended movements. Interpositus cells, however, are active after the onset and during movement, and correlate with EMG activity. They signal kinematic parameters of the actual, rather than the intended movement.[62,63]

Motor Learning

The notion that the cerebellum stores motor memory traces to aid in learning new movement patterns originated from studies of vestibulo-ocular reflex adaptation.[55,64] Learning motor skills with the extremities is also within the realm of cerebellar function. Evidence for these assertions comes from several sources. Task-related neuronal discharges progressively strengthen as skills are gained. For example, simple and complex spike patterns change during the process of learning a hand skill task, suggesting that relevant synapses become more efficient.[65] Their relative interactions are thought to provide the cerebellum's contribution to motor learning, exemplified by adaptation of movements to unexpected perturbations.[66] When trained monkeys move a handle to an assigned position against a constant load or force, complex and simple spike rates are steady. When the load on the handle is unexpectedly changed, the monkeys' attempts to reposition the handle are at first inaccurate, but eventually are corrected. During the learning period, characterized by inaccurate movements, the normally high simple spike rates decrease and the normally low complex spike rates increase. As the task is learned, the complex spike rate

returns to normal, but the simple spike rate remains reduced. Thus, modulation of climbing fiber input during learning resets the level of mossy fiber activation of Purkinje cells. The reduced mossy fiber input decreases Purkinje cell firing and disinhibits the deep cerebellar nuclei. Cerebellar output is increased and leads to the adapted response.

Novel motor behaviors require a lot of cocontraction of agonist and antagonist muscle groups; this pattern affords the moving parts greater stability. As a movement is practiced by normal subjects, agonists gradually contract more forcefully and antagonists contract less forcefully, resulting in smoother, more efficient movements. The cerebellum may control this coordination by resetting the alpha and gamma motor neuron coactivation of opposing muscle groups to adjust timing and amplitude of muscle cocontractions. Patients with cerebellar lesions who try to learn a new task maintain the strong cocontraction pattern. The damaged cerebellum cannot adjust the relative activities of agonists and antagonists, and this particular contribution to motor learning is lost.

Clinical Correlations

Cerebellar lesions cause distinctive motor symptoms. A myriad of deficits described generally as ataxia are observed. Errors occur in **kinematic** parameters of movement. For example, dysmetria is the inability to control the range of movement and is manifested as overshoots or undershoots of intended movements. Even with visual cues, patients miss intended targets. **Dysynergy** is the inability to control timing and sequencing of movement subroutines into complex sequential movements and is manifested as deterioration of smooth, complex movements. The single smooth, coordinated act of reaching and grasping for an object is replaced by several small, poorly timed substitute movements. Loss of the fast internal cerebellar updates forces the system to depend on slow, long-loop feedback from the periphery in response to the movement, and results in degradation of normal smooth sequences of movement. **Disdiadochokinesia** is the loss of ability to perform rapid alternating movements, such as quickly turning the palms upward and downward. Tremors may occur during active movements because of the loss of synergy between postural muscles that support gait or volitional movement of the extremities. Thus, the tremors can affect the trunk or extremities. Impairment of postural balance and stability occurs and is manifested as an unsteady, wide-stance gait and inability to maintain balance or posture after an unexpected change in the intended movement (e.g., uneven floor, change of target location). Adaptation of functional postural stretch reflexes is impaired and the intensity and timing of muscle cocontraction can no longer be scaled properly.[67,68] Physiologic findings associated with cerebellar lesions include disorganization of EMG, inappropriate amplitude and acceleration of muscle contractions, prolonged reaction time, and poor pursuit tracking.

Localized Lesions

Restricted lesions highlight regionalized cerebellar function. For example, the anterior lobe is selectively affected by alcohol abuse. This syndrome affects primarily the legs. Patients exhibit an ataxic, wide-stance gait. Midline and intermediate cortical or fastigial and interpositus lesions cause disorders of postural stability and gait. Hypotonia also results because of reduced gamma motor neuron activity. Lateral lesions cause difficulty with coordination of volitional movements of the extremities. Lesions restricted to the dentate lead to difficulty integrating complex tasks, poor temporal eye–hand coordination, and **hypermetria**.[69] The lateral cerebellum has been temporarily inactivated by cooling to simulate the effects of lesions. Clinically, such lesions lead to intention tremor, decomposition of complex movements, and decreased postural tone, and physiologically to errors in velocity, direction, and force.[70] Flocculonodular lesions cause vestibular deficits and abnormalities of eye movements. Symptoms include staggering, broad-based gait, and hypermetric eye movements and nystagmus. More discrete functional localization may lie in the topographic organization of longitudinally arranged afferent and efferent zones of the cortex.

Brainstem Motor Centers

Spinal motor neurons are influenced not only by the CST, but also by other descending pathways. The red nucleus, the vestibular nuclei, and the medial pontomedullary reticular formation give rise to descending spinal cord pathways. These brainstem pathways appear to play a major role in motor control. These three pathways, together with the basal ganglia, used to be termed the "extrapyramidal system," which was described as having a role in motor control distinct from that of the pyramidal system. Extrapyramidal symptoms used to be considered to constitute separate disorders. The concept of two distinct systems is no longer widely accepted because of the difficulty in clearly delineating two anatomically and functionally separate motor control systems. We now realize the existence of extensive interconnections and complex functional interrelationships. For example, although the descending pathways arise from brainstem nuclei, they are strongly influenced by cortical input. In fact, input from the motor cortex to the red nucleus and the reticular formation is by direct pathways. Some aspects of the brainstem pathways are functionally similar to those of the CST. Stimulation of the motor cortex produces similar movements regardless of whether the CST is intact, although higher stimulus intensity is required and the system fatigues more easily after CST damage.[71] Cortical activation of the brainstem pathways is thought to produce such movements.

The Red Nucleus and the Rubrospinal Tract

The red nucleus is a conspicuous, pinkish-colored structure that lies within the mesencephalic portion of the reticular formation. It consists of a caudal magnocellular (large cells) and a rostral parvicellular (small cells) division. The former has a direct projection to the spinal cord that is somatotopically organized and terminates in a pattern similar to the CST. The latter is by far the largest in humans. Input and output to both parts are somatotopically organized.

The red nucleus receives somatotopically arranged afferents primarily from the ipsilateral motor cortex and the deep cerebellar nuclei.[72] The input from the motor cortex consists of collaterals of CST neurons and axons from non-CST neurons.[73] The major cortical input is from non-CST fibers, and they cause an initial facilitation followed by an inhibition of red nucleus target neurons. Cortical afferents have selective targets in the red nucleus. The M1 and PM target the parvicellular division. The M1 and SMA project to the magnocellular division, from which the rubrospinal tract has its primary origin. In the absence of the CST, the rubrospinal tract may convey impulses from the cortex to the spinal cord to produce movements in response to electrical stimulation, as described earlier. The input from the cerebellum is more potent. Fibers from the dentate and interpositus nucleus terminate in different parts of the red nucleus.

Output from the red nucleus is diverse and includes such targets as the interpositus nucleus of the cerebellum, the trigeminal nuclei, and the spinal cord. The spinal cord is reached by way of the rubrospinal tract, which is a crossed pathway. The rubrospinal tract has a powerful influence on spinal cord reflex activity. Electrical stimulation of the path produces monosynaptic facilitation of alpha motor neurons of the distal flexor muscle group and inhibition of alpha motor neurons of the extensor muscles. Lesions to this tract lead to contralateral motor impairment of distal limb extension. The rubrospinal system, although much smaller than the CST, works closely with the corticospinal system to control the distal musculature, especially the flexors. Both tracts terminate on overlapping populations of interneurons and affect overlapping populations of motor neurons. They both facilitate the same spinal reflexes, and both facilitate distal flexors.

The Vestibular Nuclei and the Vestibulospinal Tracts

The vestibular complex is located in the medulla and is divided into four nuclei: superior, medial, lateral, and inferior. It is involved in oculomotor and skeletomotor control. Most afferents to the complex arise from cranial nerve VIII, but the cerebellum and reticular formation also contribute input. In fact, labyrinthine receptors in the utricle, saccule, and semicircular canals send information through a branch of cranial nerve VIII nearly exclusively to the vestibular complex. The cerebellum sends a large and organized projection to all four nuclei; inhibitory input comes from the Purkinje cells and excitatory input comes form the fastigial nucleus.[74] The reticular formation sends a diffuse projection to all four nuclei.

Neurons in the vestibular complex function as tight relays of labyrinthine signals on linear and angular acceleration to the spinal cord and extraocular muscles. The lateral vestibular nucleus, also known as Deiter's nucleus, is somatotopically organized and gives rise to the large lateral vestibulospinal tract. The medial and inferior vestibular nuclei give rise to a secondary spinal path, the medial vestibulospinal tract, which goes only to cervical and thoracic levels. Descending vestibulospinal fibers branch extensively to terminate across many spinal cord segments. The lateral vestibulospinal tract inhibits flexor and excites extensor motor neurons. It is responsible for extensor tonus in decerebrate animals. The reflex functions of the vestibular complex, as reflected by its anatomic connections and physiologic activity, are most directly related to the axial musculature. Vestibulospinal projections to the neck and back are direct. Activation of the medial vestibulospinal tract has similar effects on neck extensors and vertebral column extensors. It elicits precise control of the axial musculature, and some control of limb musculature, even distal musculature. For the most part, this input is polysynaptic and weak, but the overall effects are similar in that extensors are facilitated and flexors are inhibited. These less direct pathways to the limb musculature are likely to carry integrated motor commands rather than rapidly relayed labyrinthine signals.

The Medial Pontomedullary Reticular Formation and the Reticulospinal Projections

The reticular formation is a collection of diffusely arranged nuclei that extends across the pons, medulla, and midbrain. The reticulospinal tracts, however, arise only from cells in the pontine and medullary portions. The reticular formation is characterized by an intermingling of large and small cells with fibers that travel in various directions. Cells that form the reticulospinal projections receive input from many areas of the brain, including cutaneous and proprioceptive signals. Input comes to the reticular formation from the sensorimotor cortex, vestibular complex, and superior colliculus. The cortical afferents converge from many areas of the cortex, and most are monosynaptic and excitatory. The superior colliculus afferents are potent, fast, and excitatory. The superior colliculus input primarily targets neurons that travel in the reticulospinal tract to reach neck motor neurons. Many output cells give rise to axons that branch on exiting the reticular formation and form ascending and descending pathways. The pontine reticulospinal tract projection travels in the ventromedial fasciculus of the spinal cord, whereas the medullary reticulospinal tract travels in the ventrolateral fasciculus. In both, the lumbar projection cells give off cervical collaterals. Therefore, the same signals reach the forelimb and hindlimb musculature. For the most part, the pontine reticulospinal tract facilitates axial and proximal limb muscles, whereas the medullary reticulospinal tract exerts a more generalized inhibition of all muscles of the body. The long descending pathways are summarized in Figure 14–12.

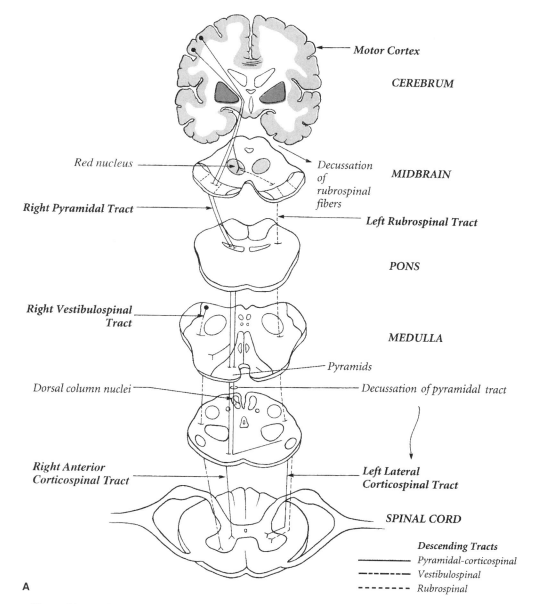

Figure 14–12. The long descending pathways. The origins and courses of the corticospinal, the vestibulospinal, and the rubrospinal tracts are shown in **(A).** The origins and courses of the medial and lateral reticulospinal tracts are shown in **(B).** (continued)

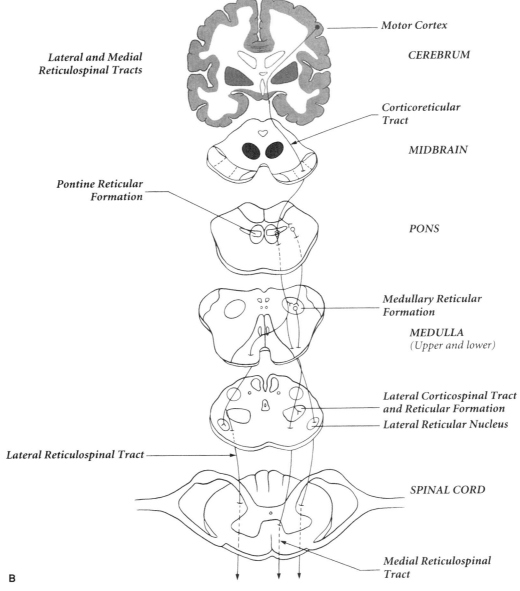

Lateral and Medial
Reticulospinal Tracts

Pontine Reticular
Formation

Lateral Reticulospinal Tract —————

B

Motor Cortex

CEREBRUM

Corticoreticular
Tract

MIDBRAIN

PONS

Medullary Reticular
Formation

MEDULLA
(Upper and lower)

Lateral Corticospinal Tract
and Reticular Formation
Lateral Reticular Nucleus

SPINAL CORD

Medial Reticulospinal
Tract

Figure 14–12. (continued)

Conclusions

Evolution of the Human Motor System

Two major changes have evolved in the motor system in higher mammals. Both of these evolutionary developments are reflected particularly in the exquisite control over hand function in nonhuman primates and even more so in humans. First, the motor areas of the cerebral cortex have increased tremendously in size and in importance compared with those of lower mammals. Signals from other motor centers are directed primarily to the cortex, which has powerful control over the descending pathways. Concurrent with this development, the CST has increased in size and influence, at the expense of other paths, such as the relatively small rubrospinal system. Second, the cortex provides direct input to motor neurons that innervate the distal hand musculature in the form of CST axons.

Parallel or Serial Processing in the Motor System

Cortical function has often been described in terms of a motor hierarchy, in that one area triggers activity in another area in control of "higher" motor function, which in turn triggers further activation of another area. Many investigators, however, dislike classifying the motor centers, especially cortical areas, as higher or lower centers and believe that they operate in a parallel manner. A relevant question would be if the SMA, traditionally considered a "higher" motor center, is needed to trigger MI activity. Although M1 neurons are activated later than those in the SMA during movements, its neurons still discharge and still elicit movements after SMA lesions. This finding would argue against serial processing of cortical signals. Furthermore, the reciprocal connections typical of cortical regions, and their separate access in and out of subcortical centers, such as the basal ganglia, support a system of parallel processing. In turn, the basal ganglia and the cerebellum exert independent influences on motor output by way of their projections to separate cortical regions. These pathways run in parallel to one another and are, for the most part, independent pathways, although some overlap exists. The extensive intrinsic circuitry of the cortex itself offers the opportunity for extensive interaction between subcortical and cortical inputs. Thus, brain regions involved with control of voluntary movement probably work cooperatively and in a parallel manner to produce smooth purposeful movements.

REFERENCES

1. Jackson JH. A study of convulsions. In: Taylor J, ed. *Selected writings of John Hughlings Jackson.* Vol 1. London: Hodder & Stoughton, 1931:162–207.
2. Fritsch G, Hitzig E. Ueber die elektrische erregbarkeit des grosshirns. *Arch Anat Physiol Wiss Med* 1870;37:300–332.
3. Ferrier D. Experiments on the brain of monkeys. *Proc R Soc Lond (Biol)* 1875;23:409–430.
4. Sherrington CS. *The integrative action of the nervous system.* New Haven, CT: Yale University Press, 1906.
5. Penfield W. *The excitable cortex in conscious man.* Liverpool: Liverpool University Press, 1958.
6. Dum RP, Strick PL. Premotor areas: nodal points for parallel efferent systems involved in the central control of movement. In: Humphrey DR, Freund H-J, eds. *Motor control: concepts and issues.* New York: John Wiley & Sons, 1991:383–397.
7. Brodmann K. *Vergleichende Lokalisationslehre der Grosshirnrinde in ihren prinzipien Dargestellt auf Grund des Zellenbaues.* Leipzig: JA Brath, 1909.
8. Huerta MF, Pons TP. Primary motor cortex receives input from area 3a in macaques. *Brain Res* 1990;537:367–371.
9. Shell GR, Strick PL. The origin of thalamic inputs to the arcuate premotor and supplementary motor areas. *J Neurosci* 1984;4:539–560.
10. Alexander GE, DeLong MR, Strick PL. Parallel organization of functionally segregated circuits linking basal ganglia and cortex. *Annu Rev Neurosci* 1986;9:357–381.
11. Asanuma C, Thach WT, Jones EG. Anatomical evidence for segregated focal groupings of efferent cells and their terminal ramifications in the cerebellothalamic pathway of the monkey. *Brain Res Brain Res Rev* 1983;5:267–297.
12. Olive E, Edgy SA, Armand J, Lemon RN. An electrophysiological study of the postnatal development of the corticospinal system in the macaque monkey. *J Neurosci* 1997;17:267–276.
13. Evarts EV. Pyramidal tract activity associated with a conditioned hand movement in the monkey. *J Neurophysiol* 1966;29:1011–1027.
14. Fetz EE, Cheney PD. Postspike facilitation of forelimb muscle activity by primate corticomotoneuronal cells. *J Neurophysiol* 1980;44:751–772.

15. Georgopoulos AP, Kalaska JF, Crutcher MD, Caminiti R, Massey JT. The representation of movement direction in the motor cortex: single cell and population studies. In: Edelman GM, Gall WE, Cowan WM, eds. *Dynamic aspects of neocortical function.* New York: John Wiley & Sons, 1984:501–524.

16. Fromm C, Wise SP, Evarts EV. Sensory response properties of pyramidal tract neurons in the precentral motor cortex and postcentral gyrus of the rhesus monkey. *Exp Brain Res* 1984;54:177–185.

17. Fetz EE, Finocchio DV, Baker MA, Soso MJ. Sensory and motor responses of precentral cortex cells during comparable active and passive joint movements. *J Neurophysiol* 1980;43:1070–1089.

18. Waters RS, Favorov O, Asanuma H. Physiological properties and pattern of projection of cortico-cortical connections from the anterior bank of the ansate sulcus to the motor cortex, area 4g, in the cat. *Exp Brain Res* 1982;461:403–412.

19. Asanuma H. *The motor cortex.* New York: Raven Press, 1989.

20. Schieber MH. Muscular production of individuated finger movements: the roles of extrinsic finger muscles. *J Neurosci* 1995;15:284–297.

21. Tanji J, Taniguchi K, Saga T. Supplementary motor area: neuronal response to motor instructions. *J Neurophysiol* 1980;43:60–68.

22. Tanji J, Kurata K. Contrasting neuronal activity in supplementary and precentral motor cortex of monkeys: I. responses to instructions determining motor responses to forthcoming signals of different modalities. *J Neurophysiol* 1985;53:129–141.

23. Roland PE, Larsen B, Lassen NA, Shihoj E. Supplementary and other cortical areas in organization of voluntary movements in man. *J Neurophysiol* 1980;43:118–136.

24. Tanji J, Okano K, Sato KC. Neuronal activity in cortical motor areas related to ipsilateral, contralateral, and bilateral digit movements of the monkey. *J Neurophysiol* 1988;60:325–342.

25. Wise SP, Mauritz K-H. Set-related neuronal activity in the premotor cortex of rhesus monkeys: Effects of changes in motor set. *Proc R Soc Lond B* 1985;223:331–354.

26. Rizzolatti G, Gentilucci M. Motor and visual-motor functions of the premotor cortex. In: Rakic P, Singer W, eds. *Neurobiology of neocortex.* Dahlem Konferenzen. New York: John Wiley & Sons, 1988:269–284.

27. He S-Q, Dum RP, Strick PL. Topographic organization of corticospinal projections from the frontal lobe: motor areas on the lateral surface of the hemisphere. *J Neurosci* 1993;13:952–980.

28. Greenough WT, Larson JR, Withers GS. Effects of unilateral and bilateral training in a reaching task on den-

dritic branching of neurons in the rat motor-sensory forelimb cortex. *Behav Neurol Biol* 1985;44:301–314.

29. Nudo RJ, Jenkins WM, Merzenich MM. Repetitive microstimulation alters the cortical representation of movement in adult rats. *Somatosens Mot Res* 1990;7:463–483.

30. Sanes JN, Suner S, Lando JF, Donoghue JP. Rapid reorganization of adult rat motor cortex somatic representation patterns after motor nerve injury. *Proc Natl Acad Sci U S A* 1988;85:2003–2007.

31. Nudo RJ, Milliken GW, Jenkins WM, Merzenich MM. Use-dependent alterations of movement representations in primary motor cortex of adult squirrel monkeys. *J Neurosci* 1996;16:785–807.

32. Nudo RJ, Wise BM, SiFuentes F, Milliken GW. Neural substrates for the effects of rehabilitative training on motor recovery after ischemic infarct. *Science* 1996;272:1791–1794.

33. Carpenter MB. Anatomical organization of the corpus striatum and related nuclei. *Res Publ Assoc Res Nerv Ment Dis* 1976;55:5–12.

34. Kitai ST, Kocsis JD, Wood J. Origin and characteristics of the cortico-caudate afferents: an anatomical and electrophysiological study. *Brain Res* 1976;118:137–141.

35. Graybiel AM, Sciascia TR. Origin and distribution of nigrotectal fibers in the cat. *Soc Neurosci Abstr* 1975;1:174.

36. Gaspar P, Berger B, Febvert A, Vigny A, Henry JP. Catecholamine innervation of the human cerebral cortex as revealed by comparative immunohistochemistry of tyrosine hydroxylase and dopamine-beta-hydroxylase. *J Comp Neurol* 1989;279:249–271.

37. Levitt P, Rakic P, Goldman-Rakic P. Region-specific distribution of catecholamine afferents in primate cerebral cortex: a fluorescence histochemical analysis. *J Comp Neurol* 1984;227:23–36.

38. Gerfen CR. The neostriatal mosaic: multiple levels of compartmental organization. *Trends Neurosci* 1992;2:133–139.

39. Graybiel AM. Neurochemically specified subsystems in the basal ganglia. *Functions of the Basal Ganglia* 1984;107:114–149.

40. Mushiake H, Strick PL. Pallidal neuron activity during sequential arm movements. *J Neurophysiol* 1995;74:2754–2758.

41. Berholz A. *Multisensory control of movement.* Oxford: Oxford University Press, 1993

42. Flowers K. "Visual closed-loop" and "open-loop" characteristics of voluntary movement in patients with parkinsonism and intention tremor. *Brain* 1976;99:260–310.

43. Turner B. Pathology of paralysis agitans. In: Vinken P, Bruyn G, eds. *Handbook of clinical neurology. Vol 6: Diseases of the basal ganglia.* New York: John Wiley & Sons, 1968:77–93.

44. Weisendanger M, Ruegg DG. Electromyographic assessment of central motor disorders. *Muscle Nerve* 1978;5:407–412.

45. Carpenter MB, Whittier J, Mettler FA. Analysis of choreoid hyperkinesia in the rhesus monkey. *J Comp Neurol* 1950;92:293–331.

46. Holmes G. The symptoms of acute cerebellar injuries due to gunshot injuries. *Brain* 1917;40:461–535.

47. Eccles JC, Llinas R, Sasaki K. The excitatory synaptic action of climbing fibres on the Purkinje cells of the cerebellum. *J Physiol* 1966;182:268–296.

48. Rubia FJ, Kolb FP. Responses of cerebellar units to a passive movement in the decerebrate cat. *Exp Brain Res* 1978;31:387–401.

49. Cajal SR. *Histologie du systeme nerveux de l'homme et des vertebres*. Madrid: Instituto Ramon y Cajal, 1972.

50. Eccles JC, Ito M, Szentagothai J. *The cerebellum as a neuronal machine*. New York: Springer-Verlag, 1967.

51. Oscarsson O. Functional organization of the spino- and cuneo-cerebellar tracts. *Physiol Rev* 1965;45:495–522.

52. Mann MD. Clarke's column and the dorsal spinocerebellar tract: a review. *Brain Behav Evol* 1973;7:34–83.

53. Oscarsson O. Functional organization of spinocerebellar paths. In: Iggo A, ed. *Handbook of sensory physiology: Vol 2. Somatosensory system*. New York: Springer-Verlag, 1973:339–380.

54. Llinas RR, Simpson JI. Cerebellar control of movement. In: Towe AL, Luschei ES, eds. *Handbook of behavioral neurobiology: Vol 5. Motor coordination*. New York: Plenum Press, 1981:231–302.

55. Ito M. *The cerebellum and neural control*. New York: Raven Press, 1984.

56. Batton RR III, Jayaraman A, Ruggiero D, Carpenter MB. Fastigial efferent projections in the monkey: an autoradiographic study. *J Comp Neurol* 1977;174:281–306.

57. McCrea RA, Bishop GA, Kitai ST. Morphological and electrophysiological characteristics of projecting neurons in the nucleus interpositus of the cat cerebellum. *J Comp Neurol* 1978;181:397–420.

58. Chambers WW, Sprague JM. Functional localization in the cerebellum: II. somatotopic organization in cortex and nuclei. *Arch Neurol Psych* 1955;74:653–680.

59. Dichgans J, Diener HC. Clinical evidence for functional compartmentalization of the cerebellum. In:

Bloedel JR, Dichgans JD, and Precht W, eds. *Cerebellar functions*. Berlin: Springer-Verlag, 1985:101–137.

60. Ivry RB, Keele SW, Diener HC. Dissociation of the lateral and medial cerebellum in movement timing and movement execution. *Exp Brain Res* 1988;73:167–180.

61. Bloedel JR, Kelly TM. The dynamic selection hypothesis: a proposed function for cerebellar sagittal zones. In: Llinas R, Sotelo C, eds. *The cerebellum revisited*. Berlin: Springer-Verlag, 1992:219–282.

62. Thach WT. Discharge of cerebellar neurons related to two maintained postures and two prompt movements: I. nuclear cell output. *J Neurophysiol* 1970;33:527–536.

63. Thach WT. Correlation of neural discharge with pattern and force of muscular activity, joint position and direction of intended next movement in motor cortex and cerebellum. *J Neurophysiol* 1978;41:654–676.

64. Robinson DA. Adaptive gain control of vestibulo-ocular reflex by the cerebellum. *J Neurophysiol* 1976;39:954–969.

65. Gilbert PFC, Thach WT. Purkinje cell activity during motor learning. *Brain Res* 1977;128:309–328.

66. Thach WT, Goodkin HG, Keating JG. Cerebellum and the adaptive coordination of movement. *Annu Rev Neurosci* 1992;15:403–442.

67. Nashner LM, Grimm RJ. Analysis of multiloop dyscontrols in standing cerebellar patients. *Progress in Clinical Neurophysiology* 1978;4:300–319.

68. Bloedel JR, Bracha V, Kelly TM, Wu J-Z. Substrates for motor learning: does the cerebellum do it all? *Ann NY Acad Sci* 1991;627:305–318.

69. Gilman S, Bloedel JR, Lechtenberg R. *Disorders of the cerebellum*. Philadelphia: FA Davis, 1981.

70. Hore J, Vilis T. Loss of set in muscle responses to limb perturbations during cerebellar dysfunction. *J Neurophysiol* 1984;51:1137–1148.

71. Hongo T, Jankowska E. Effects from the sensorimotor cortex on the spinal cord in cats with transsected pyramids. *Exp Brain Res* 1967;3:117–134.

72. Mason J. The mammalian red nucleus. *Physiol Rev* 1967;47:383–436.

73. Tsukahara N, Fuller DRG. Conductance changes during pyramidally induced postsynaptic potentials in red nucleus neurons. *J Neurophysiol* 1969;32:34–42.

74. Ito M. Cerebellar control of vestibular neurons: physiology and pharmacology. *Prog Brain Res* 1972;37:377–390.

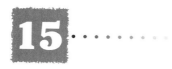

Motor 3: The Autonomic Nervous System

KIRK W. BARRON, PhD
ROBERT W. BLAIR, PhD

• • •

The term **homeostasis** was proposed by Cannon[1] and describes the maintenance of the steady-state environment of the internal organs and tissues of the body. To state this idea another way, homeostatic mechanisms keep physiological functions, such as body temperature, blood pressure, and respiration, within appropriate ranges. The autonomic nervous system contributes to the maintenance of homeostasis through neural influences on smooth muscle, cardiac muscle, and glands. The autonomic nervous system has also been referred to as the vegetative, visceral, or involuntary nervous system. Each name describes an important aspect of autonomic neural function. The term **vegetative** refers to autonomic control of nutritive function, whereas the term **visceral** denotes control of visceral organs, like the heart and the gastrointestinal tract. **Involuntary** refers to the fact that the autonomic nervous system is not normally under conscious control, in contrast to the somatic nervous system. The term **autonomic nervous system** was originally proposed in 1898 by

Langley and Dickinson[2] to describe the fact that the autonomic nervous system was "self-governing," or independent of conscious control. This autonomy is important in sustaining vital physiological functions, such as temperature regulation, blood pressure regulation, and fluid balance.

The autonomic nervous system, however, does not necessarily function as independently or as autonomously as the name suggests. For example, the eye is focused by autonomic nerves innervating the ciliary muscle, which controls the focal length of the lens. Normally, focusing is an involuntary response, but it is possible consciously to alter the focal length of the eye. Another form of interaction between the autonomic and somatic nervous systems is respiration, where the lumen size of bronchial smooth muscle in the airways of the lungs is controlled by the autonomic nervous system, but chest wall movements are produced by somatic nervous system control of skeletal muscle. These examples of the interplay between the autonomic and the somatic nervous systems demonstrate that the autonomic nervous system acts as an integrated unit within the entire nervous system to help maintain homeostasis.

Anatomy of the Autonomic Nervous System

The nervous system can be divided into two main parts, the central nervous system and the peripheral nervous system. The central nervous system is composed of the brain and the spinal cord. The peripheral nervous system can be separated into the somatic nervous system and the autonomic nervous

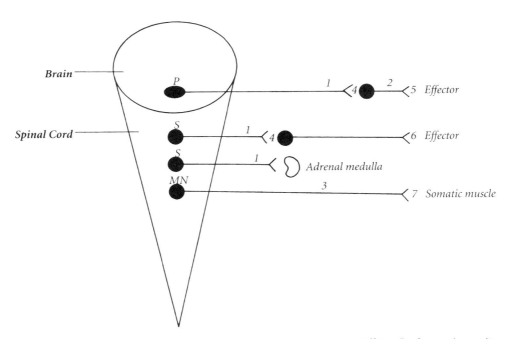

Figure 15–1. Functional anatomy of the autonomic nervous system. "Effector" refers to the cardiac muscle, smooth muscle, or glands innervated by the autonomic nervous system. P, parasympathetic preganglionic neuron; S, sympathetic preganglionic neuron; 1, preganglionic neuron; 2, postganglionic neuron; 3, somatic motor neuron; 4, acetylcholine released at this junction excites ganglionic nicotinic receptors; 5, acetylcholine released here excites muscarinic receptors; 6, norepinephrine released at this junction excites alpha and beta receptors; 7, acetylcholine released here excites neuromuscular junction nicotinic receptors.

system. The autonomic nervous system has been traditionally considered primarily an efferent, or motor system. That is, information is transmitted by autonomic nerves from the central nervous system to cardiac muscle, smooth muscle, and glands, which comprise the **effector** or **target organs**. Autonomic nerves also contain sensory or afferent nerves that course from the organs to the central nervous system. This chapter emphasizes the motor, or efferent function of the autonomic nervous system, but you should recognize that sensory information from the effector organs is also relayed to the central nervous

system by autonomic nerves. The significance of sensory nerves will become more clear in the discussion of autonomic reflexes.

The autonomic nervous system is divided into two major divisions: the **sympathetic** and **parasympathetic nervous systems**.[3-7] The organizations of these divisions have similarities as well as differences. Comparisons between different aspects of the anatomy and physiology of sympathetic and parasympathetic nervous systems are discussed in the following paragraphs, and are also shown in Figures 15–1 and 15–2, and in Table 15–1.

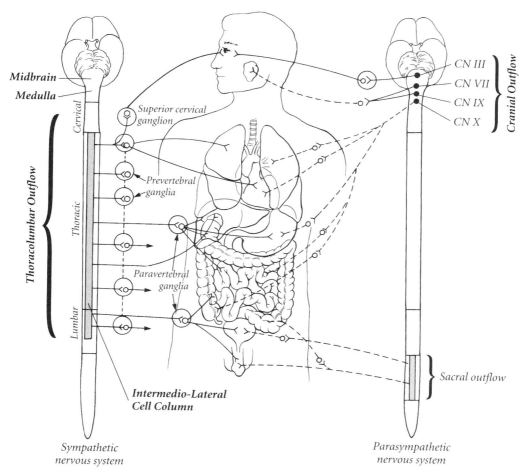

Figure 15–2. *Left side* demonstrates origin of sympathetic or thoracolumbar outflow and organs innervated by the sympathetic nervous system. *Right side* shows origin of parasympathetic, or craniosacral, outflow and organs innervated by the parasympathetic nervous system.

TABLE 15–1		
Comparison of Sympathetic (SNS) and Parasympathetic (PNS) Nervous Systems		
	SNS	**PNS**
Origin of outflow	Thoracolumbar region of the spinal cord	Craniosacral regions of the spinal cord
Location of ganglia	Near spinal cord in paravertebral ganglia or relatively remote from target organ	On or in close proximity to target organ
Preganglionic neuron	Myelinated, short	Myelinated, long
Neurotransmitter released from preganglionic neuron	Acetylcholine	Acetylcholine
Receptor for preganglionic neurotransmitter	Nicotinic	Nicotinic
Postganglionic neuron	Unmyelinated, long	Unmyelinated, short
Neurotransmitter released from postganglionic neuron	Norepinephrine	Acetylcholine
Receptor for postganglionic neurotransmitter	Adrenergic: alpha (α) or beta (β)	Muscarinic
Specificity of outflow	Can be widespread Can be specific	Specific
Condition of maximal function	Emergency, stress, "fight or flight"	Sedentary activities, voiding
Effect on energy stores	Use of energy and mobilization of energy stores; inhibition of digestion	Conservation and restoration of digestion

The general organization of the autonomic nervous system is shown in Figure 15–1. The sympathetic and parasympathetic divisions of the autonomic nervous system have several features in common. The innervation of effectors is composed of two neurons connected in series: a **preganglionic** neuron (labeled "1" in Fig. 15–1) and a **postganglionic** neuron (labeled "2" in Fig. 15–1). The cell bodies of the preganglionic neurons are located in the brain or spinal cord. The axons, which are myelinated, exit the central nervous system and project to ganglia, which are collections of postganglionic neuronal cell bodies. Preganglionic neurons form synapses on postganglionic neurons, and postganglionic neurons send unmyelinated axons to the effector organs.[3–7]

The connections of preganglionic axons to postganglionic cell bodies in autonomic ganglia are not one-to-one; that is, a single preganglionic neuron synapses with multiple postganglionic neurons. The connections show both **divergence** and **convergence**. One preganglionic axon can form synapses on several postganglionic neurons; this arrangement is termed "divergence." A preganglionic neuron can diverge to affect multiple postganglionic neurons in the same ganglion, or it can send branches up and down the sympathetic chain to affect postganglionic neurons in other ganglia. With convergence, one postganglionic neuron receives synaptic input from several preganglionic neurons. The sympathetic nervous system exhibits a greater degree of divergence than the parasympathetic nervous system. Divergence is the basis for the mass action effect of sympathetic nervous system activation—that is, a simultaneous activation of a large proportion of sympathetic efferent nerves. Evidence also indicates that sympathetic outflow can be specific, in that nerves innervating specific effector organs or tissues can be selectively excited.[8]

In the parasympathetic nervous system, one preganglionic neuron usually forms synapses on relatively few postganglionic neurons, which provides for an overall greater specificity of activation of the parasympathetic nervous system.

In the sympathetic nervous system (labeled "S" in Fig. 15–1), preganglionic cell bodies are located in the intermediolateral cell column, in spinal cord segments T1 to L2 or L3. Because preganglionic neurons exit from the thoracic and lumbar portions of the spinal cord, the sympathetic nervous system is also termed the thoracolumbar division of the autonomic nervous system (see Fig. 15–2). Axons of preganglionic neurons are relatively short and terminate in the sympathetic chain (or paravertebral) ganglia, which lie along the spinal column bilaterally, and appear like beads on a string. Sympathetic preganglionic neurons also terminate in the prevertebral ganglia (the celiac, superior mesenteric, and inferior mesenteric ganglia), which are located in the abdomen. Axons of sympathetic postganglionic neurons are relatively long and innervate effector organs.[3–7] The adrenal medulla is a special case. It is considered to be part of the sympathetic nervous system, and is functionally similar to a postganglionic neuron, except that it does not have an axon. Instead, excitation of adrenal medullary chromaffin cells by sympathetic preganglionic neurons causes the release of the catecholamines **epinephrine** (80%) and **norepinephrine** (20%) into the bloodstream.

Figure 15–2 presents a more detailed illustration of the innervation of the viscera by the sympathetic nervous system. The important aspects of sympathetic innervation in the body are shown on the left. As noted previously, the entire sympathetic innervation originates from preganglionic neurons, with cell bodies located in the intermediolateral cell column of the thoracic and upper lumbar spinal cord. One consequence of this arrangement is that sympathetic innervation to the head and face comes from preganglionic neurons in the upper thoracic spinal cord, and these neurons synapse with postganglionic sympathetic neurons in the superior cervical ganglia. Damage to either the preganglionic cell bodies that innervate the superior cervical ganglia, or directly to the superior cervical ganglia, can disrupt sympathetic innervation to the head and face. This clinical condition is known as **Horner's syndrome** and is discussed later in this chapter.

The parasympathetic nervous system is also known as the **craniosacral** division of the autonomic nervous system because the preganglionic neurons exit from the brain and sacral segments of the spinal cord[3–7] (labeled "P" in Fig. 15–1). Figure 15–1 also demonstrates a key feature of the parasympathetic nervous system: parasympathetic preganglionic axons are long and travel from the cell bodies to the effector organ. The parasympathetic ganglia are located on or near the effector organ; hence, the postganglionic axons innervating the organ are relatively short. Specific examples of parasympathetic innervation are also shown in Figure 15–2. Cranial outflow from the parasympathetic system comes from cranial nerves III, VII, IX, and X. The preganglionic parasympathetic cell bodies of the oculomotor nerve are located in the nucleus of Edinger-Westphal and send axons to innervate short postganglionic neurons located in the ciliary ganglia. The postganglionic parasympathetic neurons of the oculomotor nerve innervate the ciliary muscle of the iris. The outflow of cranial nerves VII (the facial nerve) and IX (glossopharyngeal nerve) innervates lacrimal and salivary glands of the head. The largest proportion of cranial parasympathetic outflow derives from the vagus nerve (cranial nerve X), which contains approximately 75% of the parasympathetic preganglionic neurons. The vagus provides the parasympathetic innervation to the organs in the thorax and abdomen. The sacral component of parasympathetic outflow refers to preganglionic cell bodies in spinal cord segments S2 to S4, which innervate the urinary system, the lower colon, anal sphincter, and the reproductive system. Collectively, one approach to understanding function of the sacral parasympathetic nervous system is to recognize that this component is largely involved in voiding mechanisms such as defecation and micturition.

The **somatic motor system** (labeled "3" in Fig. 15–1) innervates skeletal muscle, and this system is under conscious or voluntary control.[3,4,6] Somatic motor neurons exit the spinal cord and travel directly to skeletal muscle with no intervening synapses. Somatic motor neurons are all myelinated, like preganglionic autonomic neurons.

Autonomic Neurotransmission

Synaptic transmission in the autonomic nervous system is basically identical to that described in Chapters 3 and 4. Much of what we understand about synaptic transmission in the peripheral and central nervous system was originally demonstrated through the study of the autonomic nervous system. Although the general concepts are similar, understanding the specific points of autonomic neurotransmission is an important first approach to understanding how the autonomic nervous system functions. Chemical neurotransmission was demonstrated in 1921 by Otto Loewi.[9] Loewi used two isolated and artificially perfused frog hearts and left the vagus nerve (i.e., the parasympathetic efferent innervation) intact to one of the hearts. He took the fluid perfusing the innervated heart and transferred it to the second heart. Thus, the only contact between the two hearts was by the perfusate. When he electrically stimulated the vagus nerve, he observed a slower rate in the first heart, but the second heart slowed only when fluid perfusing the first heart was transferred to the second heart. He also showed that the effect of the vagal stimulation could be blocked with the drug atropine. Loewi proposed that the responses of the second heart must have been due to the release of a chemical from the vagus nerve. To state this another way, he demonstrated that nerves release chemicals as neurotransmitters, which, in turn, produce effects on effector organs.

Criteria for Identification of Neurotransmitters

For a chemical to be accepted as a neurotransmitter, several criteria must be met:

1 Perhaps the most basic requirement is that the neurotransmitter be released from the nerve during stimulation. A good example of this criterion is the experiment performed by Loewi, demonstrating cholinergic transmission in the heart.
2 The putative or proposed neurotransmitter substance must be localized to the nerve terminal region.
3 The neuron must contain an enzyme system capable of synthesis of the neurotransmitter.
4 There must be some mechanism for inactivation of the transmitter once it is released from the terminal.
5 Exogenous application of the suspected transmitter must mimic the response observed with release of the substance in response to stimulating the nerve.

6 Drugs that block or potentiate the effect of nerve stimulation must also block or potentiate the effects of exogenous administration of the suspected transmitter.

The original concept of neurotransmission, called "Dale's principle," held that only one neurotransmitter substance was released from a given neuron; however, a wealth of information now indicates that additional substances are also found within synaptic terminals. Examples of neuromodulatory substances include substance P, neuropeptide Y, somatostatin, enkephalins, vasoactive intestinal peptide (VIP), and calcitonin gene-related peptide, to mention only a few. Although these substances may not yet meet all the criteria for neurotransmitters, they do exert modulatory influences on the actions of the primary neurotransmitters with which they coexist in nerve terminals.[10,11]

Synaptic Neurotransmission

The autonomic nervous system has essentially two types of neurotransmitter systems: cholinergic and adrenergic.[3,4,6] Nerves from which acetylcholine is released as a neurotransmitter include all preganglionic autonomic neurons, postganglionic parasympathetic neurons, postganglionic sympathetic neurons to sweat glands, and somatic motor neurons. Adrenergic transmission is found in most postganglionic sympathetic neurons. Cholinergic neurotransmission uses acetylcholine as the neurotransmitter, whereas adrenergic transmission uses norepinephrine (also called noradrenaline) as the transmitter, except at the adrenal medulla, where epinephrine (also called adrenaline) is also released. Many of the steps in synaptic transmission in both the cholinergic and adrenergic systems are similar to the processes described in Chapters 3 and 4. Common aspects of neurotransmission include arrival of the action potential at the axon terminal; depolarization of the nerve terminal; influx of Ca^{++} into the nerve terminal; internal binding of **synaptic vesicles** to the axon terminal; fusion of the vesicles to the terminal membrane; release of transmitter; interaction between the transmitter and the postjunctional receptor; and termination of action of the free extracellular neurotransmitter. In addition to similarities, differences between adrenergic and cholinergic transmission also are important in understanding autonomic nervous system function.

Adrenergic Neurotransmission

Norepinephrine is the neurotransmitter released from most postganglionic sympathetic nerves.[3,6,12] The major components of adrenergic neurotransmission are shown in Figure 15–3. In the peripheral sympathetic nervous system, the sites of transmitter release are actually enlargements of the axon called **varicosities**. The synthesis of norepinephrine begins inside the neuron with the amino acid tyrosine, which is transported into the nerve terminal and enzymatically converted first to dihydroxyphenylalanine, also called L-dopa, then to dopamine. Dopamine in the cytosol of the neuron is transported inside the synaptic vesicles, where it is enzymatically converted to norepinephrine. Norepinephrine is stored in the vesicles until release. In the adrenal medulla, an additional enzymatic step converts norepinephrine to epinephrine. L-

Dopa, dopamine, norepinephrine, and epinephrine are **catecholamines** because they all have a characteristic catechol group, which is two hydroxyl groups (−OH) attached to an aromatic ring.[3,4,12] In the central nervous system, certain neurons use dopamine as a neurotransmitter, using the same set of enzymes as in adrenergic transmission, with the exception that dopamine is not converted to norepinephrine.

Neurotransmitter release is initiated when the nerve terminal is depolarized by an action potential, causing vesicles to fuse with the presynaptic membrane and releasing norepinephrine. Once norepinephrine is released into the synaptic junction, it diffuses across the synaptic junction and attaches to a receptor. The interaction between norepinephrine and the receptor elicits an end-organ response. Figure 15–3 shows the receptors for norepinephrine on

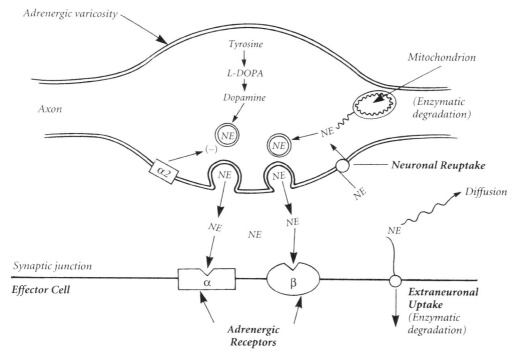

Figure 15–3. Adrenergic synapse. Norepinephrine (NE) is synthesized, stored, and released at the presynaptic sympathetic nerve terminal, which is shown here as an adrenergic *varicosity,* an enlarged area on the sympathetic efferent nerve. After release, NE diffuses across the synaptic junction and interacts with either alpha (α)- or beta (β)-adrenergic receptors. The action of NE is terminated by reuptake into the sympathetic nerve terminal, diffusion from the receptor site, or uptake by nonneuronal mechanisms.

the end-organ, or effector tissue. These receptors are divided into two major classes: alpha (α)- and beta (β)-adrenergic receptors. Autonomic receptors on target organs are discussed in more detail later in this chapter.

Once norepinephrine has produced an effect, its action must be terminated. Termination of norepinephrine's action occurs through two methods. The first and most important is by an active reuptake of norepinephrine back into the presynaptic nerve terminal.[3,4,6,12] This process is called **neuronal reuptake**, or uptake-1. The neuronal reuptake system transports norepinephrine out of the synaptic junction and returns it back into the presynaptic nerve terminal. The norepinephrine that has undergone the neuronal reuptake process can then be repackaged in synaptic vesicles and is available for subsequent release. The reuptake mechanism is also notable because certain drugs, such as cocaine and tricyclic antidepressants (e.g., desipramine and amitriptyline), inhibit the reuptake mechanism, thereby permitting extended interaction of norepinephrine at the receptor, and prolonging norepinephrine's effects.[3,4,6,12] Sympathetic neuronal reuptake has a greater preference for norepinephrine, but other structurally related molecules, such as epinephrine, may also be taken up by this mechanism. Norepinephrine that is not repackaged into vesicles is available for enzymatic destruction by the enzyme monoamine oxidase.[12]

The second method for inactivation of norepinephrine is through diffusion from the synaptic junction, followed by removal by a secondary uptake system in nonneuronal tissues; this is referred to as **extraneuronal reuptake**, or uptake-2. After nonneuronal uptake, enzymatic degradation can then metabolize and inactivate norepinephrine and other catecholamines, such as epinephrine.

Cholinergic Neurotransmission

Acetylcholine is the neurotransmitter released from preganglionic sympathetic and parasympathetic neurons, postganglionic parasympathetic neurons, somatic motor neurons, and sympathetic postganglionic neurons innervating sweat glands.[3,4,6] The principles of cholinergic transmission are similar for each site (Fig. 15–4). Acetylcholine is enzymatically synthesized from choline and acetyl-coenzyme A in the cytoplasm of the nerve terminal, and then transported into and stored in the synaptic vesicles.[3,4,6,12] Each nerve terminal may contain as many as 300,000 vesicles, and each vesicle may hold 10,000 molecules of acetylcholine.[3,4,6] After vesicular release, acetylcholine diffuses across the synaptic junction and interacts with a cholinergic receptor to elicit a response. There are two major classifications of cholinergic receptors, **nicotinic** and **muscarinic**. Nicotinic receptors are located on the dendrites of postganglionic sympathetic and parasympathetic neurons and at the neuromuscular junctions of skeletal muscle. Muscarinic receptors are located on target organs such as the heart and gastrointestinal tract.

The action of acetylcholine is terminated by enzymes called **cholinesterases**, which split the acetyl group from choline. Choline cannot be resynthesized in neural tissue, and so is conserved by transport back inside the nerve terminal, to be reused in forming new acetylcholine (labeled "choline reuptake" in Fig. 15–4). Fifty percent of the hydrolyzed choline may undergo reuptake into the synaptic terminal. Acetylcholinesterase is found in high concentrations in neural tissue, especially cholinergic synapses and the neuromuscular junction. Because acetylcholinesterase provides the mechanism for inactivation of acetylcholine, it is not surprising that inhibition of acetylcholinesterase produces widespread effects by overstimulation of cholinergic receptors. Poisons such as malathion, physostigmine, and nerve gases all produce effects through inhibition of acetylcholinesterase.[3,13] The lethal action of these poisons occurs through overstimulation and then inactivation of nicotinic receptors on skeletal muscles, which produces paralysis of skeletal muscle involved in respiration.

Autonomic Receptors

Adrenergic Receptors

The preceding discussion has examined the anatomy and synaptic transmission mechanisms of the autonomic nervous system. Before examining the physiology of the autonomic nervous system, you should understand how neurotransmitters released from nerves produce responses. As mentioned previously, neurotransmitters must attach to a receptor on the end-organ to produce an effect. The term "receptor" refers to the molecular structure to which an agent—such as a neurotransmitter—binds to produce a response.[14] For example, an increased heart rate, or **tachycardia**, occurs as the result of release

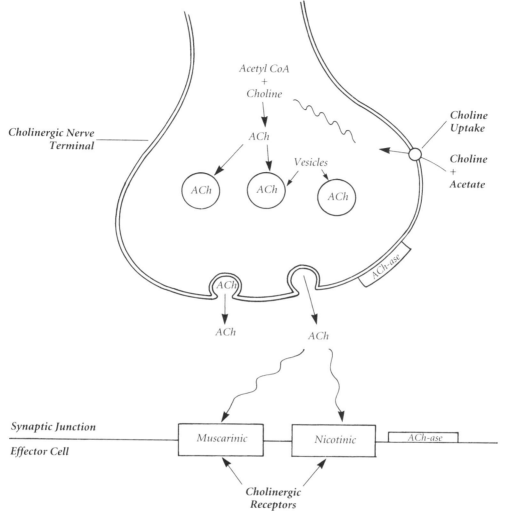

Figure 15–4. Cholinergic synapse. Acetylcholine (ACh) is synthesized in the nerve terminal and then stored in vesicles until release. Released ACh diffuses across the synaptic junction and produces an effect through activating either muscarinic or nicotinic receptors. The action of ACh is terminated by the enzyme acetylcholinesterase. Choline, a by-product of ACh destruction, can be taken up into the nerve terminal for subsequent resynthesis to ACh.

of norepinephrine from the postganglionic sympathetic nerves. Norepinephrine affects heart rate by binding to and stimulating one type of adrenergic receptor, called a **beta$_1$-adrenergic receptor.** In this example, norepinephrine would be considered an **agonist** of the beta$_1$-receptor because it attaches to the receptor and produces a response.

The term "agonist" is used not only in reference to neurotransmitters, but also with regard to exogenously administered drugs that produce effects by binding to receptors. Isoproterenol is an example of an exogenous agent, or drug, that is an agonist to the beta receptor. **Antagonist** is a related term that refers to a substance that binds to a receptor but produces no response, thereby blocking access to the receptor by the agonist. Antagonists reduce, and at high concentrations block, the effects of agonists. Propranolol is an example of a commonly encountered antagonist of the beta receptor.

Adrenergic receptors are subclassified into two main groups, alpha and beta.[4,6,15] Figure 15–5 shows the classes and subclasses of autonomic receptors. The initial categorization of alpha- and beta-adrenergic receptors was proposed by Ahlquist[16] to explain and classify the excitatory and inhibitory effects of norepinephrine and epinephrine. An easy initial approach to understanding adrenergic receptors is that activation of alpha-adrenergic receptors produces physiological excitatory responses, except in the gastrointestinal tract, where inhibition occurs. Activation of beta-adrenergic receptors primarily elicits inhibitory effects, except in the heart, where excitatory effects occur.

Figure 15–5 also shows that alpha- and beta-adrenergic receptors have been subclassified. **Alpha$_1$-adrenergic receptors** are normally stimulated by sympathetic nervous system release of norepinephrine. Alpha$_1$-adrenergic receptors are important in smooth muscle contraction, and consequently have significant influences in conditions such as contraction of vascular smooth muscle and in nasal decongestion.[17,18] Molecular and pharmacological studies indicate that there are at least four subtypes of alpha$_1$-adrenergic receptors. The relative importance of muscarinic subtypes is still under investigation.[17,18] **Alpha$_2$-adrenergic receptors** are located on the presynaptic nerve terminal, and stimulation of these receptors inhibits release of norepinephrine from the presynaptic nerve terminal[6,18,19] (see Fig. 15–3). The primary physiological effects of alpha-adrenergic receptors are attributable to activation of alpha$_1$-adrenergic receptors.

The separation of beta-adrenergic receptors into two subclasses provides a convenient way to understand them, rather than by remembering that some are inhibitory and others are excitatory. A subclassification of beta-adrenergic receptors was described by Lands et al. in 1967.[20] According to that classification, beta$_1$-adrenergic receptors are primarily found in the heart and mediate the excitatory effects of norepinephrine and epinephrine on the myocardium. Although beta$_1$-adrenergic receptors are activated by both norepinephrine and epinephrine, epinephrine is more potent that norepinephrine; that is, a lower concentration of epinephrine is required to produce a similar effect. Beta$_1$-adrenergic receptor activation increases heart rate and the ability of cardiac muscle to contract. The "inhibitory" effects of beta-adrenergic receptors are produced through activation of beta$_2$-adrenergic receptors. Beta$_2$-adrenergic recep-

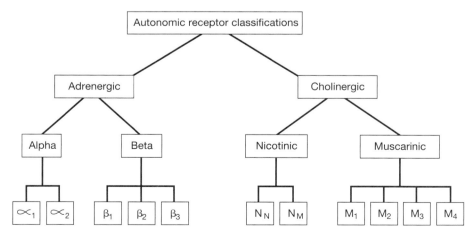

Figure 15–5. Classification of autonomic receptors. α_x, alpha-adrenergic receptor subtypes; β_x, beta-adrenergic receptor subtypes; N_N, nicotinic ganglionic receptor (i.e., neuronal); N_M, nicotinic receptors at the neuromuscular junction; M_x, subtypes of muscarinic receptors.

tors are involved in a wide range of physiological effects, such as bronchial smooth muscle dilation, inhibition of gastrointestinal tract, dilation of vascular smooth muscle, and inhibition of the uterus. Epinephrine is a potent agonist for $beta_2$-adrenergic receptors, whereas norepinephrine has much less influence on $beta_2$-receptors. Studies have identified a third form of the beta receptor, which is classified as the $beta_3$-adrenergic receptor. $Beta_3$-adrenergic receptors have also been identified in humans,[21] and are found most notably in adipose tissue, but may be located in other tissues as well. The function of the $beta_3$-adrenergic receptor in humans is still under debate[22]; these receptors may play a role in obesity

Cholinergic Receptors

As previously mentioned, cholinergic receptors are divided into two major groups—nicotinic and muscarinic receptors.[3,4,6,23,24] Both groups are stimulated by the neurotransmitter, acetylcholine. Nicotinic cholinergic receptors were originally defined by the observation that low doses of the alkaloid, nicotine, stimulates these receptors. High concentrations of nicotine inhibit nicotinic receptors. Nicotinic receptors are divided into two categories and are found at 1) autonomic ganglia, and 2) the neuromuscular junction.[3,4,6] The distinction between the two subtypes is based on the effects of antagonists. Nicotinic receptors at autonomic ganglia are known as **nicotinic ganglionic receptors** and are located on postganglionic neurons of both the sympathetic and parasympathetic nervous systems. Nicotinic ganglionic receptors are excited by acetylcholine released from both sympathetic and parasympathetic preganglionic neurons. Thus, nicotinic ganglionic receptor antagonists, such as hexamethonium or trimethaphan, block the effects of stimulation of both sympathetic and parasympathetic postganglionic neurons.

The other subtype of nicotinic receptor is located at the motor end-plate region of the skeletal muscle and mediates the effects of the voluntary, or somatic motor system. Activation of neuromuscular nicotinic receptors produces skeletal muscle contraction. Nicotinic receptors at the neuromuscular junction are blocked by antagonists, such as curare or succinylcholine.[3,4,6]

Muscarinic cholinergic receptors mediate the effects of the parasympathetic nervous system. Acetyl-choline is released from postganglionic parasympathetic nerves and activates muscarinic receptors on postjunctional membranes of effector cells.[3,4,6,23,24] As previously noted, the vagus nerve (cranial nerve X) carries most of the parasympathetic motor, or efferent, innervation to the visceral organs, such as the heart and gastrointestinal tract, where muscarinic receptors are activated. Muscarinic receptors also mediate parasympathetic effects on the eye and the urinary bladder. Atropine, a type of belladonna alkaloid, is the prototype for muscarinic receptor antagonists, and is also known as a **parasympatholytic** agent, because it blocks the effects of the parasympathetic nervous system.

Molecular biology studies have identified five subtypes of the muscarinic receptor.[6,24] Physiological or pharmacological information is available on four of these subtypes.[6,24] M_1 receptors have been found on autonomic ganglia, certain secretory glands, and the stomach. Pirenzepine is an M_1 antagonist and has been used to inhibit acid secretion in the stomach and to reduce increased motility of the gastrointestinal tract.[25] M_2 receptors are located in the heart. M_3 and M_4 receptors are on secretory glands and smooth muscle. Atropine is in general an effective antagonist to each of the muscarinic receptor subtypes.

Physiology of the Autonomic Nervous System

Important Concepts

The sympathetic and the parasympathetic nervous systems are active under different conditions.[26] Some generalities are useful in understanding the physiological functions of the two divisions of the autonomic nervous system. For instance, the sympathetic nervous system increases utilization of bodily energy resources, and is most active during stress or exercise. The sympathetic nervous system prepares us for "fight or flight" by increasing energy use in organs such as the heart, which in turn uses the energy to pump more blood through the body. In contrast, the parasympathetic nervous system is most active when a person is resting. The parasympathetic nervous system promotes restoration of body energy stores by increasing digestion and absorption. An easy way to remember parasympathetic nervous system function is to associate the parasympathetic nervous system with the concept "rest and digest."

By understanding these concepts, much of the physiological responses to activation of the sympathetic and parasympathetic nervous systems can be predicted without memorizing large amounts of detail. For example, when an individual is under stress or in a "fight or flight" situation, the irises of the eyes dilate to allow more light to the retina, and the heart beats faster (tachycardia) and more vigorously (increased contractility). During stress, blood flow to skeletal muscle increases to improve the ability to fight or run away, whereas blood flow is shifted away from organs not immediately essential in fleeing or defense, such as the small intestine or stomach.

In contrast, the activity of the parasympathetic nervous system is greatest at rest, especially when digesting a meal. In this situation, motility of the gastrointestinal tract is heightened to facilitate digestion, and the irises of the pupils are constricted, because the individual is at rest and perhaps drowsy. Heart rate is reduced, thereby conserving energy utilization, because there is little demand for additional cardiac output. These concepts offer an initial base from which to understand the working of the autonomic nervous system; as with all generalities, however, there are exceptions. A detailed explanation of physiological actions of the autonomic nervous system is presented later in this chapter.

Several additional concepts are essential in understanding the physiology of the autonomic nervous system. Many organs or tissues receive **dual innervation** from both sympathetic and parasympathetic nervous systems. As illustrated in Figure 15–2, the heart, lungs, and small intestines all receive dual innervation. Other organs such as blood vessels and the kidney receive innervation from only one of the two autonomic divisions. In organs or tissues receiving dual innervation, the functions of the sympathetic and parasympathetic nervous systems may at first appear to produce opposite, or antagonistic, effects, but these effects are really complementary. For example, activation of the sympathetic nervous system increases heart rate, whereas stimulation of the parasympathetic nervous system decreases heart rate. In physiological control of heart rate, the two systems are not turned on simultaneously; instead, one division is stimulated while the other is inhibited. For example, to increase heart rate, the excitatory effects

of the sympathetic nervous system are activated, while the inhibitory effects of the parasympathetic nervous system are inhibited, or withdrawn. The term **functional synergism** is used to describe this autonomic function in which the two divisions work together to produce a common, physiological effect.

Another important concept in autonomic physiology is **tone** or resting activity. The concept of tone describes the resting, background or basal outflow from either the sympathetic or parasympathetic nervous systems to peripheral organs or tissues. Autonomic tone is important because it allows physiological control of an organ or tissue through reduction in background neural activity. For example, because of continuous background sympathetic neural outflow (i.e., sympathetic tone) to vascular smooth muscle, vascular resistance can be reduced by a decrease in tonic sympathetic outflow. Thus, an important implication of autonomic tone is that the function of an organ can be controlled by only one autonomic division, which can decrease (reduce tone) or increase outflow to control the activity of an organ or tissue. Tone is also observed in organs receiving dual innervation. Tone occurs with most autonomic innervation, although some tissues receive little or no tonic innervation under certain physiological conditions. For example, when a person is cold, sympathetic outflow to eccrine sweat glands is very low.

Autonomic Control of Organs

Table 15–2 summarizes the physiological responses to stimulation of the sympathetic and parasympathetic nervous systems. More detailed effects of autonomic control of the specific organ systems are discussed in the following sections. For additional details, consult the physiology textbooks listed in the references.[27–30]

Eye

The radial (or dilator muscle) of the iris is stimulated by parasympathetic activity to produce **miosis**, which is a decrease in pupillary diameter (see Chapter 11). Parasympathetic control of pupil diameter is accomplished through the oculomotor nerve (cranial nerve III) and originates from preganglionic neurons in the nucleus of Edinger-Westphal (see Fig. 15–2). The oculomotor nerve also provides parasympathetic innervation to the ciliary muscle, which produces

TABLE 15-2

Responses to Stimulation of Autonomic Nervous System

Tissue or Organ	SNS	PNS
Eye		
Radial muscle of iris	Contraction leading to pupillary dilation (mydriasis)	NI
Circular muscle of iris	NI	Contraction leading to pupillary constriction (miosis)
Ciliary muscle	NI	Contraction that allows accommodation of lens for near vision
Salivary glands	Stimulation, producing thick, viscous secretion	Stimulation, producing large volume of watery secretion
Sweat glands		
Eccrine	Increased sweat production (muscarinic receptors)	NI
Heart		
Sinoatrial node	Increased heart rate (tachycardia)	Decreased hear rate (bradycardia)
Myocardial muscle	Increased contractility	Little, if any effect
Blood vessels		
Arteries		
Skin (cutaneous)	Constriction	NI
Heart (coronary)	Constriction	NI
Brain (cerebral)	Constriction	NI
Gastrointestinal tract	Constriction	NI
Veins	Constriction	NI
Lung		
Bronchial smooth muscle	Relaxation	Constriction
Glands	NI	Secretion
Liver	Glycogenolysis, gluconeogenesis (glucose from amino acids and lactate)	NI
Skeletal muscle	Glycogenolysis	NI
Adipose tissue	Lipolysis	NI
Kidney	Secretion of renin	NI
Bladder		
Detrusor muscle	Little, if any effect	Contraction
Sphincters	Contraction	Relaxation
Stomach		
Motility	Inhibition	Stimulation
Secretions	NI	Increased acid secretion

NI, not innervated; PNS, parasympathetic nervous system; SNS, sympathetic nervous system.

TABLE 15–2		
Responses to Stimulation of Autonomic Nervous System (continued)		
Tissue or Organ	**SNS**	**PNS**
Intestines		
Motility	Inhibition	Stimulation
Sphincters	Contraction	Relaxation
Secretions	NI	Stimulation
Gall bladder and ducts	Inhibition	Contraction
Genital organs		
Female—uterus	Pregnant—contraction, variable	
	Nonpregnant—relaxation	
Male	Ejaculation	Erection

NI, not innervated; PNS, parasympathetic nervous system; SNS, sympathetic nervous system.

thickening of the lens to allow for visual **accommodation**, which is focusing of the lens for near vision. To understand control of the ciliary muscle and hence the lens, it is important to recognize that the lens is elastic and suspended by ligaments. When the ciliary muscle is relaxed, the ligaments pull on the lens, causing it to be stretched outward, which makes the lens less round (or more flat). In this situation, the lens is best focused to view distant objects. Stimulation of the parasympathetic nervous system also activates muscarinic receptors in ciliary muscle, which causes the ciliary muscle to contract, resulting in reduced tension on the lens. With less tension, the natural elasticity of the lens causes it to bulge, or become more round, thereby allowing the lens to reduce its focal length to allow for near vision.

Sympathetic innervation to the eye traverses the superior cervical ganglion. Stimulation of sympathetic innervation to the circular or sphincter muscle of the iris increases the diameter of the pupil (i.e., causes **mydriasis**); however, regulation of light into the eye by control of pupillary diameter primarily involves parasympathetic control.

Heart

The autonomic nervous system influences the pumping ability of the heart. The volume of blood the heart pumps over a given period of time is termed **cardiac output**, which is an important determinant of blood pressure. The pumping rate, or

heart rate, is increased by sympathetic stimulation of the sinoatrial pacemaker in the right atrium. The contractile ability of the atria and ventricles, or **contractility**, is also increased by sympathetic stimulation. The sympathetic nervous system can increase cardiac output by increasing the heart rate, as well as by increasing cardiac contractility. The adrenergic receptors in the heart mediating the effects of the sympathetic nervous system are $beta_1$-adrenergic receptors. The vagus nerve provides parasympathetic innervation to the sinoatrial node, and during stimulation reduces heart rate (i.e., **bradycardia**). Parasympathetic innervation has no direct effect on contractility of cardiac ventricular muscle. Parasympathetic effects on the heart are mediated by muscarinic receptors.

Vascular Smooth Muscle

Both arterial and venous smooth muscle are influenced by the sympathetic nervous system. In general, sympathetic stimulation of blood vessels causes vascular smooth muscle to constrict, whereas withdrawal of sympathetic tone leads to dilation of blood vessels. The diameter of arterial blood vessels is important in control of blood pressure because vascular diameter determines the resistance to blood flow through the arterial system, which is termed **peripheral resistance**.

The response of an individual blood vessel to sympathetic stimulation depends on the vascular bed in which it is located. For instance, blood vessels in the heart, kidney, and brain are regulated by local tissue mechanisms—such as pO_2, adenosine, and pH—and are minimally influenced by the sympathetic nervous system. Blood vessels in the skin, skeletal muscle, and gastrointestinal tract vasoconstrict during sympathetic stimulation, and this vasoconstriction is produced through activation of alpha-adrenergic receptors. Epinephrine, which is secreted from the adrenal medulla, also causes arterial blood vessels in skeletal muscle to dilate, which is mediated by $beta_2$-adrenergic receptors. The parasympathetic nervous system has minimal influence on blood vessels involved in blood pressure control. As you may recall from the previous discussion, reductions in vascular muscle diameter are produced through reductions in sympathetic tone to blood vessels.

Lungs

Bronchial smooth muscle dilates in response to release of norepinephrine from sympathetic nerves. The receptor mechanism is not clear, but may involve activation of $beta_2$-adrenergic receptors, or inhibition of release of acetylcholine from parasympathetic nerves. The predominant type of adrenergic receptor in airway smooth muscle is the $beta_2$-adrenergic receptor. The primary method of stimulating $beta_2$-adrenergic receptors is from the effects of circulating epinephrine released from the adrenal medulla. Parasympathetic innervation of bronchial muscle comes from the vagus. Parasympathetic stimulation leads to bronchoconstriction through activation of muscarinic receptors by acetylcholine.

Stomach and Intestines (Gastrointestinal Tract)

The gastrointestinal tract is unique among visceral organs in that it contains its own nervous system, known as the **enteric nervous system**, which has approximately the same number of neurons as the spinal cord. Many sympathetic and parasympathetic influences on the gastrointestinal tract take place through actions on the enteric nervous system. Movements of gastric smooth muscle (i.e., gastric motility) as well as the pyloric sphincter between the stomach and duodenum are inhibited by the sympathetic nervous system. The net result of increased sympathetic activity to the stomach is a decreased rate of emptying. Both alpha- and $beta_2$-adrenergic receptors mediate sympathetic effects in the stomach, as well as in the intestine. Sympathetic stimulation produces inhibitory effects on the intestines through inhibition of intestinal smooth muscle and constriction of sphincters.

Preganglionic parasympathetic nerves travel in the vagus nerve to innervate parasympathetic postganglionic cells in the enteric nervous system in the stomach. Stimulation of the parasympathetic innervation to the stomach directly increases secretion of acid in the stomach through activation of muscarinic receptors, and indirectly increases gastric acid secretion by stimulation of release of the peptide hormone gastrin from the stomach. The parasympathetic nervous system stimulates digestion by stimulating gastric and intestinal motility and opening sphincters to allow passage of the food material (i.e., chyme) down the gastrointestinal tract. Autonomic control of the stomach and the intestine is easy to understand by keeping in mind that the parasympathetic system promotes restoration of body energy stores and aids in digestion. Parasympathetic effects in the gastrointestinal tract are mediated by muscarinic receptors located on smooth muscle and glands.

Sweat Glands

The rate of sweat secretion from the **eccrine sweat glands** is controlled by the sympathetic nervous system. Eccrine sweat glands are important in evaporative cooling for regulation of body temperature. A notable feature of autonomic control of eccrine sweat gland secretion is that the postganglionic sympathetic nerves release acetylcholine, which excites muscarinic receptors on the sweat glands. Apocrine sweat glands, which are concentrated in areas of the body such as the armpits, are involved in body odor secretions rather than in temperature regulation, and are not under autonomic control.

Salivary Glands

Salivary gland secretions lubricate food for swallowing, dissolve food so it can be tasted, and start digestion of starches with the enzyme alpha-amylase. The salivary glands are innervated by both sympathetic and parasympathetic nerves. Preganglionic sympathetic innervation to salivary glands comes from cells in the intermediolateral cell column of the spinal cord, and these neurons project to postganglionic neurons in the superior cervical ganglion. Parasympathetic innervation to salivary glands comes from the facial nerve (cranial nerve VII), which innervates the sublingual and submandibular glands, and from the glossopharyngeal nerve (cranial nerve IX), which innervates the parotid gland.[7] Activation of the parasympathetic nervous system innervation to salivary glands produces larger volumes of salivary secretion, with a more watery consistency, whereas activation of sympathetic neurons produces a more viscous secretion.

Energy Metabolism

One approach to understanding autonomic control of energy metabolism is the concept that the sympathetic nervous system promotes **catabolism**, or the use of energy stores in the body; in contrast, the parasympathetic nervous system promotes **anabolism**, which replenishes and restores energy stores. Accordingly, the sympathetic nervous system increases blood levels of the energy substrate, glucose, primarily through release of epinephrine. Epinephrine promotes the breakdown of glycogen and increases synthesis of glucose from noncarbohydrate precursors, such as amino acids (i.e., gluconeogenesis). Epinephrine also increases the release of free fatty acids from adipose tissue for use as an energy substrate. The anabolic effects of the parasympathetic nervous system are produced through stimulation of digestion and coordination of gastrointestinal activity during digestion.

Autonomic Reflexes

General Concepts

The preceding parts of this chapter emphasized efferent control of organ function by the autonomic nervous system. You should keep in mind that most, if not all, visceral organs are also innervated by sensory fibers (afferents) coursing in the same nerves containing motor (efferent) autonomic fibers. Up to 80% of the fibers in autonomic nerves are sensory, strongly suggesting that the central nervous system receives substantial input concerning the status of the viscera.

Many autonomic reflexes are important for normal physiological function. The baroreceptor reflex provides moment-to-moment control of blood pressure. Renal reflexes maintain appropriate fluid balance in the body. **Micturition**, **defecation**, and sexual function are controlled by reflexes. Constant body temperature is also maintained by reflexes. Thus, many of the body's homeostatic mechanisms are controlled or influenced by autonomic reflexes. Three reflexes are used to illustrate autonomic reflex function in the following sections.

The Baroreceptor Reflex

Autonomic reflexes, and all reflexes in general, consist of 1) sensory receptors that detect changes in the system; 2) a comparator, or integrator region that receives sensory input and decides whether changes need to be made; and 3) motor fibers that are controlled by the comparator and that modulate effector (e.g., organ) function. The baroreceptor reflex controls short-term changes in blood pressure.[27–31] One way of understanding the baroreceptor reflex is to recognize that it tries to minimize changes in blood pressure much like a thermostat in your house tries to maintain temperature at a constant level. The baroreceptor reflex is diagrammed in Figure 15–6. The sensors, or **baroreceptors**, that sense blood pressure are located in the carotid sinus region (where the internal carotid artery branches from the external carotid artery) and in the aortic arch. Baroreceptors in the carotid sinus are connected by nerve fibers that combine to form the carotid sinus nerve; this nerve then joins the glossopharyngeal nerve (cranial nerve IX), which courses to the brainstem. Aortic arch receptors are connected to nerve fibers that form the aortic nerve, which then joins the vagus nerve (cranial nerve X). Again, these afferents course to the brainstem. The comparator, or integrator, region is located in two major sites in the medulla—the nucleus tractus solitarius (NTS) and the ventrolateral reticular formation. Baroreceptor afferents terminate in the NTS. Fibers from the NTS course to the ventrolateral reticular formation. Neurons in the latter send axons to the intermediolateral cell column, where they terminate on sympathetic preganglionic neurons. The latter provide motor innervation to smooth muscle on blood vessels; this innervation regulates the diameter of the vessels, thereby influencing vascular resistance and, thus, blood pressure.

The baroreceptor reflex operates in the following manner (see Fig. 15–6). An increase in arterial blood pressure causes increased stretch on the arteries; this stretch increases the stretch on sensory receptors in the carotid sinus and aortic arch, causing the baroreceptors to generate a greater number of action poten-

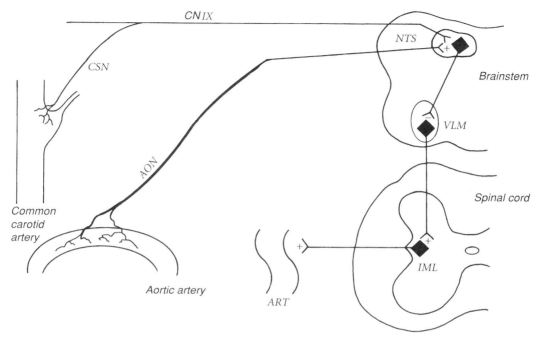

Figure 15–6. Pathways mediating the baroreceptor reflex. AON, aortic nerve with fibers innervating the ascending aorta; CSN, carotid sinus nerve with fibers innervating the carotid sinus; CN IX, glossopharyngeal nerve (cranial nerve IX); X, vagus nerve (cranial nerve X); NTS, nucleus of the solitary tract; VLM, ventrolateral reticular formation in medulla; IML, intermediolateral nucleus; ART, arteriole; +, excitatory.

tials. Thus, increased blood pressure increases the number of action potentials in the carotid sinus and aortic nerves, signalling the NTS that blood pressure is elevated. Neurons in the NTS increase their firing rate in response to the increased activity in the carotid sinus and aortic nerves. This increased baroreceptor input causes a reduced firing rate of neurons in the ventrolateral reticular formation. Hence, the excitatory drive to sympathetic preganglionic neurons is reduced, leading to reduced contraction of the smooth muscle in arteries. The arteries then dilate, reducing blood pressure back to normal. Note that the ventrolateral reticular formation provides a tonic excitatory drive to sympathetic preganglionic neurons; this drive can either be increased or decreased by the NTS, depending on whether blood pressure decreases or increases, respectively.

The NTS and ventrolateral reticular formation also receive information from many other regions of the brain and spinal cord. This input is integrated with the information coming from baroreceptors to fine-tune the degree of control of blood pressure. In summary, the baroreceptor reflex is a homeostatic reflex that continuously operates to minimize changes in blood pressure, thereby helping to ensure that all organs receive an appropriate amount of blood flow.

The Micturition Reflex

The micturition reflex[32,33] controls the filling and emptying of the urinary bladder. It is an interesting reflex because it must first allow the bladder to fill, it must sense when the bladder is full, and then it must cause the bladder to empty. This reflex also has a strong voluntary component that permits conscious control of reflex function.

The major components of the micturition reflex are shown in Figure 15–7. The parasympathetic ner-

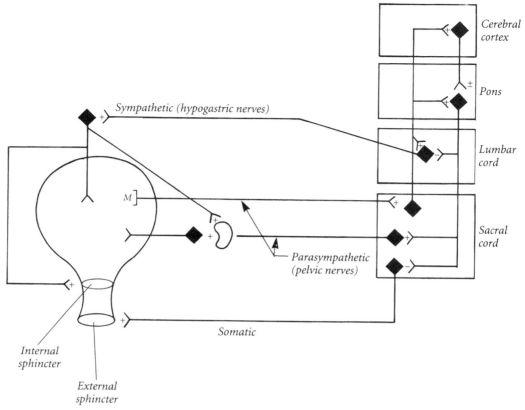

Figure 15–7. Pathways mediating micturition. At left, the main body of the bladder (detrusor muscle) is shown with the internal and external sphincters. Different regions of the central nervous system are shown on the right. M, mechanoreceptor afferents; +, excitatory connection; –, inhibitory connection. The pathway from the cerebral cortex to pons can be excitatory or inhibitory, depending on the circumstances. If the spinal cord is damaged above the sacral cord, another functional connection will develop between mechanoreceptor afferents and parasympathetic preganglionic neurons.

vous system provides innervation to the bladder, which causes it to contract. The preganglionic cell bodies lie in the sacral portions (segments S2–S4) of the spinal gray matter. The axons course by way of the pelvic nerves to the parasympathetic ganglia located in the pelvic plexus and on the wall of the bladder. Preganglionic neurons excite the postganglionic cell bodies, which innervate the detrusor muscle (i.e. the main body) of the bladder, and cause it to contract.

The bladder is also innervated by the sympathetic nervous system. The sympathetic preganglionic neu-

rons lie in the lumbar portion of the spinal cord. Some sympathetic preganglionic neurons project to the sympathetic chain ganglia, whereas others continue on to the inferior mesenteric ganglion, where they synapse on postganglionic neurons. Postganglionic neurons project to the bladder by way of the hypogastric nerves, and produce inhibition of contraction (e.g., relaxation). Postganglionic fibers also project to parasympathetic preganglionic terminals in the parasympathetic ganglia. These sympathetic fibers innervate parasympathetic preganglionic nerve terminals, producing **presynaptic inhibition** of the parasympathetic preganglionic nerve terminals. Finally, sympathetic fibers innervate the internal urethral sphincter, causing the sphincter to contract.

Mechanoreceptors in the wall of the bladder sense the degree that the bladder is stretched, and this sensory information is relayed by the pelvic nerves to the spinal cord. The greater the stretch due to filling, the greater the number of action potentials carried in the pelvic sensory nerves. Mechanoreceptor information arriving at the spinal cord has an excitatory effect on spinal cord neurons that project (ascend) to the micturition region in the dorsolateral pons. The ascending fibers excite the pontine neurons, and the pontine neurons send their axons all the way back down the sacral spinal cord to excite parasympathetic preganglionic neurons.

For the bladder to fill with urine, it must be relaxed. During the filling phase, the properties of the smooth muscle of the bladder permit it to relax and stretch as it is filled with urine. In addition, the nervous system acts to relax the bladder, permitting it to fill. As an empty bladder fills, the amount of stretch on the bladder wall is low; therefore the mechanoreceptors have little activity. This low activity level is insufficient significantly to activate the descending pathway to excite parasympathetic preganglionic neurons. Thus, parasympathetic activation is not strong enough to cause bladder contraction. The ability of the bladder itself to expand and the relative lack of parasympathetic activation are the major factors permitting the bladder to fill.

The sympathetic nervous system also contributes to bladder filling. The low activity level in mechanoreceptors is adequate for the spinal neurons to excite sympathetic preganglionic neurons in the lumbar spinal cord. This situation causes sympathetic postganglionic neurons innervating the bladder to release norepinephrine, which produces bladder relaxation due to activation of beta$_2$-adrenergic receptors on the bladder smooth muscle. In addition, excitation of the sympathetic fibers to the parasympathetic ganglia causes depolarization of parasympathetic preganglionic nerve terminals. This depolarization (presynaptic inhibition) reduces the amount of neurotransmitter (acetylcholine) released by the preganglionic fibers. This effect reduces the extent of excitation of parasympathetic postganglionic fibers. As a result, the bladder relaxes, which permits it to fill with urine. Finally, the activity of sympathetic fibers causes contraction of the internal urethral sphincter, preventing urine from flowing out of the bladder.

Thus, part of the mechanism that permits bladder filling is the result of a close interaction between the parasympathetic and sympathetic nervous systems. Remember, neurons always have some tonic activity; they are turned neither on nor off. Instead, there is a gradation of neuronal activity. As the bladder fills, the activity in mechanoreceptors is relatively low. Under these conditions, the predominant effect is excitation of sympathetic efferent nerves, although the parasympathetic neurons also have a low activity rate. Excitation of sympathetic efferent nerves causes direct relaxation of the bladder, as well as reduction of parasympathetic excitatory drive to the bladder. The combination of these effects relaxes the bladder, permitting it to fill to capacity.

When the bladder is full, the activity in the mechanoreceptors is maximally increased. This information is relayed not only to the pons but to the cerebral cortex, where conscious awareness of the desire to void is controlled. With high activity in the mechanoreceptors, the major effect is excitation of pontine neurons. The descending activity from the pons inhibits sympathetic preganglionic neurons. This effect overcomes the excitation of these neurons coming from the ascending neurons. Thus, the net result is decreased activity of sympathetic efferent nerves, which reduces direct bladder relaxation, removes the presynaptic inhibition of parasympathetic preganglionic neurons, and allows the internal urethral sphincter to relax. As noted previously, excitation of pontine neurons excites the sacral parasympathetic preganglionic neurons, which then excite the postganglionic neurons to cause bladder contraction. Then, micturition occurs.

For voiding to happen, the external urethral sphincter must also relax. This sphincter is made up of skeletal muscle fibers innervated by the somatic nervous system. The somatic fibers have tonic activity that causes contraction of the sphincter as the bladder is filling. Activation of pontine neurons inhibits these somatic fibers, causing relaxation of the sphincter.

As noted, the degree of fullness in the bladder is relayed to the cerebral cortex. The cortex can influence the activity of pontine neurons to either excite or inhibit them, depending on the circumstances. Thus, the micturition reflex can be modulated consciously.

Normally, the bladder voiding reflex must be relayed through the pons. There is no means for a shorter, more "direct" pathway. If the spinal cord is damaged anywhere above the sacral cord, such that the ascending and descending pathways connecting pons to sacral cord are cut, bladder control is lost. Initially, voiding the bladder is impossible, because the excitatory drive to the parasympathetic preganglionic neurons is lost. In about 2 weeks, some recovery of bladder control may occur. This limited recovery of function is due to the development of another functional pathway. Now the mechanoreceptor afferents can excite parasympathetic preganglionic neurons without first going to the brain. This pathway does not develop *de novo*; it is present at birth, but as the nervous system matures, it is turned off. This pathway becomes functional only some time after damage to the cord occurs; bladder function, however, is not normal with this new pathway. The bladder operates on reflex control only, with no influence from the brain; it is thus termed a "reflex bladder." The bladder in general has an increased tone, and it cannot fill up as much before it voids. Because the connections from the spinal cord to the brain are damaged, there is no conscious sensation from the bladder, and the ability consciously to control the bladder is lost.

The Erection Reflex

Erection occurs when the erectile tissue in the male penis fills with blood; this is considered a classic parasympathetic function. The process of erection is another example of functional synergism involving a complex interaction between the parasympathetic and sympathetic nervous systems.[32,34] In addition, erection illustrates one of the newer advances in knowledge of peripheral neurobiology: the involvement of peptides in autonomic function. Since the mid-1980s, many different peptides have been found to be located in autonomic neurons. Although the exact function of these peptides has not yet been discovered, one of them, VIP, is known to be the primary mediator of the dilating response required for erection.

The functional anatomy involved in the erection reflex is shown in Figure 15–8. Sympathetic preganglionic neurons exit from the T12 to L3 segments of the spinal cord and course to the inferior mesenteric ganglion. Postganglionic fibers innervate the erectile tissue (corpus cavernosum and corpus spongiosum) through the pudendal nerve. The details presented in this discussion apply mainly to the corpus cavernosum (penile shaft).

The neurotransmitter in postganglionic sympathetic neurons is norepinephrine. Excitation of these fibers releases norepinephrine to excite alpha$_1$-adrenergic receptors on the erectile tissue (indicated by the number "1" in Fig. 15–8). Activation of alpha$_1$-adrenergic receptors constricts erectile tissue. Norepinephrine can also excite alpha$_2$-receptors on the presynaptic membrane (indicated by the number "2" in Fig. 15–8). Activation of alpha$_2$-adrenergic receptors reduces the release of norepinephrine, and provides fine-tuning of the amount of norepinephrine released during nerve excitation.

Parasympathetic preganglionic neurons exit the cord from the S2 to S4 segments and course in the pelvic nerve to parasympathetic ganglia. As usual, they excite parasympathetic postganglionic fibers. Some sympathetic postganglionic fibers also excite parasympathetic postganglionic neurons. Parasympathetic postganglionic fibers innervate erectile tissue. Excitation of these fibers causes dilation (relaxation) of the erectile tissue, permitting it to fill with blood. Most, if not all, parasympathetic postganglionic cells contain acetylcholine and VIP. VIP not acetylcholine, is probably the primary mediator responsible for dilating erectile tissue; however, release of acetylcholine does excite muscarinic ("M" in Fig. 15–8) receptors, which also dilate erectile tissue. VIP stimulates VIP receptors ("V" in the Fig. 15–8). Parasympathetic postganglionic fibers also innervate sympathetic presynaptic terminals. Release of acetylcholine, and possibly VIP, depolarizes these terminals, producing presynaptic inhibition.

Afferents course from the penis to the sacral portion of the cord. These afferents excite interneurons that synapse with parasympathetic preganglionic neurons. The afferents also innervate a group of neurons (not shown in Fig. 15–8) that course to the brain, and allow sensation.

The process of erection has a strong psychological component. Limbic regions of the hypothalamus send projections to the spinal cord. These projections inhibit sympathetic preganglionic neurons and excite parasympathetic preganglionic neurons.

Erection is caused by relaxation of the erectile tissue, which permits engorgement of the penis with

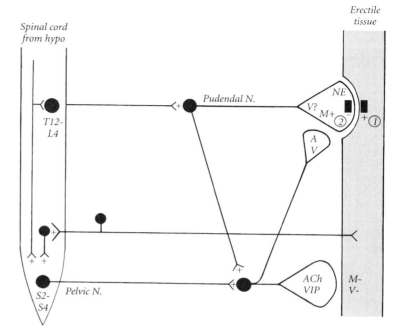

Figure 15–8. Pathways mediating erection. "Erectile tissue" refers to the corpus spongiosum. Hypo, hypothalamus; NE, norepinephrine; ACh, acetylcholine; VIP, vasoactive intestinal peptide; M, muscarinic receptor; V, VIP receptor; +, excitatory connection; −, inhibitory connection; ?, unconfirmed. Line from erectile tissue to spinal cord represents penile sensory fibers.

blood. When the penis is flaccid, sympathetic efferent nerves have a tonic excitation, causing constriction of erectile tissue. Thus, sympathetic preganglionic neurons are spontaneously active, and they excite sympathetic postganglionic fibers innervating erectile tissue. The latter fibers release norepinephrine to excite alpha$_1$-adrenergic receptors, producing constriction of erectile tissue. Not much blood flows through the penis in the flaccid state.

For erection to occur normally, parasympathetic preganglionic neurons must be activated. This activation can be accomplished in two ways. First, stimulation of penile afferent nerves can excite these neurons. Second, excitation of the descending hypothalamic pathway, due to emotional responses, can also excite parasympathetic preganglionic neurons. Excitation of parasympathetic preganglionic neurons causes excitation of parasympathetic postganglionic neurons innervating the erectile tissue. On excitation, these neurons release acetylcholine, but, more important, they also release VIP. Both VIP and acetylcholine dilate erectile tissue; however, erection can still occur

in the presence of drugs that block muscarinic receptors. For many years, this observation was puzzling; although parasympathetic innervation is required for a normal erection, acetylcholine in postganglionic fibers did not seem to be required. Beginning in the mid-1980s, we have learned that most, if not all, postganglionic parasympathetic neurons contain VIP and acetylcholine, and it is the release of VIP that provides most of the dilation of the erectile tissue.

Postganglionic parasympathetic fibers also innervate postganglionic sympathetic nerve terminals. Release of acetylcholine, and possibly VIP, depolarizes the sympathetic terminals, reducing the amount of norepinephrine released. This action of acetylcholine and VIP diminishes the influence of the sympathetic constriction response. The hypothalamic pathway can also inhibit sympathetic outflow.

The result of all these interactions is enhancement of parasympathetic dilator influences, along with diminution of sympathetic constricting influences on erectile tissue. The penis then becomes engorged with blood, producing an erection.

The outflow from the corpus cavernosum (penile shaft) has no venous constriction. Erection is maintained by the increased inflow of blood, and a decrease in outflow of blood is not required. Venous constriction does occur in the outflow from the corpus spongiosum (penile head). Some sympathetic fibers can cause an erection. These fibers presumably account for erections in some men who have had their sacral cords, or parasympathetic neurons, destroyed. These fibers are not necessarily present in all men. Impotence is a common side effect of many drugs. Any drug that alters sympathetic or parasympathetic function, or that alters mood, can potentially interfere with erectile (and thus sexual) function.

The same basic process seems to occur in women. VIP is probably responsible for the vasodilation of vessels perfusing the vagina, which permits the exudation of plasma responsible in part for vaginal lubrication. Clitoral erection is functionally comparable with erection of the penile head.

Vestibular System Interactions With the Autonomic Nervous System

The vestibular system plays a critical role in the regulation of head and eye position as well as balance (see Chapter 10). The vestibular system has long been understood to interact with the autonomic nervous system.[35,36] Perhaps the most easily recognized interaction occurs with dysfunction of the vestibular system, which can lead to nausea and **emesis** (or vomiting). Emesis involves a complex series of autonomic efferent effects on the gastrointestinal tract as well as activation of somatic muscle in the diaphragm and thorax. Similarly, motion sickness is associated with alteration in vestibular function, resulting in nausea and, if intense enough, vomiting. These observations show a close relation between the vestibular system and the autonomic nervous system.

Studies have demonstrated that interactions between the vestibular system and the autonomic nervous system occur on a more physiological or "moment-to-moment" basis.[35,36] These homeostatic mechanisms involve rapid responses in blood pressure control and breathing that are initiated by the vestibular system and result in autonomic and somatic motor responses. As an example, these reflex mechanisms are initiated

when a person stands up from a supine position. When such an event happens, gravity acts to pool blood in the legs and to exert a downward pull on the diaphragm. Pooling of blood in the lower extremities is problematic because it can lead to **postural hypotension**. Changes in the diaphragm position can hinder respiratory function. As the postural challenge occurs, otolith organs (see Chapter 10) respond to movements of the head during changes in body position. Information about these postural stimuli are relayed from otolith vestibular sensory organs to vestibular nuclei in the brainstem, which in turn relay information to the sympathetic nervous system and to the somatic nervous system. The sympathetic nervous system responds with an increase in sympathetic efferent nerve activity, which helps to elevate arterial pressure by vasoconstricting blood vessels in the legs and increasing cardiac output. The somatic nervous system responds to augment breathing by activating somatic motor nerves to the diaphragm, intercostal muscles, and abdominal muscles. The sum of these vestibular responses allows us better to adjust physiologically to changes in posture. These vestibuloautonomic interactions also work in concert with other autonomic reflexes such as the arterial baroreceptor reflex in the control of blood pressure. Ultimately, all of these reflexes act together to help maintain homeostasis.

Autonomic Denervation

An interesting phenomenon occurs when autonomic innervation to an organ is interrupted—that is, when an organ is **denervated**.[37,38] Denervated organs are said to become **supersensitive**, which means that they acquire an increased responsiveness to stimulation, such as can result from circulating substances. Conceptually, you can look at supersensitivity as a way for a denervated organ to maintain function in the face of markedly diminished or absent autonomic stimulation. The development of supersensitivity in autonomically innervated tissues—such as smooth muscle and glands—is an important distinction from what occurs in skeletal muscle, where denervation of somatic nerves eventually leads to persistent flaccid paralysis and atrophy of the muscle.

Because all autonomic innervation involves both preganglionic and postganglionic neurons, functional denervation may result from impairment of either preganglionic or postganglionic neurons. With denervation of preganglionic neurons, the postganglionic neuron remains intact and still spontaneously releases small amounts of the neurotransmitter, which reduces the degree of supersensitivity because the target organ is still stimulated, although at a much lower level. Denervation of postganglionic neurons leads to a greater degree of supersensitivity because the target organ receives no stimulation, other than possibly from circulating hormones.

Supersensitivity can be observed with parasympathetic denervation in a variety of tissues, such as lacrimal and salivary glands. An example of supersensitivity after sympathetic denervation can be found in control of pupillary diameter as a result of damage to the superior cervical ganglion (see section on Horner's Syndrome, later). Immediately after the damage, miosis occurs because of lack of dilator effects of sympathetic innervation coupled with the unopposed pupillary constrictor effect of parasympathetic activity. After several weeks, the pupil begins to dilate, and this dilation becomes more evident in stressful or emotional situations. The explanation for the development of pupil dilation is that the dilator muscle of the iris becomes supersensitive to catecholamines (e.g., to epinephrine and norepinephrine) circulating in the blood. A major source of circulating epinephrine and norepinephrine is the adrenal medulla, which increases secretion of catecholamines under stressful or emotional conditions.

Clinical Correlations

Horner's Syndrome

Horner's syndrome is caused by loss of sympathetic innervation to the head.[7,39,40] The effects of Horner's syndrome include small pupillary diameter, drooping of the eyelid, loss of sweating to the head, and vasodilation in the skin of the face. The small pupillary diameter, or miosis, occurs because the sympathetic nervous system tonically innervates the radial, or dilator, muscle of the iris. Loss of the tonic pupillary dilator influence allows the circular muscle of the iris, which is innervated by the parasympathetic nervous system, to act unopposed to promote pupillary constriction (i.e., miosis). The eyelid drooping or **ptosis** occurs because of interruption of sympa-

thetic innervation to Müller's muscle, a smooth muscle that helps raise the eyelid. **Anhidrosis**, the absence of sweating, and vasodilation of the facial skin are also consequences of interruption of sympathetic innervation to sweat glands and arterial blood vessels in the head. Horner's syndrome can occur on only one side of the face and head, depending on the nature of the cause (i.e., an injury or a tumor).

Hypertension

Hypertension, which is commonly known as high blood pressure, is the most common problem associated with the cardiovascular system.[41,42] The number of hypertensive people in the United States may be as high as 60 million, with one third of these people as yet undetected. Hypertension contributes to at least a quarter of a million deaths per year through damage to important organs such as the brain, heart, and kidneys. Hypertension can lead to cerebrovascular accidents. Coronary heart disease, leading to problems such as heart attacks, occurs three to five times more frequently in hypertensive people. Thirty percent of the deaths due to kidney failure are associated with hypertension.

Hypertension has many causes, combinations of which are responsible for the continued increase in blood pressure. Increased sympathetic outflow is one important factor that aids in the development and maintenance of high blood pressure. To understand how an increased level of sympathetic nervous system activity causes hypertension, you must first understand how the cardiovascular system operates. Basically, the heart provides the energy for circulating the blood through the body. When the heart contracts, it pumps blood into the aorta, which then forces blood into the large arteries and then into smaller and smaller blood vessels. Ultimately, blood goes into the capillaries, where an exchange of nutrients and waste products occurs, and finally, the blood is collected by the venous system, which returns it to the heart. In this system, two major factors determine the level of blood pressure. These factors are the amount of blood pumped by the heart—or cardiac output—and peripheral vascular resistance.

As previously noted, the sympathetic nervous system influences both cardiac output and vascular resistance. Under short-term, stressful situations, arterial blood pressure must be increased to keep enough blood flowing to the essential organs, such as the brain and heart. The most common way to increase arterial pressure on a short-term basis is through activation of the sympathetic nervous system, which increases cardiac output and peripheral vascular resistance. Thus, the sympathetic nervous system is important because it allows us to respond to emergency situations; a problem arises, however, when sympathetic outflow remains elevated and thus keeps arterial pressure high. This sustained increase in sympathetic outflow probably does not occur at one single time but, for reasons that are still not clear, develops gradually over years to help cause and maintain high blood pressure. The importance of the sympathetic nervous system in hypertension is easily demonstrated through the large number of drugs used to treat hypertension that act through interfering with the sympathetic nervous system. Examples of these agents are beta-adrenergic blocking drugs, such as propranolol (a combined beta$_1$- and beta$_2$-adrenergic receptor antagonist agent) and atenolol (a specific beta$_1$ antagonist agent). Beta-adrenergic blocking agents are thought to produce at least part of their actions by reducing the sympathetic drive to the heart, leading to a fall in cardiac output. Other antagonist agents, such as prazosin (an alpha$_1$-adrenergic blocking agent) act by reducing vascular muscle constriction (vasoconstriction) by interfering with the effects of norepinephrine released from sympathetic nerves.

An interesting form of hypertension that is associated with activation of adrenergic receptors is caused by **pheochromocytoma**. Pheochromocytomas are tumors of the cells in the adrenal medulla that secrete catecholamines. The effects of pheochromocytomas are due to the release of very large amounts of catecholamines, which enter the circulation and cause hypertension by activating alpha- and beta-adrenergic receptors. Although pheochromocytomas are rare, occurring in 0.1% of hypertensive people, this form of hypertension demonstrates the significance of an increased level of catecholamine release.

Postural Hypotension

Hypotension is simply low blood pressure. Postural or orthostatic hypotension is a condition in which a person feels lightheaded or faint as a result of rapidly standing up from a recumbent or sitting position.[3,40] The dizziness results from insufficient perfusion of the brain. One cause involving the autonomic nervous system is an impairment of the arterial baroreceptor reflex, which, as previously discussed, normally helps to maintain blood flow to the brain. Baroreflex impairment could in theory result from a dysfunction anywhere in the baroreflex loop, including the sensory receptors, central nervous system integration, peripheral sympathetic or parasympathetic nerves, or the end-organ responses in the heart or blood vessels. In quadriplegic or paraplegic patients, significant hypotension and pooling of blood in the extremities may occur because of interruption of sympathetic control from higher brain centers. Problems are also found with peripheral autonomic efferent nerves in diabetes, a subject discussed in the next section. Postural hypotension may result as a side effect of drugs, as in the condition observed when patients are administered antihypertensive agents that interfere with efferent sympathetic neurotransmission.

Diabetic Autonomic Neuropathy

Diabetes mellitus produces widespread problems throughout the body. One important complication of diabetes occurs as the result of damage to the peripheral nervous system, which is evident in the somatic sensory nerves and the autonomic nervous system. The earliest problems appear primarily to involve small, myelinated and unmyelinated neurons. The clinical symptoms of **diabetic autonomic neuropathy** can be widespread, but abnormalities are often associated with cardiovascular control and gastrointestinal motility.[40,43] One problem frequently observed is postural hypotension, which is primarily due to an impairment of baroreceptor reflex-mediated vasoconstriction. This problem appears to result from reduced reflex vasoconstriction, which likely is due to damage to sympathetic nerves innervating the arterial blood vessels controlling peripheral resistance. Diminished sympathetic control of blood vessels in the splanchnic and subcutaneous vascular beds is often observed in diabetes. Reduced sympathetic control of subcutaneous blood flow contributes to decreased sweating in the extremities and to development of neuropathic foot problems in patients with diabetes.

Damage to parasympathetic nerves also occurs, and is evident in control of heart rate. For example, under normal resting conditions, one of the indications of parasympathetic dominance over control of heart rate is a slight irregular interval between heart beats. In diabetes, parasympathetic innervation to the heart is damaged, resulting in a more regular heart beat; in other words, there is less variability in heart rate. Thus, one clinical indication of diabetic autonomic neuropathy is a reduced heart rate variability. Reflex reductions in heart rate due to parasympathetic activation are also impaired.

In addition to cardiovascular alterations, diabetic autonomic neuropathy may also be associated with other clinical symptoms, such as impotence, bladder dysfunction, diarrhea, impaired motility of the gastrointestinal tract, and gallbladder dysfunction.

Autonomic Dysreflexia

Autonomic dysreflexia (also termed autonomic hyperreflexia, paroxysmal hypertension, paroxysmal neurogenic hypertension, autonomic spasticity, **sympathetic hyperreflexia**, and mass reflex) is an acute condition commonly seen in patients with cervical and upper thoracic spinal cord injuries.[44–46] This syndrome is characterized by a massive, generalized sympathetic discharge in response to stimuli that are largely innocuous in spinal-intact humans. Examples of stimuli that can cause autonomic dysreflexia include increased pressure in the bladder or colon, constrictive clothing in the lower extremities, labor contractions, or even light pinpricks of the legs. Although the onset of symptoms is highly variable, as many as 85% of quadriplegics and high paraplegics may experience this potentially life-threatening situation. The onset of symptoms usually occurs after the spinal shock phase associated with the initial trauma, but the first signs of autonomic dysreflexia have been reported as long as 15 years after the injury. Many of the characteristic symptoms involve the autonomic nervous system. For example, hypertension and excessive sweating occur above the lesion and are attributable to increased sympathetic efferent nerve activity. Similarly, bradycardia occurs in response to the increased blood pressure and is due to a baroreceptor reflex-mediated increase in parasympathetic efferent nerve activity to the heart. Other symptoms that involve the autonomic nervous system include flushing of the face, cutaneous vasodilation above the lesion and vasoconstriction below the lesion, nasal obstruction, severe, throbbing headache, and piloerection. Autonomic dysreflexia

is primarily experienced in patients with lesions above T6, but has been reported in patients with lesions below T6 as well.

Because quadriplegic patients are often hypotensive under resting conditions, the high blood pressures that develop during autonomic dysreflexia represent pressure changes of a magnitude that can result in cerebrovascular hemorrhage and death. This elevation in arterial pressure is a special concern because cerebrovascular accidents are a common cause of death in patients with spinal cord injury.

REFERENCES

1. Cannon WB. Organization for physiological homeostasis. *Physiol Rev* 1929;9:399–431.
2. Langley JN, Dickinson WL. On the local paralysis of the peripheral ganglia and on the connections of different classes of nerve fibers with them. *Proc R Soc Lond* 1889;46:423–431.
3. Bowman WC, Rand MJ. *Textbook of pharmacology.* 2nd ed. London: Blackwell Scientific Publications, 1980.
4. Carrier O Jr. *Pharmacology of the peripheral autonomic nervous system.* Chicago: Year Book Medical Publishers, Inc., 1972.
5. Appenzeller O. Anatomy and histology. In: *The autonomic nervous system: an introduction to basic and clinical concepts.* 4th ed. Amsterdam: Elsevier Science Publishers B.V. (Biomedical Division), 1990:1–33.
6. Lefkowitz RJ, Hoffman BR, Taylor P. Neurotransmission: the autonomic and somatic nervous systems. In: Hardman JG, Limbird LE, Molinoff PB, Ruddon RW, Goodman GA, eds. *The pharmacological basis of therapeutics.* 9th ed. New York: McGraw-Hill, 1996:105–140.
7. Carpenter MB, Sutin J. *Human neuroanatomy.* 8th ed. Baltimore: Williams & Wilkins, 1983.
8. Jänig W, Sundlöf G, Wallin BG. Discharge patterns of sympathetic neurons supplying skeletal muscle and skin in man and cat. *J Auton Nerv Syst* 1983;7:239–256.
9. Loewi O. Über humorale Übertragbarkeit der Herznervenwirkung. *Pflugers Arch* 1921;239–242.
10. Burnstock G. The changing face of autonomic neurotransmission. *Acta Physiol Scand* 1986;126:67–91.
11. Lundberg JM, Hökfelt T. Multiple coexistence of peptides and classical transmitters in peripheral autonomic and sensory neuron: functional and pharmacological. *Prog Brain Res* 1986;68:241–262.
12. Cooper JR, Bloom FE, Roth RH. *The biochemical basis of neuropharmacology.* 6th ed. New York: Oxford University Press, 1991.
13. Taylor P. Anticholinesterase agents. In: Hardman JG, Limbird LE, Molinoff PB, Ruddon RW, Goodman GA,

eds. *The pharmacological basis of therapeutics*. 9th ed. New York: McGraw-Hill, 1996:161–176.

14. Kenakin TP, Bond RA, Bonner TI. II. Definition of pharmacological receptors. *Pharmacol Rev* 1992;44:351–362.

15. Insel PA. Adrenergic receptors: evolving concepts and clinical implications. *N Engl J Med* 1996;334:580–585.

16. Ahlquist RA. A study of adrenotropic receptors. *Am J Physiol* 1948;153:589–599.

17. Minneman KP, Esbenshade TA. α_1-Adrenergic receptor subtypes. *Annu Rev Pharmacol* 1994;34:117–133.

18. Hoffman BB, Lefkowitz RJ. Catecholamines, sympathetic drugs, and adrenergic receptor antagonists. In: Hardman JG, Limbird LE, Molinoff PB, Ruddon RW, Goodman GA, eds. *The pharmacological basis of therapeutics*. 9th ed. New York: McGraw-Hill, 1996:199–248.

19. Bylund DB, Eikenberg DC, Hieble JP, et al. International union of pharmacology nomenclature of adrenoreceptors. *Pharmacol Rev* 1994;46:121–136.

20. Lands AM, Luduena FP, Buzzo JP. Differentiation of receptors responsive to isoproterenol. *Life Sci* 1967;6:2241–2249.

21. Emorine LJ, Marullo S, Briend-Sutren M-M, et al. Molecular characterization of the human β-3-adrenergic receptor. *Science* 1989;245:1118–1121.

22. Emorine L, Blin N, Strosberg AD. The human beta 3-adrenoreceptor: the search for a physiological function. *Trends Pharmacol Sci* 1994;15:3–7.

23. Dale HH. The beginnings and the prospects of neurohumoral transmission. *Pharmacol Rev* 1954;6:7–13.

24. Elgin RM, Reddy H, Watson N, Challiss RAJ. Muscarinic acetylcholine receptor subtypes in smooth muscle. *Trends Pharmacol Sci* 1994;15:114–119.

25. Brown JH, Taylor P. Muscarinic receptor agonists and antagonists. In: Hardman JG, Limbird LE, Molinoff PB, Ruddon RW, Goodman GA, eds. *The pharmacological basis of therapeutics*. 9th ed. New York: McGraw-Hill, 1996:141–160.

26. Cannon WB. *The wisdom of the body*. New York: WW Norton, 1932.

27. Schmidt RF, Thews G. *Human physiology*. New York: Springer-Verlag, 1983.

28. Berne RM, Levy MN. *Physiology*. 3rd ed. St. Louis: Mosby, 1993.

29. Vander AJ, Sherman JH, Luciano DS. *Human physiology: the mechanisms of body function*. 6th ed. New York: McGraw-Hill, 1994.

30. Patton HL, Fuchs AF, Hille B, Scher AM, Steiner R. *Textbook of physiology*. Philadelphia: WB Saunders, 1989.

31. Spyer KM. The central nervous organization of reflex circulatory control. In: Loewy AD, Spyer KM, eds. *Central regulation of autonomic functions*. New York: Oxford University Press, 1990:168–188.

32. DeGroat WC, Steers WD. Autonomic regulation of the urinary bladder and sexual organs. In: Loewy AD, Spyer KM, eds. *Central regulation of autonomic functions*. New York: Oxford University Press, 1990:310–333.

33. Chai TC, Steers WD. Neurophysiology of micturition and continence. *Urol Clin North Am* 1996;23:221–236.

34. Andersson KE, Wagner G. Physiology of penile erection. *Physiol Rev* 1995;75:191–236.

35. Yates BJ. Vestibular influences on the autonomic nervous system. *Ann NY Acad Sci* 1996;781:458–473.

36. Yates BJ, Jakus J, Miller AD. Vestibular effects on respiratory outflow in the decerebrate cat. *Brain Res* 1993;629:209–217.

37. Cannon WB, Rosenblueth A. *The supersensitivity of denervated structures*. New York: MacMillan, 1949.

38. Fleming WW, McPhillips JJ, Westfall DP. Postjunctional supersensitivity and subsensitivity of excitable tissues to drugs. *Rev Physiol Biochem Pharmacol* 1973;68:55–119.

39. Patten J. *Neurological differential diagnosis*. 2nd ed. London: Springer-Verlag, 1995.

40. Freeman R. Autonomic nervous system. In: Stein JH, ed. *Internal medicine*. 3rd ed. Boston: Little, Brown, & Co., 1990:1894–1903.

41. Kaplan N. Arterial hypertension. In: Stein JH, ed. *Internal medicine*. 3rd ed. Boston: Little, Brown, & Co., 1990:235–252.

42. Folkow B. Physiological aspects of primary hypertension. *Physiol Rev* 1982;62:348–504.

43. Watkins PJ. Diabetic autonomic neuropathy. *N Engl J Med* 1990;322:1078.

44. Adler C, Pedretti LW. Spinal cord injury. In: Pedretti LW, Zoltman B, eds. *Occupational therapy: practice skills for physical dysfunction*. 3rd ed. St. Louis: CV Mosby, 1990:582–602.

45. Kurnick NB. Autonomic hyperreflexia and its control in patients with spinal cord lesions. *Ann Intern Med* 1956;44:678–686.

46. Trop CS, Bennett CJ. Autonomic dysreflexia and its urological implications: a review. *J Urol* 1991;146:1461–1469.

HIGHER COGNITIVE FUNCTIONS

16

Neural Mechanisms of Normal Emotions

ALLAN SIEGEL, PhD

JOSEPH W. CHEU, DO, PhD

• • •

Aggression, Emotions, and Rehabilitation Medicine

The neuroanatomy and neurochemistry of aggression are important in rehabilitation medicine because aggression is often involved in both the cause and the result of injuries requiring rehabilitation. Because of their similarities and overall relationships to human affective disorders, investigators have used several animal models of aggression (discussed later in this chapter) to identify the underlying neural mechanisms.[1] Such disorders include episodic dyscontrol, hostility, and aggression after traumatic brain injury (TBI).

In cases of TBI, a number of central nervous system neuronal groups are likely involved in the expression and modulation of aggression. These aggressive acts may be verbal, physical, self-directed, or directed at others.[2] Thus, any process resulting in focal, multifocal, or diffuse axonal damage, especially damage to the temporal and frontal lobes, is likely to affect the mechanisms that subserve aggressive behavior. Complaints of irritability, frustration, loss of temper, and anger are common in studies of TBI survivors. In these patients, problems with modulation of aggression are frequently at the root of family complaints of "change in personality." Moreover, increases in the frequency or intensity of aggressive outbursts are common reasons for admission to rehabilitation hospitals and residential, postacute "behavioral" rehabilitation programs.[3,4]

The displays of aggression vary across TBI patients, although they are often consistent within a given patient and reflect a lowered threshold for triggering aggressive outbursts than the person had before the head injury.[3] The displays characteristically have an all-or-nothing quality, present with a paroxysmal onset, and are frequently short-lived.

Current pharmacologic therapy is unsatisfactory because of its nonspecific effects on behavior. For example, benzodiazepines and other sedatives can produce paradoxical agitation, perhaps by making the patient less capable of coherently processing the environment's events and by further impairing inhibitory mechanisms.[2] Psychostimulants given to improve alertness and attention may lead to unpredictable excessive stimulation and agitation.[3]

To understand and predict the effects of future pharmacologic intervention, understanding the neuronal circuitry, neurophysiology, and related neurochemical mechanisms underlying aggression and related emotional disorders is necessary. Accordingly, we have summarized our knowledge of the neural structures and underlying brain mechanisms that mediate and control aggressive behavior and related processes in the cat. Particular attention has been given to the roles of the limbic system, hypothalamus, and midbrain **periaqueductal gray**. The importance of the study of these structures in the cat is underscored by their remarkable similarities in structure and function to those of the human.[5] Therefore, the dramatic personality changes in patients who have frequent violent episodes can best be understood from the results derived from studies conducted in the cat. Such information may further serve as a basis for the development of therapeutic agents for the treatment of brain disorders such as hyperaggressiveness after TBI and those associated with episodic dyscontrol.

Models of Aggression

The study of the neurobiology of emotional behavior entails the analysis of the brain structures and mechanisms involved in the expression and regulation of specific patterns of behavior that are classified, for lack of better terminology, as "emotional" in nature. Investigators have attempted to develop various models of emotional behavior in different species, which required the use of techniques such as brain ablations, lesions, and electrical or chemical stimulation of the brain. This chapter presents an overview of the neurobiologic substrates underlying several models of emotional behavior, relatively well established from the animal literature, describing experiments where methods such as these have been used, principally in the cat and to a lesser extent in the rat. Accordingly, we have limited our primary discussion to an analysis of the following kinds of emotional responses: **predatory aggression**, **affective defense behavior**, and flight behavior. Some consideration is given to the neurobiology of alcohol-induced modulation of aggression and stress and the psychoneuroimmunologic concomitants of these emotional states. A brief overview of depression as well as its effects on mobility and injuries is also presented.

Neural Models of Aggressive Behavior

Over the past few decades, behavioral models have been established in different species to study the behavioral, physiologic, anatomic, and pharmacologic properties of these responses. Some of these models, described in detail by Moyer,[6] include irritable aggression, which occurs in response to a threat, intimidation, or annoying environmental condition; maternal aggression, which is displayed by a mother reacting to a threat to her recent offspring; fear-induced aggression, which occurs in the presence of an aversive stimulus in the absence of escape; sex-related aggression, which occurs in the presence of the stimulus that evokes sexual behavior (i.e., normally the female) and usually during the act of copulation; territorial aggression, which occurs in the form of a defensive attack, when an intruder enters an animal's defended area; predatory aggression, which constitutes a directed attack by a predator toward a natural prey object; and affective defense (also known as defensive rage), which encompasses the behavior and physiologic processes (and properties) associated with most of these models of aggression, with the exception of **predatory attack**. For this reason, the following discussion is limited to an analysis of affective defense behavior and predatory aggression. This discussion considers the sites in the brain where these responses can be elicited, the basic organization of the anatomic substrates necessary for the expression of these forms of aggression, the brain structures that modulate these responses, and some of their neurochemical regulatory properties.

Defensive Rage Behavior

Defensive rage behavior is a response that is associated with clear-cut, affective signs, including piloerection, retraction of the ears, arching of the back, marked pupillary dilatation, hissing (and sometimes growling), and unsheathing of the claws. Affective defense behavior can be elicited by electrical or chemical stimulation of a cat's brain, and occurs frequently under natural conditions in the environment. As noted previously, such conditions include the presence of a threatening stimulus, such as the presence of a conspecific within its territory, or a situation in which a female cat perceives that its kittens are threatened by another animal. After electrical or chemical stimulation of the appropriate sites in the brain, a cat displays affective defense responses. These responses are directed against a moving object, such as a rat, another cat, or even an experimenter.[7]

In the laboratory, this response can be elicited by electrical stimulation of wide regions of the rostrocaudal extent of the medial hypothalamus and the dorsal portion of the midbrain periaqueductal gray matter of the cat. In addition, similar response patterns have been elicited after microinjections of the cholinergic agonist carbachol were infused into the medial hypothalamus, or when glutamate or related compounds were injected into the midbrain periaqueductal gray [7,8] (Fig. 16–1A).

Anatomic Considerations. Since the early 1970s, a number of new anatomic techniques have allowed investigators to begin to identify the neural circuits involved in the regulation of affective defense behavior and other related responses. Several of the methods have enabled investigators to trace the distribution of fibers associated with a given function from the relevant cell bodies in an anterograde direction (i.e., away from the cell body) to the sites where the axons terminate. The first method uses tritiated amino acid autoradiography, in which an amino acid precursor, such as proline or leucine, is labeled with radioactivity and then microinjected into a region where stimulation can elicit the behavioral response. The cell bodies in that region convert the injected amino acid into protein, which is then transported down the axon to its terminal endings. After the animal is sacrificed, the brain tissue is processed using standard autoradiographic procedures and sectioned into thin slices. Then, by identifying the distri-

bution of label in each section, the light microscope can be used to trace the pathways of interest.[7,8]

A second method uses ^{14}C-2-deoxyglucose (2DG) **autoradiography**, a standard method for metabolic mapping of the brain. Radioactively labeled 2DG is systematically injected into brain sites from which the attack response can be elicited while the stimulation is applied. This technique works on the following principle: local variations in energy metabolism can be visualized because the radioactive glucose analog (i.e., 2DG) is phosphorylated to 2DG-6-phosphate, and is not further metabolized. At this point, the neuron retains this radioactive metabolite because the cell has become impermeable; the pattern of distribution of a radiolabeled metabolite in metabolically active neurons can be determined with autoradiographic methods (i.e., techniques that detect the radioactivity). The rate at which neurons incorporate the radioactive metabolite is related to the rate of glucose utilization, which is itself a function of energy metabolism. In other words, during stimulation of a specific site in the brain from which an attack response can be elicited, the brain regions that are normally involved in the expression of this response and that are anatomically linked to the attack site become more metabolically active. Investigators can take advantage of this activity to use autoradiography as a window into regional brain involvement while a behavior occurs.[7,8]

The third method involves the **retrograde** tracing of neurons from their terminal endings back to their cell bodies of origin. In this approach, a retrograde tracer, such as horseradish peroxidase or Fluoro-Gold, is microinjected into a behaviorally identifiable region and, after a survival period long enough to allow the label to be transported back to the cell and stain that cell, the animal is sacrificed and the brain tissue is processed to identify the labeled cells in question. Using this procedure, an investigator is able to identify the cell groups in particular brain regions that specifically project to sites associated with the attack response. Such information is extremely useful in identifying the nuclear groups of the **limbic system,** for example, which play a critical role in the modulation of these forms of aggression.

The fourth method comprises immunocytochemical procedures, which are used to identify the neurons that synthesize a particular neurotransmitter involved in the modulation of aggressive behavior. The immunocytochemical procedures initially involve sec-

AQ1

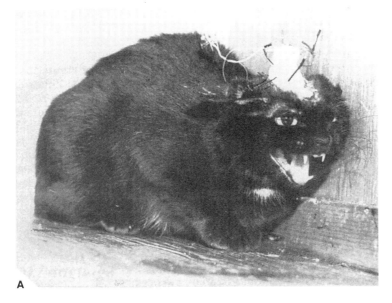

A

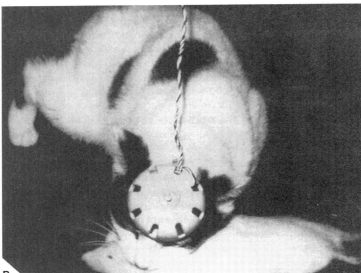

B

Figure 16–1. A: Affective defense behavior elicited by electrical stimulation of the medial hypothalamus of the cat. **B:** Quiet biting attack behavior elicited by electrical stimulation of the lateral hypothalamus of the cat. (Reproduced with permission from Siegel A, Brutus M. Substrates of aggression and rage in the cat. *Progress in Psychobiology and Physiological Psychology.* 1990;14: 135–233.

tioning of the brain tissue on a freezing microtome and then treating it with the primary antibody that binds with the neurotransmitter (neuromodulator) in question on the cell bodies of neurons. In the next step, the tissue is reacted with a secondary antibody that binds with the primary antibody. Because the secondary antibodies have a fluorescence molecule attached to them, the immunopositive cells for a particular neurotransmitter can be seen under a fluorescent microscope.[9]

In addition, a **double-labeling** technique is used to identify the origin and neurochemical properties of neurons that project to a given region and that provide the substrate for the expression or modulation of a given form of aggressive behavior. This method uses a combination of retrograde axonal tracing with the immunocytochemical procedures that are necessary for the (double) labeling of the neurons in question. Here, a retrograde label such as Fluoro-Gold is microinjected into a site in the brain from which the behavior in question could be elicited or from which modulation of a form of aggressive behavior could be obtained. After 1 to 2 weeks, the animal is sacrificed and the brain is sectioned on a freezing microtome. The tissue is immunoreacted for the putative neurotransmitter or neuromodulator in question and analyzed for the presence of double-labeled cells. Because fluorescence and ultraviolet filters on the microscope have different emission and excitation wavelengths, these investigators can identify a double-labeled cell when it is seen separately under each filter[9] (Fig. 16–2).

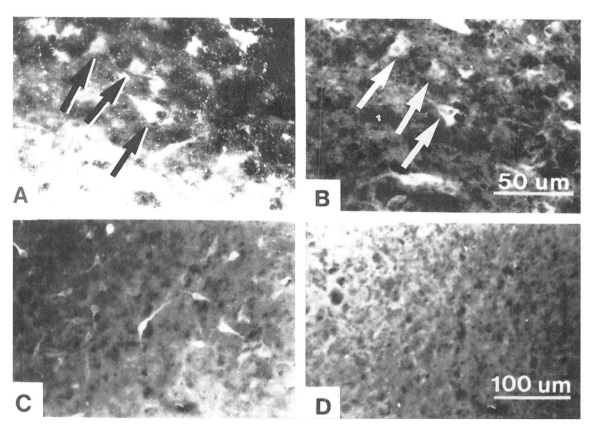

Figure 16–2. Photomicrographs indicate the presence of retrogradely labeled and immunopositive neurons in the medial hypothalamus. Retrogradely labeled cells in the medial hypothalamus were identified after microinjections of Fluoro-Gold into the lateral hypothalamus. Immunocytochemical procedures were used to identify γ-aminobutyric acid (GABA)-immunopositive neurons. Arrows indicate double-labeled neurons for both Fluoro-Gold **(A)** and GABA **(B),** whereas other neurons are labeled only for Fluoro-Gold **(C)** but not for GABA **(D).** These data provided evidence that GABAergic neurons situated in the medial hypothalamus project to the lateral hypothalamus. (Reproduced with permission from Han Y, Shaikh MB, Siegel A. Medial amygdaloid suppression of predatory attack behavior in the cat: II. role of a GABAergic pathway from the medial to the lateral hypothalamus. *Brain Res* 1996;716:72–83).

Pathways Associated With the Expression of Defensive Rage Behavior. As a result of the application of these methods, a picture of the anatomic organization of the pathways associated with affective defense behavior is emerging. These pathways are shown in Figure 16–3. Two principal regions of the brain are vital for the "normal" expression of this behavior: the medial hypothalamus and the midbrain periaqueductal gray.

A series of studies have suggested that the general direction of information flow during affective defense involves ascending groups of fibers from the region of the ventromedial hypothalamus rostrally to the anteromedial hypothalamus. From this region, fibers are then directed caudally into the midbrain periaqueductal gray. The midbrain periaqueductal gray is the most caudal aspect along the neuraxis of

the brain from which an integrated affective defense response can be clearly elicited.[7,8]

Fibers arising from those regions of the periaqueductal gray associated with the expression of affective defense behavior pass caudally into lower levels of the pons and medulla, where they synapse with both somatomotor (i.e., special visceral efferent) neurons such as motor nuclei of cranial nerve V and perhaps VII, and neurons in the brainstem reticular formation that normally are associated with autonomic functions.[10]

In this manner, components of the attack response such as vocalization, increased heart rate and blood pressure, and pupillary dilatation occur because of the anatomic organization of these descending fibers. Activation of motor nuclei of cranial nerves V and VII is probably the necessary and sufficient con-

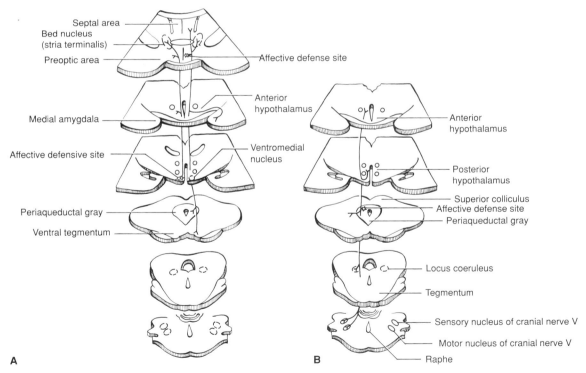

Figure 16–3. Principal projections from **(A)** medial hypothalamus and midbrain periaqueductal gray **(B)** associated with affective defense behavior in the cat. Fibers projecting to the periaqueductal gray from the hypothalamus for the expression of this behavior arise mainly from the anteromedial levels.

dition for the vocalization component of this response. Similarly, activation of selective cell groups in the lower brainstem reticular formation, which project to the autonomic nuclei of the intermediolateral cell columns of the thoracic and lumbar regions of the spinal cord, is the anatomic basis for the autonomic components of this response, such as increased heart rate and blood pressure, as well as pupillary dilatation.

Another interesting feature of the anatomic circuitry for this response is that fibers from the periaqueductal gray also pass rostrally back into the medial hypothalamus to regions from which this response is known to be elicited. Although the significance of such a "feedback loop" has yet to be elucidated, this pathway may represent a positive feedback that is necessary for the response to persist over a given time period. The increased duration of this response is of obvious survival value to the cat when it is accosted by another animal that threatens its existence.[10]

Regions That Modulate Affective Defense Behavior

1. Excitatory Regions and Their Pharmacologic Properties. A number of forebrain structures have important regulatory functions with respect to several forms of aggressive and other related responses. These regions constitute the limbic system. The most significant structure in this regard is the **amygdala**. The amygdala is composed of different groups of subnuclei. The cells in the central and lateral nuclei project caudally through a pathway known as the **ventral amygdalofugal pathway** to the lateral hypothalamus and midbrain periaqueductal gray, and powerfully inhibit the affective defense response.[7]

Other fibers arising from the medial, basomedial, and cortical nuclei of the amygdala form the well defined pathway known as the stria terminalis. Perhaps the most important projection of this system of fibers is to the rostrocaudal extent of the medial hypothalamus, where affective defense behavior can be elicited. This pathway powerfully facilitates the occurrence of this response. Other components of the limbic system that facilitate affective defense behavior include the medial aspect of the **septal area**, the **pyriform cortex**, and the **bed nucleus of the stria terminalis** (Fig. 16–4). The neurochemical mechanisms underlying regulation of defensive rage behavior

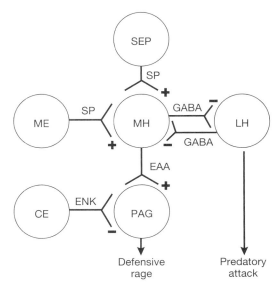

Figure 16–4. Functional circuitry governing modulation of the hypothalamus and midbrain periaqueductal gray from the amygdala and associated structures. The periaqueductal gray receives excitatory and inhibitory inputs from the medial hypothalamus, which receives excitatory inputs from medial amygdala and septal area, and the functions of these projections are mediated by substance P receptors in the medial hypothalamus. The medial hypothalamus, in turn, projects to the lateral hypothalamus. This neuron inhibits neuronal processes associated with the lateral hypothalamus, such as predatory attack behavior, and its functions are mediated by GABA A receptors. The medial hypothalamus also receives inhibitory, GABAergic inputs from the lateral hypothalamus. Thus, reciprocal inhibitory connections exist between the medial and lateral hypothalamus. Such functions would serve a useful ethologic purpose—for example, by reducing the likelihood that characteristics of defensive rage would be present when predatory attack behavior is prepotent. Likewise, the reverse also applies, namely, that when defensive rage is prepotent, characteristics of predatory attack would be suppressed. The likely neurotransmitters for the specific components of this circuitry are indicated. CE, central nucleus of amygdala; EAA, excitatory amino acids; ENK, enkephalins; GABA, γ-aminobutyric acid; LH, lateral hypothalamus; ME, medial amygdala; MH, medial hypothalamus; PAG, midbrain periaqueductal gray; SEP, septal area and its inhibitory functions mediated by GABA A receptors; SP, substance P.

from these regions, however, have yet to be discovered. Thus, a delicate balance of excitatory and inhibitory inputs from the limbic system governs the likelihood of occurrence of an affective defense response.[7,8] As noted later, the limbic system also plays a similar role in the regulation of predatory attack behavior.

A number of different neurotransmitters are important as regulatory mechanisms for this form of aggressive behavior. Several different neurotransmitters seem to have excitatory functions. Catecholamines (i.e., dopamine and norepinephrine) facilitate the occurrence of affective defense behavior, particularly at the level of the anterior medial hypothalamus, where both dopamine and norepinephrine significantly enhance this form of aggression. In view of other functions associated with them, catecholamines may have a general enhancing property that facilitates ongoing responses, so that the amplifying effects observed on affective defense are not specific to this response.

Other putative neurotransmitters that seem to play important roles in the regulation of affective defense are the excitatory amino acids and substance P. The pathway from the (anterior) medial hypothalamus to the midbrain periaqueductal gray that is essential for the expression of this response probably uses excitatory amino acids that bind with the glutamate receptor known as *N*-methyl-D-aspartate (NMDA). Some experiments have shown that substance P neurons, which are present in the medial amygdala, project directly to the medial hypothalamus, where they powerfully facilitate the occurrence of affective defense, by acting on substance P–neurokinin receptors in the medial hypothalamus.

2. Inhibitory Regions and Their Pharmacologic Properties. Neurotransmitters that inhibit affective defense behavior include gamma-aminobutyric acid (GABA) and the enkephalins. At the level of the periaqueductal gray, local injections of the GABA agonist, muscimol, powerfully suppress affective defense behavior. Although the cells of origin of these GABAergic neurons have not been identified, many of these neurons probably constitute "local" interneurons situated within the neuropil of the midbrain periaqueductal gray.

The lateral and medial hypothalamus, which mediate predatory attack and defensive rage behavior in the cat, respectively, are linked by reciprocal inhibitory pathways. These pathways have been shown

to be GABAergic and their inhibitory functions are mediated by GABA A receptors.[8,11]

We should consider the functional significance of these reciprocal GABAergic inhibitory pathways. Because defensive rage and predatory attack are mutually incompatible responses, one possible function of these inhibitory pathways is that each projection serves to block the expression of one of these forms of aggression when the other is prepotent. For example, when an animal is preparing to elicit a predatory response, the mechanism mediating vocalization must be shut down for the element of surprise in capturing the prey object to be effective. Likewise, when defensive rage behavior is required, the mechanism mediating predation must be inhibited for the expression of such components of defensive rage such as pronounced vocalization, paw strike, and arching of the back to take place. In this manner, the reciprocal inhibitory GABAergic pathways between the medial and lateral hypothalamus serve a critical ethologic function by enabling a given form of aggressive response to occur under the appropriate environmental and stimulus conditions.

Other experiments have provided evidence that GABAergic neurons are located in both the lateral and medial hypothalamus. The GABAergic neurons located in the lateral hypothalamus project to the medial hypothalamus, whereas those located in the medial hypothalamus project to the lateral hypothalamus.[11,12] The GABAergic neurons that project from the lateral to medial hypothalamus serve to inhibit affective defense behavior, whereas those that arise from the medial hypothalamus serve to inhibit predatory attack behavior (see later).

Some studies have also indicated that enkephalinergic neurons, whose cells are located in the central and lateral amygdaloid nuclei, project to the midbrain periaqueductal gray and use enkephalins as neurotransmitters. These neurotransmitters are released onto periaqueductal neurons, and their suppressive effects are mediated by μ-opioid receptors.[13]

A variety of experiments have also indicated that serotonergic neurons play an important role in modulating affective defense behavior. Although the overall pattern of results suggests that serotonin (5-hydroxytryptamine [5-HT]) has a general suppressive effect on this form of aggression, some studies have suggested that the modulating effects are receptor selective. Specifically, activation of 5-HT1A receptors in the midbrain periaqueductal gray suppresses affective defense, whereas activation of 5-HT2/1C receptors in the same region facilitates the occurrence of this response.[14] It is clear that future studies must be designed to delineate the roles of other 5-HT receptors in the regulation of different forms of aggressive behavior.

Thus, several lines of research are beginning to reveal functions of different types of receptors as well as the sites of action where different putative neurotransmitters may play highly significant roles in the regulation of this form of aggression. Future studies along these lines will be necessary to understand better the neurochemistry of aggressive behavior and to develop drugs that might control this specific form of behavior.

Predatory Attack Behavior

This form of aggression is clearly predatory in nature. It is characterized by stalking of the prey object (an anesthetized rat, when studied in the laboratory), followed by biting the back of the prey object's neck. Predatory attack behavior has also been well documented in the ethologic literature, indicating that the pattern of response observed from electrical brain stimulation is virtually identical to that which occurs under natural conditions (see Fig. 16–1B). In the laboratory, electrical stimulation of the lateral hypothalamus of the cat elicits predatory attack (on a rat). In addition, stimulation of the ventral aspect of the midbrain periaqueductal gray matter of the cat also elicits predatory attack behavior.[7,8]

Anatomic Considerations. The region of the lateral hypothalamus adjacent to the position of the descending column of the fornix (i.e., perifornical hypothalamus) is the principal site of origin for the descending pathway to the midbrain and pons, thus forming the anatomic substrate for the expression of predatory attack behavior. The fibers descend from different levels of the perifornical hypothalamus to the midbrain periaqueductal gray and to lower regions, such as the reticular formation, nucleus locus ceruleus, and motor nucleus of the trigeminal nerve[8,9] (Fig. 16–5). The integrating properties of the perifornical hypothalamus are evident from these projections for several reasons:

1 As noted for the pathways associated with affective defense behavior, the reticular formation in general, and the nucleus locus ceruleus in particular, receive these hypothalamic inputs.

These areas have significant projections to autonomic nuclei of the lower brainstem and spinal cord (intermediolateral cell columns of the thoracic and lumbar levels) that activate the sympathetic nervous system.

2 Moreover, the projection to the motor nucleus of the trigeminal system is important in producing a jaw-closing response that presumably constitutes the substrate for the biting component of the attack response.

3 Finally, fibers projecting from the midbrain periaqueductal gray that are involved in the expression of predatory attack behavior project rostrally "back" into the lateral hypothalamus. In this manner, such a circuit (i.e., lateral hypothalamus to the midbrain periaqueductal gray to the lateral hypothalamus) would comprise a positive feedback loop that could serve to increase the likelihood that the attack response persists over the period of time required for the response to be successfully completed.

Regions That Modulate Predatory Attack Behavior. The regions that modulate this form of aggressive behavior have been analyzed in considerable detail. In brief, much of the limbic system plays a major role in modulating this response. The overwhelming effect of activation of limbic structures is to inhibit this form of aggression. For example, very powerful suppression of predatory attack occurs from stimulation of the prefrontal cortex, medial amygdala, pyriform cortex, much of the septal area, the bed nucleus of the stria terminalis, the dorsal aspect of the hippocampal formation, and anterior portions of the cingulate gyrus. In contrast, facilitation of predatory attack behavior is associated with the ventral aspect of the hippocampal formation, the far lateral aspect of the septal area, and the central and lateral nuclei of the amygdala[7,8] (Fig. 16–6). Thus, it is reasonable to conclude that, in a manner similar to that described previously for affective defense, the modulatory properties of the limbic system on the lateral hypothalamus serve as a critical mechanism governing whether or not an attack response will occur under given stimulus conditions.

Relationship Between Epilepsy and Aggression. An important question is how these limbic modulating mechanisms might underlie aggressive behavior in humans. One way of assessing such limbic system processes is to observe the effects on behavior when

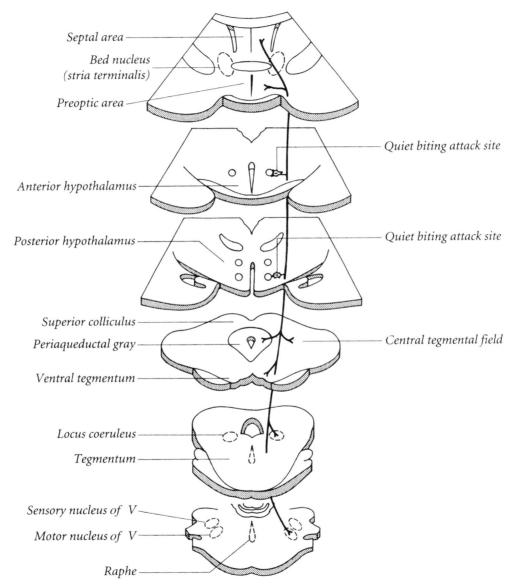

Septal area

Bed nucleus (stria terminalis)

Preoptic area

Quiet biting attack site

Anterior hypothalamus

Posterior hypothalamus

Quiet biting attack site

Superior colliculus

Periaqueductal gray

Central tegmental field

Ventral tegmentum

Locus coeruleus

Tegmentum

Sensory nucleus of V

Motor nucleus of V

Raphe

Figure 16–5. The principal projections of the lateral hypothalamus associated with predatory attack behavior in the cat. These include descending projections to the midbrain periaqueductal gray, ventral tegmentum, locus ceruleus, and the trigeminal complex. (Reproduced from Siegel A, Pott C. Neural substate of aggression and flight in the cat. *Prog Neurobiol* 1988;31:261–283.)

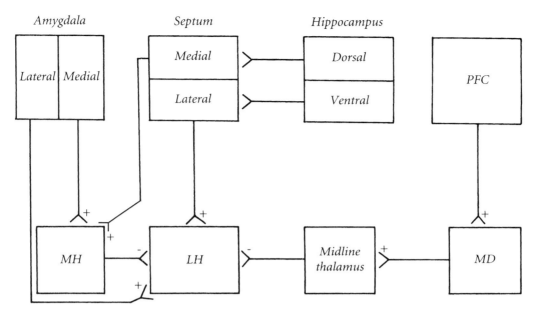

Figure 16–6. Schematic diagram indicating the functional circuitry governing limbic system modulation of predatory attack behavior associated with the lateral hypothalamus. LH, lateral hypothalamus; MD, mediodorsal thalamic nucleus; MH, medial hypothalamus; PFC, prefrontal cortex.

one or more components of this system is disrupted. Human studies have provided compelling evidence supporting the view that patients with disturbances of limbic structures, such as tumors or seizure foci of the temporal lobe (which presumably affect the amygdala and hippocampal formation), display a heightened aggressiveness. In particular, violent reactions typically occur in response to innocuous stimuli. Such responses, indeed, have been referred to as the "episodic dyscontrol syndrome." On the basis of animal studies, the intensity of aggressive responses that occur in the postictal period is probably a function of the location of the epileptic focus in the temporal lobe.

Pharmacologic Properties of Predatory Attack Behavior. In general, much less is known about the pharmacology of the predatory attack system than that of the affective defense system. A number of studies have examined the role of monoamines in this form of aggressive behavior. In brief, experiments using drugs that block the rate-limiting step in the biosynthesis of serotonin (i.e., parachlorophe-

nylalanine) have shown that predatory attack behavior is facilitated after drug administration. These data suggest that serotonin normally inhibits this response.[8] Although the location of the action of serotonin for suppressing this response is unknown, it probably acts directly at the level of the lateral hypothalamus, because fibers from the serotonin-producing neurons of the raphe complex of the midbrain and pons project to this region of hypothalamus. Other studies conducted in the rat suggest that suppression of predatory attack may be mediated by a specific type of serotonin receptor (i.e., the 5-HT1A receptor), as described earlier for affective defense.[15]

Studies have been designed to test whether other neurotransmitters play a role in the regulation of predatory attack behavior. Similar to their effects on affective defense behavior, both norepinephrine and dopamine facilitate predatory attack behavior. Again, the sites in the brain where such transmitters might act remain unknown, but both the central nucleus of the amygdala, which facilitates predatory attack, and the lateral hypothalamus, from which this response can be elicited, receive strong dopaminergic inputs. Accordingly, catecholamines may increase the likelihood that predatory attack will occur by exciting neurons in either (or both) of these structures that play such an important role in the elicitation of this behavior.

Some studies have also sought to determine the effects of other putative neurotransmitters—such as GABA, substance P, and opioid peptides—on predatory attack behavior. Some experiments have indicated that opioid peptides facilitate the occurrence of predatory attack; both substance P and GABA suppress predatory attack.[8,11,16] The anatomic substrate for this mechanism appears to be as follows: substance P neurons, located in the medial amygdala, project to the medial hypothalamus and are excitatory to neurons in this region. In turn, one group of medial hypothalamic neurons are GABAergic; they project to the lateral hypothalamus and inhibit functions associated with that structure such as predatory attack. Thus, the projections from the medial amygdala facilitate affective defense by their excitatory actions on the medial hypothalamus and suppress predatory attack because of the presence of the GABAergic connection from the medial to lateral hypothalamus.

Relevance of Affective Defense and Predatory Attack Behavior to Human Aggression. These two forms of aggression have been reported in child and adolescent psychiatric patients, and they have been classified as subcategories of human aggressive behavior. In this study, the authors described and categorized predatory aggression as controlled, planned, and goal-oriented, and defensive rage as affective (i.e., unplanned, impulsive, uncontrolled, and overt in nature). The reliability of this classification scheme was further demonstrated by cluster analysis using a questionnaire test battery.[17] The significance of these observations underscores the parallels between feline and human aggression and thus points to the value of the respective animal models of aggression in providing insights into the neural mechanisms underlying human aggression.

Effects of Alcohol on Aggression. An expanding body of literature derived from both human and animal studies has clearly demonstrated that alcohol can have a powerful potentiating effect on aggressive behavior.[18] In particular, in humans violent reactions typically follow moderate to heavy alcohol consumption among certain personality types. In others, however, alcohol seems to show little effect on aggression. This finding suggests that alcohol does not produce aggressive behavior, but enhances violent responses in those individuals who are prone to this kind of behavior. Animal studies have shown that low to moderate levels of alcohol consumption can potentiate aggressive responses, whereas very high doses of alcohol reduce aggressiveness, presumably as a result of its effects on sensory and motor systems. More recent work has shown that alcohol administration differentially modulates affective defense and predatory attack by powerfully facilitating the occurrence of affective defense while suppressing predatory attack.[19,20] Alcohol has been shown to have a potent effect on different receptor systems and, in particular, NMDA and GABA receptors.[21] Therefore, alcohol probably modulates aggressive behavior through its effects on one or both of these receptor systems. In support of this view, a most recent study has demonstrated that NMDA receptor blockade in the midbrain periaqueductal gray can block the potentiating effects of alcohol on affective defense behavior. Likewise, GABA receptor blockade in the lateral hypothalamus can also eliminate the suppressive effects of alcohol on predatory attack behavior. A further delineation of the receptor mechanisms governing alcohol's modulating effects on different forms of aggression is essential for development of a better understanding of the mechanisms underlying this process. Such data would also provide the rationale for drug development research aimed at controlling the potentiating effects of alcohol on aggressive behavior.

Flight Behavior

Another form of emotional behavior that can be elicited in both cat and rodent is flight behavior. This response is characterized as an attempt by an animal to escape from an aversive stimulus, such as a predator, competitor, or other stimulus condition that is perceived as threatening. This form of behavior is of great survival value to an animal when it is confronted with a predator in a natural setting. It can be elicited by electrical or chemical stimulation of the medial hypothalamus or midbrain periaqueductal gray matter, and results in a vigorous attempt by the animal to jump out of the experimental chamber.[8]

Anatomic Considerations. The pathways associated with flight, when it is elicited from the hypothalamus, have been described by autoradiographic methods.[8] At the level of the hypothalamus, the fiber pathways essential for elicitation of this response are much more diffuse than those associated with either affective defense behavior or predatory attack behavior. The major projections that pass caudally from the sites in the hypothalamus from which the flight response is elicited exit the medial hypothalamus and enter different aspects of the midbrain and pontine tegmentum, such as the dorsal aspect of the periaqueductal gray and central and ventral tegmental regions. Presumably, these downstream pathways constitute initial components of pathways that ultimately supply the lower brainstem and spinal cord and that are critical for the emotional and somatomotor components of this response (Fig. 16–7).

Other descending fibers from the hypothalamus enter a region of the thalamus called the centre–median–parafascicular complex. This structure plays an important role in the regulation of pain perception. Moreover, when this complex of neurons is destroyed by the placement of lesions, the capacity to elicit flight behavior by electrical stimulation is considerably diminished. It is not clear whether flight behavior actually includes a pain component.

The ascending components of the pathways arising from sites in the hypothalamus from which flight can be elicited supply principally limbic nuclei, such as medial and basal components of the amygdala, the bed nucleus of the stria terminalis, and the septal area. Each of these regions appears to have the capacity to modulate flight behavior. Thus, such projections appear to play an important feedback role in the regulation of this response by modulating the sites in the limbic system that in turn modulate the flight mechanism at the level of the hypothalamus. This kind of mechanism is similar to those involved in the regulation of other processes, such as motor functions, in which (indirect) reciprocal connections exist between cerebellum and frontal lobe, red nucleus, reticular formation, and vestibular nuclei, or between the neocortex and basal ganglia. Thus, feedback mechanisms appear to play a central role in the regulation of a wide variety of processes in the central nervous system, including those associated with affective defense and predatory attack behavior.

Pharmacologic Properties. The role of neurotransmitters in this form of emotional behavior has not been widely investigated. Earlier studies suggested that agonists of the neurotransmitter acetylcholine, injected systemically, could facilitate the occurrence of this response.[8] Later studies reported that local administration of the cholinergic compounds could produce flightlike responses.[8] These findings were confounded, however, by the fact that drug administration frequently produced convulsive seizures as well. Little or no conclusive data are available concerning the possible roles of other putative neurotransmitters in this form of emotional behavior.

Overview of Models of Stress

The models of emotional behavior described previously—affective defense behavior, predatory attack, and flight behavior—are clearly discernible and operationally defined forms of behavior that can easily be elicited in the laboratory, and that closely parallel behavioral patterns that occur normally in nature. In contrast, a number of intrinsic difficulties are inherent in attempting to establish a similar strategy for stress. The most obvious difficulty is one of definition. In humans, in everyday circumstances, stress can appear under a very wide range of conditions and intensities.

Definitions of stress involve both stimulus and response conditions. Stimuli that often induce low levels of stress include slow-moving highway traffic patterns; delays in achieving goal expectancies, such as missing food items in a grocery store that are required for making dinner; learning that you have a flat tire after getting into your car to travel somewhere to give a lecture; or waiting for someone who is late for a date to go to the theater. Illustrations of situations that induce higher levels of stress include conditions that threaten job security, or life-threatening situations, such as being accosted by an armed robber. Such stimuli are known as "stressors." Different types of stressors can produce different types of behavioral and physiologic responses.

The responses made to a given set of environmental stimuli also define stress. Normally, an organism chooses a response pattern that helps it to deal with the stressful stimuli by reducing or eliminating it. Such a behavioral response is generally referred to as "coping behavior." The various kinds of behavioral and physiologic events that occur as response patterns to the stressful stimuli can easily be cataloged. Moreover, one can also measure or evaluate how the brain processes information in the presence of stressful stimuli. Under these circumstances, investigators fre-

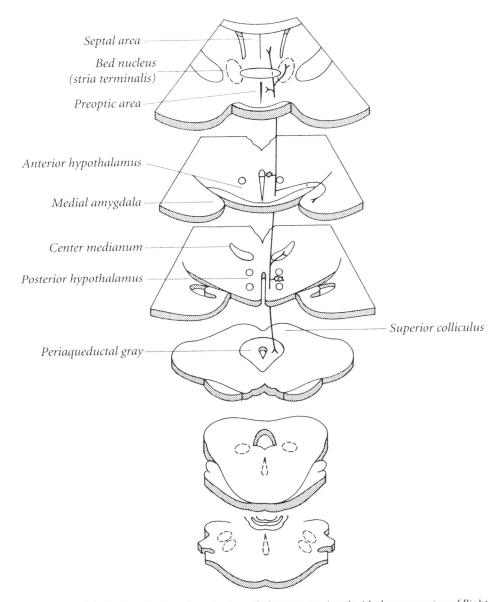

Figure 16–7. Principal projections from the hypothalamus associated with the expression of flight behavior in the cat. Descending fibers project mainly to the midbrain periaqueductal gray, whereas ascending fibers supply limbic structures that regulate emotional behavior associated with the hypothalamus. (Reproduced from Siegel A, Pott C. Neural substrate of aggression and flight in the cat. *Prog Neurobiol* 1988;31:261–283.)

quently attempt to determine what changes occur in the brain in response to stressors, or to determine the effects of activation of specific regions of the brain on the stress response. Thus, the complete definition of stress ought to include the components of stimulus conditions, brain processing mechanisms, and physiologic or behavioral response. Unfortunately, definitions of stress are not entirely uniform because different investigators may use different components as the defining properties. Moreover, our understanding of the biologic nature of stress is further complicated by the fact that different investigators frequently study different response measures as dependent variables in their analysis of stress. Accordingly, we present a brief survey of some of the experimental variables considered in the literature.

Neuroendocrine Components of Stress

Advances in neuroanatomic and neurochemical techniques have permitted investigators to begin to identify the structures and pathways in the brain associated with the ultimate expression of the stress response.[22] One of the most important regions that has been identified in this regard is the paraventricular nucleus of the hypothalamus. This group of cells is significant in synthesizing oxytocin, vasopressin, and corticotropin-releasing factor (CRF). Oxytocin and vasopressin are hormones released through the posterior pituitary. Oxytocin causes uterine contractions at birth and also promotes the milk ejection reflex. Vasopressin promotes water resorption by the kidneys and vasoconstriction. Secretion of CRF also seems to be influenced by oxytocin and vasopressin. CRF is transported down the hypothalamic axon to the anterior pituitary through vascular beds in the ventral hypothalamus to cause the release of adrenocorticotropic hormone (ACTH), which, in turn, causes the release of adrenal steroids. The relationship of this system to stress has been demonstrated in a number of paradigms, including one that focuses on the animal that is defeated in an aggressive encounter as the subject for this model. In this type of experiment, the defeated animal has been shown to have elevated cortisol levels after the fight.

Portions of the limbic system play a significant role in the regulation of ACTH through projections to the paraventricular nucleus region. Two of these limbic structures include the central nucleus of the amygdala and the bed nucleus of the stria terminalis, which receives a major opioid peptide projection from the central nucleus. Evidence that the central nucleus can modulate ACTH release is based on the observation that lesions of this structure can reduce the ACTH release that normally occurs in response to stress produced by immobilization of the animal.

Several neurotransmitter systems, such as opioid peptides and serotonin, have been shown to mediate the release of ACTH. The fact that large numbers of receptors for these neurotransmitters are located adjacent to or within the paraventricular region suggests that these transmitters act directly on this structure. Moreover, in the brain in general and the limbic system in particular, the number of adrenal steroid receptors can change as a function of endocrine manipulations, such as ACTH infusion. Thus, the brain and the endocrine system may communicate about the onset of stress using a delicate negative feedback system. In this manner, the onset of stress probably results in the activation of neurons in several regions of the limbic system, which then influence the release of ACTH from the pituitary by acting on the paraventricular nucleus (as described previously).

Because of the high concentrations of steroid receptors in the limbic system, the release of steroids from the adrenal gland selectively alters neuronal discharge patterns in the limbic system, leading to a modification of limbic system effects on the paraventricular nucleus (Fig. 16–8). The onset of stress significantly alters the effectiveness of this autoregulatory mechanism that controls the release of adrenal steroids during the period of stress. In other words, stress has a disruptive effect on the feedback regulatory mechanism that controls the release of adrenal steroids.

Effects of Peptides on Autonomic Functions Associated With Stress Responses

A variety of peptides in the brain have been shown to influence autonomic nervous system functions typically associated with stress responses. In general, such peptides presumably act either as neurotransmitters or neuromodulators at such sites as the limbic system and hypothalamus. Consistent with this view is the fact that stimulation of the medial hypothalamus results in a massive sympathoadrenal activation typical of intense stress.[22] As indicated earlier in this chapter, this type of physiologic response occurs when affective de-

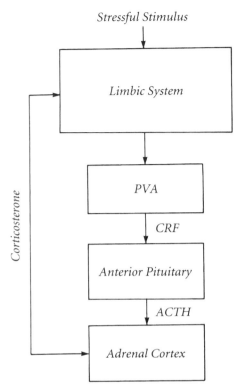

Figure 16–8. Schematic diagram indicating the possibility of negative feedback relationships between the brain and adrenal gland associated with stress. Stressful sensory stimuli may result in activation of several limbic nuclei, such as the amygdala or bed nucleus of the stria terminalis, which in turn stimulate the paraventricular nucleus (PVA) to release corticotropin-releasing factor (CRF). CRF causes the anterior pituitary to release adrenocorticotropic hormone (ACTH), which can then cause the release of corticosterone from the adrenal cortex. The feedback loop may be completed when corticosterone passes through the blood–brain barrier to bind with the corticosterone receptors in these limbic nuclei, thus altering the further release of this hormone.

fense behavior is induced, either under experimental conditions or under normal circumstances, when a cat is under stress as a result of being threatened by another species. Examples of peptides with autonomic regulatory properties include somatostatin, which can cause an increase in heart rate and respiration; β-endorphin, which results in a decreased mean arterial pressure; bombesin, which can inhibit adrenal epinephrine release and cause an increase in blood pressure; angiotensin II, which also produces an increase in mean arterial pressure; and substance P and calcitonin gene-related peptide, which are associated with increases in heart rate.

Effects of Stress on the Immune System

Some studies have begun to provide evidence that powerful stressors (such as divorce or death of a spouse) can cause significant changes in the immune system. In animals, rats subjected to stressful conditions display significant suppression of peripheral blood lymphocyte proliferation. In the brain, opioid peptides may play a significant role in the regulation of this response, acting perhaps at the level of the midbrain periaqueductal gray, the central nucleus of the amygdala, or the bed nucleus of the stria terminalis. Some studies have demonstrated that neuronal activity in the limbic system and, in particular, the amygdala and anatomically related regions, can significantly modify autonomic and immune functions. Perturbation of these regions can produce neuroimmunomodulation by altering, for example, cytokine production, nonkiller cell activity, CRF activity, and T-cell mitogen responses.[23,24] Little is known about the specific mechanisms by which the brain controls immune function, or how brain mechanisms are altered by changes in immune function. An understanding of these mechanisms will be obtained only when the specific receptors and related neuronal circuitry have been identified.

Neural Correlates of an Animal Model of Depression

Human depression is a very complex disorder. Therefore, investigators have developed several models in the rat. Each model is characterized by reduced exploratory behavior, such as locomotion in the open field, and reduced rearing behaviors. This form of behavior is a valid model because in human depression patients display withdrawal and inactivity. In one approach, α-methyl-paratyrosine, a drug that inhibits tyrosine hydroxylase (the rate-limiting enzyme in the biosynthesis of both dopamine and norepinephrine), is administered to the rat systemically at various times during the day. A second approach is to administer amphetamine base (extracted from amphetamine sulfate) together with a nonoxidizing vehicle, polyethylene glycol, subcutaneously. A third approach is to subject the animal to chronic stress in which the stressors are administered in a semirandom fashion over several weeks. Examples of these stressors include electrical foot shock, food or water deprivation, cold swim at 7°C, or shaking in a rotational device for 30 minutes.

Using these models of depression, 2DG autoradiography was used to identify the structures that become metabolically reduced or activated in these rats.[25] Regional glucose utilization measurements, which indicate changes in brain metabolism, revealed that regional glucose metabolism was elevated in the lateral habenula nucleus in each of the three models. Regional metabolic rates were reduced, however, in the medial prefrontal cortex, in the anterior ventral nucleus of the thalamus, and in the inferior colliculus. Moreover, general forebrain levels of glucose utilization were decreased in a global fashion. Although studies of this kind are in a relatively preliminary stage, newer techniques make possible similar kinds of metabolic mapping in the human that could then be compared with evolving data in lower forms. These animal models of depression hold out the possibility that future studies will be able to unravel more precisely the specific anatomic substrates and mechanisms that underlie this clinical state.

Clinical Correlations

This chapter has presented an overview of the literature about the neural bases of different forms of emotional behavior. This review is by no means exhaustive. Instead, it focuses on selective forms of emotional behavior because our present understanding of the neurobiology of emotions has evolved in part from models based on these forms of behavior. These models include affective defense behavior, predatory attack behavior, and flight behavior, with some additional consideration given to the topics of stress and depression. It should be obvious that much of our knowledge of the neurobiology of emotions remains incomplete. It is hoped that we will gain a better understanding of this subject as more sophisticated research tools, which can be applied to the existing models of emotional behavior, become available. Such accomplishments will provide greater insights into the mechanisms underlying re-

lated emotional processes and associated disturbances in humans, which can ultimately lead to rational therapeutic treatments for these conditions.

REFERENCES

1. Siegel A. Aggression in epilepsy: animal models. In: Devinsky O, Theodore WH, eds. *Epilepsy and behavior.* New York: Alan R. Liss, 1991:390–404.
2. McAllister TW. Neuropsychiatric sequelae of head injuries. *Psychiatr Clin North Am* 1992;15:395–413.
3. Whyte J, Rosenthal M. Rehabilitation of the patient with head injury. In: DeLisa JA, ed. *Rehabilitation medicine: principles and practice.* Philadelphia: JB Lippincott, 1992:585–608.
4. Brooke MM, Questad KA, Patterson DR, Bashak KJ. Agitation and restlessness after closed head injury: a prospective study of 100 consecutive admissions. *Arch Phys Med Rehabil* 1992;73:320–323.
5. Carpenter MB, Sutin J. *Human neuroanatomy.* Baltimore: Williams & Wilkins, 1983.
6. Moyer KE. *The psychology of aggression.* New York: Harper and Row, 1976.
7. Siegel A, Brutus M. Neural substrates of aggression and rage in the cat. *Progress in Psychobiology and Physiological Psychology* 1990;14:135–233.
8. Siegel A, Pott C. Neural substrate of aggression and flight in the cat. *Prog Neurobiol* 1988;31:261–283.
9. Schubert K, Shaikh MB, Siegel A. NMDA receptors in the midbrain periaqueductal gray mediate hypothalamically evoked hissing behavior in the cat, *Brain Res* 1996;762:80–90.
10. Shaikh MB, Barrett JA, Siegel A. The pathways mediating affective defense and quiet biting attack behavior from the midbrain central gray: an autoradiographic study. *Brain Res* 1987;437:9–25.
11. Han Y, Shaikh MB, Siegel A. Medial amygdaloid suppression of predatory attack behavior in the cat: I. role of a substance P pathway from the medial amygdala to the medial hypothalamus. *Brain Res* 1996;716:59–71.
12. Cheu JW, Siegel A. GABA A receptor mediated suppression of feline defensive rage behavior: role of the lateral hypothalamus. *Brain Res* 1998;783:293–304.
13. Shaikh MB, Lu CL, Siegel A. An enkephalinergic mechanism involved in amygdaloid suppression of affective defense behavior elicited from the midbrain periaqueductal gray in the cat. *Brain Res* 1991;559:109–117.
14. Shaikh MB, De Lanerolle N, Siegel A. Serotonin 5-HT1A and 5-HT2/1C receptors in the midbrain periaqueductal gray differentially modulate defensive rage behavior elicited from the medial hypothalamus of the cat. *Brain Res* 1997;765:198–207.
15. Miczek KA, Haney M, Tidey J, Vivian J, Weerts E. Neurochemistry and pharmacotherapeutic management of

aggression and violence. In: Reiss AJ Jr, Miczek KA, Roth JA, eds. *Understanding and preventing violence.* Vol. 2. Washington: National Academy Press, 1994:245–514.

16. Han Y, Shaikh MB, Siegel A. Medial amygdaloid suppression of predatory attack behavior in the cat: II. role of a GABAergic pathway from the medial to the lateral hypothalamus. *Brain Res* 1996;716:72–83.

17. Vitiello B, Behar D, Hunt J, Stoff D, Ricciuti A. Subtyping aggression in children and adolescents. *J Neuropsychiatry Clin Neurosci* 1990;2:189–192.

18. Miczek KA, DeBold JF, Haney M, Tidey J, Vivian J, Weerts EM. Alcohol, drugs of abuse, aggression and violence. In: Reiss AJ Jr, Miczek KA, Roth JA, eds. *Understanding and preventing violence*. Vol. 2. Washington: National Academy Press, 1994:377–570.

19. Schubert K, Shaikh MB, Han Y, Pohorecky L, Siegel A. Differential effect of ethanol upon feline rage and predatory attack behavior: an underlying neural mechanism. *Alcohol Clin Exp Res* 1996;20:882–889.

20. Siegel A, Schubert K, Shaikh MB. Neurotransmitters regulating defensive rage behavior in the cat. *Neurosci Biobehav Rev* 1997;21:733–742.

21. Crews F, Morrow AL, Criswell H, Breese G. Effects of ethanol on ion channels. *Int Rev Neurobiol* 1996;39:283–367.

22. Brown MR, Koob JF, Rivier C, eds. *Stress: neurobiology and neuroendocrinology*. New York: Marcel Dekker, Inc., 1991.

23. Demetrikopoulos MK, Siegel A, Schleifer SJ, Obede J, Keller SE. Electrical stimulation of the dorsal midbrain periaqueductal gray suppresses peripheral blood natural killer cell activity. *Brain Behav Immun* 1994;8:218–228.

24. Haas HS, Schauenstein K. Neuroimmunomodulation via limbic structures: the neuroanatomy of psychoimmunology. *Prog Neurobiol* 1997;51:195–222.

25. Caldecott-Hazard S, Mazziotta J, Phelps M. Cerebral correlates of depressed behavior in rats, visualized using 14C-2-deoxyglucose autoradiography. *J Neurosci* 1988;8:1951–1961.

Neural Mechanisms of Learning and Memory

MARY FRANCES BAXTER, MA, OTR
DOUGLAS A. BAXTER, PhD

• • •

In rehabilitation, many patients have conditions in which learning and memory deficits are primary or secondary characteristics of their diagnoses, such as Alzheimer's disease (for reviews, see Albert,[1] Gabrieli,[2] and Weiner et al.[3]). Many other conditions and diagnoses have known deficits in learning and memory, including **traumatic brain injury**, cerebral vascular accident (CVA), tumors of the central nervous system (CNS), autism, schizophrenia, and many of the chromosomal disorders.[4]

A fundamental tenet of rehabilitation is that the brain is plastic and that therapists can affect functions of the brain, as demonstrated by changes in the behaviors and skills of clients. Thus, an important aspect of training to be a rehabilitation therapist must include an understanding of the mechanisms underlying neural plasticity, learning, and memory. Such an understanding helps foster a better comprehension of diseases or conditions that affect learning and memory and provides insights into therapeutic techniques that exploit the intrinsic, plastic properties of the nervous system.

We introduce some of the well established general concepts and basic principles that underlie the research on synaptic plasticity and cellular mechanisms of learning and memory, which is an exciting and rapidly changing area of research in neuroscience. We also touch on some of the data linking the results from cellular studies of synaptic plasticity to techniques of behavioral modification and learning. The chapter ends with a discussion of how, using certain techniques and principles derived from simple forms of learning, motor tasks can be relearned after injury to the nervous system.

Definitions

The concepts of learning and memory are inextricably related; memory is the persistence of learning that can be expressed later as needed.

Learning

A traditional definition of learning is a change in behavior as a result of experience, and memory is the ability to store and recall learned experiences. These definitions are less than ideal, however, because some examples of learning do not involve overt behavioral changes. For example, learning may represent a change in an internal state that is behaviorally "silent" and therefore represents a process that is a "potential" for a change in behavior, rather than an immediate change in behavior. In addition, any definition of learning should distinguish learning from maturational changes and from changes in behavior produced by injury or fatigue. A fairly general definition of learning has been provided by Yadin Dudai[5]: *learning* is an experience-dependent generation of enduring internal representations, or modification in such representations. *Experience* excludes changes related to maturation, injury, and fatigue.

Memory

Memory is the retention of these experience-dependent changes over time. The temporal domains of memory vary considerably, from short-term forms lasting minutes, such as the memory of a telephone number, to long-term forms lasting days, weeks, or lifetimes, such as the memory of a childhood experience. In some cases, a short-term memory can be stabilized into an enduring long-term form. This process is known as *consolidation*. Finally, the process that allows memory to be accessed is *retrieval*, the use of memory in neuronal and behavioral operations.

Different Types of Learning Paradigms

Discussion of the cellular neurophysiology of learning and memory should include a brief review of some of the most common examples of simple learning paradigms that have been described at the behavioral level. The cellular analogues and mechanisms are being investigated for these examples of learning. Neurobiologists studying the cellular basis of learning and memory use paradigms that were initially developed to condition motor responses. These examples of learning are defined by the procedures (i.e., paradigms) used to produce them. Two broad categories of learning paradigms are the nonassociative and associative learning paradigms (Fig. 17–1).

Nonassociative Learning

Associative learning paradigms include **classical conditioning** (also known as Pavlovian conditioning) and **operant conditioning** (also know as instrumental conditioning). In both of these examples of associative learning, two events or stimuli are temporally paired. Associative learning allows an animal to draw conclusions about causal relationships in its environment. In contrast, nonassociative learning paradigms do not involve any temporal relationship between stimuli. Examples of this form of learning are **habituation** and **sensitization**. These two paradigms are attractive to scientists because the stimuli can be precisely controlled and there is usually a well defined behavioral response. Moreover, through nonassociative learning paradigms, the neural pathways of many reflexive behaviors have been described. This knowledge of the circuit enables powerful cell biologic approaches to be applied to the analysis of the underlying mechanisms.

Habituation

Habituation, perhaps the simplest example of nonassociative learning, refers to a decrement of a behav-

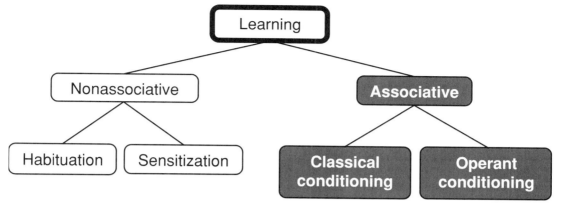

Figure 17–1. Categories of learning. In behavioral experiments, different examples of learning are distinguished by the paradigms used to present stimuli. Associative paradigms involve a close temporal relation between two stimuli (e.g., classical conditioning) or between a behavior and a reinforcement (e.g., operant conditioning) for learning to occur. In contrast, nonassociative paradigms do not involve a specific temporal relationship among stimuli. The two simplest and most common examples of nonassociative learning are habituation and sensitization, both of which occur in a wide variety of response systems and, therefore, are fundamental properties of behavior. The two most common examples of associative learning are classical (or Pavlovian) conditioning and operant (or instrumental) conditioning.

ioral response during repetitive application of an innocuous or benign stimulus. For example, a person learns to ignore the ticking of a mechanical clock. Habituation is a universal phenomenon and the term can be applied to many isolated components of behavior. Habituation is distinguished from simple fatigue because responsiveness can be rapidly restored (i.e., dishabituated) by the presentation of a strong or novel stimulus to the animal. The duration of habituation can be from minutes (i.e., short term) to weeks (i.e., long term). Thompson and Spencer have described the parametric features of habituation.[6]

Sensitization
Sensitization (also known as pseudoconditioning) is another example of nonassociative learning. The term refers to the strengthening of a response after an intense or noxious stimulus. For example, the unexpected explosion of a firecracker can make a person "jumpy," and after this intense stimulus any small noise can elicit a heightened response. The sensitizing stimulus activates general arousal mechanisms. Thus, the response has no specificity and responses to a wide variety of stimuli are enhanced. A single sensitizing stimulus can induce short-term sensitization (i.e., a behavioral enhancement lasting min-

utes), whereas repeated training can induce long-term sensitization (i.e., a heightened responsiveness lasting weeks).

Associative Learning

Classical Conditioning
Classical conditioning is a type of associative learning in which presentation of a reinforcing (unconditional) stimulus is contingent on the presentation of a preceding (conditional) stimulus. The change in behavior produced by repeated pairing of the two stimuli can be measured in a number of ways. An example of classical conditioning involves the training procedure originally described by Pavlov to condition salivation in dogs.[7] Before training, meat powder, the unconditional stimulus (US), reliably elicits salivation, the unconditional response (UR). The signal for the presentation of the US is called the conditional stimulus (CS), and, in the original experiments of Pavlov, the CS was a bell. Traditionally, the CS does not evoke a response similar to the UR, and is typically known as a "neutral" stimulus. During training, the US was made contingent on the CS by repeatedly pairing the presentations of CS and US. After training, the response to the CS alone had

changed such that the bell elicited salivation (the conditional response, CR). The persistence of a CR after training is called *retention*. When the contingency between CS and US was eliminated by repeatedly presenting the bell in the absence of the meat powder (US), the ability of the CS to elicit the CR (salivation) gradually diminished. This process is called *extinction*.

In Pavlovian (classical) conditioning, contingency is usually established by the close temporal pairing (contiguity) of CS and US. (For a more detailed discussion, see Mackintosh[8,9] and Rescorla[10]). Delivering the CS before the US is known as *forward conditioning*, whereas delivery of the CS after the US is known as *backward conditioning*. In classical conditioning, the temporal relationship between the presentation of the CS and US is graded such that an optimum time period exists for conditioning (~0.5 second). Shorter or longer intervals between the two stimuli result in less effective conditioning. The relationship between duration and onset of the CS and US can also be critical for the effectiveness of the conditioning procedure. The condition in which the CS terminates before the US onset is known as *delayed conditioning*. The interval between CS onset and US onset is called the CS-US interval or the *interstimulus interval*. Most conditioning procedures involve repeated pairings of the CS and US. The interval between these pairings is called the *intertrial interval*.

Specificity of behavioral change due to pairing can be most clearly shown by using a differential conditioning procedure. In this procedure, two different conditional stimuli are used in the same animal; one is specifically paired with the US and is therefore called the CS+, whereas the other, the CS−, is specifically unpaired. Comparing the response to the CS+ with the response of the CS− can assess learned changes in behavior.

In Pavlov's experiments, the bell (the CS) initially presented alone did not produce salivation. In some types of conditioning procedures, the CS initially produces a small response similar to that evoked by the US. After pairing, the response to the CS is enhanced. This type of conditioning is known as alpha-conditioning. Both alpha- and classical conditioning are similar in that they require close temporal relationships between the CS and the US. In classical conditioning, however, the neutral CS does not produce a response similar to the UR initially. In alpha-conditioning, the CS produces a weak response that is subsequently enhanced. Some investigators have

argued that the distinction between alpha- and classical conditioning is somewhat descriptive because in principle the two types could be mediated by identical cellular mechanisms.

Sensitization and alpha-conditioning also resemble each other. They both involve modification of a previously existing response to a stimulus. They differ, however, in their temporal requirements: alpha-conditioning require a close temporal association between the CS and US, and sensitization does not.

Operant Conditioning

Operant conditioning (also known as *instrumental conditioning* or trial-and-error learning) is the second type of associative learning. It differs from classical conditioning in that the reinforcing stimulus is contingent on the performance of a behavior (i.e., operant) produced by the animal rather than on a CS delivered by the experimenter. As a result, the animal learns the consequences of its own behavior and alters the behavior as a result of training. Skinner described an illustrative paradigm.[11] Before training, a pigeon confined in a small compartment pecks randomly at the walls. During training, delivery of food (i.e., reinforcement) is made contingent on the animal pecking a single location in the compartment (such as a small disk). Because food and the peck are paired, the pigeon continues to peck at the disk after training even in the absence of food reinforcement. As in classical conditioning, the learned behavior is extinguished when repeated pecks are no longer followed by food reinforcement.

As with classical conditioning, operant conditioning requires a close temporal association. Operant conditioning differs from classical conditioning, however, in that the reinforcement is contingent on the animal's response rather than on the presentation of the CS. Cellular analogues of operant conditioning are much more difficult to study because the behavioral responses involved are not usually under experimental control. Some studies have demonstrated that operant conditioning paradigms can influence activity in neural circuits in vitro. Changes in cellular properties that are induced by the operant conditioning paradigm are under investigation.[12]

The types of learning discussed previously have received the greatest attention from behaviorists and have been most amenable to experimental analysis by neurobiologists, but many other types of learning occur (e.g., **priming**, imprinting, latent learning, observational learning, aversion learning). The definitions given previously are operational and describe a behavioral level of analysis (see Chap. 1). When presented at a mechanistic level (e.g., at the level of the single neuron), some of the distinctions among various examples of conditioning may not hold. Instead, at the cellular level, basic mechanisms underlying these different examples of learning may be similar.[13,14]

Memory Systems

Psychologists have found that human memory is composed of multiple memory systems[15–17] (Fig. 17–2). Although the precise categorization of these systems is still under debate, they can generally be divided into two broad categories: **declarative memory** and **nondeclarative memory.**

Definitions

Declarative memory, also known as explicit memory, encompasses the memory for facts and concepts (semantic memory) as well as the memory for events (episodic or autobiographical memory). In humans, declarative memories are associated with conscious recollections of facts and events. Nondeclarative memory, also known as **implicit** memory, operates at an unconscious level. Nondeclarative memory encompasses the memory for skills and habits, priming, examples of associative learning

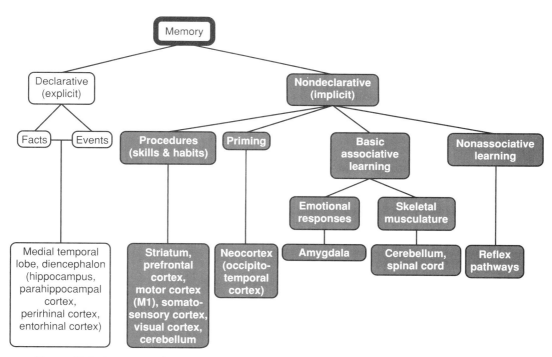

Figure 17–2. Categories of memory systems and associated brain structures. Memory is not a single entity, but consists of several separate entities that depend on different systems in the central nervous system. A key distinction is between the capacity for conscious recollection of facts and events (declarative memory) and unconscious learning capabilities (nondeclarative memory), which are manifest as changes in performance. Evidence for distinguishing between memory systems has come primarily from studies of amnesic patients who perform poorly on declarative memory tasks but retain the ability to learn new skills. (Summary of data from Squire LR, Zola SM. Structure and function of declarative and nondeclarative memory systems. *Proc Natl Acad Sci USA* 1996;93:13515–13522; and Ungerleider LG. Functional brain imaging studies of cortical mechanisms for memory. *Science* 1995;270:769–775.)

such as classical conditioning, operant conditioning, and types of nonassociative learning such as sensitization and habituation.

Evidence of Memory Systems

A considerable body of evidence indicates that the various memory systems are supported by distinct anatomic structures. These conclusions have been derived from a number of strategies. Among these strategies is the use of modern imaging techniques such as positron emission tomography and functional magnetic resonance imaging. These imaging techniques can show regions of the brain engaged by specific memory tasks (see Fig. 17–2). Studies of learning and memory deficits in experimental animals with lesions have also helped identify areas of the brain that are involved in learning and memory processes. Finally, brain regions involved in learning and memory have been identified through detailed behavioral assessments of patients with learning and memory deficits produced either by injury (e.g., traumatic brain injury, tumors, CVA) or by surgical removal of regions of the brain, which became necessary to treat disorders such as epilepsy.

An early case study was particularly revealing and has had a major impact on the development of modern views on the distributed representation of memory systems. Brenda Milner and her colleagues studied a patient known as H.M. who, in 1953, underwent surgery to treat severe epileptic seizures. The surgery included removal of the medial temporal region of the brain, which included the amygdala, the anterior two thirds of the hippocampus, and the hippocampal gyrus. After the surgery, H.M. appeared normal in many respects except for severe anterograde amnesia. Specifically, he could not form any new long-term declarative memories. For example, on the day after an interview, he had no recollection that the previous day's interview had occurred nor memory of any events associated with the interview. H.M. also could not add new words to his vocabulary. Thus, he appeared to be unable to form any new memories for events, facts, or concepts. Although he could not form any new long-term episodic or semantic memories, his early childhood memories were intact. Presumably, these memories are stored in a region of the brain outside the medial temporal region, which was removed during surgery. Of particular interest was the finding that H.M. retained the ability to acquire new skills at a level comparable with normal people. For example H.M. was able to learn to trace a star while looking only in a mirror. He also learned to work the Tower of Hanoi puzzle. Although he could acquire these new skills (i.e., nondeclarative memory), he had no conscious recollection of ever acquiring them (i.e., no declarative memory).

Anatomic Loci

Studies of the type described previously indicate that the medial temporal lobe and diencephalon are critical for declarative memories (see Fig. 17–2). Anatomic loci for nondeclarative memories are more diverse and seem to depend on the particular brain structure or structures engaged by the task. Thus, the learning of certain skills and habits involves the striatum, whereas the learning of certain movements can involve the cerebellum or spinal cord. Conditioning of emotional responses depends on the amygdala (see Fig. 17–2).

Processes Contributing to Learning and Memory

Memories are probably stored through highly selective changes in the strength of synaptic connections between neurons in the brain. As such, storage of information in the brain appears to involve persistent, use-dependent alteration in the efficacy of synaptic transmission. The cellular and molecular bases of synaptic plasticity have been studied extensively for many years (for reviews, see Byrne,[18] Fagnou and Tuchek,[19] and Hawkins et al.[20]). An overview of some of the types of synaptic plasticity that have been implicated in the processes of learning and memory is presented in the following sections. Several animal models are considered, including the **defensive withdrawal reflex** of the marine mollusk *Aplysia*, long-term potentiation in the rodent hippocampus, and long-term depression in the rabbit cerebellum.

Cellular Bases of Nonassociative Learning

Neural Mechanisms

To investigate the neural mechanisms of learning, ideally the study should include a simple response, a carefully controlled stimulus, and a well characterized neural circuit that is amenable to detailed cellular, biophysical, and biochemical analysis. These conditions are met in simple organisms such as the marine mollusk *Aplysia* (a type of sea slug), which has large, identifiable neurons. The neural circuitry that mediates the defensive withdrawal reflexes of *Aplysia* has been used extensively as a model system for studies of nonassociative learning (for reviews, see Byrne,[18] Byrne and Kandel,[21] Kandel, and Schwartz[22]).

The essential neuronal circuitry that mediates the defensive withdrawal reflexes is illustrated in Figure 17–3A. Stimuli activate sensory neurons that innervate the skin. In the CNS, the sensory neurons make monosynaptic excitatory connections with motor neurons that mediate the withdrawal. The simple reflexive withdrawal that is mediated by such a circuit can undergo habituation and sensitization, as well as associative conditioning. When a weak stimulus (e.g., a gentle tactile stimulus or mild electrical shock) is presented repeatedly to the skin, the reflex withdrawal is initially robust, but becomes weaker with each successive stimulus (see Fig. 17–3B). That is, the response habituates. If a strong noxious stimulus is given to another part of the animal (e.g., a strong pinch or a powerful electric shock), a large increase in the withdrawal reflex occurs. If the reflex has been habituated previously, this increase is called dishabituation. If the reflex was not habituated, an increase in the response is called sensitization.

Electrophysiology of Neural Circuitry
An examination of the electrophysiolgic properties of the neural circuitry reveals that a decrement in the amplitude of the excitatory **postsynaptic potential** (EPSP) at the sensory-to-motor neuron synapse accompanies, and might account for, the habituation (see Fig. 17–3C). This form of synaptic plasticity is known as *homosynaptic depression*. It is termed "homosynaptic" because the synaptic depression appears to be a property of the sensorimotor pathway itself and can be evoked simply by repeated stimulation of the presynaptic sensory neuron. The decrease in the amplitude of the EPSP results from a decrease in the release of neurotransmitter from the presynaptic terminal. At least two subcellular processes are believed to underlie this decrease in neurotransmitter release (Fig. 17–4). First, a use-dependent decrease in Ca^{++} influx during repetitive presynaptic activity is believed to contribute to homosynaptic depression. As described in Chapter 3,

Ca^{++} influx during the presynaptic action potential is a critical factor controlling the release of neurotransmitter. Two types of Ca^{++} currents have been identified in the sensory neurons of *Aplysia*,[23] which are known as **L-type** and **N-type Ca^{++} currents** ($I_{Ca;L-type}$ and $I_{Ca;N-type}$, respectively). Only $I_{Ca;N-type}$ directly contributes to the release of neurotransmitter, however. The magnitude of $I_{Ca;N-type}$ decreases in parallel with habituation and decreased neurotransmitter release.[24] Second, a modeling study indicated that a decrease in the availability of releasable neurotransmitter (or functional release sites) may also contribute to synaptic depression.[25,26] During repetitive activity, the presynaptic stores of releasable neurotransmitter become depleted. Thus, the combination of a decrease in Ca^{++} influx and a depletion of neurotransmitter is believed to underlie synaptic depression, the cellular correlate of habituation.

Conversely, an increase in transmission at the sensory-to-motor neuron synapse accompanies, and might account for, the sensitization/dishabituation (see Fig. 17–3C). This facilitation of synaptic transmission, the cellular correlate of the enhanced reflex, is heterosynaptic. The sensitizing stimulus activates a **facilitatory neuron** that forms synapses on the sensory neuron (see Fig. 17–3A). These facilitatory neurons, some of which are serotonergic, enhance the release of neurotransmitter from the sensory neurons by activating a complex array of second messenger systems within the sensory neuron (see Fig. 17–4; for recent reviews, see Byrne and Kandel[21] and Byrne et al.[27]).

Molecular Mechanisms
The sequence of biochemical steps in sensitization involves, first, **serotonin** (5-hydroxytryptamine [5-HT]), which is released by the facilitatory neuron and binds to receptors on the sensory neurons. At least two types of receptors have been identified. One receptor is coupled to an **adenylyl cyclase**, an enzyme that catalyzes the production of the second messenger **3′,5′-cyclic adenosine monophosphate** (cAMP). The other receptor is believed to be coupled to **phospholipase C**, an enzyme that cleaves membrane lipid chains, producing the second messengers inositol triphosphate (IP3) and diacylglycerol (DAG). Then, the second messengers activate an array of **protein kinases**, which catalyze the transfer of the phosphate group of **adenosine triphosphate** to the hydroxyl moiety of a specific amino acid, thereby regulating the functions of proteins.

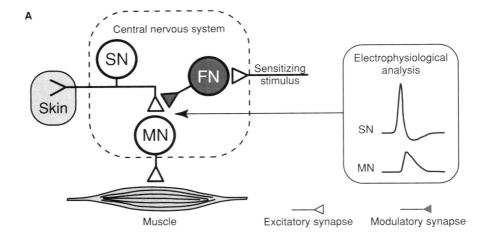

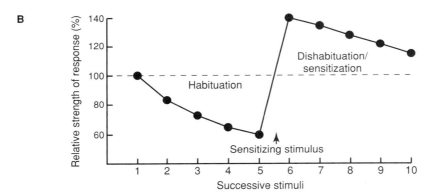

Figure 17–3. Withdrawal reflexes of _Aplysia_ can be used to study the cellular mechanisms that may underlie nonassociative learning. **A:** Simplified neural circuit illustrating the key elements involved in a defensive withdrawal reflex. Sensory neurons (SN) innervate peripheral structures, such as the skin. A stimulus applied within the receptive field of a sensory neuron elicits an action potential, which is conducted along the axon toward the central nervous system (CNS). In the CNS, the sensory neuron makes an excitatory synaptic connection onto a motor neuron (MN). The motor neuron, in turn, innervates the muscles that mediate withdrawal. Thus, this circuit is similar to the simple monosynaptic reflex arcs found in vertebrates, including humans. Sensitizing stimuli activate a general arousal system, which is believed to induce the release of serotonin (5-HT) from facilitatory neurons (FN). The electrophysiologic properties of the circuit can be monitored by intracellular recordings of the presynaptic and postsynaptic cells (i.e., the SNs and MNs, respectively). An action potential in the sensory neuron elicits an excitatory postsynaptic potenital (EPSP) in the motor neurons. **B:** Hypothetical behavioral experiment. Habituation of the reflex can be induced by repeated presentation of a mild stimulus. Initially, the stimulus elicits a robust withdrawal. The response to the successive four stimuli progressively declines such that by the fifth stimulus, the withdrawal has declined to only 60% of its original amplitude. Between the fifth and sixth test stimuli, a strong sensitizing stimulus was applied to the animal. The subsequent responses to the test stimuli are significantly enhanced. This enhancement of a previously habituated response is known as dishabituation. If the response had not been previously habituated, the enhancement would have been referred to as sensitization. (continued)

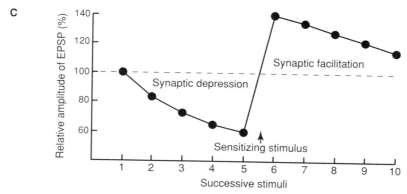

Figure 17–3 (continued). C: Hypothetical examples of intracellular correlates of nonassociative learning. Simultaneous intracellular recordings from sensory neurons and motor neurons were used to monitor synaptic efficacy during nonassociative learning. During habituation, the amplitude of EPSPs is observed to decrease (i.e., synaptic depression). Thus, activity in the sensory neuron is less likely to elicit a response (i.e., habituation). Conversely, during sensitization, the amplitude of the EPSPs is observed to increase (i.e., synaptic facilitation). Thus, activity in the sensory neuron is more likely to elicit a response (i.e., sensitization).

Protein kinase A (PKA) is activated by cAMP and protein kinase C (PKC) is activated by DAG. A role for Ca^{++}/calmodulin-dependent kinase II also has been suggested, and it may be activated by the IP3-dependent release of Ca^{++} from intracellular stores.[28] Next, the kinases phosphorylate a number of ionic channels (or associated proteins), thereby modulating the biophysical properties of the sensory neuron. In general, the membrane's conductance to K^+ is decreased. Reduction of this K^+ conductance, which normally repolarizes the action potential (see Chap. 3), prolongs the action potential in the sensory neuron and allows the N-type Ca^{++} channels to be activated for longer periods. More Ca^{++} is able to enter the terminal, thereby enhancing the release of neurotransmitter. In addition, the kinases are believed to modulate processes that directly contribute to neurotransmitter release, such as increasing the flux of neurotransmitter from a storage pool to the releasable pool (i.e., mobilization). Finally, the kinases enhance the L-type Ca^{++} channels, which do not directly regulate the release of neurotransmitter but act to increase mobilization of neurotransmitter.

In summary, homosynaptic depression is believed to be a cellular mechanism underlying habituation. The molecular mechanisms of homosynaptic depres-sion are believed to involve an activity-dependent decrease in Ca^{++} current in the presynaptic terminal and a depletion of neurotransmitter that is available for release. Heterosynaptic facilitation is believed to be a cellular mechanism underlying dishabituation and sensitization. The molecular mechanisms of heterosynaptic facilitation are more complex and involve numerous second messenger systems (e.g., cAMP and DAG), **protein kinases** (e.g., PKA and PKC), and protein substrates (e.g., ion channels and processes mediating mobilization). The general consequence of this complex array, however, is an increase in the duration of the presynaptic action potential, which in turn allows greater Ca^{++} influx and greater release of neurotransmitter.

Cellular Bases of Associative Learning

Associative modifications of synaptic efficacy, which are believed to underlie associative learning, depend on the temporal correlation between activities in two neurons (for a review, see Baxter and Byrne[29]). Possibly the best known mechanism for associative learning was proposed by Hebb.[30] His postulate for learning states: "When an axon of cell A is near enough to

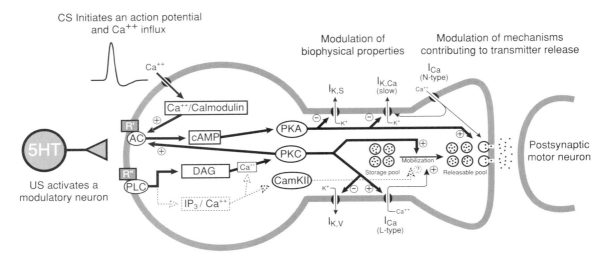

Figure 17–4. Cellular and molecular events believed to underlie nonassociative and associative synaptic plasticity in sensory neurons of *Aplysia*. A facilitatory neuron (see Figs. 17–3 and 17–5) releases the modulator neurotransmitter serotonin (5-HT), which binds to receptors (R) in the membrane of the sensory neuron. At least two distinct types of receptors exist. One type (R′) is coupled to adenylyl cyclase (AC), an enzyme that catalyzes the synthesis of cyclic adenosine 3′5′-monophosphate (cAMP). A second type is believed to be coupled to phospholipase C (PLC), an enzyme that catalyzes the degradation of phospholipids in the membrane into diacylglycerol (DAG) and inositol triphosphate (IP3). IP3, in turn, can induce the release of Ca^{++} from intracellular stores. These second messengers (cAMP, DAG, and Ca^{++}), acting through their respective kinases (protein kinase A[PKA] and protein kinase C[PKC], affect multiple cellular processes (e.g., ionic conductances and process contributing to the release of neurotransmitter), the combined effects of which enhance the release of neurotransmitter. Nonassociative synaptic enhancement (such as might occur during sensitization) can be induced by the release of 5-HT alone, which is sufficient to activate the enzymatic cascade. Associative synaptic enhancement (such as might occur during classical conditioning) emerges from the dual regulation of adenylyl cyclase by 5-HT and Ca++/calmodulin. If spiking activity, and thus Ca^{++} influx, occurs in the sensory neuron in close temporal proximity to the release of 5-HT, then significantly more cAMP is generated and significantly greater synaptic enhancement occurs (see Fig. 17–5).

excite a cell B and repeatedly or persistently takes part in firing it, some growth process or metabolic changes takes place in one or both cells such that A's efficiency as one of the cells firing B is increased."

The key feature of what has become known as the "Hebbian Learning Rule" is that increases in synaptic efficacy depend on concurrent activity in the presynaptic and postsynaptic cells—that is, a close temporal correlation between activities in two cells.

The three most prominent forms of associative synaptic plasticity are **activity-dependent neuromodulation** (ADM), **long-term potentiation** (LTP), and **long-term depression** (LTD). Each ex-

ample of associative synaptic plasticity is discussed in turn in the following sections. The essence of the mechanisms that underlie each of these three examples of associative synaptic plasticity is the discovery of dually regulated molecules (for reviews, see Abrams and Kandel[31] and Casabona[32]). For example, studies of classical conditioning in *Aplysia* indicate that the enzyme adenylyl cyclase may serve as a molecular site of convergence between two signals: Ca^{++} influx (i.e., the signal from the CS) and the binding of molecules of neurotransmitter to their receptors (i.e., the signal from the US). The dually regulated molecule that underlies associative synaptic plasticity can be an enzyme (as is the case for ADM and LTD), or it can be a receptor for a neurotransmitter (as is the case for LTP).

Activity-Dependent Neuromodulation

An enzyme-dependent cellular mechanism called ADM may contribute to associative learning in *Aplysia*.[33,34] As described previously, the withdrawal reflexes of *Aplysia* have been used as a model system to study the cellular mechanisms underlying nonassociative learning (e.g., habituation, dishabituation, and sensitization). These behaviors and their underlying neural circuitry have also been used to study the cellular processes contributing to associative learning, such as classical conditioning.[18,35–39] A general cellular scheme of associative learning is illustrated in Figure 17–5A. In the within-subject version of a classical conditioning (i.e., differential conditioning), the same subject receives two CSs, one paired with the US (i.e., CS+). The other is explicitly unpaired with the US (i.e., CS−) and is presented during the intertrial interval (see Fig. 17–5B). Initially, the two sensory neurons (SN_1 and SN_2) that constitute pathways for CSs make weak subthreshold connections to a motor neuron (see Fig. 17–5C). Delivering the reinforcing stimulus or US has two effects. First, the US alone activates the motor neuron and produces the UR. Second, the US activates a diffuse modulatory system (the facilitatory neuron) that enhances the release of neurotransmitter from all sensory neurons. This nonspecific enhancement contributes to sensitization of the CS− sensory neuron (see earlier discussion). Temporal specificity, a defining characteristic of associative learning, occurs when the CS+ (spiking activity in SN_1) is paired with the US. This temporally specific pairing causes a selective amplification of the modulatory effects in the sensory neuron whose activity was paired with the US (see Fig. 17–5C). The pair-specific amplification of the modulatory effects in the CS+ sensory neuron leads to an enhanced ability of SN_1 to activate the motor neuron, and thereby to produce the CR.

At the molecular level, the mechanisms underlying ADM are believed to be similar to those for heterosynaptic facilitation, which underlies sensitization (see Fig. 17–5). The neuromodulator that is released by the US (i.e., 5-HT) acts, in part, by activating the adenylyl cyclase and thereby increasing the synthesis of cAMP, which activates PKA. The subsequent protein phosphorylations lead to a re-

duction of K^+ currents. Consequently, action potentials elicited after the reinforcing stimulus are broader (because the repolarizing K^+ current is reduced). The broader spikes allow greater influx of Ca^{++} and greater release of neurotransmitter, and thus, sensitization of the response (see Fig. 17–5C). The temporal specificity of the associative conditioning is due, in part, to an increase in the level of cAMP beyond that produced by the modulator (i.e., 5-HT) alone.[40,41] The influx of Ca^{++} associated with the CS+ (spike activity) appears to amplify the US-mediated modulatory effects. The Ca^{++} binds to calmodulin, and the Ca^{++}/calmodulin complex amplifies the activation of the adenylyl cyclase by 5-HT.[42,43] The levels of cAMP in the unpaired sensory neuron (i.e., CS−) were not amplified above the levels induced by the US alone, because the Ca^{++} that entered during the CS− had decayed before the US arrived. Thus, the conditioned terminals (i.e., CS+) produced more cAMP, leading to greater activation of PKA. Increased activation of PKA produces more phosphorylation of K^+ channels, greater spike broadening, enhanced Ca^{++} influx, more neurotransmitter release, and a larger postsynaptic response[44] (see Fig. 17–5C).

An important conclusion is that this mechanism for associative learning is an elaboration of mechanisms already in place that mediate sensitization, a simpler example of learning. Both nonassociative (i.e., heterosynaptic facilitation) and associative (i.e., ADM) examples of synaptic plasticity are mediated, in part, by 5-HT–dependent activation of adenylyl cyclase. The associative aspects of ADM are derived from the dual regulation of the adenylyl cyclase by 5-HT and Ca^{++}/calmodulin. The observation that simple and complex forms of neuronal plasticity can share some aspects of molecular mechanisms raises the interesting possibility that complex forms of learning may use simpler mechanisms as building blocks.[12] This idea has been suggested by some psychologists for many years. Until now, it has not been testable at the cellular level.

A final point is that the mechanisms described previously for ADM all take place in the presynaptic cells. Activity in the postsynaptic motor neurons was not considered, and the model presented in Figure 17–4 does not require the involvement of the postsynaptic cell. It would appear, therefore, that classical conditioning of the withdrawal reflex is based entirely on a presynaptic mechanism. This differs

A

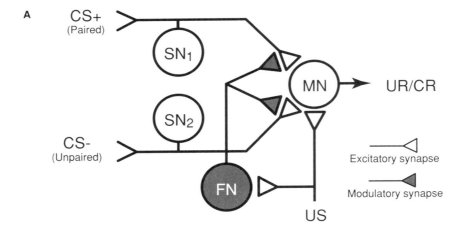

B

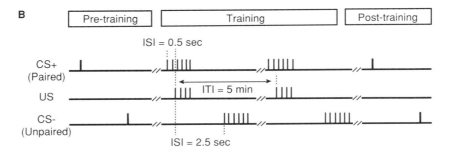

Figure 17–5. Withdrawal reflexes of *Aplysia* can be used to study the cellular mechanisms that may underlie associative learning. **A:** Schematic diagram illustrating how a differential conditioning paradigm can be applied to the neural circuit that mediates a defensive withdrawal reflex. In a differential conditioning paradigm two conditional stimulus (CS) pathways are stimulated in addition to the unconditional stimulus (US) pathway. FN, facilitatory neuron; MN, motor neuron; SN, sensory neuron; CR, conditional response; UR, unconditional response. **B:** Schematic diagram (not to scale) of a differential conditioning paradigm. The conditional stimuli (CSs) are mediated by activity in the sensory neurons and the conditional response (CR) is mediated by activity in the motor neuron (see **A**). Before training, test stimuli are applied to measure the amplitude of the CR. During training, activity in one sensory neuron (CS+) is paired with a strong unconditional stimulus (US) that activates a facilitatory neuron. The facilitatory neuron releases a modulatory neurotransmitter, which is believed to be serotonin, onto the sensory neurons. Activity in a second sensory neuron (CS−) is unpaired with the US. The interstimulus interval (ISI; i.e., the time between the onsets of the CS and the US) was 0.5 second for the CS+ and 2.5 minutes for the CS−. The intertrail interval (ITI; i.e., interval between presentations of the US) was 5 minutes. (continued)

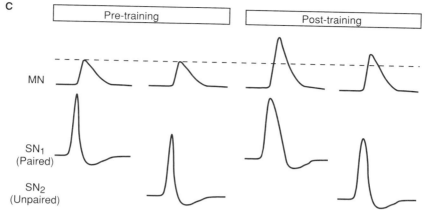

C

| Pre-training | Post-training |

MN

SN₁
(Paired)

SN₂
(Unpaired)

Figure 17–5 (continued). C: Hypothetical experiment illustrating the results from a differential conditioning paradigm. The strength of the CR is measured as the amplitude of the excitatory post-synaptic potential (EPSP) that is elicited by stimulating a sensory neuron. Before training, single action potentials in each of two sensory neurons (SN) elicit EPSPs of comparable amplitude in the motor neuron. During training, the activity in SN_1 is paired with the US, whereas the activity in SN_2 is unpaired. After training, the amplitude of both EPSPs is increased. The amplitude of EPSP generated by SN_1 (i.e., the paired cell) is much larger, however. The small increase in the amplitude of the EPSP generated by SN_2 is nonassociative and is believed to represent sensitization induced by the US. The large increase in the amplitude of the EPSP generated by SN_1 represents a pairing-specific enhancement (i.e., an associative synaptic enhancement) that is believed to contribute to classical conditioning. Note that the duration of the action potentials in the sensory neurons was increased after training. This increase in spike duration is an important contributing factor to the increase in EPSP amplitude (see Fig. 17–4).

from a Hebb-type mechanism, in which activity in both presynaptic and postsynaptic cells is required (see previous discussion). Some evidence, however, suggests that postsynaptic activity (i.e., depolarization and spiking in the motor neuron) contributes to ADM (e.g., Bao et al.[45]; for review, see Lechner and Byrne[46]). Thus, elements of the Hebbian rule may also contribute to associative learning in *Aplysia*. More direct examples of the Hebbian rule underlying associative synaptic plasticity are presented in the discussions of LTP and LTD (see later).

Long-Term Potentiation

Investigations of the cellular bases of learning and memory in vertebrate systems have focused largely on the hippocampus because of its involvement in both human and animal memory processing (for reviews, see Schacter[47] and Shen et al.[48]). Much of this research has focused on LTP. LTP is a sustained increase in synaptic strength elicited by brief, high-

frequency stimulation of excitatory afferents (for recent reviews, see Fagnou and Tuchek,[19] Maren and Baudry,[45] Martinez and Derrick,[50] and Wang et al.[51]). LTP was first described in the hippocampus.[52] It has subsequently been observed at many excitatory synapses in the CNS, such as in the amygdala[53,54] and visual cortex.[55,56] The idea that many neural systems are capable of exhibiting long-term synaptic plasticity is consistent with the emerging view that the brain has multiple memory systems. The most intensively studied form of LTP is that expressed at the synaptic connections from the Schaffer collateral fiber pathway onto pyramidal neurons in region CA1 of the hippocampus (Fig. 17–6).

Figure 17–6 schematically illustrates an experimental arrangement for inducing and analyzing LTP. An intracellular recording is made from a postsynaptic neuron (e.g., a pyramidal cell in the CA1 region) that receives monosynaptic excitatory inputs from presynaptic neurons (e.g., pyramidal cells in the CA3

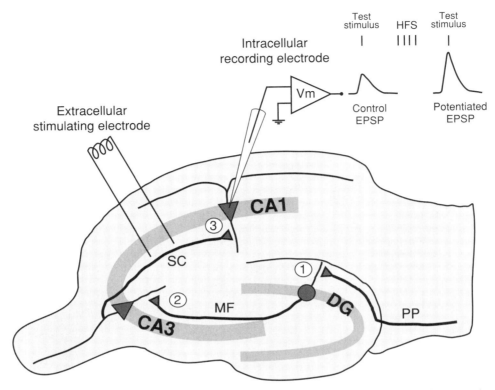

Figure 17–6. Trisynaptic circuit of the hippocampus. There are three major afferent pathways in the hippocampus: 1) the perforant pathway (PP) from the entorhinal cortex forms excitatory synaptic connections onto granule cells of the dentate gyrus (DG); 2) the granule cells give rise to axons that form the mossy fiber (MF) pathway, which makes excitatory connections onto pyramidal cells in area CA3 of the hippocampus; and 3) the CA3 pyramidal cells project to pyramidal cells in area CA1 by way of the Schaffer collaterals (SC). All three excitatory synaptic pathways use glutamate as a neurotransmitter and all three can manifest long-term potentiation. For example, intracellular recordings can be used to monitor the membrane potential (Vm) of an individual CA1 pyramidal cell and excitatory postsynaptic potentials (EPSPs) can be elicited by placing an extracellular stimulating electrode among the Schaffer collaterals. After a brief high-frequency stimulus (HFS; e.g., 1 second burst of stimuli at 100 Hz), the amplitude of the subsequent test EPSPs is significantly enhanced. This potentiation can last many hours, and is known as long-term potentiation.

region that project to the CA1 region by the Schaffer collateral fiber pathway). Brief electrical shocks delivered to the afferent pathway (i.e., the Schaffer collateral fiber pathway) elicit action potentials in the axons of the pathway. The release of neurotransmitter from the presynaptic terminals produces an EPSP in the postsynaptic cell. Individual test stimuli are used to monitor the strength of the synaptic connections. After a stable baseline period (i.e., control EPSP), a brief high-frequency stimulus is delivered to

the input pathway. Subsequent test stimuli produce enhanced EPSPs (i.e., the potentiated EPSP). This potentiation can last for several hours in vitro and for several weeks in vivo. Thus, LTP has generated a great deal of interest as a putative cellular memory mechanism.

If LTP represents a cellular mechanism for associative learning and memory, then you might expect a cellular analogue of classical conditioning involving LTP; that is, the induction of LTP should require the close temporal association of two stimuli. Figure 17–7 is a schematic representation of an experimental protocol developed by Barrionuevo and Brown[57] to investigate the associative properties of LTP in vitro. Three stimulating electrodes were used to activate three separate presynaptic pathways to the single postsynaptic cell (see Fig. 17–7A). For two of the pathways (W_1 and W_2), the intensity of stimulation was very weak. These weak stimuli elicited small, subthreshold EPSPs in the postsynaptic cell. For the third pathway (S), the intensity of stimulation was strong and this strong stimulus was sufficient to elicit action potentials in the postsynaptic cell. The weakly stimulated pathways were considered analogous to the two CSs in a differential conditioning protocol and the strongly stimulated pathway was analogous to the US. During the pretraining period, the weakly stimulated pathways were activated alternately at a low frequency to establish a stable baseline (see Fig. 17–7B). During training, a brief burst of stimuli in one of the weakly stimulated pathways (W_1) was paired with a high-frequency burst in the strongly stimulated pathway. The brief burst of stimuli in the second weak pathway (W_2) was explicitly unpaired with activity in the strong pathway during training. As illustrated in the posttraining period (see Fig. 17–7C), LTP (i.e., a sustained enhancement in the amplitude of individual test EPSPs) was induced only in the weak pathway that was paired with strong afferent input during training (i.e., W_1). The key contributing factor of the strong stimulus pathway was its ability to induce a large depolarization and spiking activity in the postsynaptic cell. Thus, it is also possible to induce LTP by pairing activity in the weakly stimulated pathway with depolarization current pulses injected directly into the postsynaptic cells.[58,59] The LTP induced in these types of experiments is referred to as associative LTP; the general phenomenon is called *associativity*. Thus, the induction of LTP expressed an essential feature of associative learning: namely the requirement for close temporal contiguity between two stimuli (i.e., the CS and the US). Moreover, it would appear that associative LTP follows the Hebbian learning rule because it is induced by pairing presynaptic and postsynaptic activity.

The general phenomenon of LTP has been observed in a number of synapses, but the underlying mechanisms for these different examples of LTP may differ. For example, each of the three major afferent pathways in the hippocampus express LTP, but asso-

ciative LTP is expressed only in the perforant pathway and the Schaffer collateral fiber pathway. The LTP in the mossy fiber pathway is nonassociative. The following discussion focuses on the mechanisms of associative LTP in the Schaffer collateral fiber pathway (Fig. 17–8).

The Hebbian nature of LTP in the CA1 area of the hippocampus is probably derived from the unusual properties of the N-methyl-D-aspartate (**NMDA**) subtype of the **glutamate receptor**: its dual regulation by neurotransmitter and membrane voltage (for reviews, see Collingridge and Bliss,[60,61] Madison et al.,[62] Nicoll et al.,[63] and Rison and Stanton[64]). The Schaffer collateral axons from the CA3 region of the hippocampus that terminate on the pyramidal cells of the CA1 region use glutamate as their neurotransmitter. Glutamate acts on its target cells in the CA1 region by binding to three types of glutamate receptors: alpha-amino-3-hydroxy-5-methyl-4-isoxazolepropionate receptors (AMPA-R), NMDA receptors (NMDA-R), and metabotropic glutamate receptors (M-GluR). These glutamate receptors activate second messenger systems such as the phospholipase C/IP3/DAG system[65–67] (see Fig. 17–8). Under normal conditions, hippocampal synaptic responses elicited by low-frequency stimulation are mediated primarily by the interaction of glutamate with AMPA-R, an ionotropic subclass of glutamate receptors that gates a fast cationic (i.e., Na^+, K^+) conductance. Glutamate also binds to the NMDA-R, but because of a block by Mg^{++} of their associated ionic channels, no permeability changes occur. This Mg^{++} block of the NMDA-R channel is voltage dependent and, as the postsynaptic membrane is depolarized, the Mg^{++} is forced out of the channel, which relieves the block. Thus, during high-frequency stimulation of excitatory afferents, the resultant strong postsynaptic depolarization coupled with presynaptic release of glutamate activates the NMDA-R by releasing the voltage-dependent Mg^{++} block. NMDA-R activation results in Ca^{++} influx into the postsynaptic cell. The elevated levels of intracellular Ca^{++} in combination with other second messenger systems activated by the M-GluR trigger a series of enzymatic cascades that lead to persistent modification of synaptic efficacy.[68,69]

The nature of enzymatic cascades is still poorly understood, but some evidence suggests the involvement of PKC and Ca^{++}/calmodulin kinase II (for reviews, see Fagnou and Tuchek,[19] Maren and Baudry,[49]

(text continues on page 338)

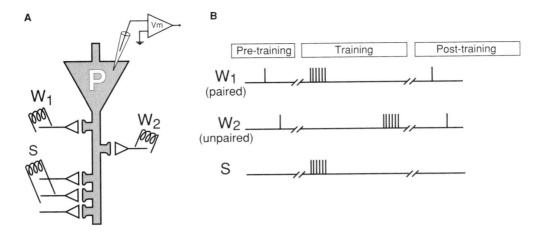

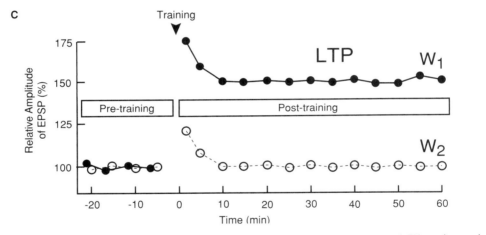

Figure 17–7. Hypothetical experiment to illustrate how long-term potentiation (LTP) can be used to study cellular mechanisms that may underlie classical conditioning. **A:** Arrangement of stimulating electrodes. A single pyramidal cell (P) can receive thousands of excitatory inputs, most of which are located on small dendritic spines. Three stimulating electrodes are used to activate three distinct subsets of the excitatory inputs to a single cell. The intensities of two of the stimuli are weak (W_1 and W_2) and therefore activate very few presynaptic fibers. The intensity of the third stimulus is much stronger (S) and activates a large population of presynaptic fibers. **B:** Stimulus paradigm (not to scale). Individual weak stimuli are used to measure the synaptic strength before and after training (pre- and post-training). During training, the W_1 and S pathways are stimulated simultaneously with brief, high-frequency bursts of activity (e.g., 1 second, 100 Hz). About 3 seconds later, a similar burst of activity is elicited in the W_2 pathway, but this activity is not paired with the S stimulus. **C:** Long-term potentiation. Before training (pre-training) the synaptic strengths of W_1 and W_2 change little in response to repeated test stimuli. Immediately after training, both synaptic pathways are enhanced. The strength of the W_2 pathway, however, rapidly returns to its control (i.e., pre-training) level. This transient enhancement immediately after a high-frequency stimulation is referred to as post-tetanic potentiation. In the W_1 pathway, however, the synaptic strength remains elevated throughout the remainder of the experiment. This sustained enhancement is referred to as long-term potentiation.

Figure 17–8. Molecular processes believed to underlie the induction and expression of long-term plasticity in synaptic connections from Schaffer collaterals to CA1 cells. A single presynaptic terminal and postsynaptic spine complex is illustrated. Synaptic transmission is mediated by the release of glutamate (Glu), which binds to receptors in the postsynaptic membrane. At least three types of glutamate receptors can be distinguished. The AMPA-type receptor (AMPA-R), an iontophore, mediates normal excitatory transmission (i.e., when glutamate binds to the receptor, a pore is opened and ions flow across the membrane and change the membrane potential). The metabotropic receptor (M-GluR) is probably coupled to phospholipase C (PLC), an enzyme that catalyzes the degradation of phospholipids in the membrane into diacylglycerol (DAG) and inositol triphosphate (IP3), which in turn can elicit release of Ca^{++} from intracellular stores. The NMDA-R is also an iontophore, but at potentials near the resting membrane potential of the cell, no ions flow through the NMDA-R because of a voltage-dependent block of the pore by Mg^{++}. If the postsynaptic membrane is sufficiently depolarized to remove the Mg^{++} block, then the NMDA-R allows Ca^{++} influx while glutamate is bound to the receptor. Changes in the levels of intracellular Ca^{++}, in combination with the Ca^{++} binding protein calmodulin, activate a number of protein kinases and phosphatases. Moderate increases in Ca^{++}/calmodulin levels probably activate protein phosphatase 2B (PP2B), which in turn, leads to activation of protein phosphatase 1 (PP1). One target of PP1 is probably the AMPA-R. Dephosphorylation of the receptor decreases its conductance and thereby reduces the amplitude of subsequent excitatory postsynaptic potentials (EPSPs). This example of synaptic plasticity is known as long-term depression. In contrast, larger increases in Ca^{++}/calmodulin levels probably activate protein kinase C (PKC; in combination with DAG) and Ca^{++}/calmodulin-dependent protein kinase II (CamKII). PKC and CamKII, in turn, are believed to phosphorylate NMDA-R and AMPA-R and thereby increase their conductance. In addition, the kinases may elicit the synthesis and release of retrograde messenger that enhances the release of neurotransmitter from presynaptic terminals. The increases in presynaptic neurotransmitter release and in postsynaptic sensitivity to glutamate act to increase amplitude of the EPSP. This example of synaptic plasticity is referred to as long-term potentiation.

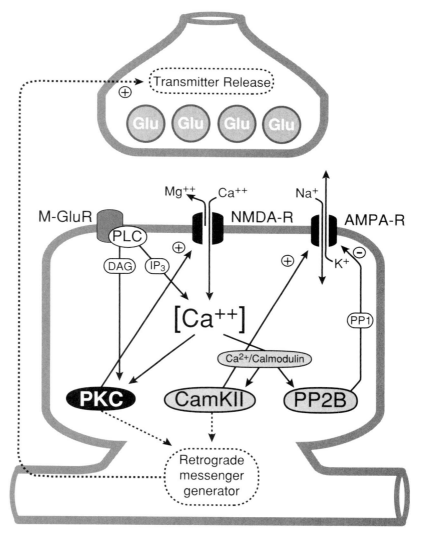

Wang et al.[51] Fukuraga et al.,[70] and Riedel,[71]). The Ca^{++} that enters through the NMDA-R is critical for activating both of these protein kinases. Moreover, the nature of the synaptic modification that expresses and maintains LTP is a matter of controversy. Currently, there is evidence for both postsynaptic changes in the glutamate receptors and presynaptic increases in the release of neurotransmitter. Presumably, the presynaptic changes are mediated by retrograde messengers, such as nitric oxide. Retrograde messengers are generated and released by the postsynaptic cell and then diffuse to presynaptic sites of action.

No discussion of hippocampal LTP would be complete without considering LTD and how their mechanisms may overlap (for reviews, see Ramakers et al.,[66] Bear and Abraham,[72] Bear and Malenka,[73] Debanne and Thompson,[74] Stanton,[75] Wagner and Alger,[76] and Zhuo and Hawkins[77]). In addition to activating protein kinases, NMDA-R–mediated influx of Ca^{++} can activate an opposing class of enzymes known as protein phosphatases (see Fig. 17–8). Protein phosphatases oppose the actions of protein kinase by removing the phosphate group from amino acid residues (i.e., dephosphorylation). Intermediate levels of postsynaptic depolarization may lead to moderate increases in the levels of intracellular Ca^{++}. These moderate levels of Ca^{++} fail to activate the protein kinase cascade, but are sufficient to activate the Ca^{++}/calmodulin-dependent protein phosphatase known as protein phosphatase 2B (also referred to as "calcineurin").[78,79] The activation of protein phosphatase 2B indirectly (i.e., through its ability to regulate the activity of protein phosphatase 1) downregulates the postsynaptic glutamate receptors. This leads to an enduring depression of synaptic efficacy (i.e., LTD). It has long been believed that for learning to occur there must be some type of LTD-like process. Otherwise, if only LTP were involved, synaptic efficacy would soon saturate and learning would be impossible. Theoretic studies indicate that greater amounts of information can be stored in neural networks with bidirectional control of synaptic strength (i.e., where both increases and decreases in synaptic strength are possible). Just as LTP has been observed at synapses throughout the CNS, so has LTD, and the mechanisms underlying LTP and LTD vary in these different regions of the CNS. For example, LTD has been studied extensively in the cerebellum. The findings indicate that cerebellar LTD is not mediated by NMDA-R or by protein phosphatases (see later).

In summary, associative LTP exhibits many properties typical of memory. For example, its induction requires close temporal contiguity between two signals, it is rapidly induced, and, once stabilized, it is quite resistant to disruption. Further support for a role for LTP in memory is indicated by the high correspondence between the optimal LTP induction conditions and endogenous patterns of neural activity that accompany learning. Specifically, LTP is induced optimally by afferent stimulation that is patterned at theta frequency,[80] a frequency that dominates in the hippocampus during information-gathering behaviors. Finally, the associative aspects of LTP are mediated, in part, by the unusual properties of the NMDA-R. This channel is dually regulated. It becomes functional only when glutamate binds to the receptor and the membrane is depolarized. Thus, the NMDA-R is ideally suited as a coincidence detector of simultaneous presynaptic and postsynaptic activity (for reviews of the role of LTP in learning and memory, see Shen et al.,[48] Maren and Baudry,[49] Martinez and Derrick,[50] and Izquierdo and Medina[81]; see, however, Holscher[82]).

Long-Term Depression

Increasing evidence suggests that, in addition to its major functional role in the regulation of fine motor control, the cerebellum is involved in other important functions. These functions include sensorimotor learning and memory (for reviews, see Kim and Thompson,[83] Llinas and Walsh,[84] Raymond et al.,[85] and Schreurs et al.[86]). Studies suggest that LTD, a process of synaptic plasticity occurring in Purkinje cells, is involved in associative learning and memory. Like LTP in the hippocampus, LTD in the cerebellar cortex is a widely studied form of synaptic plasticity in the mammalian brain (for reviews, see Maren and Baudry,[49] Zhuo and Hawkins,[77] Ito,[87] Linden,[88] and Linden and Conner[89]). Cerebellar LTD shares many of the memory-like properties of hippocampal LTP. LTD is long-lasting (it lasts for hours in vitro), it obeys Hebbian rules (i.e., it is associative), and it is specific to stimulated synapses (for discussions of the role of cerebellar LTD in learning and memory, see Maren and Baudry,[49] Holscher,[82] Raymond et al.,[85] Thompson,[90] and Thompson and Kim[91]).

The basic circuitry of the cerebellar cortex is illustrated schematically in Figure 17–9A. Purkinje neurons, which are inhibitory and function as the sole

A

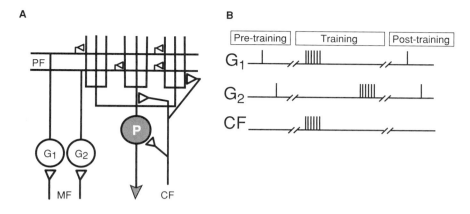

B

C

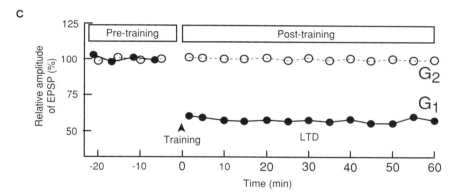

Figure 17–9. Associative long-term depression (LTD) in the cortex of the cerebellum. **A:** Microcircuitry of the cerebellar cortex: a schematic of the basic cerebellar circuit. The entire cerebellum shares a common architecture. Purkinje neurons (P), the only outputs from the cerebellar cortex, project by inhibitory connections to the deep cerebellar nuclei (not shown), which provide outputs to other brain regions. Inputs are transmitted to the cerebellum over climbing fibers (CF) and mossy fibers (MF). The climbing fiber input arises from the inferior olivary nuclei. Each Purkinje neuron receives monosynaptic excitatory inputs from just one climbing fiber, and each climbing fiber projects to approximately 10 Purkinje cells. The climbing fiber inputs are restricted to the soma and proximal dendritic branches. The mossy fiber inputs arise from several brainstem nuclei and from the spinal cord. Mossy fibers synapse on granule cells (G), which in turn form parallel fibers (PF) and make excitatory contacts with numerous Purkinje neurons. The parallel fiber inputs are restricted to the distal dendritic branches. The cerebellar cortex also contains a number of inhibitory interneurons (e.g., Golgi, basket, and stellate cells; not shown). **B:** Stimulus paradigm (not to scale). Two granule cells (G_1 and G_2) and a climbing fiber (CF) were stimulated independently. All three cells converged onto a single postsynaptic Purkinje cell. The strength of the granule cell inputs was tested by individual test stimuli before and after training (pre-training and post-training, respectively). During training, the activity in one of the granule cells (G_1) was paired with stimulation of the climbing fiber input. The activity in the other granule cell (G_2) was explicitly unpaired with climbing fiber activity. **C:** Hypothetical experiment to illustrate associative LTD. Before training (pre-training), the synaptic strength of G_1 and G_2 changes little in response to repeated test stimuli. After training, the strength of the G_2 pathway remained depressed throughout the remainder of the experiment. This sustained synaptic depression is known as LTD. The depression was specific to the granule cell that paired with climbing fiber activity during training. Thus, this represents an associative form of synaptic depression. EPSP, excitatory postsynaptic potential.

output of the cerebellar cortex, receive two excitatory inputs that are organized in very different ways. The parallel fibers (PF), which are axons of cerebellar granule cells, make highly divergent synapses on the more distal portions of the Purkinje neuron dendritic arbor (i.e., a single Purkinje neuron receives approximately 150,000 synaptic inputs from PFs). In contrast, each Purkinje neuron receives a powerful input from a *single* climbing fiber (CF), which is an axon from an inferior olive neuron, on the soma and proximal dendritic arbor. Fast excitatory synaptic transmission at both PF and CF synapses is mediated primarily by postsynaptic AMPA-R (Fig. 17–10). Figure 17–9B and C schematically illustrates an experi-

mental protocol developed by Schreurs et al.[84] to investigate the associative properties of LTD in vitro and to illustrate how LTD can be induced using a protocol similar to that of differential conditioning. Two independent PF inputs to a single postsynaptic Purkinje neuron were stimulated. To monitor the strength of the independent PF inputs, individual test stimuli were applied before and after training. During training, a brief burst of stimuli in one PF pathway (G_1) was paired with a high-frequency burst in the CF input to the same Purkinje neuron. The brief burst of stimuli in the second PF pathway (G_2) was explicitly unpaired with activity in the CF during training. The two PF pathways were analogous to the

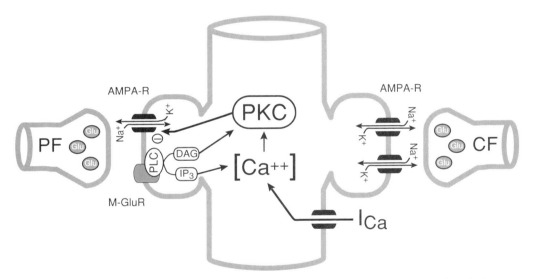

Figure 17–10. Molecular processes believed to underlie the induction and expression of cerebellar long-term depression. Two postsynaptic spine complexes on the dendritic arbor of a Purkinje cell are illustrated. One of the spines receives a synaptic input from a parallel fiber (PF) and the other spine receives a synaptic input from a climbing fiber (CF). Note that although the PF and CF inputs are illustrated as occurring on the same dendritic branch, this is not accurate. Rather, PF inputs are restricted to the more distal segments of the dendritic arbor, and CF inputs occur on the soma and proximal dendrites (see Figure 17–9A). EPSPs at both PF and CF inputs are mediated by the AMPA-receptor (AMPA-R). The strength of CF input, however, is much larger and is capable of eliciting strong postsynaptic depolarizations and spiking activity. Thus, the CF inputs can activate voltage-gated Ca^{++} currents (I_{Ca}), which in turn, elevate intracellular levels of Ca^{++} in the Purkinje cells. Glutamate release from PF inputs also activates the metabotropic glutamate receptors (M-GluR), which are coupled to phospholipase C (PLC). The activation of PLC liberates inositol triphosphate (IP3) and diacylglycerol (DAG), which in combination with CF-mediated increased levels of Ca^{++} activate protein kinase C (PKC). One of the substrates of PKC is believed to be the AMPA-R (or associated proteins), and the phosphorylation of the AMPA-R decreases its conductance or ability to bind glutamate. Thus, synaptic transmission of the PF input is depressed.

two CSs in a differential conditioning protocol, and the CF input was analogous to the US. As illustrated in the posttraining period (see Fig. 17–9C), LTD (i.e., a sustained decrease in the amplitude of individual test EPSPs) was induced only in the PF pathway that was paired with CF activity input during training (i.e., G_1). The LTD induced in these types of experiments is referred to as associative LTD. Note, as with associative LTP (see Fig. 17–7), the change in synaptic efficacy is input specific; it is restricted to the PF pathway whose activity was closely associated with activity in the CF. The key contributing factor of the CF pathway was its ability to induce a postsynaptic depolarization sufficient to activate voltage-gated Ca^{++} channels in the Purkinje neuron. Thus, LTD can also be induced by pairing activity in a PF with direct depolarization of the postsynaptic cells.[92]

The critical events in the induction of LTD involve the coupling of a potent Ca^{++} signal, which is generated by CF discharges, with activation of M-GluR at PF to Purkinje cell synapses (see Fig. 17–10). The elevation of intracellular Ca^{++} is probably mediated by both voltage-gated Ca^{++} channels activated by the CF-induced depolarization, and by the release of Ca^{++} from intracellular stores by an M-GluR–mediated second messenger cascade (i.e., IP3). Several intracellular second messengers and protein kinases are critical for cerebellar LTD, including DAG and PKC. The modification that underlies LTD at PF synapses appears to be a sustained desensitization of AMPA-R responses.[93,94] Thus, the final common pathway for the induction and expression of both hippocampal LTP and cerebellar LTD is an elevation of intracellular Ca^{++}, an activation of enzymatic cascades, and a modification of postsynaptic AMPA-R. In contrast, in LTP, the NMDA-R represents the integrating device for the two signals (i.e., presynaptic and postsynaptic activity), whereas the dual regulation of PKC by DAG and Ca^{++} appears to detect the temporal contiguity between presynaptic and postsynaptic activity that leads to the induction of cerebellar LTD.

Stages in Memory Storage

The duration of memory for both implicit and explicit forms of learning (see Fig. 17–2) is graded and is related to the number of training trials. In general, memory is divided into at least two temporally distinct components: short-term, which lasts a few

minutes to hours and is labile and highly sensitive to disruption, and long-term, which is stable, self-maintained, and lasts days, weeks, and in some cases a lifetime. Studies have led to the development of a three-phase molecular model for memory formation. These phases are sequentially dependent (Fig. 17–11; for reviews, see Fagnou and Tuchek,[19] Bailey et al.,[95] Brunelli et al.,[96] Carew,[97] Dragunow,[98] Hiroi and Nestler,[99] Montminy,[100] Ponomarenko and Kamyshev,[101] and Tsuda[102]). The basic model consists of short-term memory, intermediate-term memory, and, finally, long-term memory. Second messenger and protein kinase cascades play a pivotal role in initiating the separate memory processes (i.e., induction) of different durations, and protein synthesis is accepted as underlying the formation of long-term memory (see later).

Short-Term Memory

Short-term memory (i.e., phase 1) processes are subserved by covalent modifications of preexisting proteins (e.g., phosphorylation and dephosphorylation). Such proteins include ionic channels or associated proteins, or proteins within the machinery that mediates synaptic transmission (e.g., mobilization of receptors for neurotransmitters). Short-term memory involves an alteration of preexisting synaptic connections and does not require ongoing macromolecular synthesis, such as gene transcription or protein synthesis (i.e., translation). The conversion of a transient short-term memory into a more stable long-term memory (i.e., consolidation) is accompanied by the growth of new synaptic connections and requires a cellular program of gene expression and increased protein synthesis.

Intermediate- and Long-Term Memory

In general, long-term memories are induced only after multiple training trials. With repeated or prolonged training, protein kinases translocate to the nucleus, where they act on nuclear substrates that include transcription factors (i.e., proteins that bind to DNA and regulate the rate of gene transcription). The transcription factors regulate, in part, a family of genes known as immediate-early genes. The proteins encoded by immediate-early genes include both effector proteins (e.g., enzymes) and additional transcription factors that, in turn, regulate the expression

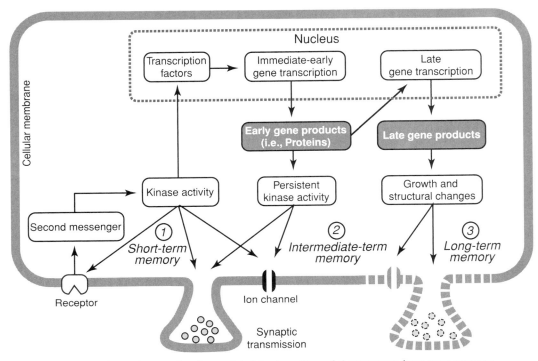

Figure 17–11. Three-phase molecular model of the transition of short-term to long-term memory. The storage of long-term memory is associated with a cellular program of second messenger/kinase system activation, gene transcription in the nucleus, altered protein synthesis, and the growth of new synaptic connections (dashed component of cellular membrane). The first phase of memory (i.e., short-term memory) is mediated by kinases and the modification of preexisting proteins and synaptic connections. A second phase (i.e., intermediate-term memory) is mediated by persistent activation of kinases, which prolongs the modification of preexisting proteins. With sufficient training, the kinases translocate to the nucleus and phosphorylate nuclear substrates, some of which are transcription factors. The transcription factors, in turn, regulate the transcription of immediate-early genes (IEGs). Some of the translated products of IEGs (ie., proteins) are also transcription factors that regulate the transcription of late genes, and presumably the translated products of the late genes mediate growth processes. Thus, consolidation of memory requires activation of a complex molecular network.

of late genes. Among the early effector proteins are enzymes that may function to help maintain the activity of kinases and prolong the covalent modification of preexisting proteins. This modification mediates an intermediate phase of memory. The duration of such an intermediate-term memory would depend on the half-life of the effector proteins, which usually is on the order of several hours. (Note that persistent kinase activity and intermediate-term memory may also occur through alternate mechanisms, such as autophosphorylation, which do not require

transcription and translation.) The proteins encoded by later genes are presumably structural and are responsible for stabilizing the long-term memory through the growth of new synaptic connections. The storage of memory is associated with a program of enzymatic activity, gene expression, altered protein synthesis, and growth. Short- and intermediate-term memory are mediated by covalent modification of preexisting proteins, whereas long-term memory is initiated by early regulator genes, whose protein products trigger the induction of new proteins.

General Principles

Extensive behavioral, anatomic, physiologic, and molecular analyses since the late 1980s have revealed what appear to be some general principles of learning and memory. These principles include the following:

1 Learning and memory have multiple forms.
2 Multiple, but distinct, regions of the brain serve as loci for learning and memory.
3 At least short-term forms of memory involve changes in existing neural circuits.
4 These changes may involve multiple cellular mechanisms in single neurons.
5 Second messenger systems appear to play a role in mediating cellular changes.
6 Changes in the properties of membrane channels are commonly correlated with learning and memory.
7 Long-term memory requires new protein synthesis and growth, whereas short-term memory does not.

Clinical Correlations

How does the understanding of cellular and molecular mechanisms underlying synaptic plasticity bring us closer to an understanding of the mechanisms underlying rehabilitation? This review of cellular and molecular processes underlying learning and memory suggests two general principles that might be applied to rehabilitation therapy:[103]

1 The brain changes its functional configuration in response to internal and environmental stimuli. Moreover, some optimal induction conditions and patterns can take advantage of the intrinsic properties of the cellular and molecular processes that underlie neuronal plasticity.
2 Cellular and molecular processes that underlie neuronal plasticity are ubiquitous properties of neural systems, and thus, functional changes can be induced in all levels of neural organization.

The application of these general principles is probably best illustrated by examples of applying learning paradigms in the rehabilitation context.

Applying Associative Learning Paradigms to Recovery After Brain Injury

The motor cortex is intimately involved in the initiation of voluntary motor action, especially fine manipulative abilities. Surprisingly, however, a gradual return of motor abilities often occurs in the weeks and months after injury. Neurophysiologic and neuroanatomic bases have long been sought to account for functional recovery after cortical injury. Research using rats and monkeys has demonstrated the electrical and structural changes in the brain as a result of "rehabilitation" techniques.[104–106] After introducing an infarct (similar to a CVA) into the brain of the animals, operant conditioning paradigms were used to retrain the animals. The investigators had two major findings. First, lack of use of the affected side caused changes in the brain, and atrophy of brain structures occurred, resulting in increased disuse of the limb. Second, results indicated that forced use of the affected limb resulted in electrical remapping of the brain. In other words, adjacent cells took over function from the damaged cells, resulting in improvement in limb abilities. Moreover, recent neurophysiologic studies also indicated that the motor cortex is alterable throughout life, and that functional reorganization in cortical areas can occur after damage that occurred up to 12 years previously (see Chap. 21).

Learning-induced functional plasticity is not restricted to the cortex. For example, the spinal cord itself appears to be capable of learning specific motor tasks.[107–115] Both classical and operant conditioning paradigms have been used to "train" neural circuits in the spinal cord. The ability of the spinal cord to learn complex motor tasks has been clearly demonstrated by the maintenance of locomotor function in animals (including humans) whose spinal cord has been transected. Both short- and long-term adaptations can occur and the ability to acquire motor skills is present for years after the spinal cord injury. Thus, the capacity for functional plasticity may be substantially more extensive than previously thought. The life-long capacity for functional reorganization and plasticity is probably a common feature of all levels of neural organization, from the cortex to the spinal cord.

Dementia and Alzheimer's Disease

Dementia is defined by the *Diagnostic and Statistical Manual for Mental Disorders* (DSM-IV) as the development of cognitive deficits and at least one of the following disturbances: aphasia, apraxia, agnosia, or a disturbance in executive function. The cognitive deficits must be sufficiently severe to cause impairments in occupational or social functioning or must represent a decline from a previous level of functioning. Dementia is a group of symptoms that may occur with certain diseases or physical conditions. The most common of these is Alzheimer's disease (AD), but others include infectious disorders, congenital deficits, head injury, multiple sclerosis, and endocrine conditions.

Alzheimer's disease is a disorder of the CNS first identified by Alois Alzheimer, a German neurologist, in 1906. This degenerative disease affects cognitive functioning and leads to a decline in functional and social skills. It is estimated that 58% of residents in nursing homes have AD. The cause of AD remains unclear, but the physical and chemical alterations in brain structure that cause the cognitive deficits in AD are well known (see Chap. 20).

The structural changes in the brain include neurofibrillary tangles, neuritic plaques, and granulovascular degeneration. Each of these changes affects neuronal function. The changes occur primarily in the cerebral cortex and limbic system, specifically the hippocampus and the amygdala. The behaviors of a person with AD directly reflect the cognitive changes that occur as a result of the damage to these brain centers. An understanding of the function of the hippocampus, amygdala, and cerebral cortex in learning and memory helps to clarify the memory and cognitive deficits common in AD and other conditions.

Clinical Manifestations of Alzheimer's Disease

A client diagnosed with AD may have any or all of the following behaviors related to cognitive decline: 1) repetition of the same question or movement; 2) a change in personality, usually becoming more angry and agitated; 3) the use of inaccurate or incorrect statements, often trying to "fill in the blanks" of the missing memory; 4) the experience of hallucinations or paranoia as a result of the brain's inability to interpret sensory information correctly; 5) regression of social skills and inappropriate interactions with family, friends, and loved ones; significant others and parts of conversations and interactions may not be remembered; 6) refusal to groom and bathe

as a result of the lack of meaning associated with social interaction and societal mores; 7) wandering; and 8) as memory and cognitive functions decline, the affected person may begin looking for something real or imaginary, only to forget the object of the search in the process, thus appearing to wander aimlessly.

Treatments for Alzheimer's Disease

The development of treatments for AD is being pursued along many diverse lines. Primary treatment is aimed at the core elements of AD: memory and other cognitive loss at the symptomatic level. An understanding of the cellular and molecular mechanisms of learning and memory are providing a framework that is guiding the development of new pharmacologic tools.[116–121] In this regard, several attempts have been made to develop cognitive enhancers based on the properties of synaptic plasticity mechanisms. For example, one approach has been directed toward developing pharmacologic agents that modulate the properties of AMPA-R and thereby enhance in the induction of LTP and memory.[122] In general, the strategy is to identify molecular deficiencies in patients with AD that are associated with memory function (e.g., neurotransmitter receptors or kinases) and develop intervention that increases synaptic efficacy under conditions that would normally remain subthreshold for triggering the enzymatic cascades necessary for learning and memory.

In conclusion, neuroscience research is providing intriguing insights into the neuronal processes that underlie learning and memory. Understanding this research may lead to new therapeutic approaches that are based on both the basic rules of motor coordination and the rules governing functional plasticity in the nervous system.

Acknowledgment
Dr. D. A. Baxter was supported, in part, by National Institutes of Health grant R01-RR-11626.

REFERENCES

1. Albert MS. Cognitive and neurobiologic markers of early Alzheimer disease. *Proc Natl Acad Sci U S A* 1996; 93: 13547–13551.
2. Gabrieli JDE. Memory systems analyses of mnemonic disorders in aging and age-related diseases. *Proc Natl Acad Sci U S A* 1996;93:13534–13540.

3. Weiner MF, Koss E, Wild KV, et al. Measures of psychiatric symptoms in Alzheimer patients: a review. *Alzheimer Dis Assoc Disord* 1996;10:20–30.

4. DeLisa JA, Gans BM. *Rehabilitation medicine: principles and practice.* 2nd ed. Philadelphia: JB Lippincott, 1988.

5. Dudai Y. *The neurobiology of memory: concepts, findings, trends.* New York: Oxford University Press, 1989.

6. Thompson RF, Spencer WA. Habituation: a model phenomenon for the study of neuronal substrates of behavior. *Psychol Rev* 1966;73:16–43.

7. Pavlov IP. *Conditioned reflexes: an investigation of the physiological activity of the cerebral cortex.* London: Oxford University Press, 1927.

8. Mackintosh NJ. *Conditioning and associative learning.* New York: Oxford University Press, 1974.

9. Mackintosh NJ. *The psychology of animal learning.* New York: Academic Press, 1983.

10. Rescorla RA. Pavlovian conditioning and its proper control procedures. *Psychol Rev* 1967;74:71–80.

11. Skinner BF. *The behavior of organisms.* New York: Appleton-Century, 1938.

12. Nargeot R, Baxter DA, Byrne JH. Contingent-dependent enhancement of rhythmic motor patterns: an in vitro analog of operant conditioning. *J Neurosci* 1997;17:8093–8105.

13. Hawkins RD, Kandel ER. Is there a cell-biological alphabet for simple forms of learning? *Psychol Rev* 1984;91:375–391.

14. Raymond JL, Baxter DA, Buonomano DV, Byrne JH. A learning rule based on empirically-derived activity-dependent neuromodulation supports operant conditioning in a small network. *Neural Networks* 1992;5:789–803.

15. Squire LR, Knowlton BJ. Memory, hippocampus, and brain systems. In: Gazzinga M, ed. *The cognitive neurosciences.* Cambridge, MA: The MIT Press, 1994:825–838.

16. Squire LR, Zola SM. Structure and function of declarative and nondeclarative memory systems. *Proc Natl Acad Sci U S A* 1996;93:13515–13522.

17. Ungerleider LG. Functional brain imaging studies of cortical mechanisms for memory. *Science* 1995;270:769–775.

18. Byrne JH. Cellular analysis of associative learning. *Physiol Rev* 1987;67:329–439.

19. Fagnou DD, Tuchek JM.. The biochemistry of learning and memory. *Mol Cell Biochem* 1995;149–150:279–286.

20. Hawkins RD, Kandel ER, Siegelbaum S. Learning to modulate transmitter release: themes and variations in synaptic plasticity. *Annu Rev Neurosci* 1993;16:625–665.

21. Byrne JH, Kandel ER. Presynaptic facilitation revisited: state and time dependence. *J Neurosci* 1996;16:425–435.

22. Kandel ER, Schwartz JH. Molecular biology of learning: modulation of transmitter release. *Science* 1982;218:433–443.

23. Edmonds B, Klein M, Dale N, Kandel ER. Contributions of two types of calcium channels to synaptic transmission and plasticity. *Science* 1990;250:1142–1147.

24. Klein M, Shapiro E, Kandel ER. Synaptic plasticity and the modulation of the Ca^{2+} current. *J Exp Biol* 1980;89:117–157.

25. Gingrich KJ, Byrne JH. Simulation of synaptic depression, posttetanic potentiation, and presynaptic facilitation of synaptic potentials from sensory neurons mediating gill-withdrawal reflex in *Aplysia. J Neurophysiol* 1985;53:652–669.

26. Bailey CH, Chen M. Morphological basis of short-term habituation in *Aplysia. J Neurosci* 1988;8:2452–2459.

27. Byrne JH, Zwartjes R, Homayouni R, Critz S, Eskin A. Roles of second messenger pathways in neuronal plasticity and in learning and memory: insights gained from *Aplysia. Adv Second Messenger Phosphoprotein Res* 1993;27:47–108.

28. Nakanishi K, Zhang F, Baxter DA, Eskin A, Byrne JH. Role of calcium-calmodulin-dependent protein kinase II in modulation of sensorimotor synapses in *Aplysia. J Neurophysiol* 1997;78:409–416.

29. Baxter DA, Byrne JH. Learning rules from neurobiology. In: Gardner D, ed. *The neurobiology of neural networks.* Cambridge, MA: The MIT Press, 1992:71–106.

30. Hebb DO. *The organization of behavior.* New York: Wiley, 1949.

31. Abrams TW, Kandel ER. Is contiguity detection in classical conditioning a system or a cellular property? Learning in *Aplysia* suggest a possible molecular site. *Trends Neurosci* 1988;4:128–135.

32. Casabona G. Intracellular signal modulation: a pivotal role for protein kinase C. *Prog Neuropsychopharmacol Biol Psychiatry* 1997;21:407–425.

33. Hawkins RD, Abrams TW, Carew TJ, Kandel ER. A cellular mechanism of classical conditioning in *Aplysia*: activity-dependent amplification of presynaptic facilitation. *Science* 1983;219:400–405.

34. Walters ET, Byrne JH. Associative conditioning of single sensory neurons suggest a cellular mechanism for learning. *Science* 1983;219:405–408.

35. Carew TJ, Hawkins RD, Kandel ER. Differential classical conditioning of a defensive withdrawal reflex in *Aplysia californica. Science* 1983;219:397–400.

36. Carew TJ, Walters ET, Kandel ER. Classical conditioning in a simple withdrawal reflex in *Aplysia californica. J Neurosci* 1981;1:1426–1437.

37. Hawkins RD, Carew TJ, Kandel ER. Effects of interstimulus interval and contingency on classical conditioning of *Aplysia* siphon withdrawal reflex. *J Neurosci* 1986;6:1695–1701.

38. Abrams TW. Activity-dependent presynaptic facilitation: an associative mechanism in *Aplysia. Cell Mol Neurobiol* 1985;5:123–145.

39. Byrne JH. Neural and molecular mechanisms underlying information storage in *Aplysia*: implications for learning and memory. *Trends Neurosci* 1985;8:478–482.

40. Abrams TW, Karl KA, Kandel ER. Biochemical studies of stimulus convergence during classical conditioning in *Aplysia*: dual regulation of adenylate cyclase by Ca^{2+}/calmodulin and transmitter. *J Neurosci* 1991;11:655–2665.

41. Ocorr KA, Walter ET, Byrne JH. Associative conditioning analog selectively increases cAMP levels of tail sensory neurons in *Aplysia*. *Proc Natl Acad Sci U S A* 1985;82:2548–2552.

42. Eliot LS, Dudia Y, Kandel ER, Abrams TW. Ca^{2+}/calmodulin sensitivity may be common to all forms of neural adenylate cyclase. *Proc Natl Acad Sci U S A* 1989;86:9564–9568.

43. Xia Z, Strom DR. Calmodulin-regulated adenylyl cyclase and neuromodulation. *Curr Opin Neurobiol* 1997;7:391–396.

44. Eliot LS, Hawkins RD, Kandel ER, Schacher S. Pairing-specific, activity-dependent presynaptic facilitation at *Aplysia* sensory-motor synapses in isolated cell culture. *J Neurosci* 1994;14:368–383.

45. Bao J-X, Kandel ER, Hawkins RD. Involvement of presynaptic and postsynaptic mechanisms in a cellular analog of classical conditioning at *Aplysia* sensory-motor neuron synapses in isolated cell culture. *J Neurosci* 1998;18:458–466.

46. Lechner HA, Byrne JH. New perspective on classical conditioning: a synthesis of Hebbian and non-Hebbian mechanisms. *Neuron* 1998;20:1–4.

47. Schacter DL. *Searching for memory: the brain, the mind and the past*. New York: HarperCollins, 1997.

48. Shen Y, Specht SM, Ghislain ID, Li R. The hippocampus: a biological model for studying learning and memory. *Prog Neurobiol* 1994;44:485–496.

49. Maren S, Baudry M. Properties and mechanisms of long-term synaptic plasticity in the mammalian brain: relationships to learning and memory. *Neurobiol Learn Mem* 1995;63:1–18.

50. Martinez JL, Derrick BE. Long-term potentiation and learning. *Annu Rev Psychol* 1996;47:173–203.

51. Wang JH, Ko GY, Kelly PT. Cellular and molecular bases of memory: synaptic and neuronal plasticity. *J Clin Neurophysiol* 1997;14:264–293.

52. Bliss TVP, Lomo WT. Long-lasting potentiation of synaptic transmission in the dentate area of the anesthetized rabbit following stimulation of the perforant path. *J Physiol (Lond)* 1973;232:331–356.

53. Chapman PF, Kairiss EW, Keenan CL, Brown TH. Long-term synaptic potentiation in the amygdala. *Synapse* 1990;6:271–278.

54. Maren S. Synaptic transmission and plasticity in the amygdala: an emerging physiology of fear conditioning circuits. *Mol Neurobiol* 1996;13:1–22.

55. Artola A, Brocher S, Singer W. Different voltage-dependent thresholds for inducing long-term depression and long-term potentiation in slices of rat visual cortex. *Nature* 1990;347:69–72.

56. Kirkwood A, Bear MF. Elementary forms of synaptic plasticity in the visual cortex. *Biol Res* 1995;28:73–80.

57. Barrionuevo G, Brown TH. Associative long-term potentiation in hippocampal slices. *Proc Natl Acad Sci U S A* 1983;80:7347–7351.

58. Kelso SR, Gangong AH, Brown TH. Hebbian synapses in hippocampus. *Proc Natl Acad Sci U S A* 1986;83:5326–5330.

59. Wigstrom H, Gustafsson B, Huang Y-Y, Abraham WC. Hippocampal long-term potentiation induced by pairing single afferent volleys with intracellularly injected depolarizing pulses. *Acta Physiol Scand* 1986;126:317–319.

60. Collingridge GL, Bliss TVP. NMDA receptors: their role in long-term potentiation. *Trends Neurosci* 1987;7:288–293.

61. Collingridge GL, Bliss TVP. Memories of NMDA receptors and long-term potentiation. *Trends Neurosci* 1995;18:54–56.

62. Madison DV, Malenka RC, Nicoll RA. Mechanisms underlying long-term potentiation of synaptic transmission. *Annu Rev Neurosci* 1991;14:379–397.

63. Nicoll RA, Kauer JA, Malenka RC. The current excitement in long-term potentiation. *Neuron* 1988;1:97–103.

64. Rison RA, Stanton PK. Long-term potentiation and N-methyl-D-aspartate receptors: foundations of memory and neurologic disease? *Neurosci Biobehav Rev* 1995; 19:533–552.

65. Angenstein F, Staak S. Receptor-mediated activation of protein kinase C in hippocampal long-term potentiation: facts, problems and implications. *Prog Neuropsychopharmacol Biol Psychiatry* 1997;21:427–454.

66. Ramakers GMJ, Pasinelli P, Hens JJH, Gispen WH, De Graan PNE. Protein kinase C in synaptic plasticity: changes in the in situ phosphorylation state of identified pre- and postsynaptic substrates. *Prog Neuropsychopharmacol Biol Psychiatry* 1997;21:455–486.

67. van der Zee EA, Luiten PG, Disterhoft JR. Learning-induced alterations in hippocampal PKC-immunoreactivity: a review and hypothesis of its functional significance. *Prog Neuropsychopharmacol Biol Psychiatry* 1997;21:531–572.

68. Riedel G. Function of metabotropic glutamate receptors in learning and memory. *Trends Neurosci* 1996; 19:219–224.

69. Riedel G, Reymann KG. Metabotropic glutamate receptors in hippocampal long-term potentiation and learning and memory. *Acta Physiol Scand* 1996;157:1–19.

70. Fukuraga K, Miller D, Miyamoto E. CaMKinase II in long-term potentiation. *Neurochem Int* 1996;28:343–358.

71. Riedel G. Protein kinase C: a memory kinase? *Prog Neuropsychopharmacol Biol Psychiatry* 1997;21:373–378.

72. Bear MF, Abraham WC. Long-term depression in hippocampus. *Annu Rev Neurosci* 1996;19:437–462.
73. Bear MF, Malenka RC. Synaptic plasticity: LTP and LTD. *Curr Opin Neurobiol* 1994;4:389–399.
74. Debanne D, Thompson SM. Associative long-term depression in the hippocampus in vitro. *Hippocampus* 1996;6:9–16.
75. Stanton PK. LTD, LTP, and the sliding threshold for long-term synaptic plasticity. *Hippocampus* 1996;6:35–42.
76. Wagner JJ, Alger BE. Homosynaptic LTD and depotentiation: do they differ in name only? *Hippocampus* 1996;6:24–29.
77. Zhuo M, Hawkins RD. Long-term depression: a learning-related type of synaptic plasticity in the mammalian central nervous system. *Rev Neurosci* 1995;6:259–277.
78. Artola A, Singer W. Long-term depression of excitatory synaptic transmission and its relationship to long-term potentiation. *Trends Neurosci* 1993;16:480–487.
79. Lisman J. A mechanism for the Hebb and the anti-Hebb processes underlying learning and memory. *Proc Natl Acad Sci U S A* 1989;86:9574–9578.
80. Larson J, Lynch G. Theta pattern stimulation and the induction of LTP: the sequence in which synapses are stimulated determines the degree to which they potentiate. *Brain Res* 1989;489:49–58.
81. Izquierdo I, Medina JH. Correlation between the pharmacology of long-term potentiation and the pharmacology of memory. *Neurobiol Learn Mem* 1995;63:19–32.
82. Holscher C. Long-term potentiation: a good model for learning and memory? *Prog Neuropsychopharmacol Biol Psychiatry* 1997;21:47–68.
83. Kim JJ, Thompson RF. Cerebellar circuits and synaptic mechanisms involved in classical eyeblink conditioning. *Trends Neurosci* 1997;20:177–181.
84. Llinas R, Walsh JP. On the cerebellum and motor learning. *Curr Opin Neurobiol* 1993;3:958–965.
85. Raymond JL, Lisberger SG, Mauk MD. The cerebellum: a neuronal learning machine? *Science* 1996;272:1126–1131.
86. Schreurs BG, Oh MM, Alkon DL. Pairing specific long-term depression of Purkinje cell excitatory postsynaptic potentials results from a classical conditioning procedure in the rabbit cerebellar slice. *J Neurophysiol* 1996;75:1051–1060.
87. Ito M. Long-term depression. *Annu Rev Neurosci* 1989;12:85–102.
88. Linden DJ. Long-term synaptic depression in the mammalian brain. *Neuron* 1994;12:457–472.
89. Linden DJ, Conner JA. Long-term synaptic depression. *Annu Rev Neurosci* 1995;18:319–357.
90. Thompson RF. The neurobiology of learning and memory. *Science* 1986;233:941–947.
91. Thompson RF, Kim J. Memory systems in the brain and localization of a memory. *Proc Natl Acad Sci U S A* 1996;93:13438–13444.
92. Narasimhan K, Linden DJ. Defining a minimal computational unit for cerebellar long-term depression. *Neuron* 1996;17:333–341.
93. Hemart N, Daniel H, Jaillard D, Crepel F. Properties of glutamate receptors are modified during long-term depression in rat cerebellar Purkinje cells. *Neurosci Res* 1995;19:213–221.
94. Linden DJ, Dichinson MH, Smeyne M, Connor JA. A long-term depression of AMPA currents in cultured cerebellar Purkinje cells. *Neuron* 1991;7:81–89.
95. Bailey CH, Bartsch D, Kandel ER. Toward a molecular definition of long-term memory storage. *Proc Natl Acad Sci U S A* 1996;93:13445–13452.
96. Brunelli M, Barcia-Gill M, Mozzachiodi R, Scuri R, Zaccardi ML. Neurobiological principles of learning and memory. *Arch Ital Biol* 1997;135:15–36.
97. Carew TJ. Molecular enhancement of memory formation. *Neuron* 1996;16:5–8.
98. Dragunow M. A role for immediate-early transcription factors in learning and memory. *Behav Genet* 1996;26:293–299.
99. Hiroi N, Nestler EJ. Nuclear memory: gene transcription and behavior. *Adv Pharmacol* 1998;42:1037–1041.
100. Montminy M. Transcriptional regulation by cyclic AMP. *Annu Rev Biochem* 1997;66:807–822.
101. Ponomarenko VV, Kamyshev NG. Genetic aspects of the mechanisms of learning. *Neurosci Behav Physiol* 1997;27:245–249.
102. Tsuda M. Cascade of gene expression induced by Ca^{2+} signals in neurons. *Neurochem Int* 1996;29:443–451.
103. Neistadt ME. The neurobiology of learning: implications for treatment of adults with brain injury. *Am J Occup Ther* 1994;48:421–430.
104. Nudo RJ, Milliken GW. Reorganizations of movement representations in primary motor cortex following focal ischemic infarcts in adult squirrel monkeys. *J Neurophysiol* 1996;5:2144–2149.
105. Nudo RJ, Milliken GW, Jenkins WM, Merzenich MM. Use-dependent alterations of movement representations in primary motor cortex of adult squirrel monkeys. *J Neurosci* 1996;16:785–807.
106. Nudo RJ, Wise BM, SiFuentes F, Millliken GW. Neural substrates for the effects of rehabilitation training on motor recovery after ischemic infarct. *Science* 1996;272:1791–1794.
107. Buerger AA, Fennessy A. Learning of leg position in chronic spinal rats. *Nature* 1970;225:751–752.
108. Edgertor VR, de Leon RD, Tillakaratne N, Recktenwald MR, Hodgson JA. Use-dependent plasticity in spinal stepping and standing. *Adv Neurol* 1997;72:233–247.
109. Hodgson JA, Roy RR, deLeon R, Dobkin B, Edgeton VR. Can the mammalian lumbar spinal cord learn a motor task? *Med Sci Sports Exerc* 1994;26:1491–1497.

110. Illich PA, Salinas JA, Grau JW. Latent inhibition, overshadowing, and blocking of a conditioned antinociceptive response in spinalized rats. *Behav Neural Biol* 1994;62:140–150.

111. Joynes RL, Grau JW. Mechanisms of Pavlovian conditioning: role of protections from habituation in spinal conditioning. *Behav Neurosci* 1996;110:1375–1387.

112. Joynes RL, Illich PA, Grau JW. Evidence for spinal conditioning in intact rats. *Neurobiol Learn Mem* 1997;67:64–68.

113. Schalow G, Blanc Y, Jeltsch W, Zach GA. Electromyographic identification of spinal oscillator patterns and recouplings in a patient with incomplete spinal cord lesion: oscillator formation training as a method to improve motor activities. *Gen Physiol Biophys* 1996;15:121–220.

114. Whelan J. Control of locomotion in the decerebrate cat. *Prog Neurobiol* 1996;49:481–515.

115. Wolpaw JR. Acquisition and maintenance of the simplest motor skills: investigation of CNS mechanisms. *Med Sci Sports Exerc* 1994;26:1475–1479.

116. Etcheberrigary E, Gibson GE, Alkon DL. Molecular mechanisms of memory and the pathophysiology of Alzheimer's disease. *Ann N Y Acad Sci* 1994;747:245–255.

117. Ingram DK, Shimada A, Spangler EL, et al. Cognitive enhancement: new strategies for stimulating cholinergic, glutamatergic, and nitric oxide systems. *Ann N Y Acad Sci* 1996;786:348–361.

118. Jin LW, Saitoh T. Changes in protein kinases in brain aging and Alzheimer's disease: implications for drug therapy. *Drugs Aging* 1995;6:136–149.

119. Knopman DS, Morris JC. An update on primary drug therapies for Alzheimer disease. *Arch Neurol* 1997;54:1406–1409.

120. Nicoletti F, Bruno V, Copani A, Casabona G, Knopfel T. Metabotropic glutamate receptors: a new target for the therapy of neurodegenerative disorders? *Trends Neurosci* 1996;19:267–271.

121. Olney JW, Wozniak DF, Farber NB. Excitotoxic neurodegeneration in Alzheimer disease: new hypothesis and new therapeutic strategies. *Arch Neurol* 1997;54:1234–1240.

122. Ingvar M, Ambros-Ingerson J, Davis M, et al. Enhancement by an ampakine of memory encoding in humans. *Exp Neurol* 1997;146:553–559.

18

Neural Mechanisms of Language

CHRISTIANA M. LEONARD, PhD

• • •

Language is a symbolic system that humans use for communicating thoughts. No other organism spontaneously develops such a system. Although chimpanzees can learn to use American Sign Language or systems of tokens, teaching must be explicit and the chimp never develops the comprehension level of most 2-year-old children.[1] The ability to develop language must depend on anatomic and physiologic specializations in the human brain. The techniques that have been used to study these specializations include the clinical description of patients with brain damage, cortical stimulation of patients evaluated for epilepsy surgery, anatomic and neurophysiologic study of the auditory cortex, evaluation of the effects on language development of early brain damage, and structural and functional brain imaging.

349

Although studies with these techniques have revealed many interesting phenomena, our understanding of the neural substrate of language is still primitive because there is no generally accepted animal model. The absence of work on animal models is the result of the influence of a brilliant linguist, Noam Chomsky, who maintains that there is a discontinuity between animal and human communication: that humans have a special-purpose language acquisition device that develops relatively independently of experience.[2] This influential theory has had a deadening effect on work on mammalian neuroanatomic and neurophysiologic characteristics that might underlie information processing in primitive forms of language. The influence of this theory is waning, however, and the next 20 years will probably see a dramatic increase in our understanding of the neural specializations for language.

Language

The processes required for generating and comprehending language are organized on many levels, including that of phonology (the sound structure), syntax (the structure of words and sentences), semantics (meaning), and pragmatics (how language is used for communication). Neither imaging nor clinical data support a simple correspondence of these levels with different neural systems.[3]

Language as a Specialized Form of Information Processing

Neurobiologists tend to conceptualize language function in terms of information processing.[4] The primary and secondary cortical sensory areas in the occipital, parietal, and temporal lobes form an intricate mosaic of repeated maps of the peripheral receptor sheets on the retina, cochlea, and body surface.[5] Each map amplifies stimulus energy differences along a particular dimension (e.g., frequency, intensity, or location). Visual area MT (middle temporal) in the superior temporal sulcus specializes in discriminating rates and direction of object motion, for example. The frontal lobe also contains a mosaic of maps, but in this case, the maps represent temporal and spatial characteristics of intended response targets.[6] Complex sequences of behavior are generated by the frontal response selection regions on the basis of sensory information represented in the posterior sensory maps. The sensory in-

formation reaches the frontal areas through elaborate converging and diverging topographic fiber projections from the parietal and temporal lobes.

Topographically ordered maps of acoustic features and articulatory targets are probably important components of the neural processes underlying elementary mechanisms of speech perception and production. Whether complex processes like sentence generation and comprehension can also be explained in terms of the interaction of neurons in topographically ordered maps remains to be investigated. In the absence of a conceptually organized scientific neurolinguistics, this chapter starts with a historical introduction.

Functional Lateralization

In the middle of the last century, Marc Dax and Paul Broca, two French physicians, reported that **aphasia** (a disturbance of language) was much more likely to follow brain damage in the left hemisphere than the right.[7] After postmortem examination of a series of brains, Broca localized the cause of the disturbance to the left frontal lobe, an area that has come to be known as **Broca's area** (Fig. 18–1). This was the first suggestion that the left and right hemispheres might have different functional specializations, a division of labor called **functional lateralization.** Broca later identified a left-handed patient with aphasia after right hemisphere damage. From this one case, he predicted that all left-handed people would have language function localized to the right—an overgeneralization, as it turned out. The organization of the left-handed brain is rarely the reverse of that of the right-hander because right-sided dominance for language is rare in both left- and right-handers. This fact suggests that there are fundamental differences in the neural organization of the left and right hemispheres.

Broca's most famous patient was called "Tan" because that was the only word he could speak. A remarkable feature was that he still understood both spoken and written language. This was the first reported instance of "expressive aphasia," an inability to generate fluent discourse in the presence of good comprehension. A few years later, Karl Wernicke described a complementary syndrome arising from damage to the left posterior perisylvian area in which verbal output was fluent but filled with meaningless words and substitutions that corrupted the meaning. The anterior and posterior regions, respectively, of the cortex surrounding the Sylvian fissure in

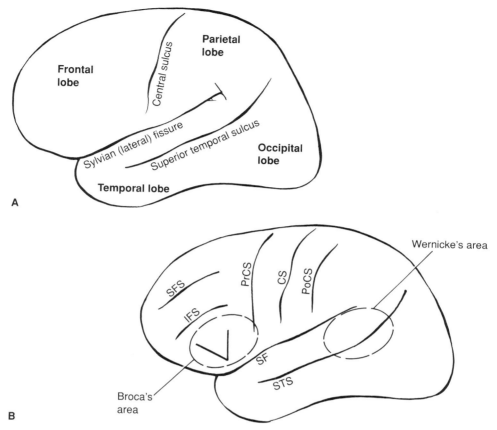

Figure 18–1. A: Schematic view of anatomy of the left hemisphere, showing lobes and major landmarks. **B:** Schematic view of the location of Broca's and Wernicke's areas. CS, central sulcus; IFS, inferior frontal sulcus; PoCS, postcentral sulcus; PrCS, precentral sulcus; STS, superior temporal sulcus; SF, Sylvian fissure.

the *left* hemisphere soon became known as Broca's and Wernicke's areas.

How Universal Is Left Hemisphere Dominance for Language?

The Wada Test

The hemispheric localization of language in living people can be determined using a test devised by Juan Wada for presurgical planning in epilepsy patients.[8] This test, commonly called the **Wada test** or the Amytal test, requires the injection of a short-acting barbiturate into the left and right carotid arteries while the patient is asked to count backward. When the barbiturate reaches the hemisphere that supports lan-

guage, the patient stops counting briefly. Rasmussen and Milner found that 96% of right-handed patients and 70% of left-handed patients stop counting when the left hemisphere is anesthetized, whereas 15% of left-handed patients do not stop counting at all, suggesting that they have bilateral control of language.[9] The remaining 15% of left-handers stop counting when the right hemisphere is anesthetized. These data, combined with similar evidence from the brain lesion literature, demonstrate how rare it is for the right hemisphere to support language.

The Dichotic Listening Test

Because injection of barbiturate into the carotid artery carries a finite risk, it cannot be used as a research procedure in normal people. Therefore, investigators have been interested in developing a noninvasive method for determining functional lateralization in healthy people who have not suffered brain damage. In 1961, Doreen Kimura, a Canadian psychologist, published the **dichotic listening** procedure.[10] In this test, subjects receive different stimuli simultaneously in the two ears and report what they hear. In general, right-handers report verbal information (words and numbers) heard through the *right* ear more accurately than that heard through the *left* ear (referred to as right ear superiority). This effect depends on the fact that information from the right ear reaches the left hemisphere slightly more rapidly than that from the left ear. Right ear superiority is not absolute because the auditory pathways from each ear (unlike the visual and somatosensory pathways) are largely bilaterally distributed in the cortex. The dichotic listening procedure does not, therefore, provide reliable information about hemispheric dominance for language in individuals.[11]

Neurobiologic Basis for Left Hemisphere Language Dominance

Right ear superiority is specific for consonants, not vowels.[12] The most obvious difference between consonants and vowels is their modulation in time. The acoustic signal for a consonant changes much more rapidly in time than that for a vowel. The fact that consonants are perceived more accurately when presented to the right ear is one of many pieces of evidence that the left hemisphere has specialized mechanisms for processing rapid auditory signals.[13] In adults, temporal information is critical for speech detection. Spectral (pitch) information can be considerably degraded as long as temporal information is retained.[14] In terms of our information processing model, then, it seems likely that there are auditory processing maps in the left hemisphere that specialize in discriminating temporal features of auditory stimuli, whereas maps in the right hemisphere specialize in processing spectral information.

Patients with aphasia frequently have problems in identifying temporal patterns and detecting small temporal gaps between auditory stimuli.[15,16] Spectral differences, on the other hand, appear to be more efficiently processed in the right hemisphere.[17,18] Children with language impairment also have difficulty in discriminating and detecting short sounds.[19–21] Both congenital and acquired language difficulties

appear to be associated with problems in specialized temporal processing mechanisms that may be housed in the left hemisphere.

Anatomic Location of Left Hemisphere Language Specializations

Where are language functions located within the left hemisphere? Evidence for language localization comes mainly from three sources: 1) the analysis of the areas destroyed by strokes that cause aphasia[22,23]; 2) cortical recording and stimulation in patients being evaluated for epilepsy surgery[7,24]; and 3) brain activation using **positron emission tomography (PET)** or **functional magnetic resonance imaging (MRI)**.[3] Experimental methods that can be used in humans have severe limitations. Brain damage after stroke is diffuse and involves the cortex, subcortical white matter, and the insula. Premorbid language competence is usually unknown. Brain stimulation can be performed only in people with long-standing brain damage and is generally confined to regions that are planned to be included in surgery (i.e., not normal cortex). Imaging methods have a very low signal/noise ratio and poor spatial and temporal resolution. Convergent findings from all three methods, however, provide powerful evidence concerning localization.

All methods agree in localizing most language functions to the cortical regions surrounding the Sylvian fissure (lateral sulcus) in the territory of the left middle cerebral artery. An exhaustive study of patients with aphasia[23] confirmed the identification of two focal regions (Broca's and Wernicke's areas) on the banks of the left Sylvian fissure. The only other cortical region that appears essential is the medial frontal region supplied by the anterior cerebral artery. After anterior cerebral artery or anterior communicating artery infarcts, patients initiate very little behavior, a syndrome called akinetic mutism.[25] After recovery they have little spontaneous speech. The intention to speak is apparently regulated in the medial prefrontal cortex anterior to the supplementary motor cortex. This region is superior to the anterior cingulate cortex, which is part of the limbic system. In animals, stimulation of the cingulate cortex causes calls and emotional vocalizations, whereas lesions eliminate this behavior. The relative contributions of the anterior cingulate and medial prefrontal cortices to language generation are under investigation.

Disturbances in language can also follow stimulation and lesions in the thalamus and basal ganglia. Language deficits seen after basal ganglia damage are probably due to associated cortical damage.[26] The role of the thalamus in language is not understood. After thalamic lesions, patients can repeat, and seem to have good comprehension. They have naming problems and make semantic errors, however. Because the thalamus provides a major excitatory drive to the cortex, language disturbances after thalamic damage may reflect degradation of cortical function due to deafferentation. In this chapter, attention is focused on the traditional language regions surrounding the Sylvian fissure.

Definition of Broca's and Wernicke's Areas

Broca's and Wernicke's areas are abstract concepts, not anatomic structures. Each area consists of a focal region and a surround. The focal region for Broca's area is the inferior frontal gyrus. The surround region includes the premotor cortex in the precentral gyrus, the dorsolateral prefrontal cortex in the middle frontal gyrus, and the insula. (Figure 18–2 and Table 18–1 provide a descriptive summary of the anatomic regions that are referred to in this chapter.) The focal region for Wernicke's area is the posterior superior temporal gyrus. The surround region includes the anterior superior temporal gyrus, the middle and inferior temporal gyri, the supramarginal and angular gyri in the parietal lobe, and the insula. The different aphasia syndromes that are described in the literature do not map cleanly onto different regions.[16]

The core of Broca's area lies in the inferior frontal gyrus in the left hemisphere. It is formed by three **cytoarchitectonic** areas: Brodmann's areas 44, 45, and 47. The Latin names for these regions are pars opercularis, pars triangularis, and pars orbitalis. The pars opercularis lies anterior to the premotor cortex for the mouth (area 6). The pars triangularis is shaped like a triangle and is formed by two branches of the lateral fissure, the anterior horizontal **ramus** (branch) and the anterior ascending ramus. The pars orbitalis lies anterior to the anterior horizontal ramus, adjacent to the orbital surface of the frontal lobe. These three regions can be distinguished from more posterior "motor" areas by the cell size and packing density in layer IV, the layer that receives thalamic af-

ferents. Layer IV in Broca's area, like the rest of the nonmotor frontal lobe (termed *prefrontal cortex*), is called "granular" because it is full of very tiny neurons. Granular cortex is characteristic of the primary sensory areas in all mammals. Only primates have a granular layer IV in the prefrontal cortex, however. Because primates are unique in the complexity and flexibility of their response selection mechanisms, it seems likely that a granular layer IV is associated with an enhancement of prefrontal function.

On medial MRI sections, the pars triangularis is located just lateral and dorsal to the insula (Fig. 18–3). It enlarges laterally. In some people, two triangular regions are visible medially. In some cases the two triangles merge laterally, whereas in others one or both enlarge. Another common anatomic variant that appears laterally in the pars opercularis is called "sulcus diagonalis." Sulcus diagonalis can arise from the anterior ascending ramus or the lateral fissure itself. Differences in the shape and size of cortical gyri may reflect differences in intrinsic and extrinsic connections[27] that could underlie individual differences in language function. People from families of language-impaired children are more likely to have a sulcus diagonalis, for example.[28]

Wernicke's area is even less well defined than Broca's area.[29] Wernicke placed it at the junction between the superior temporal gyrus and the middle temporal gyrus (see Fig. 18–1B; Fig. 18–4). Subsequently, the region expanded to include the banks of the lateral fissure and even the parietal lobe because aphasia is seen after lesions in many different parts of this territory. Anatomic structures that have been included in Wernicke's area include the posterior horizontal and posterior ascending rami of the lateral fissure, and the temporal and parietal branches of the superior temporal sulcus. The gyrus surrounding the posterior ascending ramus is commonly referred to as the supramarginal gyrus (Brodmann's area 40), whereas the gyrus surrounding the parietal branch of the superior temporal sulcus is called the angular gyrus (Brodmann's area 39; see Fig 18–2).

Relation of Wernicke's Area to the Auditory Cortex

The Transverse Gyrus of Heschl

The posterior horizontal ramus of the lateral fissure is marked by a prominent anatomic specialization unique to humans: the transverse gyrus of Heschl

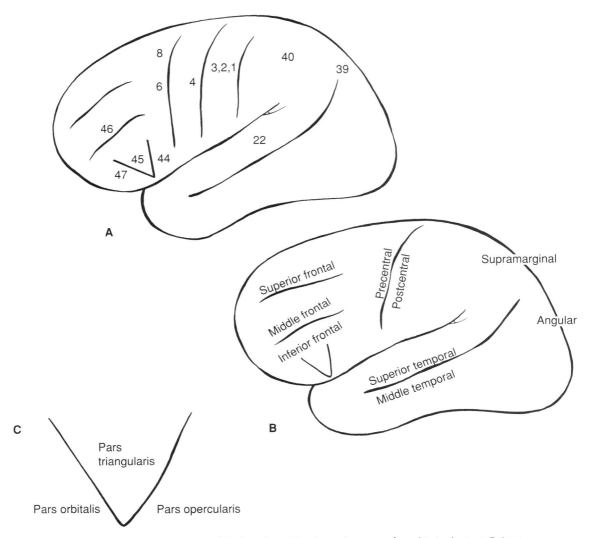

Figure 18-2. A: Schematic view of the location of Brodmann's areas referred to in the text. **B:** Location of major gyri visible on the lateral surface of the brain. **C:** Blown-up view of inferior frontal gyrus. See Table 18-1 for a list of gyri and their corresponding Brodmann's areas.

(frequently referred to as "Heschl's gyrus"). This gyrus contains one or two tonotopic maps of the primary auditory cortex (Brodmann's areas 41 and 42). Although most textbooks paint these Brodmann's areas on the exterior surface of the temporal lobe in concentric circles, it is important to realize that the primary auditory cortex is entirely hidden, and lies on the superior bank of the lateral fissure. The trans-

verse gyrus angles forward at an angle of approximately 45 degrees (see Fig. 18–4B, C). High frequencies are localized caudomedially and low frequencies anterolaterally.[30]

The Planum Temporale
Caudal to the primary auditory cortex on the transverse gyrus lies the planum temporale (part of Brod-

TABLE 18-1

Summary of Major Anatomic Regions Discussed in this Chapter

Lobe	Gyrus	Subdivision or Regional Name	Brodmann's Area No.	Proposed Function
Frontal	Middle frontal	Dorsolateral prefrontal cortex	46	Spatial working memory
	Inferior frontal	Pars opercularis	44	Oromotor function
		Pars triangularis	45	Working memory for language assembly
		Pars orbitalis	47	
	Precentral	Premotor	6	Integrated motor sequences
	Medial frontal	Supplementary motor	6	Planning motor behavior
	Anterior cingulate		24	Emotional behavior, attention
Parietal	Postcentral		3, 2, 1	Primary somatosensory
	Supramarginal		40	Praxis, phonologic store
	Angular		39	Reading
Temporal	Heschl's transverse		41, 42	Primary auditory
	Planum temporale		22	Secondary auditory
	Superior temporal		22	Language
	Middle temporal		21	Language
	Inferior temporal		37	Naming
Occipital	Gyral terms not in common use	Striate	17	Primary visual cortex
		Extrastriate	18, 19	Visual association cortex

MS, multiple sclerosis.

mann's area 22). Brodmann's area 22 contains the auditory association cortex. It extends laterally onto the surface of the superior temporal gyrus. This region is always activated in imaging experiments with auditory stimuli.[31-34] The relation between auditory processing and language comprehension is not well understood. An information processing view would suggest that the planum of the left hemisphere should contain auditory maps of spectral and temporal features specific to language, such as the voice onset times that characterize different consonants. In view of left hemisphere dominance for language, it seems reasonable to expect that there would be anatomic and physiologic differences in the maps in the two hemispheres.

Although it is generally assumed that the secondary auditory cortex on the planum temporale processes one or more specific dimensions of auditory information that are critical for encoding representations of phonemes, syllables, and words, there is little experimental evidence to support this localization. In fact, a recent functional imaging experiment found that the only region of Wernicke's area that appeared specifically activated by spoken words was the superior temporal sulcus, not the planum

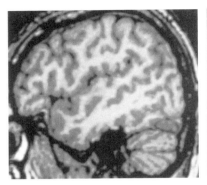
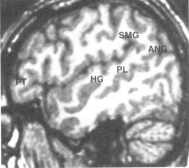

Figure 18–3. Location of cortical areas specialized for language as visualized on a sagittal magnetic resonance image. ANG, angular gyrus; HG, Heschl's gyrus; primary auditory cortex; PL, planum temporale: auditory association cortext; PT, pars triangularis (Broca's area); SMG, supramarginal gyrus. PT, ANG, and SMG are cortical areas associated with Wernicke's area.

temporale.[33] An enormous amount of work needs to be done to characterize the spatial distribution of auditory and linguistic functions in Broca's and Wernicke's areas.

Animal Experiments

The cortical basis for vision has been much more thoroughly researched than that for audition. There are a few informative animal experiments, however. There is a severe, long-lasting deficit in short-term auditory memory after removal of the superior bank of the superior temporal sulcus in monkeys.[35] The animals were able to remember visual stimuli, but not tones. The investigators demonstrated that this was not due to a simple sensory or perceptual problem because although the animals could discriminate the stimuli, they simply could not remember them long enough to match them to a sample. Problems with auditory memory characterize many patients with speech and language problems.[16]

There have been a few isolated experiments that have suggested that auditory processing is laterally asymmetric in monkeys. Petersen et al.[36] played species-specific calls to macaques through earphones and found that the monkeys demonstrated a right ear bias for responding to the calls of their own species but not for responding to unfamiliar calls of other species. Hauser[37] demonstrated that adults but not infants are more likely to turn their right ear in the direction of a monkey call. These findings are interpreted as demonstrating an underlying lateralized neural specialization for responding to biologic communication signals that could be an evolution-

ary precursor to our own left hemisphere language specialization. Both studies were purely behavioral, however, and few studies have attempted to follow up the findings by looking at lateralized effects of auditory cortical lesions.[38–40] Monkeys are, however, more impaired in responding to species-specific vocalizations after lesions of the left superior temporal gyrus. This finding suggests that left hemisphere specializations for species-specific auditory communication have a long evolutionary history.

There have been no reports of anatomic or neurophysiologic asymmetries that might underlie these behavioral results. Chimpanzees, but not monkeys, tend to have a longer Sylvian fissure on the left.[41] The most blatant functional asymmetry in a vocal control system is in the oscine songbirds.[42] In canaries and other finches that learn their songs, the vocal control system is almost completely lateralized to the left side. Song is lost after left but not right hypoglossal section, an intervention that denervates the syrinx, the peripheral organ that controls vocal output. Subsequently, Nottebohm et al.[43] found that lesions in the left hemisphere of the forebrain eliminate the production of most song syllables. They suggested that song learning might be a good model for cerebral localization for language. Unfortunately, no anatomic asymmetries were found above the level of the hypoglossal nucleus.[43] It was concluded that the reason that left and not right lesions eliminated song was that the descending pathways are entirely unilateral, and because there is peripheral lateralization, central lateralization is an obligatory result.

It has been found that rats, a species that depends on olfaction, not audition for most of its species-

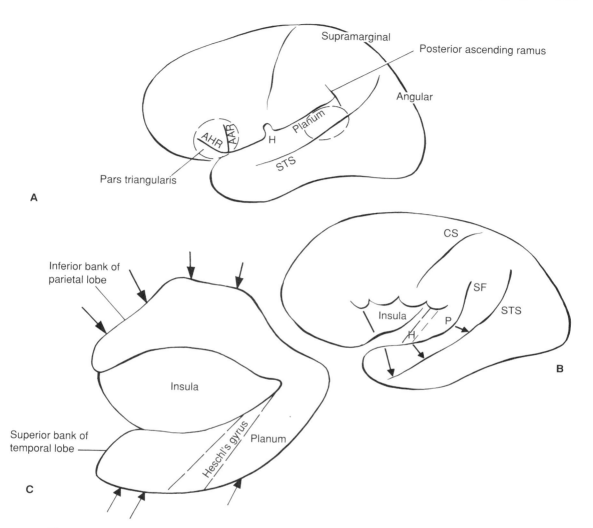

Figure 18-4. A: Schematic view of the location of the gyri and sulci implicated in the generation and comprehension of language. AAR, anterior ascending ramus; AHR, anterior horizontal ramus; H, first transverse gyrus of Heschl; STS, superior temporal sulcus. **B:** An artist's rendering of the relation between the insula and the superior surface of the temporal lobe. The Sylvian fissure (SF) has been opened to expose the insula and the structures of the lower bank. Heschl's gyrus (H) is separated from the planum temporale (P) by a prominent sulcus (Heschl's sulcus, represented by the more posterior dashed line). CS, central sulcus; STS, superior temporal sulcus. **C:** An enlarged view with both banks of the Sylvian fissure pulled apart to expose their inner surfaces and their junction with the insula. The lines indicated by arrows would normally be apposed to form the upper and lower banks of the Sylvian fissure.

specific communication, have a left hemisphere bias for detecting auditory temporal sequences.[44] This suggests that a left lateralized specialization for rapid temporal processing is remarkably widespread in the animal kingdom. Functional lateralization must have developed early in the evolution of complex organisms. The neurophysiologic mechanisms responsible for this specialization remain completely mysterious.

Language Localization

The Geschwind-Wernicke Model

The middle cerebral artery is a terminal branch of the internal carotid artery. It originates at the ventromedial tip of the insula and then divides into many "candelabra" branches that climb dorsally over the insula and then double back in a sheaf of hairpin turns to cover the frontal, parietal, and temporal opercula (lids) of the insula. The facing surfaces of the opercula form the banks of the Sylvian fissure. Vascular defects or clots can occur at any point in the distribution of the middle cerebral artery. The classic model of language originated with Karl Wernicke and was popularized in this country by Norman Geschwind, the father of American **behavioral neurology**. This model divides the aphasias into two main types: receptive, caused by damage in the posterior territory of the middle cerebral artery; and expressive, caused by anterior damage. Figure 18–5 shows this model diagrammatically. Visual information about letter shape and spacing is processed in the visual association cortex (extrastriate cortex). Auditory information about word sounds is processed in the auditory association cortex on the superior bank of the temporal lobe. Word meanings are stored diffusely in the temporal and parietal lobes. Wernicke's area is conceptualized as a nodal switching station where word meanings are connected to auditory and visual word images. When an utterance is generated, the phonologically and semantically encoded message is sent to Broca's area, where it is translated into an articulatory code that can be expressed by the vocal musculature. The fiber bundle postulated to carry the phonologic-semantic message forward from Wernicke's to Broca's area is called the arcuate fasciculus. It travels forward in the white matter medial to the insula.

The reason that damage to Wernicke's area is thought to cause aphasia is that the road map connecting the lexicon (storehouse of meanings) to the phonologic code is disrupted and appropriate meanings are no longer activated by hearing, seeing, or imaging words. In addition, the ability to use meaning to guide the creation of appropriate phonologic

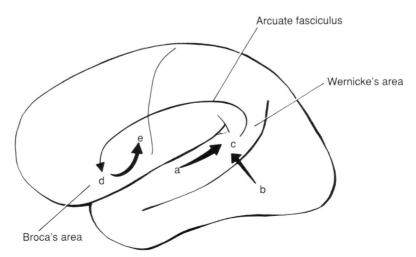

Figure 18–5. Schematic view of the classic Geschwind-Wernicke model of language generation. Key: a, auditory word image; b, visual word image; c, attachment of meaning in Wernicke's area; d, sentence assembly in Broca's area; e, motor pattern generation in premotor cortex for mouth and larynx.

codes is compromised. Receptive aphasics, who have impaired comprehension, are frequently referred to as "Wernicke's aphasics," whereas expressive aphasics (impaired fluency) are called "Broca's aphasics." This dichotomy implies that expressive language is localized to the left frontal lobe and comprehension is localized to more posterior regions. This division of labor fits with our general concepts of brain localization in that information processing regions are located in the parietal and temporal lobes, whereas response selection is located anterior to the central sulcus.[6] Unfortunately, recent studies suggest that the Geschwind-Wernicke model is an oversimplified view of language organization.[16] Neither the aphasia syndromes nor the language areas are so neatly organized into expressive and receptive components.[34] Comprehension or speech production can be impaired after lesions or stimulation anywhere in the distribution of the middle cerebral artery.[45]

Individual Differences

George Ojemann, a neurosurgeon, has been studying the functions of the language cortex in patients with epilepsy, by stimulating their cortices before surgery.[24] He is following a tradition started by Wilder Penfield, a Canadian neurosurgeon who pioneered the technique.[7] There is a wide spatial distribution of regions where stimulation can interrupt the same language function (Fig. 18–6). In the same person,

stimulation of two widely spaced spots can disrupt naming, word repetition, or recall. The only consistency between people is that the spots that interfere with language tend to lie close to the Sylvian fissure or in the middle temporal gyrus. There does, however, appear to be a cortical "gatekeeper" for language output that is similarly located in all people. Stimulation in the left frontal operculum (the posterior part of Broca's area) arrested speech in all people tested.[46] With this exception, there appear to be large individual differences in the distribution of areas involved in language function.

The data from patients with brain damage support Ojemann's position. Patients with brain damage in what appear to be similar areas demonstrate large individual differences in language function. Ojemann suggests that these differences might stem from anatomic and physiologic differences in brain localization for language between people.[24] One class of individual differences that has received particular attention is the issue of sex differences. Many different lines of evidence suggest that language is less lateralized in women than in men. They are less likely to have aphasia after posterior damage than men,[22] their brains are more likely to be symmetric,[47] the volume of the superior temporal cortex is relatively larger,[48] and imaging studies demonstrate bilateral activation.[49] In spite of this individual variability, however, there are some generalizations that can be made about the cortical localization of language function.

Figure 18–6. Cortical areas where stimulation interferes with verbal production or oromotor function. Key: G, errors on a syntax task; N, naming errors; NR, naming and reading errors; VM, short-term verbal memory deficit; X, speech arrest, errors in single oral movements. (Adapted from Ojemann G. Brain organization for language from the perspective of electrical stimulation mapping. *Brain and Behavioral Sciences* 1983;6:189–230.)

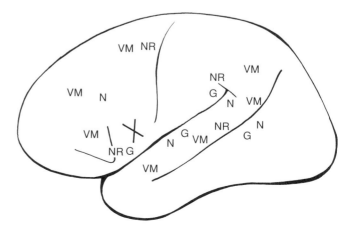

Broca's Area and Language Generation

The designation of Broca's area as the motor speech region implies that speech should be initiated by stimulation in Broca's area. But, in fact, *speech arrest*, not speech, is produced by cortical stimulation.

Fluency

The one aspect of aphasia that reliably differentiates anterior and posterior damage in the perisylvian region is **fluency**.[22] After anterior damage (to Broca's area), patients no longer produce fluent speech. They are impaired at repeating single syllables and making single oral movements. Speech is "telegraphic," that is, words are omitted that are not essential for the communication of meaning. In English, that means that the **closed class** "pivot words" or *functors* (e.g., to, with, or, and) are omitted.[50] In the past, this symptom was sometimes referred to as "agrammatism," on the assumption that patients spoke telegraphically because they had lost their knowledge of grammar. However, experimental work has demonstrated that patients with telegraphic speech maintain their knowledge of grammar and can identify ungrammatical sentences.[51] A modern explanation hypothesizes that Broca's aphasics have lost the ability to retrieve sentence components efficiently when trying to formulate an utterance. To speed up sentence generation while keeping meaning intact, patients drop expendable sentence parts. In English, the most expendable parts are the pivot words or functors. (Telegrams can be understood without these small words.)

The Turkish language does not include free-standing functional morphemes. In Turkish, grammatical inflections are added to words and are essential for conveying meaning.[52] Turkish-speaking Broca's aphasics are nonfluent but they do not speak telegraphically, because this concept does not exist—it is not possible to convey the same meaning with fewer words. Because patients with Broca's aphasia have a good idea of the meaning they wish to convey, they do not omit words or grammatical inflections. Their speech is nonfluent because they make false starts, pauses, and repetitions of the same word.

Working Memory

Current concepts of how language is formulated involve a concept called **working memory**.[53] Working memory is a short-term representational system used for preparing responses. Information is not stored in working memory, but the system has access to items stored in long-term memory as well as current perceptual information. In the left hemisphere, the working memory system is composed of an articulatory loop made up of a subvocal rehearsal system and a phonologic store. If a subject is presented with a string of words and then given a distracting task, the words are remembered better if the task is a drawing task than the task of counting numbers backward. This is because the drawing task calls on the visuospatial working memory system of the right hemisphere and does not interfere with rehearsal in the articulatory loop.

The idea that Broca's area might be involved in representational memory for the purpose of guiding verbal responses is supported by a large body of work in nonhuman primates by Patricia Goldman-Rakic. She has demonstrated that the dorsolateral prefrontal cortex (monkeys do not have an inferior frontal gyrus) is essential for working memory.[54] Monkeys with damage in this region cannot perform a delayed-response task. They cannot remember where a reward has been hidden when they are required to hold this information "in mind" during a delay. Electrophysiologic recording in this region has demonstrated cells that fire during the delay, leading to the inference that these cells are maintaining a temporary memory of where the animal should search when the delay is over. Goldman-Rakic has shown that the dorsolateral prefrontal cortex actually contains a map of anticipated locations—that is, cells in particular locations in the brain fire when the monkey must remember to look in a particular location. This is called *spatial* working memory. Goldman-Rakic has suggested that Broca's area is a human homologue of the monkey dorsolateral prefrontal cortex. In the human case, syllables and words (rather than spatial locations) are "held in mind" while phrases and sentences are assembled.[55] As expected, recent imaging experiments place the subvocal rehearsal system in Broca's area and the long-term phonologic store in Wernicke's area.[56]

Functions of Wernicke's Area

Damage to posterior branches of the middle cerebral artery or its distribution in Wernicke's area also cause aphasia, but they rarely affect fluency. Speech output has normal prosody and rhythm but is filled with errors, and in extreme cases can be meaningless. Wernicke hypothesized that brain damage in this region destroys the link between the auditory images of words and their semantic representations. Bates et al.[57] suggest that posterior damage affects self-monitoring. Speech is filled with errors because the system that normally checks acoustic output for meaning has become corrupted. Kimura and Watson have shown that the ability to initiate and mimic sequences of movements is impaired after posterior lesions.[58] In their study, there was a double dissociation in the effects of anterior and posterior lesions. Patients with anterior lesions were more impaired on repeating single movements and syllables, whereas patients with posterior damage were impaired on repeating phrases and sequences of movements.

The first PET studies that were performed of single-word processing[59] surprised many neurologists because activation in Wernicke's and Broca's areas was not prominent. For a time, it was conventional to discount the 100 years' work on aphasia and accept the findings of the more modern techniques. More recently, however, methods with improved sensitivity have convincingly demonstrated specialized regions for spoken and written word recognition within Wernicke's area.[32] In this study, spoken words activated the posterior superior temporal gyrus, whereas words presented visually activated the middle temporal gyrus.[32] Another study, which was directed at determining whether there was spatial separation of phonologic and semantic processing, found activation in the superior temporal gyrus when subjects were identifying phonemes in aurally presented nonsense words. When they were listening for words designating small animals (a semantic task), the center of activation shifted ventrally, into the middle temporal gyrus.[31] More work remains to be done to determine how language processing mechanisms are distributed in Wernicke's area.

Most imaging studies demonstrate more activation in the left hemisphere than the right during language tasks. This left-sided advantage may be due to the fact that language structures on the right are smaller and there is thus less tissue to be activated, or that structures on the right side are simply less active. The right hemisphere does, however, participate in comprehension. Studies of patients whose corpus callosa have been sectioned because of intractable epilepsy have demonstrated considerable language

comprehension by the right hemisphere.[60] The right hemisphere is better at processing emotional prosody (the pitch, stress, and rhythm changes that convey fear, anger, happiness, or urgency). Right hemisphere mechanisms are also thought to play a crucial role in pragmatics—the use of language as a social tool and the interpretation of metaphor and jokes.[16] It has been suggested that spatial mechanisms in the right hemisphere may facilitate constructing and interpreting coherent discourse. Pragmatics and discourse are hard to study experimentally, however. The advent of modern imaging techniques should make some of these issues more accessible to neurobiologic study.

Anatomic Asymmetry

The Sylvian Fissure

What are the anatomic specializations that might be related to language lateralization? A hundred years ago, the Sylvian fissure was reported to be longer on the left in 63% of a large series of brains. This asymmetry is less prominent in the chimpanzee and virtually absent in the monkey. A more recent study by Rubens et al.[61] found that the Sylvian fissure is shaped differently on the left and the right (Fig. 18–7). In 25 of 36 brains (69%), the left fissure was long and straight, ending in a short terminal bifurcation. On the right, the fissure angled up sharply into the parietal lobe. In the remaining 11 brains there was no marked asymmetry. In no case was the asymmetry reversed (a sharply angled left fissure and straight right fissure). These results have been replicated in postmortem and MRI experiments.[62,63] Ruben et al. speculated that a sharply angled right fissure could be caused by an expansion of the posterior parietal cortex on the right and that this rightward asymmetry might underlie lateral specializations for visuospatial functions.

Geschwind and the Planum Temporale

Early reports of leftward asymmetries in the planum temporale were discounted by American scientists before Geschwind and Levitsky[64] measured planar length in 100 postmortem brains. They found that 65% of the plana were longer on the left, 24% were symmetric, and only 11% were longer on the right.

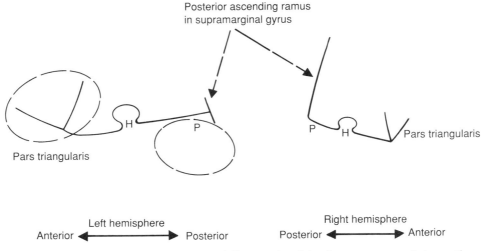

Figure 18–7. Schematic view of the anatomic differences in sylvian fissure structures between the left and right hemispheres. Dotted areas indicate the general location of Broca's and Wernicke's areas. The planum (P) and pars triangularis are larger on the left, whereas the posterior ascending ramus is larger on the right. H, Heschl's gyrus.

Interestingly, that is exactly the average asymmetry that had been previously found between the length of the left and right Sylvian fissures. This leftward asymmetry was soon confirmed in newborn and infant brains. Asymmetry was found to be present by 7 months of fetal life, thus predating the emergence of language capacity (see review by Witelson[65]). Subsequent postmortem studies have demonstrated that the areas devoted to both the primary and secondary auditory cortices are larger on the left[66,67] and have a more defined columnar architecture.[68] Nonauditory asymmetries have also been described that may be related to right hemisphere specialization for spatial attention. For example, the posterior ascending ramus in the supramarginal gyrus is larger in the right hemisphere.[63,69–71] This rightward asymmetry in the parietal lobe is consistent with the right hemisphere dominance for visuospatial function.

Language Lateralization and Planar Asymmetry

Planar asymmetry is a robust phenomenon. Although subsequent studies used different methods of measurement as well as somewhat different criteria to define the borders of the planum, the original results were repeatedly confirmed. What is the relationship between this asymmetry and language lateralization?

Recently, Geschwind's prediction that asymmetry of the planum is associated with lateralization for language has been verified in a small sample. Foundas et al.[72] studied 12 epileptic patients with known, unilateral language localization identified by the Wada procedure. All 12 had longer plana in their "eloquent" hemisphere (the hemisphere silenced by the barbiturate injection). Eleven were right-handed and had language localized in the left hemisphere and typical *leftward* planar asymmetry. The one left-handed patient had right hemisphere language and reversed *rightward* asymmetry. Subsequently, measurements on two additional patients with right hemisphere language have been reported. Both had reversed asymmetry. These findings are important because they provide evidence that the relative sizes of homologous structures in the two hemispheres may play a role in the emergence and anatomic localization of language function.

Structural Correlates of Planar Asymmetry

Several types of auditory association cortex have been described that differ very slightly in their cytoarchitectonic characteristics. The two groups that have studied the cytoarchitecture of the planum temporale have described different patterns for the location, extent, and nature of the auditory association cortex.[68] Neither group found that the planum temporale was coextensive with a particular type of cortex, or that the origin of the posterior ascending ramus marked a cytoarchitectonic boundary. Because both groups studied small samples, it is possible that sampling variations are responsible for the differences.

One study of four brains reported that anatomic asymmetry in the planum is due to a larger expanse of a particular type of cytoarchitectonic field on the left.[66] By implication, this particular type of cortex could be specialized to perform some unique function specific for language (perhaps providing a map of distinctive features or phonemes characteristic of the speaker's native language). This possibility remains to be investigated. Another anatomic asymmetry between the cortices of the left and right hemisphere has been described. Cellular columns are more widely spaced in both the primary and association cortices on the left side.[73] Wider spacing means that the neuropil/cell ratio is higher on the left, an anatomic feature suggestive of more sophisticated processing mechanisms. Both these studies should be replicated in larger samples.

Planar Asymmetry and Language Disabilities

Three strategies have been used to link planar asymmetry and functional lateralization: 1) anatomic analyses of the structure of the planum temporale described previously; 2) direct comparisons using the Wada test; and 3) study of the planum temporale in people with language impairments such as **dyslexia**. Galaburda et al. performed postmortem analysis of planar asymmetry in people with compromised language function, using brains from people described as dyslexic provided to him by the Orton (now, International) Dyslexia Society. Some of the people also had seizures, articulation difficulties, and more generalized language disorders. In 1985,

they reported the surprising finding that four cases all had an absence of planar asymmetry.[74] Because only 25% of Geschwind's sample of 100 brains had demonstrated symmetric plana, symmetry in four of four cases exceeded that expected by chance.

In addition, Galaburda et al. found heterotopia (unusual cell collections) in widespread regions of the white matter and under the pial surface of the dyslexic brains. A heterotopia is a neuropathologic abnormality that arises in the early stages of neural development, when neurons are migrating to their final position in the cortex. Later, Galaburda[75] found symmetry of the planum as well as heterotopias in four additional brains. In every case, planar symmetry was due to the presence of a large right planum. Galaburda hypothesized that a developmental failure of pruning, possibly due to excess testosterone, was responsible for the enlarged right planum.

Imaging Studies of Hemisphere Asymmetries

No other group has studied planar symmetry in postmortem brains, but many imaging studies have addressed this question. Because the planum was not visible on computed tomography scans or in early MRI studies, early attempts adopted the strategy of measuring hemisphere asymmetries. Marjorie LeMay, a radiologist, and her colleagues were the first to report that brain asymmetry could be measured in living people.[76,77] She found that the left hemisphere extends further posteriorly than the right (called the occipital petalia), and that the Sylvian point (the location of the bends in the middle cerebral artery that occur posterior to the insula) is higher on the right. These asymmetries are thought to be related to underlying brain asymmetries, but to date there have been no studies aimed at verifying this relationship by correlating skull, blood vessel, and brain asymmetries in the same people.

Typically, skull asymmetries are measured in axial sections. Many of these studies have demonstrated statistically that learning-disabled groups and women tend to be more symmetric. Although the plane of the axial section is assumed to be similar across scans, small variations in head position can cause large variations in the skull region measured, affecting the comparability of the structures on the right and left sides. The large error involved in these studies has made it impossible to make any individual correlations between language and brain anatomy.

Structural Imaging Studies of the Planum Temporale

Early computed tomography scan data and two more recent MRI studies confirmed that dyslexics were more likely to have symmetry or reversed (rightward) asymmetry.[78,79] Surprisingly, however, both MRI studies reported that symmetry was due to small *left* plana, rather than to increased size on the right. The two MRI studies imaged the brain in the sagittal and coronal plane, respectively, and identified the planum using anatomic landmarks, but did not distinguish between the temporal and parietal banks of the planum. Other MRI studies using the more traditional axial plane have compared widths or volumes of the parietooccipital cortices in the two hemispheres. These studies have also reported anomalous or reversed symmetry in dyslexics.[80,81]

Dramatic improvements in MRI technology now allow visualization of serial sections of the brain on gapless series of thin sections, using volumetric acquisitions. Furthermore, these images have anatomic validity. Measurements of the planum on sagittal images of postmortem specimens correlate highly with planar size measured on photographs of the same specimens.[82] Studies of dyslexic subjects using modern imaging techniques have not confirmed the earlier findings of atypical asymmetry in dyslexia.[70,83] Functional imaging studies, by contrast, have shown differences between brain activation in dyslexics and control subjects during rhyming and tonal memory tasks.[84,85] Thus, a functional rather than a structural impairment is suggested in this disease.

Specific language impairment, which is a more serious disorder than pure dyslexia, and which often includes reading disability, does, however, seem to be associated with atypical planar asymmetry. Three studies all agree in finding reduced size in a region that includes the left planum.[86–88] In addition, a study of normal 5- to 9-year-old children has found that the degree of planar asymmetry predicts skill in **phonemic awareness**.[89] Young children with symmetric plana had poor phonemic awareness, whereas their same-age peers with better skills had marked asymmetry. Phonemic awareness, the ability to conceptualize the sound structure of language, is closely related to reading ability, although the causal direction

is not clear. It may be that the size of auditory maps is reduced in children with symmetric plana, leading to a developmental lag in the acquisition of phonemic awareness.

Asymmetry in Broca's Area

The asymmetries of structures in the inferior frontal gyrus are much less robust than posterior asymmetries. One review of the literature concluded that there was no convincing evidence for anatomical asymmetry,[90] although several authors had reported asymmetry of different subregions in small samples of postmortem tissue. One postmortem report that studied the cellular structure of the pars triangularis found that the average size of the largest pyramidal cells was larger on the left.[91] Foundas et al.[92] measured the pars triangularis in 11 of the same epilepsy patients with Wada tests from their planum study. They found that 10 of the right-handers with language localization on the left had leftward asymmetry of the pars triangularis.[92] The left-handed patient with language localized on the right had a robust reversed asymmetry. Thus, the one patient with right hemisphere dominance for language had reversed asymmetry in both Wernicke's and Broca's areas. Another small study of normal right- and left-handers found that pars triangularis asymmetry was reduced in left-handers, consistent with the reduced likelihood of left hemisphere dominance for language in the left-handed population.

Developmental Changes in Functional Localization

Aphasia rarely follows brain damage in the right hemisphere. Does this mean that the right hemisphere does not have the neural software and hardware to support language? In the case of the adult, only a minority are able to recover functionally satisfactory communication skills. Clearly, the adult right hemisphere is not able to assume the functions abandoned by the left hemisphere. It is paradoxical, then, to find that most children with brain damage in the left hemisphere develop perfectly adequate language.[93–95] Many theorists interpreted the phenomenon of normal language development in the face of early brain damage to mean that the two hemispheres are equipotential at birth and that the potential of the right hemisphere to support language wanes slowly during development.

Some put the end of neuroplasticity (called the end of the *critical* or *sensitive period*) at 2 years, some at 6 years, and some at puberty. There simply were not enough good data to decide between these alternatives. Brain damage in childhood is rare, rarely unilateral, and in general poorly documented. Because there are wide individual differences in the rate of normal language development and the size of adult vocabulary and language skill, it is difficult to define the boundaries between normal and abnormal language function.[96] For example, at the age of 16 months, comprehended vocabulary can range from 30 to 300 words in children who are otherwise normal. Against a background of normal variation as wide as this, it is obviously difficult to demonstrate a convincing effect of brain damage.

A recent longitudinal study has shed some light on what has been a very confused and confusing issue. Bates et al.[95] have coordinated work at three medical centers to identify all children with perinatal (within 6 months of birth) unilateral brain damage. The children have already been followed up, to 7 years of age, and the study is still continuing. As expected, most children are within the normal range on measures of vocabulary and syntax development, whether their lesions are on the left or on the right. On the average, however, the children are in the lower range of normal. Brain damage takes a toll even if language develops.

Bates' study demonstrated a few differential but transient effects of brain damage in different regions. Children with left posterior damage were slower to develop vocabulary and grammar, and children with either left or right frontal damage were delayed in vocabulary and grammar development during the period of the **vocabulary burst** (19 to 31 months). By the age of 7 years, however, no site-specific effects could be demonstrated. Bates hypothesizes that cortical specialization is the result of competition among regions for control over tasks. She believes that the left hemisphere normally gains control over language because it contains general mechanisms that are specialized for the extraction of perceptual detail, not because of innately specified language acquisition modules, per se. When the left hemisphere has been compromised by damage, the right hemisphere or neighboring regions can take over the operations necessary to acquire vocabulary and syntax. Neural mechanisms may not be performing at peak efficiency, and a Shakespearean mastery of

language may be improbable in the presence of left hemisphere disease, but an adequate mastery of language will develop, nonetheless.

For the Future

Individual differences in the organization of language function may correspond to anatomic differences in the organization of the Sylvian fissure. The language regions surrounding the lateral fissure are best visualized in sagittal sections. Routine MRI studies rarely include sagittal views of the cortex because they are not designed to localize brain damage in terms of sulcal morphology. If accurate description of the anatomy of the lesion is of interest, then the scan protocol should include laterally placed sagittal images. Moreover, the images should be analyzed in collaboration with an expert neuroanatomist or neurologist, because neuroradiologists do not routinely receive training in sulcal morphology and the lateral fissure demonstrates a wide range of morphology on MRI. In many cases, the transverse gyrus of Heschl is duplicated, either because a second bulge appears in the planum immediately posterior to the transverse sulcus, or because the primary gyrus is split by a sulcus of variable length, the sulcus intermedius. The primary auditory cortex occupies only the portion of the transverse gyrus anterior to the sulcus intermedius or transverse sulcus.[97] Whether duplication of the transverse gyrus affects information processing by the region should be investigated. Multiple gyri may represent areas of extra growth—in particular, cytoarchitectonic or functional regions. Variation in branching angles may also be significant. The posterior ascending ramus may ascend in a superior direction because of developmental differences in connectivity, or mechanical forces such as pressure from parietal lobe structures.[27] It is possible that the morphologic variants seen in this region may give insight into normal and deviant developmental trajectories and predict the degree of plasticity that is possible after early and late lesions.

Clinical Correlations

The generation and comprehension of language involve the interaction of many complex mechanisms. Many of these mechanisms appear to be regulated by systems located in and around the banks of the

Sylvian fissure. An area located anterior to the premotor cortex in the left frontal operculum plays a crucial role, in that stimulation or damage there interferes with fluent production of speech. The left posterior superior and middle temporal gyri contain mechanisms for the perceptual analysis of phonologic, semantic, and syntactic characteristics. Conflicting results from imaging experiments and clinical analyses may be due to individual differences in the spatial distribution and segregation of language processing mechanisms. Development of the neural systems responsible for language may show a large degree of individual variability because of interactions between genetic and environmental factors. Sparing of language function is seen after early lesions, whereas permanent loss follows adult damage. Analysis and rehabilitation in aphasic patients should be individualized, concentrating on specific strengths and weaknesses in an attempt to substitute healthy alternative mechanisms for damaged processes. Technical improvements in imaging techniques and the development of animal models should lead to a tremendous increase in our understanding of the neuroscience of language.

REFERENCES

1. Savage-Rumbaugh E, Murphy J, Sevcik R, Brakke K, Williams S, Rumbaugh D. Language acquisition in ape and child. *Monographs of the Society for Research in Child Development* 1993;58:1–221.
2. Pinker S. *The language instinct.* New York: William Morrow, 1994.
3. Frackowiak RSJ. Functional mapping of verbal memory and language. *Trends Neurosci* 1994;17:109–115.
4. Elman J, Bates E, Johnson M, Karmiloff-Smith A, Parisi D, Plunkett K. *Rethinking innateness: a connectionist perspective on development.* Cambridge, MA: MIT Press, 1996.
5. Allman J. Maps in context: some analogies between visual cortical and genetic maps. In: Vaina L, ed. *Matters of intelligence.* Dordrecht, The Netherlands: D. Reidel, 1987:369–393.
6. Passingham R. *The frontal lobes and voluntary behavior.* Oxford: Oxford University Press, 1993.
7. Penfield W, Roberts L. *Speech and brain-mechanisms.* Princeton, NJ: Princeton University Press, 1959.
8. Wada J. A new method for the determination of the side of cerebral speech dominance: a preliminary report on the intracarotid injection of sodium Amytal in man. *Med Biol* 1949;14:221–222.
9. Rasmussen T, Milner B. Clinical and surgical studies of the cerebral speech areas in man. In: Zulch KJ,

Creutzfeldt O, Galbraith GC, eds. *Otfrid Foerster symposium on cerebral localization.* New York: Springer-Verlag, 1975:238–257.
10. Kimura D. Cerebral dominance and the perception of verbal stimuli. *Can J Psychol* 1961;15:166–171.
11. Strauss E, Gaddes W, Wada J. Performance on a free-recall verbal dichotic listening task and cerebral dominance determined by the carotid Amytal test. *Neuropsychologia* 1987;25:747–753.
12. Shankweiler D, Studdert-Kennedy M. Identification of consonants and vowels presented to left and right ears. *Q J Exp Psychol* 1967;19:59–63.
13. Tallal P, Miller S, Fitch RH. Temporal processing in the nervous system: implications for the development of phonological systems. *Ann NY Acad Sci* 1993;682:27–47.
14. Shannon R, Zeng F, Kamath V, Wygonski J, Ekelid M. Speech recognition with primarily temporal cues. *Science* 1995;270:303–304.
15. Robin D, Tranel D, Damasio H. Auditory perception of temporal and spectral events in patients with focal left and right cerebral lesions. *Brain Lang* 1990;39:539–555.
16. Caplan D. *Language: structuring, processing and disorders.* Cambridge, MA: MIT Press, 1992.
17. Zatorre R. Pitch perception of complex tones and human temporal-lobe function. *J Acoust Soc Am* 1988;84: 566–572.
18. Zatorre R, Evans A, Meyer E, Gjedde A. Lateralization of phonetic and pitch discrimination in speech processing. *Science* 1992;256:846–849.
19. Tallal P, Stark R, Mellits D. Identification of language-impaired children on the basis of rapid perception and production skills. *Brain Lang* 1985;25:314–322.
20. Kraus N, McGee TJ, Carrell TD, Zecker SG, Nicol TG, Koch DB. Auditory neurophysiologic responses and discrimination deficits in children with learning problems. *Science* 1996;273:971–973.
21. Wright B, Lombardino L, King W, Puranik C, Leonard C, Merzenich M. Deficits in auditory temporal and spectral processing in language-impaired children. *Nature* 1996;387:176–178.
22. Kimura D, Carson M. Cognitive pattern and directional asymmetry of finger-ridge count. *University of Western Ontario Department of Psychology Research Bulletin* 1993;716.
23. Kertesz A. *Aphasia and associated disorders.* New York: Grune & Stratton, 1979.
24. Ojemann G. Brain organization for language from the perspective of electrical stimulation mapping. *Brain and Behavioral Sciences* 1983;6:189–230.
25. Benson D. Aphasia. In: Heilman K, Valenstein E, eds. *Clinical neuropsychology.* New York: Oxford University Press, 1993:17–36.
26. Crosson B, Nadeau S. The role of subcortical structures in linguistic processes: recent developments. In: Stemmer B, Whitaker H, eds. *Handbook of neurolinguistics.* San Diego: Academic Press, 1997.

27. Van Essen D. A tension-based theory of morphogenesis and compact wiring in the central nervous system. *Nature* 1997;385:313–318.
28. Clark M, Plante E. Morphology of the inferior frontal lobe in language impaired adults. *Cognitive Neuroscience Society Annual Meeting* 1995;2:9.
29. Bogen J, Bogen G. Wernicke's region: where is it? *Ann NY Acad Sci* 1976;280:834–843.
30. Liegeois-Chauvel C, Musolino A, Chavel P. Localization of the primary auditory area in man. *Brain* 1991;114:139–153.
31. Demonet J, Chollet F, Ramsay S, et al. The anatomy of phonological and semantic processing in normal subjects. *Brain* 1992;115:1753–1768.
32. Howard D, Patterson K, Wise R, et al. The cortical localization of the lexicons: positron emission tomography evidence. *Brain* 1992;1115:1769–1782.
33. Binder JR, Frost JA, Hammeke TA, Rao SM, Cox RW. Function of the left planum temporale in auditory and linguistic processing. *Brain* 1996;119:1239–1247.
34. Binder J. Human brain language areas identified by functional magnetic resonance imaging. *J Neurosci* 1997;17:353–362.
35. Colombo M, Rodman H, Gross C. The effects of superior temporal lesions on the processing and retention of auditory information in monkeys Cebus apella. *J Neurosci* 1996:4501–4517.
36. Petersen M, Beecher M, Zoloth S, Moody D, Stebbins W. Neural lateralization of species-specific vocalizations by Japanese macaques. *Science* 1978;202:324–326.
37. Hauser M. *Evolution of human communication*. Cambridge, MA: Harvard University Press, 1995.
38. Dewson J, Cowey A, Weiskrantz L. Disruptions of auditory sequence discrimination by unilateral and bilateral cortical ablations of superior temporal gyrus in the monkey. *Exp Neurol* 1970;28:529–549.
39. Heffner H, Heffner R. Temporal lobe lesions and perception of species-specific vocalizations by macaques. *Science* 1984;226:75–76.
40. Heffner H, Heffer R. Effects of restricted lesions on absolute thresholds and aphasia-like deficits in Japanese macaques. *J Neurophysiol* 1986;56:683–701.
41. Yemi-Komshian G, Benson D. Anatomical study of cerebral asymmetry in the temporal lobe of humans, chimpanzees, and rhesus monkeys. *Science* 1976;192:387–389.
42. Nottebohm F, Nottebohm M. Left hypoglossal dominance in the control of canary and white-crowned sparrow song. *J Comp Physiol [A]* 1976;108:171–192.
43. Nottebohm FF, Stokes TM, Leonard CM. Central control of song in the canary. *J Comp Neurol* 1976;165:457–486.
44. Fitch R, Brown C, O'Connor K, Tallal P. Functional lateralization for auditory temporal processing in male and female rats. *Behav Neurosci* 1993;107:844–850.
45. Blumstein S. Impairments of speech production and speech perception in aphasia. *Philos Trans R Soc Lond B Biol Sci* 1994;346:29–36.
46. Ojemann G, Mateer C. Human language cortex: localization of memory, syntax, and sequential motor-phoneme identification systems. *Science* 1979;205:1401–1403.
47. Kulynych J, Vladar K, Jones D, Weinberger D. Gender differences in the normal lateralization of the supratemporal cortex-MRI surface-rendering morphometry of Heschl's gyrus and the planum temporale. *Cereb Cortex* 1994;4:107–118.
48. Harasty J, Double K, Halliday G, Kril J, McRitchie D. Language-associated cortical regions are proportionally larger in the female brain. *Arch Neurol* 1997;54:171–176.
49. Shaywitz B, Shaywitz S, Pugh K, et al. Sex differences in the functional organization of the brain for language. *Nature* 1995;373:607–609.
50. Bates E, Thal D. Associations and dissociations in child language development. In: Miller J, ed. *Research on child language disorders*. Austin, TX: Pro-ed, 1991:147–168.
51. Linebarger M, Schwartz M, Saffran E. Sensitive to grammatical structure in so-called agrammatic aphasics. *Cognition* 1983;13:361–392.
52. Slobin D. Aphasia in Turkish: Speech production in Broca's and Wernicke's patients. *Brain Lang* 1991;41:149–164.
53. Baddeley A. *Working memory*. New York, Oxford University Press, 1986.
54. Goldman-Rakic P. Cellular basis of working memory. *Neuron* 1995;14:477–485.
55. Goldman-Rakic P. Development of cortical circuitry and cognitive function. *Child Dev* 1987;58:642–691.
56. Paulesu E, Frith D, Frackowiak R. The neural correlates of the verbal component of working memory. *Nature* 1993;362:342–345.
57. Bates E, Wulfeck B, MacWhinney B. Cross-linguistic research in aphasia: an overview. *Brain Lang* 1991;41:123–148.
58. Kimura D, Watson N. The relation between oral movement control and speech. *Brain Lang* 1989;37:565–590.
59. Petersen S, Fox P, Posner M, Mintum M, Raichle M. Positron emission tomographic studies of the cortical anatomy of single-word processing. *Nature* 1988;331:585–589.
60. Gazzaniga M. Right hemisphere language following brain bisection: a 20 year perspective. *Am Psychol* 1983;38:525–549.
61. Rubens A, Mahwold M, Hutton J. Asymmetry of the lateral Sylvian fissures in man. *Neurology* 1976;26:620–624.
62. Steinmetz H, Ebeling U, Huang Y, Kahn T. Sulcus topography of the parietal opercular region: an anatomic and MR study. *Brain Lang* 1990;38:515–533.
63. Witelson S, Kigar D. Sylvian fissure morphology and asymmetry in men and women: bilateral differences in relation to handedness in men. *J Comp Neurol* 1992;323:326–340.

64. Geschwind N, Levitsky W. Human brain: left–right asymmetries in temporal speech region. *Science* 1968; 161:186–187.

65. Witelson S. Bumps on the brain: right–left asymmetries in temporal speech region. In: Segalowitz S, ed. *Language functions and brain organization*. Orlando, FL: Academic Press, 1982:117–144.

66. Galaburda A, Sanides F, Geschwind N. Human brain: cytoarchitectonic left–right asymmetries in the temporal speech region. *Arch Neurol* 1978;35:812–817.

67. Musiek F, Reeves A. Asymmetries of the auditory areas of the cerebrum. *J Am Acad Audiol* 1990;1:240–245.

68. Seldon H. The anatomy of speech perception: human auditory cortex. In: Peters A, Jones E, eds. *Cerebral cortex*. New York: Plenum, 1985:273–327.

69. Steinmetz H, Rademacher J, Jancke L, Huang Y, Thron A, Zilles K. Total surface of temporoparietal intrasylvian cortex: diverging left–right asymmetries. *Brain Lang* 1990;39:357–372.

70. Leonard C, Voeller KS, Lombardino L, et al. Anomalous cerebral structure in dyslexia revealed with magnetic resonance imaging. *Arch Neurol* 1993;50:461–469.

71. Jancke L, Schlaug G, Huang Y, Steinmetz H. Asymmetry of the planum parietale. *NeuroReport* 1994;5:1161–1163.

72. Foundas A, Leonard C, Gilmore R, Fennell E, Heilman K. Planum temporale asymmetry and language dominance. *Neuropsychologia* 1994;32:1225–1231.

73. Seldon H. Structure of human auditory cortex: I. cytoarchitectonics and dendritic distributions. *Brain Res* 1981;229:277–294.

74. Galaburda A, Sherman G, Rosen G, Aboitiz F, Geschwind N. Developmental dyslexia: four consecutive cases with cortical anomalies. *Ann Neurol* 1985;18: 222–233.

75. Galaburda A. Ordinary and extraordinary brain development: anatomical variation in developmental dyslexia. *Annals of Dyslexia* 1989;39:67–79.

76. LeMay M, Culebras A. Human brain: morphological differences in the hemispheres demonstrable by carotid angiography. *N Engl J Med* 1972;287:168–170.

77. LeMay M, Kido D. Asymmetries of the cerebral hemispheres on computed tomogram. *J Comput Assist Tomogr* 1978;2:471–478.

78. Larsen J, Hoien T, Lundberg I, Odegaard H. MRI evaluation of the size and symmetry of the planum temporale in adolescents with developmental dyslexia. *Brain Lang* 1990;39:289–301.

79. Hynd G, Semrud-Clikeman M, Lorys A, Novey E, Eliopulos D. Brain morphology in developmental dyslexia and attention deficit disorder/hyperactivity. *Arch Neurol* 1990;47:919–926.

80. Hynd GW, Semrud-Clikeman M. Dyslexia and brain morphology. *Psychol Bull* 1989;106:447–482.

81. Duara R, Kusch A, Gross-Glenn K, et al. Neuroanatomic differences between dyslexic and normal readers on magnetic resonance imaging scans. *Arch Neurol* 1991; 48:410–416.

82. Steinmetz H, Rademacher J, Huang Y. Cerebral asymmetry: MR planimetry of the human planum temporale. *J Comput Assist Tomogr* 1989;13:996–1005.

83. Filipek P. Neurobiological correlates of developmental dyslexia: how do dyslexic brains differ from those of normal readers? *J Child Neurol* 1995;10:62–69.

84. Rumsey J, Andreason P, Zametkin A, et al. Failure to activate the left temporoparietal cortex in dyslexia. *Arch Neurol* 1992;49:527–534.

85. Rumsey J, Andreason P, Zametkin A, et al. Right frontotemporal activation by tonal memory in dyslexia, an O-15 PET study. *Biol Psychiatry* 1994;36:171–180.

86. Plante E, Swisher L, Vance R, Rapcsak S. MRI findings in boys with specific language impairment. *Brain Lang* 1991;41:52–66.

87. Jernigan T, Hesselink J, Sowell E, Tallal P. Cerebral morphology on MRI in language and learning-impaired children. *Arch Neurol* 1990;48:539–545.

88. Gauger L, Lombardino L, Leonard C. Brain morphology in children with specific language impairment. *Journal of Speech and Language Research* 1997;40:1272–1284.

89. Leonard C, Lombardino L, Mercado L, Browd S, Breier J, Agee O. Cerebral asymmetry and cognitive development in children: a magnetic resonance imaging study. *Psychological Science* 1996;7:79–85.

90. Witelson S, Kigar D. Asymmetry in brain function follows asymmetry in anatomical form: gross, microscopic, postmortem and imaging studies. In: Boller F, Grafman J, Rizzolatti G, Goodglass H, eds. *Handbook of neuropsychology*. Amsterdam: Elsevier, 1988:111–142.

91. Hayes T, Lewis D. Anatomical specializations of the anterior motor speech area. *Brain Lang* 1995;49:289–308.

92. Foundas A, Leonard C, Gilmore R, Fennell E, Heilman K. Pars triangularis asymmetry and language dominance. *Proc Natl Acad Sci U S A* 1996;93:719–722.

93. Lenneberg E. *Biological foundations of language*. New York: John Wiley & Sons, 1967.

94. Aram D. Language sequelae of unilateral brain lesions in children. In: Plum F, ed. *Language, communication and the brain*. New York: Raven Press, 1988:171–198.

95. Bates E, Thal D, Aram D, Eisele J, Nass R, Trauner D. From first words to grammar in children with focal brain injury. *Developmental Neuropsychology* 1997;13: 275–343.

96. Bates E, Dale P, Thal D. Individual differences and their implications for theories of language development. In: Fletcher P, MacWhinney B, eds. *Handbook of child language*. Oxford: Blackwell, 1995:96–163.

97. Rademacher J, Caviness V, Steinmetz H, Galaburda A. Topographical variation of the human primary cortices: implications for neuroimaging, brain mapping and neurobiology. *Cereb Cortex* 1993;3:313–329.

19

Development of the Nervous System

THÉRÈSE CABANA, PhD

As you have learned from the previous chapters of this book, the nervous system is a very complicated machine, comprising an impressive number of cells organized in an intricate network of connections. It controls the complete repertoire of a person's behavior: internal functions, such as digestion or heartbeat; basic and complex interactions with the environment, such as perception of temperature or hearing a birdsong; interactions of all sorts with other people; learning, such as reading or the motor act of playing the piano; and emotions, such as love or fear. Moreover, all of these behaviors must also be coordinated to ensure the fitness of the person at every moment.

In most animals, and particularly in mammals, the development of the nervous system is considerably protracted, but still occurs to a large extent before many of the behaviors mentioned previously are expressed. Other body organs and systems begin forming at about the same time, or later, than the nervous system but terminate earlier (except for pure size increase); they become functional in the embryo as soon as their rudiments are in place—for example, the heart, the blood vessels, and, as a whole, the cardiovascular system. A large part of the development of the nervous system depends on strictly determined criteria to prepare an exceedingly complicated connection network that will be ready for use when needed— so strict, in fact, that it may seem paradoxical for a system whose function is communication. You will see in the course of this chapter how, indeed, a large part of neural development is determined, and how, at the same time, it can be controlled in a number of ways to adjust to the environment.

The development of the nervous system comprises a series of events that more or less follow a temporal sequence: 1) neurulation, or the formation of the neural tube and neural crest from a part of the embryonic ectoderm; 2) cell proliferation within the neural tube; 3) migration of postmitotic cells and their aggregation in definitive locations; 4) cytodifferentiation, or formation of the axonal and dendritic processes characteristic of nerve cells; and 5)

formation of the connections between nerve cells and either other nerve cells or muscle cells. Partly overlapping these events, reorganization, elimination, and stabilization of elements also occur.

This chapter tries to combine a descriptive approach with a functional one, as well as combining a holistic, systemic approach with a reductionist, cellular and molecular one. It is impossible, in just one chapter, to cover all aspects of the development of this most complicated and fascinating system in detail; this topic alone has been the object of numerous review articles and textbooks in the last decade or so. Nonetheless, it is hoped that it will allow you not only to appreciate how the nervous system is formed, but to comprehend better its adult organization.

Neurulation

The nervous system starts forming at a time when the human embryo is approximately 21 to 22 days of age and measures less than 4 mm in length. The embryo, called a **gastrula**, is made up of three superimposed sheets of cells (excluding the extraembryonic structures, such as the amnion and the yolk sac): the ectoderm, mesoderm, and endoderm (Fig. 19–1). The entire nervous system, including the peripheral nervous system, derives from the dorsomedial part of the embryonic ectoderm.

Formation of the Neural Tube and Neural Crest

The very first event in the formation of the nervous system consists of a thickening of the dorsomedial part of the ectoderm, corresponding to an elongation of the cells that, from squamous or cuboidal, become columnar (Fig. 19–2A). That part of the ectoderm is now called the **neuroectoderm**, whereas the rest of the embryonic ectoderm, wherein cells remain flat, is known as general ectoderm. Because the neuroectoderm is thicker than the general ectoderm, it is also called the **neural plate**.

The formation of the neural plate does not occur simultaneously along the entire craniocaudal length of the embryo. Instead, it begins approximately at the mid-level of the embryo, which corresponds to the mid-cervical level in the adult, and gradually proceeds both cranially and caudally from that point. This spatiotemporal sequence also generally holds true for the subsequent stages of neural devel-

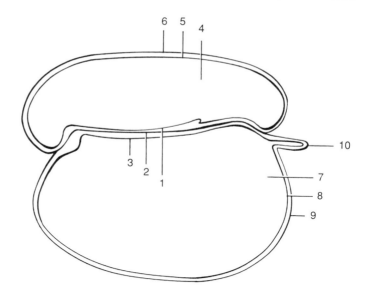

To Identify:

1. Embryonic ectoderm
2. Embryonic mesoderm
3. Embryonic endoderm
4. Amniotic cavity
5. Amniotic ectoderm
6. Amniotic mesoderm
7. Yolk sac cavity
8. Yolk sac endoderm
9. Yolk sac mesoderm
10. Allantois

Figure 19–1. The human embryo toward the end of gastrulation and before neurulation. It is composed of the three primordial germ layers and develops into the amniotic cavity, itself filled with amniotic fluid.

opment. The neural plate is fairly wide rostrally and somewhat narrow caudally. Nearly 50% of all ectodermal cells eventually become neuroectodermal.

Under the ectoderm of the gastrula lies the loose sheet of mesoderm, the most medial part of which consists of a denser aggregation of cells forming a longitudinal rod distinct from the rest of the mesoderm. This structure, called the **notochord**, serves transiently as a kind of vertebral skeleton for the embryo. The part of the ectoderm dorsal to the notochord actually becomes the neural plate. Thanks largely to the work of the German embryologist Hans Spemann in the 1920s and 1930s, we have known for some time that the notochord must be present for the neural plate to form. Indeed, if the notochord is surgically removed, the neural plate does not form.

Likewise, if the notochord is transplanted, such as under the flank ectoderm, the neural plate forms in that ectopic site. Thus, the notochord induces the overlying ectoderm to differentiate into neuroectoderm. This embryonic **induction** is chemically mediated, acts over a concentration gradient, and does not require contact of notochord and ectoderm.

The lateral margins of the neural plate elevate, pulling with them the attached general ectoderm and creating a depression between them (see Fig. 19–2B). The neural plate margins are thus called **neural folds**, and delimit the **neural groove**. As the neural folds elevate, they also move medially, toward each other (see Fig. 19–2C). Eventually, they make contact and fuse, forming a closed tube, the **neural tube**, the lumen of which is called the **neu-**

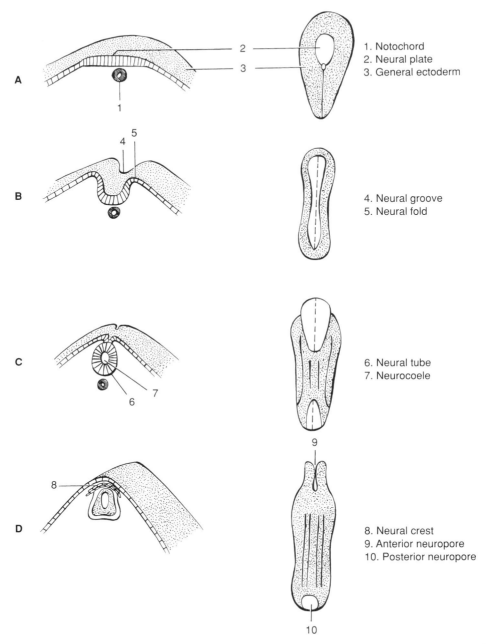

A

2
3

1. Notochord
2. Neural plate
3. General ectoderm

B

5
4

4. Neural groove
5. Neural fold

C

7
6

6. Neural tube
7. Neurocoele

9

D

8

8. Neural crest
9. Anterior neuropore
10. Posterior neuropore

10

Figure 19-2. Neurulation: left, three-dimensional cross sections; right, dorsal views. **A:** Formation of the neural plate. **B:** Elevation of the neural folds. **C:** Fusion of the neural folds on the midline and closure of the neural tube. **D:** Separation of the neural fold cells from both the neural tube and the general ectoderm and formation of the neural crest.

rocele (see Fig. 19–2D). The general ectoderm detaches from the closing neural tube and fuses on the midline, now covering the neural tube. Thus, the neural tube becomes positioned between the notochord and the dorsal (general) ectoderm.[1]

The portions of the neural folds immediately attached to the general ectoderm are not incorporated into the neural tube, but neither do they remain part of the ectoderm. Rather, at the closure of the neural tube, they detach from both general ectoderm and neural tube and become interposed between them, forming a unique structure in the shape of the French circumflex mark (^), called the **neural crest** (see Fig. 19–2D).

Neurulation is thus the first step in the formation of the nervous system, and is usually defined as the formation of the neural tube, but also encompasses the concomitant formation of the neural crest. The central nervous system—the neuraxis, comprising the spinal cord and the brain—derives from the neural tube. Most of the peripheral nervous system—sensory ganglia, autonomic ganglia and plexuses, adrenal medulla, neuroendocrine cells found among the epithelia lining the digestive tract and respiratory tubes, melanocytes of the skin, and a number of other structures, including some skeletal components of the head—derive from the neural crest. Not all sensory ganglia, however, originate in the neural crest. Cranial sensory ganglia derive largely, if not entirely, from the ectodermal sensory placodes. Spinal sensory ganglia (dorsal root ganglia) have traditionally been thought to derive from the neural crest, or perhaps partly from the neural tube, but evidence also suggests that they may form from the medialmost part of the mesodermal somites.[2]

Defects of Neurulation

As stated previously, the spatiotemporal sequence of neural tube formation follows that of the neural plate. The ends of the neural tube, however, remain open over a relatively long period of time. These openings at both ends of the neural tube, the posterior and anterior **neuropores**, allow circulation of the amniotic fluid in the neurocele. Hence, the **cerebrospinal fluid (CSF)** initially consists of amniotic fluid. Failure of the posterior neuropore to close in its due course results in a lesion known as **spina bifida**. The severity of this condition depends on the amount of neural tube (presumptive spinal cord) left open. Failure of the anterior neuropore to close, which normally occurs even later than that of the

posterior, leads to **anencephaly**. An important proportion of the brain does not develop, and, consequently, the overlying, protective cranium does not form, which makes the fetus nonviable. Anencephaly characterizes approximately 0.1% of pregnancies. Obviously, closure of the neuropores must coincide with the development of vascularization and the choroid plexuses to ensure CSF metabolism.

Local Variations: Spinal Cord and Encephalic Vesicles

Not only does the neural plate vary in width at different levels, but local variations occur during the process in which it is folding into a tube, so that the neural tube differs in size and shape along the craniocaudal axis of the embryo. It is greatly enlarged cranially, inside the emerging head bud, with a wide neurocele, and has more the shape of a vesicle than of a tube; it gives rise to the brain, and is appropriately called the "encephalic vesicle." The rest of the neural tube remains narrow and tubular in shape, and is at the origin of the spinal cord.

Although neurulation marks the beginning of organogenesis, organs other than the nervous system begin to form as well. The embryo as a whole increases in size; it lengthens and bends in on itself ventrally. The neural tube does not remain straight but follows this bend. A ventral fold, the **cervical flexure**, marks the junction of the presumptive brain and spinal cord. Another ventral flexure, the **cephalic flexure**, appears about midway in the encephalon. Furthermore, two lateral constrictions subdivide the latter into three primordial vesicles: **rhombencephalon**, continuous with the presumptive spinal cord, **mesencephalon**, and **prosencephalon** (Fig. 19–3). From the lateral wall of the prosencephalon, bilaterally, the **optic vesicles** emerge. These vesicles are the origin of the neural component of the eye, the retina.

Additional constrictions subdivide the three primordial encephalic vesicles: the rhombencephalon subdivides into the **myelencephalon**, the presumptive medulla oblongata, and the **metencephalon**, the presumptive pons and cerebellum; the mesencephalon makes no subdivisions and gives rise to the midbrain tegmentum and tectum; the prosencephalon subdivides into the **diencephalon**, the future epithalamus, thalamus, and hypothalamus, and the **telencephalon**, at the origin of the basal forebrain and cerebral hemispheres. The telencephalon is in the form of paired vesicles, the telencephalic vesicles. The optic stalks,

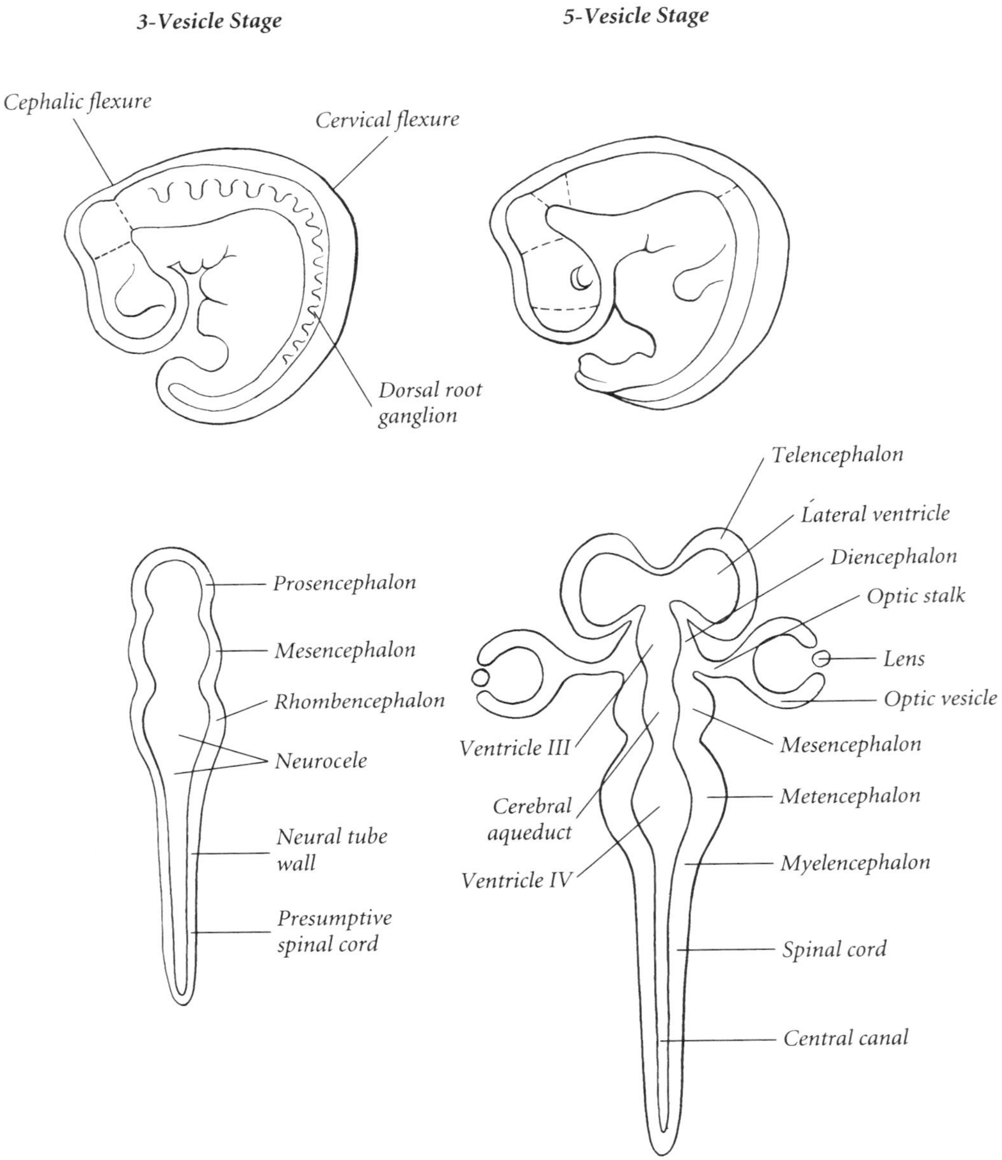

3-Vesicle Stage   *5-Vesicle Stage*

Figure 19–3. The neural tube at the three-vesicle stage (left) and five-vesicle stage (right). *Top:* Side views of the embryo showing the neural tube by transparency (note the flexures). *Bottom:* Longitudinal (horizontal) section showing the neural tube as if stretched.

containing the optic nerves, link the growing optic vesicles to the diencephalon.

As the presumptive spinal cord and brain begin to differentiate, the neurocele adapts its shape to the local variations. In the spinal cord, it takes the name of **central canal**, and in the brain, the name of various **ventricles** located there. In the rhombencephalon (myelencephalon and metencephalon together), the fourth ventricle is wide and, viewed dorsally, has a rhombic shape; in the diencephalon, the third ventricle is narrow but elongated dorsoventrally; the greatly reduced cerebral aqueduct traverses the midbrain and links the fourth and third ventricles; the lateral ventricles (or second and first ventricles) occupy the cerebral hemispheres.

Cell Proliferation

The epithelium of the neural plate, as well as of the newly closed neural tube, is pseudostratified, comprising one layer of columnar cells. The nuclei of those cells do not all occupy the same position in the cells, giving the epithelium a stratified appearance. The base of this **neuroepithelium**, its external portion, is toward the mesodermal structures, whereas the apex, or internal portion, is toward the neural groove or the neurocele. As for other epithelia, a basal lamina lines it. Deriving from the mesoderm, the **meninges** (pia mater, arachnoid, and dura mater) will form around the neural tube.

The Germinal Zone: Dividing Cells

After closure of the neural tube, a developmental period occurs during which neuroepithelial cells divide actively, leading to the addition of a great number of cells to the tube and to stratification of its epithelium (Fig. 19–4A,B). Neuroepithelial cells divide at a rapid rate and the interphase is short.

The Intermediate Zone: Postmitotic Neuroblasts

Eventually, some daughter cells leave the mitotic cycle, that is, become **postmitotic**. Such cells are pushed externally in the epithelium, superficial to the dividing cells. The wall of the neural tube thus becomes subdivided into two zones: a **germinal zone** of dividing cells and an **intermediate zone**, or mantle, of postmitotic cells (see Fig. 19–4C,D). A

marginal zone forms later (see Fig. 19–4D). The intermediate zone gradually becomes thicker, by addition of postmitotic cells, whereas the germinal zone decreases and eventually is reduced to a single cell layer—the **ependymal** epithelium (see Fig. 19–4E)—where cells develop cilia beating into the ependymal canal (central canal or ventricles).

Newly postmitotic cells are morphologically undifferentiated: small and either round or ovoid. Most of them, in the early stages, are **neuroblasts**. Although the suffix *blast* implies a precursor cell that can divide, the term *neuroblast* often refers to postmitotic, undifferentiated nerve cells. Neurons are terminal cells; they will not divide in later life. Neurons lost over time are not replaced. During the period of intense neuronal production, **glioblasts** of the type that serve as a substrate for postmitotic neuroblasts to migrate out of the germinal epithelium (as will be seen in the next section) are present in relatively small numbers. Glial cells (astrocytes and oligodendrocytes) are produced mostly toward the end of the period of cell proliferation. Contrary to neurons, glioblasts can be produced throughout life, as needed and with the proper signal.

The moment (date) a neuron becomes postmitotic is considered as its "production" (its "birthdate"). Using autoradiographic techniques to label the nuclei of dividing cells, Altman and Bayer were able to determine the time of production of neuronal populations in the entire nervous system of the rat.[2–13] This work is mentioned again later. In the case of the human, prenatal development is long. Neuron production occurs early in ontogenesis for most parts of the central nervous system. Nevertheless, some regions that are phylogenetically new form relatively late and, because of the considerable development attained by these regions in the human, they account for an important proportion of the total neuron number. Neuron production may still occur around the time of birth in these regions.

Cell Number and Its Controls

At the end of the period of cell proliferation, the thickness of the neural tube varies considerably both within a level (dorsal, lateral, or ventral walls of the tube) and between levels as a result of differential proliferation in the germinal zone, of differential total duration of the proliferative period around and along the tube, and of differences in the migratory routes taken by postmitotic cells to reach the intermediate zone.

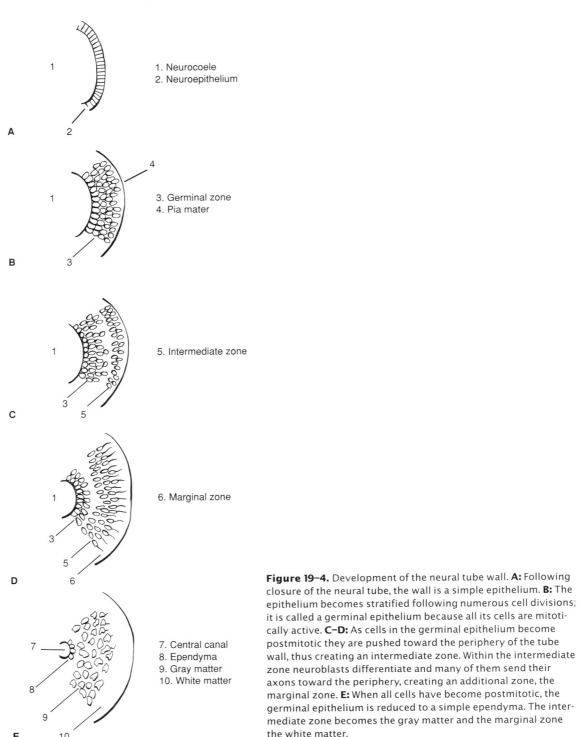

1. Neurocoele
2. Neuroepithelium

3. Germinal zone
4. Pia mater

5. Intermediate zone

6. Marginal zone

7. Central canal
8. Ependyma
9. Gray matter
10. White matter

A

B

C

D

E

Figure 19-4. Development of the neural tube wall. **A:** Following closure of the neural tube, the wall is a simple epithelium. **B:** The epithelium becomes stratified following numerous cell divisions; it is called a germinal epithelium because all its cells are mitotically active. **C-D:** As cells in the germinal epithelium become postmitotic they are pushed toward the periphery of the tube wall, thus creating an intermediate zone. Within the intermediate zone neuroblasts differentiate and many of them send their axons toward the periphery, creating an additional zone, the marginal zone. **E:** When all cells have become postmitotic, the germinal epithelium is reduced to a simple ependyma. The intermediate zone becomes the gray matter and the marginal zone the white matter.

The total number of neurons is finite, estimated at about 85 billion in the human central nervous system. Most of them are in phylogenetically new regions (12 to 15 billion telencephalic neurons and 70 billion cerebellar granule cells, but only approximately 1 billion brainstem and spinal neurons). Therefore, cell proliferation must be tightly controlled. Besides the predominant genetic control, other factors are either known or suspected to control cell proliferation: growth factors, hormones (notably the thyroid hormone, thyroxine), cell–cell interactions, and opioids (particularly at later stages of proliferation). The finite number of neurons, however, does not depend solely on additive events, that is, on cell proliferation, but also on subtractive events, that is, cell death occurring normally during ontogenesis. In certain, but not all, cell populations of the central and peripheral nervous system, a significant loss of neurons, ranging from between 20% to 80%, occurs at an early time, before synaptogenesis. This cell death does not depend solely on afferents, targets, or function, as is explained in the last section of this chapter; a certain percentage of neurons is indeed programmed to die in the normal course of development. An interesting review written by Oppenheim, the scientist most closely connected to studies of neuronal death, should be consulted for further details.[14]

Because the total number of glial cells is not fixed in early development, controls on the proliferation of these cells, or precursors, act throughout life. Glia number seems to match neuron number in various regions. A mitogenic effect of nerve cells on glial cells occurs at least during development. Other controls, however, operate at maturity in response to unforeseen needs, such as injuries. A good review of the subject of cell number and its controls in the nervous system can be found in a 1988 article by Williams and Herrup.[15]

Cell Migration and Aggregation

As mentioned previously, when neuroblasts of the central nervous system become postmitotic, they are "pushed" superficially in the wall of the neural tube. In fact, they actively migrate from the germinal to the intermediate zone, a process of the utmost importance for neurons, because their respective morphology, connectivity, and function depend, to a large extent, on the proper acquisition of their positions.

Radial Glial Cells

The active migration of neuroblasts requires the cooperation of a category of transient glial cells, the **radial glial cells**. The existence of such cells was already recognized by **Ramon y Cajal** at the turn of the century.[16] They have been extensively studied by Rakic[17], to whom we owe much of what is known about neuronal migration. As their name implies, radial glial cells are disposed radially in the neural tube. They are elongated cells extending from the neurocele to the basal lamina, with their nuclei in an apical location. Their basal cytoplasmic processes may branch. According to the thickness of the developing neural tube along its axis, the length of radial glial cells may vary from about one tenth up to several millimeters, but all of them do not extend the entire thickness of the tube.

When a neuroblast in the germinal zone exits the mitotic cycle (becomes postmitotic), it associates with a radial glial cell and elongates as it starts migrating along the latter. Such a neuroblast can now be described as having, on either side of its nucleus, a motile **leading process** extending toward the pial surface, and a **trailing process** (Fig. 19–5). Migration is saltatory and involves cytoskeletal elements of the neuroblast, in addition to molecular interactions between the neuronal and glial membranes through adhesion molecules. One such molecule is astrotactin. The speed of migration is in the range of tens of micrometers per hour. More than one neuroblast may be migrating along the same glial cell at one time. Neuroblasts thus locomote along glial processes until they reach their definitive locations in the intermediate zone, at which point adhesion between neural and glial elements is lost.

Neuroblasts need interaction with radial glia for migrating and, likewise, radial glia need interaction with neurons to provide the appropriate scaffold for neuronal migration. The interplay between neuroblasts and radial glia is complex and only partly understood. Mechanisms intrinsic to the migratory process, related to the adhesion properties, might dictate the cessation of migration and, therefore, establish the definitive location of the different neuroblasts.[18] When neuronal migration is completed, the radial glial cells may either degenerate or transform into astrocytes, often after having reentered the mitotic cycle.

Types of Migration

The neuronal migration just described, from the ependymal toward the pial surface, can be qualified

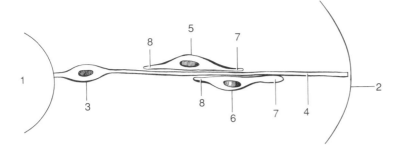

Identify:
1. Neurocoele
2. Pia mater
3. Cell body of the radial glial cell
4. Long process of the radial glial cell
5–6. Cell bodies of two migrating neuroblasts
7. Leading process
8. Trailing process

Figure 19–5. Simplified schematic representation of radial neuronal migration along a radial glial cell in the wall of the neural tube.

as **radial migration**. Radial migration occurs throughout the length of the neuraxis: in the presumptive spinal cord, in the brainstem, and in cortical structures. Also, a **tangential migration**, oblique or parallel to the surface of the neural tube, occurs and concerns mostly phylogenetically newer, late-forming regions. In this case, migrating neuroblasts pass from one radial glia to another tangentially. They may also use a different migration substrate: the earlier-formed axonal tracts, instead of glial cells. Neurons of the pontine nuclei and the inferior olive migrate tangentially, from their site of production at the lateral edge of the rhombencephalon to their ventral position in the brainstem. In the neocortex and some other regions, neurons may successively use both types of migration and substrates.

Proliferation and Migration in the Peripheral Nervous System

In the section on cell proliferation, the neural crest and the peripheral nervous system were not mentioned because, in contrast to central neuroblasts that migrate after becoming postmitotic, peripheral neuroblasts divide during and after migration. Neural crest formation obeys the same spatiotemporal sequence as that of the neural tube. As soon as the neural tube has closed and the neural crest has formed, the latter separates at the midline and metamerizes, as do the

somites of the mesoderm. Each segment forms a rather loose aggregate of cells that migrate away from their origin. Migrating crest cells divide actively and groups of cells separate from each other to undertake new migratory paths. Some groups of crest cells migrate only for short distances, such as those that will form the dorsal root ganglia or the autonomic ganglia of the paravertebral sympathetic chain. Others migrate for relatively long distances, including those forming the autonomic plexuses of the parasympathetic division inserted into the muscular walls of viscera, and the cells of the adrenal medulla. Peripheral neuroblasts or their precursors do not migrate on glial substrates, but mostly on the **extracellular matrix (ECM)**. The ECM is biochemically complex and not identical in all embryonic regions. One component of the ECM known to be essential to crest cell migration is fibronectin. In the absence of fibronectin, the neural crest cells cease migrating and aggregate.

Proliferation and Migration in the Spinal Cord

A cross-section of the developing spinal cord shows that it is nearly circular; the neurocele is narrow and elongated dorsoventrally, and the germinal and intermediate (and later the marginal) zones are organized concentrically around the canal. The dorsal and ventral walls are narrow and thin—only one layer of cells—whereas the lateral walls are thick (Fig. 19–6A). As stated earlier, using nuclear labeling techniques, Altman and Bayer[2] were able to provide detailed descriptions of the patterns of cell proliferation in the rat, and also of migration of neuroblasts from their original site of formation in the germinal zone (around the neurocele) to their definitive location in the intermediate zone. Their findings could almost certainly be applied to other mammals, including humans, except for the timetables, which are species specific and proportional to the total duration of embryogenesis.

Cell proliferation is more active in the germinal zone of the lateral walls, and migration of the postmitotic cells obeys a fairly radial pattern, whereas neuroblasts originating from the dorsal and ventral germinal epithelium migrate obliquely. Within the lateral wall of the presumptive spinal cord, the ventral half is thicker than the dorsal half during most of development, and at most levels of the cord. Thus, from the beginning, the separation of the spinal cord into ventral **basal plate** and dorsal **alar plate** is manifest (see Fig. 19–6B,C). The distinction between basal and alar plates is also marked by the **sulcus limitans** midway in the lateral lining of the neurocele. Proliferation and subsequent migration begin somewhat earlier in the basal plate, but also terminate earlier. In addition to this general ventrodorsal gradient of cell production, there is also a general, but not absolute, lateromedial or outside–in gradient. Indeed, neuroblasts that are the first to be produced migrate farther from their site of origin in the germinal epithelium than do those produced subsequently, which occupy positions closer and closer to the central canal. The neurocele then becomes gradually smaller, and is eventually reduced to the central canal (see Fig. 19–6C).

Basal plate neuroblasts differentiate into somatic motor neurons and associated interneurons. At the levels of the developing limb buds, somatic motor neurons and interneurons are added laterally, creating the two enlargements of the spinal cord. When the cord is viewed along its axis (Fig. 19–7), the two pools of motor neurons are seen to form longitudinal columns: the uninterrupted **medial motor column**, innervating the trunk musculature, and the **lateral motor column**, at the levels of the enlargements, innervating the limbs. In the brachial enlargement, motor neurons of the lateral column are produced earlier than those of the medial column, according to the lat-

eromedial gradient mentioned, but this does not seem to be the case in the lumbosacral enlargement, where the gradient is more mediolateral (inside–out). The basal plate is thus considered a motor center, the **ventral horn** in the adult. Alar plate neuroblasts differentiate into sensory interneurons, many of them receiving the dorsal root afferents. The alar plate is thus a sensory center, the **dorsal horn** in the adult. Like its ventral counterpart, it is wider at the enlargements in relation to the additional somatic mass innervated. Dorsal horn neurons are in general smaller than ventral horn neurons. This difference brings about another general, but not absolute, observation of development: large neurons are produced earlier than small neurons in comparable regions. At the junction of the basal and alar plates at thoracic and sacral levels of the cord are the visceral motor neurons. They innervate the autonomic ganglia, or plexuses, of the sympathetic division for those in thoracic segments (the intermediolateral cell column) or of the parasympathetic division for those in sacral segments. Other levels of the cord have no visceral motor neurons. The visceral portion is sometimes described as forming a **lateral horn**.

Proliferation and Migration in the Brainstem

Here too, the work of Altman and Bayer[6–10] on neurogenesis in the brainstem of the rat has served as the basis for understanding the patterns of cell proliferation in the germinal epithelium and their subsequent migration to the intermediate zone. The term "brainstem" usually designates that part of the brain in which motor nuclei of the cranial nerves are present; it is a cranial extension of the spinal cord, albeit modified by the addition of structures. It includes the rhombencephalon and mesencephalon, but excludes the prosencephalon (but the cerebellum and tectum—inferior and superior colliculi—should also be excluded from the brainstem because they in fact constitute its roof). Except for the part caudal to the obex, the shape of the developing rhombencephalon differs from that of the developing spinal cord. Indeed, the dorsal wall is one cell thick and so widened that the "lateral" walls are ventral to the fourth ventricle. The sulcus limitans in the floor of the ventricle still separates a basal plate from an alar plate, the latter being lateral to the former instead of dorsal, as in the cord (Fig. 19–8). In the mesen-

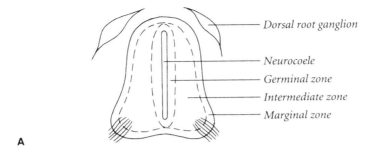

A

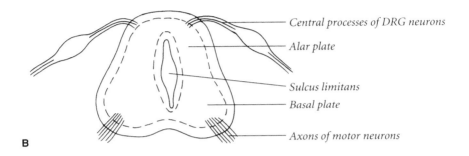

B

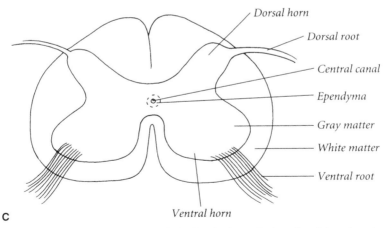

C

Figure 19–6. Schematic representation of the developing spinal cord and dorsal root ganglia (DRG) in cross sections. **A:** Early differentiation of the neural tube; period of intense proliferation and migration. **B:** Cell proliferation slows down. The intermediate and marginal zones thicken as more postmitotic cells are added and differentiate. **C:** Mature spinal cord.

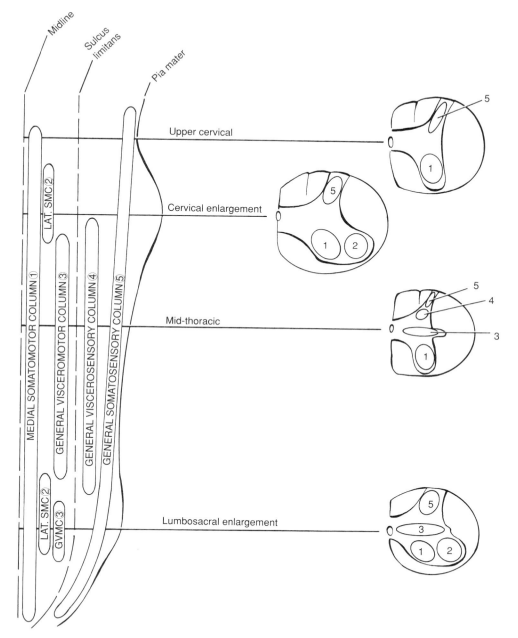

Figure 19–7. Columnal organization of the functional nuclear groups in the spinal cord. *Left:* Longitudinal dorsal view as if the columns were seen by transparency. *Right:* Cross-sectional view of the columns at four selected levels.

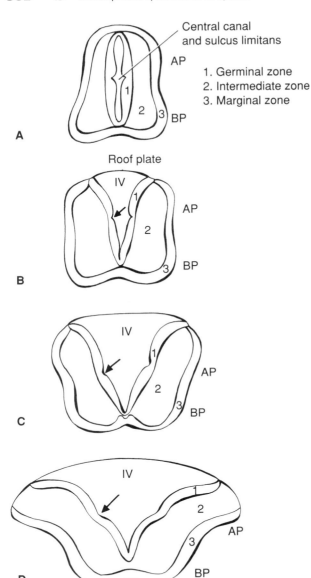

Central canal
and sulcus limitans

AP

1. Germinal zone
2. Intermediate zone
3. Marginal zone

BP

A

Roof plate

IV

AP

BP

B

IV

AP

BP

C

IV

AP

BP

D

Figure 19–8. Opening of the spinal cord central canal **(A)** into the rhombencephalon fourth ventrical **(B–D)** as seen in cross sections. **B** is from a level of the myelencephalon rostral to the obex, **D** is at the level of the junction between myelencephalon and metencephalon and **C** is at a level intermediate between B and D. The alar plate (AP) becomes more lateral in relation to the basal plate (BP) at more rostral levels of the brainstem, instead of dorsal to it as in the spinal cord. The *arrows* point to the sulcus limitans. *IV,* fourth ventricle.

cephalon, the neurocele is less wide, the sulcus limitans less obvious, and the dorsal wall is thin.

The patterns of cell proliferation and migration in the brainstem show similarities to those in the spinal cord, but there are also differences, as mentioned previously, with respect to tangential migration. In the brainstem, as in the spinal cord, the somatic mo-

tor neurons are the first to be produced; they also follow a radial migratory route from their sites of origin in the germinal epithelium, and form the medial-most longitudinal column in the floor of the fourth ventricle (Fig. 19–9). The visceral motor neurons (e.g., the preganglionic neurons of the parasympathetic division of the autonomic nervous system—

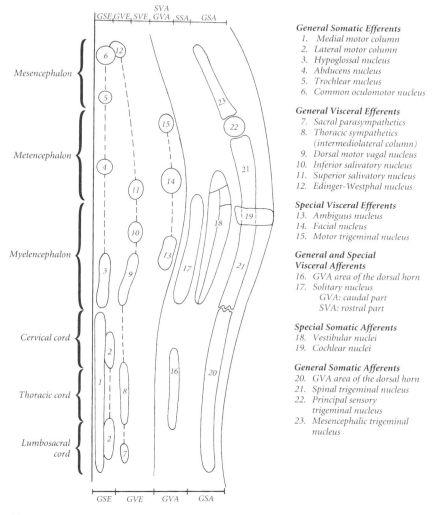

Figure 19–9. Schematic representation of the columnar organization of the functional nuclear groups in the brainstem and spinal cord as seen by transparency from a dorsal longitudinal view. GVA, general visceral afferent; SVA, special visceral afferent. (Modified and reproduced by permission from Haines D. *Neuroanatomy: an atlas of structures, sections and systems.* Baltimore: Williams & Wilkins, 1987.)

the brain, itself, has no sympathetic component), are the next group of neurons to be produced, and they occupy a location lateral to the former group of cells. Sensory neurons are generated somewhat later and over a longer period of time than motor neurons, and the somatic sensory cells are produced earlier than the visceral ones. They come to occupy

positions lateral to the motor groups, in the floor of the fourth ventricle, the separation between them marked by the sulcus limitans. Somatic sensory neurons are lateral to visceral sensory neurons. Motor neurons of the special visceral types, innervating the muscles of branchial arch origin, become postmitotic late, toward the end of the period of sensory cell production. They migrate over a longer distance from the germinal zone to occupy positions ventral to, and intermediate between, the (general) visceral motor neurons and the visceral sensory neurons. Raphe and reticular neurons are produced during nearly the entire duration of motor and sensory neuron production.

Thus, the same general topographic relationships between functional columns found in the spinal cord apply to the brainstem, but, instead of being ventrodorsal, they are mediolateral. When the brainstem is viewed longitudinally (see Fig. 19–9), the somatic motor neurons appear to form an interrupted longitudinal column, medially. More laterally, the general visceral motor neurons also form an interrupted longitudinal column. The special visceral neurons form an interrupted longitudinal column ventrolaterally. The visceral sensory column and the somatic sensory column are next, laterally. The general gradient of cell production is from medial to lateral between columns and within columns. On top of it, a general caudal-to-rostral gradient occurs within the columns, except for the special visceral column, in which the gradient is rostral to caudal. For example, within the somatic motor column, neurons of the caudal-most hypoglossal nucleus are produced earlier than those of the abducens nucleus, which predate neurons of the trochlear nucleus or the oculomotor nucleus. In the special visceral column, the rostral-most neurons of the motor trigeminal nucleus become postmitotic sooner than those of the facial nucleus, the neurons of the nucleus ambiguus being the last. In the brainstem, too, large neurons tend to be produced before small neurons, but this is not an absolute observation.

The inferior and superior colliculi as well as the deeper periaqueductal gray originate from the lateral and dorsal walls of the neuroepithelium of the mesencephalon, and are considered to be alar plate derivatives. Their neurons are produced relatively late and over an extended period of time. They migrate radially—in general from ventral to lateral to dorsal—and the superior colliculus obeys the inside–out pattern described later for the neocortex.

In relation to the development of the cerebellum, some structures in the brainstem, the precerebellar nuclei, have no equivalent in the spinal cord (although there are spinal neurons that project to the cerebellum). They include the inferior olive, the lateral reticular nucleus, the external cuneate nucleus, the pontine tegmental reticular nucleus, and the pontine nuclei.

They originate from the germinal epithelium in the lateral-most part of the rhombencephalon, the **rhombic lip**, as does the cerebellum itself, and migrate along tangential routes to reach their ventral destinations in the brainstem. They usually are not considered as belonging to either the basal or the alar plate. Neurons of the precerebellar nuclei are produced according to a general mediolateral gradient, superimposed on a general caudal-to-rostral one. Most of these phylogenetically newer structures form later than the core of the brainstem, in accordance with the later developing cerebellum.

The red nucleus and the substantia nigra are other phylogenetically new structures that have no counterparts in the spinal cord. They probably originate from the ventrolateral portion of the mesencephalic germinal epithelium, and migrate radially to their final locations. Their cells are produced over a short time span, being neither the earliest nor the latest to become postmitotic in that brain area. In the red nucleus, the gradient is caudal to rostral, the large neurons related to the brainstem and spinal cord being produced before the small neurons related to the cerebellum and neocortex. A number of other brainstem structures, such as the second- or third-order relay nuclei of the auditory pathways, which do not belong to the broad classes used in the preceding discussion, are not considered here.

Proliferation and Migration in the Diencephalon and Basal Forebrain

In the diencephalon, the neurocele is elongated dorsoventrally but is narrow in the transverse plane. The dorsal roof and ventral floor of the early neural tube are thin and narrow, and the greater development concerns its lateral walls. The major subdivisions—epithalamus, thalamus, and hypothalamus—are distinguished almost from the beginning. The sulcus delimiting the thalamus from the hypothalamus is not the sulcus limitans, and the diencephalic subdivisions are not considered rostral continuations of the basal and alar plates of the spinal cord and brainstem. No cranial nerve motor nuclei are present. The diencephalon receives one pair of nerves, the optic nerves, which belong to the special senses and distribute also to the superior colliculus. Neurons of the epithalamus and hypothalamus are generated over a relatively extended period of time and migrate mostly radially, according to a general outside–in gradient, in a lateromedial pattern. Thalamic neurons are produced over a shorter time span and have complex migration patterns, making it almost impossible to summarize them. Even within one functional group of thalamic nuclei, such as the specific sensory relay nuclei, a common pattern is difficult to discern.

The different components of the basal forebrain originate from portions of the medial, ventral, and ventrolateral wall of the paired telencephalic vesicles at caudal levels. Here, too, the patterns of neurogenesis and migration are complex.[11,12] Neurons in the septal area are produced according to a mediolateral sequence, the bilateral medial nuclei fusing on the midline at the level of the anterior commissure. Given the location of the neuroepithelium of origin, this amounts to a general outside–in pattern. Neurons in the amygdala are generated along a marked rostrocaudal gradient. As for the septum, however, no common pattern is obvious among the subdivisions of the amygdala.

Proliferation and Migration in Cortical Regions

The cerebellum, which develops from the metencephalic vesicle of the neural tube, and the cerebral hemispheres and olfactory bulbs, which develop from the telencephalon, are examined next in this context.

As stated earlier, the cerebellum originates in the lateral-most part of the rhombencephalic neuroepithelium, the rhombic lip, a region with ill-defined limits.[3,4] From that lateral situation, the germinal epithelium on both sides spreads medially on the one-cell–thick rhombencephalic roof, to eventually fuse on the midline. As this medial progression takes place, cells proliferate and, from this germinal zone, the neurons of the deep cerebellar nuclei and the Purkinje cells are generated sequentially (Fig. 19–10), forming together the equivalent of an intermediate zone termed the **mantle**, such as the one described in the spinal cord and brainstem. Some of the large cells of the future granular layer are also produced at that time. Migration occurs radially and the Purkinje cells have to cross the ranks of the earlier-formed nuclear cells to reach their destination. Because of its original source in the rhombic lip, the germinal zone is formed according to a general lateromedial gradient, and the subsequent cerebellar development follows this gradient. In this way, the medial-most fastigial nucleus, consid-

ered to be phylogenetically the oldest of the deep cerebellar nuclei, is formed last, whereas the lateral-most dentate nucleus, the newest phylogenetically, is formed first.

Toward the end of Purkinje cells production, other cells from the rhombic lip migrate medially in the roof of the metencephalon and create a second germinal epithelium superficial to the Purkinje cell layer, the **external germinal layer** (also termed the "external granular layer"), or EGL (see Fig. 19–10A, parts b and c). EGL cells proliferate at a tremendous rate to give rise to the granule cells of the granular layer. The postmitotic granule cells, therefore, migrate radially from their site of origin in the EGL and pass through the layer of Purkinje cells to attain their final destination below that layer (see Fig. 19–10A, parts c and d). Within the granule cell layer, the deeper cells are the earliest produced.

The phylogenetically new and late-forming neocortex is so voluminous in humans that it covers most of the brain dorsally and laterally, including part of the cerebellum, itself well developed. The basic histologic organization of the neocortex is similar in all areas, and comprises six layers, numbered I to VI, from the surface to the underlying medullary layer leading to the formation of the internal capsule. These areas are described in Chapter 14, in the discussion of motor cortex function. Variations are found on this pattern, concerning mostly the greater or lesser development of layers IV and V, and leading to the description of heterotypical primary areas—motor and sensory—or to homotypical association areas. Neocortical development from the germinal epithelium of the telencephalic vesicles obeys a general inside–out gradient (see Fig. 19–10B), and migration occurs mostly radially but also tangentially. The first cells to be produced come to occupy the deep layers; cells produced in the intermediate period migrate through the ranks of the latter and come to occupy intermediate layers; and those produced last migrate through the previous layers to reach the most superficial layers. An exception to this rule are the neurons found in the predominantly fibrous layer I, which are among the first to become postmitotic, together with the scattered neurons of the medullary layer located below the six numbered layers.

The phylogenetically older cortical regions, rhinal and hippocampal, may start forming earlier than the neocortex, but the neurogenesis of some components may progress until well after birth. They develop from the ventral and ventrolateral as-

Cerebellum

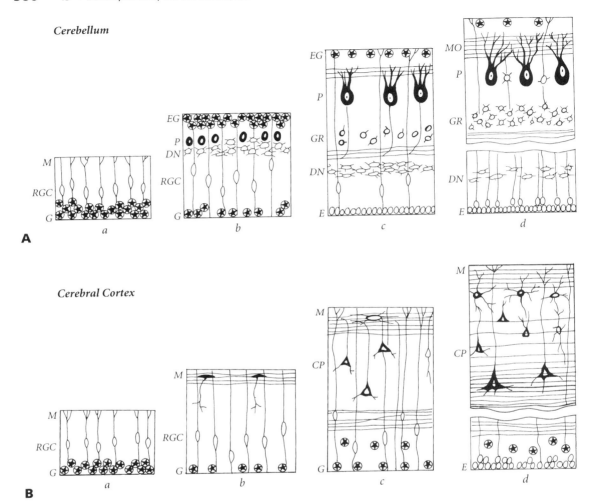

Cerebral Cortex

Figure 19–10. Neuronal migration in two cortical structures: the cerebellum **(A)** and the cerebral cortex **(B).** CP, cortical plate; DN, deep cerebellar nuclei; E, ependyma; EG, external germinal zone; G, germinal zone; Gr, granule cell layer; M, marginal zone; Mo, molecular layer; P, Purkinje cell layer; RGC, radial glial cell. (Modified and reproduced with permission from Jacobson M. *Developmental neurobiology.* New York: Plenum, 1979.)

pects of the telencephalic vesicles. The adult histologic organization, however, is reduced to three layers, but the general inside–out gradient of neuron production prevails and migration is predominantly radial. In the olfactory bulb, generation of the accessory bulb predates that of the main bulb. Good evidence suggests that one type of local neuron, the granule cell, is generated throughout a lifetime in the main olfactory bulb and in the dentate gyrus of the hippocampal formation. Such neurogenesis would be concomitant with an equal rate of cell death, however, resulting in a fairly stable cell population number.

One observation common to all cortical regions is that the long-projection neurons are generated before the local neurons. In other words, large neurons are produced before small ones because, as a general rule, the longer the axon of a neuron, the larger its soma. In nuclear regions, projection neurons also become postmitotic before interneurons.

Defects of Proliferation and Migration

Cell migration is an important step in neural ontogenesis. Defective migration may result in abnormal cell positioning and abnormal cell connections. In the human, minor defects of neuronal migration have been implicated in developmental dyslexia. Major defects of migration are usually combined with, or the consequence of, abnormal proliferation, the two being difficult to dissociate, and may result in gross malformations, such as microencephaly, lissencephaly, macrogyria, and others.[19]

Cell Aggregation

It should be obvious from the preceding descriptions that when cells cease migrating, those with common properties aggregate and form either nuclear or laminar arrangements. In this case, "common properties" does not necessarily signify identical morphology or connections but, rather, functional resemblance: a common role. A given aggregate may often contain at least two neuronal populations: large-projection neurons, whose axons leave the nucleus (or lamina) to project away; and small, local neurons with short axons. The former are generated earlier than the latter. Both types of neurons in each aggregate are, however, related to the same functions—the relay of visual information in the lateral geniculate nucleus, or the relay of auditory information in the medial geniculate nucleus, for example. Unfortunately, little is known at this time about the possible existence and mode of operation for mechanisms that may control these aggregates. It has been hypothesized that signals are sent to tell neurons—sometimes quite different from one another—to become "neighbors," and that these signals somehow dictate directional as well as temporal aspects of migration, notably its cessation.

Selective aggregation has also been explained by chemical affinities between cells mediated by membrane recognition molecules, or perhaps by adhesion molecules. In vitro experiments have shown that cells from different organs that are first dissociated and then mixed and cultured together will, given sufficient time, preferentially aggregate with cells from the same organ of origin. This finding also seems to be the case in the nervous system; dissociated cells from different brain regions indeed reaggregate with their kin after some time in culture.

Whether the same recognition mechanism operates during development, to help neurons aggregate, remains to be determined.

Cell Differentiation

Once settled in their final destinations, neurons differentiate morphologically: they elaborate the cytoplasmic processes that provide the morphologic basis for their specific functional characteristic of directional impulse transmission. Some classes of neurons, such as the granule cells of the cerebellar cortex, begin their differentiation while still migrating.

Neuronal Polarity

As you learned in Chapter 3, neurons are polarized cells with an afferent (receptor) pole, the dendrite, and an efferent (effector) pole, the axon. A given neuron usually has multiple dendrites, which branch, but a single axon, which may give collaterals to different targets along the way, and which arborizes at the terminations. The nerve impulse is transmitted along the neurolemma, or nerve cell membrane, from dendrites to soma to axon, at which terminal arborization it is transduced into a chemical signal at the synaptic junction.

The dendrites and the axon of a neuron differ at the ultrastructural level, particularly in the preferential distribution of certain organelles in each type of process: ribosomes and Golgi elements, for example, are present in dendrites but absent in axons. Such compartmentalization probably derives from an intrinsic and differential polarity of the microtubules in neuronal processes due to the asymmetry of the tubulin molecules, and microtubule polarity probably accounts for differential organelle transport. Other biochemical differences, discussed further on, also distinguish dendrites from axons.[20]

We do not yet know how such polarity is attained during development. In vivo, the axon is the first of the two types of processes to form, but in vitro, where cells are free of extrinsically imposed polarity, numerous identical processes appear, and the first one to elongate more rapidly than the others is the one that becomes the axon. Other in vitro experiments have shown permissive or inhibitory effects of certain ECM molecules, especially laminin and fibronectin, on either axonal or dendritic outgrowth.[21] ECM molecules, for which the neurolemma has receptors, have been invoked to explain the establishment of the cytoskeletal polarity mentioned previously.

In some regions of the nervous system where neuronal migration has been particularly well studied, such as the cerebral cortex or the cerebellar cortex, the **trailing processes** of migrating cells become their axon. This is not the case for all neurons, however. Where true, though, the establishment of neuronal polarity could be determined by factors directing neuronal migration, instead of, or in addition to, factors such as the length advantage of a growing process, or the ECM.

The Marginal Zone: Fiber Tracts

In the spinal cord and brainstem, many of the cells in the intermediate zone direct their axons toward the pial surface of the differentiating neural tube, creating an additional zone at the periphery of the intermediate zone, the **marginal zone** (see Fig. 19–4D). The axons of the somatic and visceral motor neurons leave the marginal zone and exit the neural tube by the ventral roots at spinal levels or by the appropriate cranial nerves at brain levels. These axons make up relatively small contingents of fibers, however. Most axons, once in the marginal zone, make a sharp turn to either ascend or descend the neuraxis and reach other levels, where they reenter the intermediate zone and establish synaptic contacts with nerve cells, as will be seen later. Target neurons may sometimes be quite distant from the cell bodies at the origin of the axons that synapse on them.

Just as cell bodies with common properties aggregate, their axons likewise bundle up in the marginal zone, hence forming fiber tracts. Numerous fiber tracts are named according to their site of origin and their site of termination. For example, the spinothalamic tract has cell bodies of origin located in the spinal cord, and terminates in the thalamus. Axons that travel short distances tend to occupy the innermost part of the marginal zone, bordering the intermediate zone, as in the propriospinal tracts in the spinal cord. Tracts connecting distant regions—for example, the pyramidal tract that originates in the cerebral cortex and terminates in the spinal cord—tend to be peripheral, because they are added to earlier-established bundles. This rule is not absolute, however, and must furthermore take into account the existence of **topography**. For instance, in the dorsal columns, which carry primary afferent fibers (the cell bodies of which are in the dorsal root gan-

glia) from all levels of the spinal cord to the dorsal column nuclei in the caudal myelencephalon, fibers appear to be added more and more laterally in the dorsal funiculus as they enter the cord and ascend. They are added in this manner because fibers originating from the caudal-most levels occupy the medial-most part of the column in the fasciculus gracilis, and those originating from the rostral-most levels are found laterally in the fasciculus cuneatus, as would be obvious in a cross-section of the upper cervical cord, as you learned earlier in the chapter on proprioception (see Chap. 8). The fasciculus gracilis terminates in the nucleus gracilis and the fasciculus cuneatus in the nucleus cuneatus, lateral to nucleus gracilis. In development, however, dorsal root fibers are not added from medial to lateral in the dorsal funiculus because, as already mentioned, the cord and the dorsal root ganglia form according to a general rostrocaudal gradient. Therefore, when fibers ascending from caudal levels reach the cervical cord, they are added medially to the rostral fibers already in place. Because dorsal column fibers convey sensory information of the somatic type, the topography in the system is called *somatotopy*.

In later stages of development, glial cells migrate from their site of origin in what remains of the germinal epithelium to colonize the marginal zone, where **oligodendrocytes** produce myelin around a number of axons. Because of its high lipid content, the myelin gives a white color to the regions of the nervous system where it abounds, an appearance that is visible in fresh and fixed tissue. The intermediate zone, where neuronal cell bodies aggregate and glial cells are predominantly **astrocytes**, does not contain a significant amount of myelin and appears gray. In the adult spinal cord, the gray matter has more or less the shape of a butterfly around the central canal, and the white matter is organized around it. In the medulla and pons, gray matter and white matter are piled up in the floor of the fourth ventricle. To this basic organization of the brainstem, the phylogenetically new nuclei and tracts are added ventrally.

In the cerebellum and rostral regions of the brain, the complexity of the proliferation and migration processes results in less uniformity in the direction of axonal elongation. In cortical structures, the equivalent of the marginal zone is often found deep to the mantle. Because the trailing processes become axons in many of these neurons, they are not directed toward the pial surface but toward the germinal zone. A cell-free zone of incoming axons is created between the thinning germinal zone and the thickening cortical plate: the medullary layer.

Axonal Growth: The Growth Cone

Neuronal processes, particularly axons, can extend over long distances from their cell bodies of origin, traversing various terrains within the nervous system or outside of it, and, to do so, develop a special "organ," the **growth cone**. The term was coined by Ramon y Cajal in 1890[22] to describe the enlarged tips of growing nerve extensions. Much—perhaps all—of the growth of neuronal processes, both axonal and dendritic, occurs at the growth cone, which serves not only as a lengthening device, but as a locomot-

ing guide to the appropriate destination.[23] The growth cone, particularly in axons, has been extensively studied in numerous systems and animals, with many studies using culture preparations.

The growth cone is the enlarged tip of a growing **neurite**, the latter referring to an undifferentiated neuronal process. Its size and shape vary, but it consists of a central core that adheres to the substrate on which the neurite grows. Extensions emerge from the cone's core—either finger-like, the **filopodia**, or veil-like, the **lamellipodia**—and these extensions do not adhere to the substrate, or adhere only weakly (Fig. 19–11). The growth cone may send out or retract its extensions, so that its shape as a whole changes constantly. The growth cone contains the

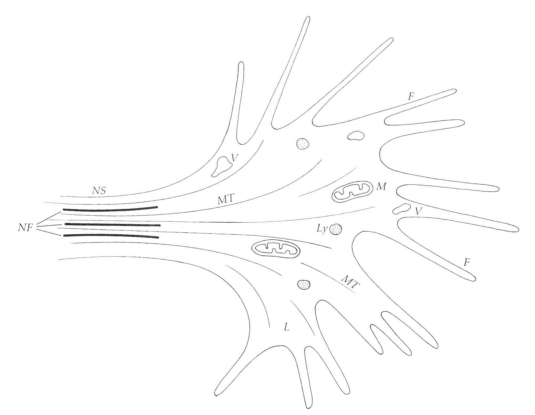

Figure 19–11. A growth cone. F, filopodia; L, lamellipodia; Ly, lysosome; M, mitochondria; MT, microtubules; NF, neurofilaments; NS, neuritic shaft; V, vesicle. (Modified and reproduced with permission from Van Hoof COM, Oestreicher AB, De Graan PNE, Gispen WH. Role of the growth cone in neuronal differentiation. *Mol Neurobiol* 1989;3:101–133.)

organelles necessary for progression on a substrate as well as for growth itself, that is, for addition of cytoplasm and membrane. Cytoskeletal elements (tubules and filaments), mitochondria, and various vesicles predominate in the central core, and contractile proteins, notably actin, abound in the extensions. The membrane of the growth cone differs from that of the neuronal soma or the neurite with respect to structural protein components, receptors, or ion channels. The growth cone membrane is simpler and more fluid. Nonetheless, compared with the rest of the neurolemma, it is enriched in some receptors, such as nerve growth factor receptors, and in calcium channels. To grow on a surface, the filopodia and lamellipodia first extend, thanks to movements made possible by the contractile proteins and to membrane insertion, and then fill with the organelle-rich cytoplasm from the core, which detaches from the substrate. What was once the core becomes incorporated into the neuritic shaft, thus lengthened, and the new core now adheres to the substrate. From it may span new extensions. Measurements in vivo reveal that growth speed ranges between 5 to 200 micrometers an hour, varying along a given path according to the complexity of the environment, and slowing down as a system matures.

The shape of growth cones is correlated with speed of locomotion, complexity of the milieu, and state of maturation. The first axons of a fascicle to grow, the **pioneer axons**, which originate in the earliest neurons of the population giving rise to the fascicle, have large and elaborate growth cones because these are the ones that "sense" the environment, often the ECM or neural tissue, as being "different" from themselves, and that "make the decisions" to direct growth. The axons that later join the tract grow in apposition to the ones already established, a process called **fasciculation**, and elaborate only very simple growth cones that may not deserve the appellation. Along a given pathway, the growth cones become more complex in rough terrains and points of "decision," such as at the chiasma for the optic nerve axons, where they also grow more slowly. It appears obvious that the growth cones of axons are almost always far more complex than those of dendrites.

Control of Growth Cone Navigation

For an axon to follow the correct path and reach the proper targets, it must constantly be guided along its route so that its growth cone "makes the right decision." Different guidance strategies may operate to put the growing axons on the right path; they are explained in another section. As indicated in the previous paragraph, guidance is mediated by the complex interactions of the growth cone itself with the environment, and this section focuses on the mechanisms of these interactions at the growth cone.[24,25]

First, the growth cone must adhere to the substrate to be able to progress on it, a phenomenon much studied in tissue culture. The nature of the substrate on which the axon grows, whether a neuron (the membrane of a neighbor axon, for example) or the ECM, provides important cues that are processed differently by the growth cone. Given substrates of different **adhesion** qualities, a neurite grows more readily on the most adhesive one, for example, on a collagen fiber. Adhesiveness alone does not suffice to explain the "choice" a neurite makes, however. A neurite may prefer a less adhesive substrate, such as laminin, if its membrane contains more binding molecules for it. Certain substrates are indeed "neurite-promoting." If selective adhesion plays a role in axonal growth, active **contact inhibition** equally intervenes. Axons of a certain length encounter different substrates during their growth, and their growth cone membrane may modify accordingly. A number of other factors also act on the growth cone, in a permissive or an inhibitory fashion, to direct and redirect (correct) its growth. Diffusible molecules in the extracellular space influence the growth cones having receptors for them. Even electrical activity may affect the rate and direction of axonal growth.

Growth cones secrete proteolytic enzymes that can degrade some components of the ECM, such as fibronectin or laminin. The result may either be to facilitate growth cone progression by removing a barrier, or to forbid it by removing an adhesive, neurite-promoting substrate. Nonneural elements present in the growing environment (central or peripheral) of neurites, such as glial cells and fibroblasts, release inhibitors for these proteases. The net growth of neurites would thus be controlled by a balance between the actions of these molecules. It may seem paradoxical that the same glial cells that produce protease inhibitors also secrete a neurite-promoting factor.

Growth factors are diffusible chemical agents that stimulate neurite outgrowth. This does not exclude the possibility of a guiding, or tropic, action on the growth of neurites, but it is not implicit. Tropic factors per se are discussed later, along with path finding and topography.

The best known of all growth factors, thanks largely to the pioneering work of Levi-Montalcini, is the trophic factor known as **nerve growth factor (NGF)**, a peptidic substance that brings life support to developing sensory and sympathetic ganglion cells, as well as promoting and even directing the growth of their peripheral neurites. The dependency of sensory neurons on NGF as a trophic agent disappears after synapse stabilization, but that is not the case for sympathetic neurons. NGF is now also known to act on some neurons of the central nervous system. NGF is produced by the targets of axonal neurites and acts on specific receptors of the growth cones, and later on the terminals for those neurons that remain dependent. NGF is internalized at the growth cone and transported retrogradely to the cell body. Other growth factors of the nervous system, like brain-derived growth factor or fibroblast growth factor, originally identified in nonneural tissues, or the neurotrophins, such as NT-3, NT-4, and NT-5, are much less understood.[26] The different actions of these agents on neuronal life and activity—growth promotion, tropism, and trophism—may be difficult to dissociate. In this context, the review article by Barde should be consulted.[27] More and more, however, abnormalities with growth factors or their receptors are being linked with neurodegenerative diseases such as Alzheimer's disease or Parkinson's disease.

Among the chemical signals that affect the growth of axons are the same ones that serve as agents of synaptic communication in the mature nervous system: the neurotransmitters. Their action on neurite outgrowth has been documented more for dendrites than for axons, but in either case, they act before synaptogenesis. They are present at low concentration in the intercellular space, presumably released from neurons without the synaptic specializations being requisite. A transmitter does not necessarily act on all the neurons in a system, nor does it have the same effect on all the neurons it influences. The general action is inhibitory. A transmitter that does not directly affect a neuron may do so indirectly, however, by counteracting the inhibitory effect of another transmitter, resulting in facilitated growth for that neuron. Depolarizing, excitatory transmitters can inhibit neurite outgrowth, whereas hyperpolarizing, inhibitory transmitters can reverse that action. Identified neurotransmitters known to influence neurite outgrowth include acetylcholine, norepi-

nephrine, serotonin, dopamine, glutamate, gamma-aminobutyric acid, and some peptides.

Calcium may be the common denominator that integrates the action of several stimuli that are known to influence neurite growth, including diffusible substances and electrical activity in the area.[28] The use of synthetic fluorescent dyes has made possible the measurement and localization of free intracellular calcium. Fluctuations in calcium concentration are correlated with growth cone motility, a significantly higher concentration being recorded in growth cones of actively elongating neurites than in stable ones. Experimental manipulations of the environmental factors mentioned previously have demonstrated that these factors modify, one way or another, the intracellular concentration of free calcium, through alteration of the growth cone membrane potential. If the temporal summation of these effects results in too large increases or decreases of intracellular calcium concentration, growth cone motility and elongation are inhibited. An optimal concentration is required for proper growth, and that concentration differs in different axonal systems. Other second messengers, such as cyclic adenosine monophosphate or protein kinase C may also regulate neurite outgrowth, but it is probable that their action depends on calcium. This issue is discussed in Chapter 4.

Calcium would permit the polymerization of cytoskeletal components found in the growth cones, notably tubulin in the form of microtubules, and the interactions of actin with actin-binding proteins. Furthermore, calcium would permit the addition of membrane at the growth cones because fusion of membranous vesicles with the plasma membrane is calcium dependent. This does not differ from the mechanism of exocytosis of neurotransmitters by synaptic vesicles in the mature state (see Chaps. 3 and 4).

One phosphoprotein called **GAP 43**—growth-associated protein, a protein with a molecular weight of 43 kD (in fact, it ranges from 43 to 57 kD)—has been consistently found in the growth cones of axons, but not in those of dendrites.[29] Because of its absence in dendrites, the molecule cannot be essential for growth itself, but because of its ubiquity in growing axons and its absence in mature ones, it must be involved in some aspects of growth particular to axons. It is interesting to note that in culture preparations such as those mentioned previously in reference to neuronal polarity, all neuronal processes initially express GAP 43. Therefore, GAP 43 cannot be invoked to explain neuronal polarity. As soon as one process grows faster and gets longer than the others—that is, as soon as one process becomes the axon—all the other processes, the ones known to become the dendrites, lose GAP 43 expression. GAP 43 occurs in the cytoplasm of growth cones, and may possibly bind to the cytoplasmic face of the membrane, as well as interact with the cytoskeleton. GAP 43 may affect the rate of membrane insertion into the growth cone, a rate much higher in growing axons than dendrites. Another important hypothesis concerning the role of GAP 43 is its involvement in the regulation of calcium. GAP 43 binds calmodulin and could serve as a calmodulin store within the growth cone. In summary, it may regulate the interactions between the varied environmental stimuli acting on the growth cone membrane and on the intracellular calcium levels.

Formation of Dendrites and Characteristic Shapes of Neurons

Usual histologic preparations reveal only a fraction of the nervous tissue. Nissl staining shows the cell bodies of neurons and proximal portion of dendrites: the pale nucleus with a prominent nucleolus and the perikaryal cytoplasm with Nissl bodies (those aggregates of rough endoplasmic reticulum so abundant in nerve cells that they appear as dark granules under the light microscope), as well as the nucleus and an occasional rim of cytoplasm of glial cells. Most neurons thus appear multipolar in shape. The major part of neuronal processes, axonal and dendritic, or of glial processes, do not contain stainable material that could reveal their organization. Thanks to the argyrophilic property of the neuronal membrane, silver impregnation techniques have unveiled the dendritic arborizations of nerve cells, but they leave the myelinated axons unstained. Better yet for demonstrating in detail the entire configuration of nerve cells are the more recent intracellular injections of dyes. But, of course, the latter procedure is not ordinarily used and cannot be applied to entire sections of tissue.

Even in common Nissl preparations, however, the multipolar shape of neurons immediately stands out, a characteristic attributable to the multiple dendrites. When describing a neuron, what are described more often than not are the dendrites. Dendrites, indeed, confer on the neuron its morphology. Neurons can differ considerably from one another in their dendrites: by number, length, degree and pattern of branching, length and diameter of each segment, orientation in three dimensions, smoothness of surface, presence or absence of spines, and their localization. The morphology of mature neurons remains constant over time, except perhaps for relatively minor modifications at the synapses. They obtain their characteristic shape during ontogeny.

The dendrites of a neuron begin to form later than its axon, as mentioned earlier in this section. In fact, they may not grow significantly until the axon nears its targets, and until afferents arrive in their vicinity. These observations suggest that dendritic growth may somehow be influenced by external factors. If the growth of dendrites is in actuality influenced by external factors, as will be seen shortly, what about their morphologic characteristics? Are they intrinsic properties of neurons or are they dictated by extrinsic forces? Experiments in adult and developing animals indicate that numerous characteristics of a dendritic tree remain after deafferentation. In spite of minor changes, the identity of a deafferented neuron can often be recognized. This statement generally holds true for neurons grown in culture. Studies of so-called "deafferentation" may not offer definite proofs of the afferents influencing dendritic growth or shape, because most neurons receive more than one type of afferent, and only rarely are all of them removed. How do we differentiate between those remaining and those sprouting from the remaining afferents? Using the Mauthner cells of the premetamorphic axolotl as a model has helped resolve that problem. These two neurons, one on each side of the brainstem, receive ipsilateral vestibular afferents. Superinnervation of a Mauthner cell by transplantation of an ear primordium on one side has produced a significant enhancement of dendritic branching, whereas deprivation of the contralateral cell has caused a decrease of dendritic surface.

Dendrites grow similarly to axons, by growth cones that interact with the environment. Some of the factors that influence axonal growth probably act on dendritic growth cones. An inhibitory effect of some neurotransmitters on dendritic outgrowth has been documented in many systems. Such an effect is manifested at about the time of synaptogenesis, however, and thus relatively late in the formation of a dendritic tree. The inhibition has been invoked as a means of signifying to a dendrite that it has reached an appropriate site for synaptogenesis, and to stabilize connections in the making. These previous factors exert their action on dendrites orthogradely (anterogradely). A retrograde control of dendritic growth has also long been suspected to occur, but was not proven until recently. It was demonstrated in a simple system—the projections from the isthmooptic nucleus to the retina—that the polarization of the dendrites of isthmooptic nucleus neurons deprived of their target, the retina, is significantly less accentuated. The cell bodies and other characteristics of the dendrites do not appear modified. How this retrograde action operates is not yet understood.

Formation of Connections Between Axons and Targets

Because the main function of the nervous system is communication, the ultimate goal of development consists in establishing the circuitry underlying that function. At the cellular level, this means the formation of synapses, or **synaptogenesis**. The appropriate elements involved, however (i.e., the presynaptic axon terminal and the postsynaptic cell), whether neuronal (generally part of a dendrite or soma) or muscular, must be brought together first. Axons may have quite remote targets; by their terminal arborization, they may contact many cells, and by their collaterals they may even contact cells in several distant regions (divergence). Numerous axons from different origins may converge onto one neuron (convergence). The very intricate yet precise circuitry of the nervous system is established during ontogenesis, and the connections thus formed remain stable afterward. The expression "stereotyped connectivity" may not be that overly simplistic. The process of matching axons with the right targets as a result of the axons following the right trajectories can be called, from the axons' point of view, **path finding**. It concerns aspects of axonal growth that were not treated as such in the previous section. The best review of the topic, including information on some of the interactions with the growth cones considered previously, remains a 1988 article by Dodd and Jessell.[24]

Path Finding

In the course of normal development, axons do something remarkable: they follow the correct trajectory, find the appropriate target, and make the proper connections, with relatively little error. In other words, the mature pattern of connectivity is attained almost from the outset. One classic illustration of such specificity is the innervation of the limb.[25] Sensory and motor fibers exit the spinal cord and dorsal root ganglion at several segments, such as C5 to T1 for the upper limb. Fibers from the five segments mix and fasciculate toward the brachial plexus, but they defasciculate distally to reorganize, as they enter the limb, into the fiber bundles innervating the different limb muscles. Spinal fibers make the right connections even if rerouted, within reasonable limits. What are the path-finding strategies available to axons?

Simple mechanical routing, called **stereotropism**, has been invoked after the observations that, in tissue culture, axons seek scratches in the culture dish and grow along them; they also choose the paths of least resistance. In vivo, physical guidance might be offered in the form of barriers, such as cartilage for peripheral fibers. Conversely, extracellular spaces could create channels through which axons grow. Dissociating this phenomenon from others, such as preferential adhesion or contact inhibition, becomes difficult.

Contact guidance, mediated by membrane molecules, plays a major role in steering axons. It includes the aforesaid preferential adhesion, which explains the mechanism of growth on a surface as much as its directionality. Most ligands present on the membrane surface of the growth cone and the neuritic shaft (e.g., N-CAM—neural cell adhesion molecule, N-cadherin, or integrin receptors) and on the substrate (e.g., laminin, if the substrate is nonneuronal, or the previously named membrane molecules, if the substrate is neuronal) are widespread. Distinct binding specificity could be obtained if axonal membranes expressed different combinations at different times. Remember that, by the release of proteases, growth cones can modify the environment locally. Contact inhibition is also mediated by molecules.

The best understood instance of selective adhesion as guidance is fasciculation. Several surface glycoproteins can serve as ligands in fasciculation: integrins, neurofascin, L1, TAG-1, and the like, in homophilic or heterophilic binding. At this point, it might be interesting to address whether pioneer axons are the only ones in a developing fascicle able to navigate to their targets, and if the followers are able only to fasciculate. The question has been answered by ablating either the pioneer axons or their cell bodies, and observing whether proper growth of the following axons ensued. It does. The axons lacking pioneers on which to fasciculate transform themselves into new pioneers by elaborating complex growth cones instead of minimal enlargements. Moreover, the transected original pioneers, provided their cell bodies are spared, can transform into followers that fasciculate.

Chemotropism, the chemical attraction of axons by their targets at a distance, was already invoked by Ramon y Cajal[16] as a mechanism that brings axons to the right targets with great accuracy. Despite circumstantial evidence, definite proof of its existence was not found until recently. The interesting experiment of Dodd and Jessell[24] must be cited. As described previously, most axons of the intermediate zone of the spinal cord are directed toward the marginal zone. Some axons from the middle third of the lateral wall, instead, take a circumvoluted path and grow toward the floor plate to cross the midline, join the marginal zone there, and ascend the cord contralaterally (Fig. 19–12). The belief that the floor plate attracts these axons is legitimate. This idea can be tested by removing the floor plate from a slice of cord in vitro and transplanting it into another location or, simply, placing it outside the cord, laterally, before the time when the axons would normally grow. After sufficient time in culture, the commissural axons grow outside the cord and toward the explanted floor plate, rather than along their normal path. Their identity was verified with neuronal tracers to exclude the possibility that they were motor neuronal axons. They do not grow toward the floor plate explanted too far away from the cord, indicating that the chemical attraction obeys a concentration gradient. The chemical agent has since been characterized biochemically, and the search for others in other systems goes on.

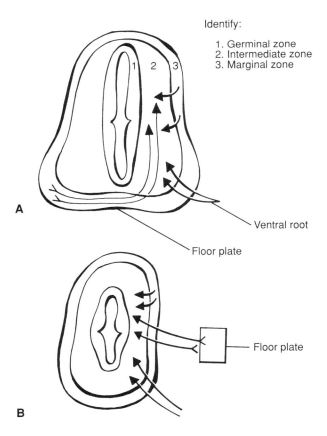

Identify:
1. Germinal zone
2. Intermediate zone
3. Marginal zone

Ventral root

Floor plate

Floor plate

Figure 19–12. A: In the course of normal spinal cord development, the axons of the neurons differentiating in the intermediate zone grow into the marginal zone toward distant targets or even exit the marginal zone to innervate muscles. The axons of some neurons, however, grow ventrally toward the floor plate, which they cross to reach the contralateral marginal zone. **B:** If the floor plate is removed and explanted lateral to the developing cord, the axons of the commissural neurons are directed toward the marginal zone and exit the latter to grow toward the explant.

As the previous example illustrates, chemoattraction need not originate from the definitive target, because these axons head to distant rostral levels once they have crossed in the floor plate. Intermediate "targets" along the way, or stepping-stones, may guide growing axons toward their terminal destination. Long, often late-developing projection axons most likely resort to intermediate targets, as do axons that form earlier than their final targets. The notion of intermediate targets has been strengthened by the discovery, in certain systems, that some of them seem to be transient, as if created specifically for the purpose of guiding axons, to be eliminated thereafter. For example, neurons located deep to the cortical plate in the developing neocortex serve as intermediate targets for incoming thalamic axons, the latter ultimately destined for layer IV. Those cells are programmed to die, but do not die before the attracted thalamic axons have reached their late-forming layer IV target. Some early cells elaborate axons that serve as pioneers in an immature, uncomplicated system, where distances are short, for the long axons growing later. This phenomenon is seen across the articulations of insect limbs. When the long projection is finally established, the early, transient cells die, eliminating with them the pioneer axons.

In some cases—for example, in the visual cortex—certain neurotransmitters are expressed transiently by permanent neurons. The timing of their expression corresponds to the arrival of afferents, and has been interpreted as intermediate chemoattraction.

Earlier in this chapter you learned that electrical activity in general inhibits axonal growth. This idea holds true for discrete, local electrical stimuli on the growth cone. Some form of electrical activity may, however, stimulate and direct axonal growth, a kind of guidance called **galvanotropism**. Experiments have shown that axons grow more rapidly toward the cathode (the negative electrode) than the anode. Measurements of voltage differences in embryonic fluids have revealed the existence of voltage gradients. Whether these gradients may take part in elaborating the complicated network of connections in the embryo remains to be determined.

Defects of Path Finding

Mutations in adhesion proteins, such as L1, can cause severe developmental defects. These proteins, and notably L1, are in fact multifunction proteins that are involved in various aspects of axonal growth

and guidance, including fasciculation, and may also play a role in earlier stages of development, such as cell migration, where contact with a substrate is also used as a mechanism. Malformations are usually numerous and implicate several long fiber tracts. For instance, the corticospinal tract and the corpus callosum may be malformed, diminished, or simply absent. Hydrocephaly and a thin cerebral cortex, spasticity, aphasia, and mental retardation have been reported consequent to L1 mutation.[30]

Topography

Most projection systems, central as well as peripheral, are organized topographically, as you learned in previous chapters. Topography may bear specific names related to the modality of the system (e.g., somatotopy, tonotopy, visuotopy), but, in all cases, relies on the same principle of orderly projections reflecting a functional organization. Within a given system, such as the visual system, the orderly projections from one source to a target, such as the retinotectal projections, often retain a topographic relationship within the fascicle conveying them—in this case, the optic nerve. This is not always the case, as can be seen in limb innervation. When either type of tract is manipulated to modify the order of the fibers within it, the latter nonetheless find their targets and establish topographic connections. Each axon again finds its exact correct address, as if each set of axon and target were "imprinted" with a common identity. How is such accuracy explained?

A common but not absolute rule of development is that the spatiotemporal sequence of formation of the target—such as neuronal production and dendritogenesis in the tectum, to continue with the preceding example—corresponds to that of the source: neuronal production and axogenesis in the retina. The sequences of development of both regions parallel topography. Therefore, the earliest retinal axons are the first to arrive in the tectum, where they face a limited choice of synaptic partners: the earliest-formed tectal cells. Those axons arriving at midtime are equally restricted to the newly available targets because the older ones are taken and the youngest ones are not yet formed, and so on. Timing alone does not suffice to explain topography,[25] however, at least not in all systems, particularly in light of the finding that displacement of earlier-formed connections occurs in certain regions, such as during muscle innervation.

In a number of projection systems, the target possesses chemical, graded **positional cues** that correspond to positional gradients within the source, such as the TOP molecules in the retinotectal projection system. The expression of these recognition molecules is restricted in time. These data provide a modern verification of the traditional chemoaffinity, or chemical imprinting, hypothesis. This finding does not invalidate the importance of timing as a factor accounting for the formation of topographic projections. The two mechanisms complement each other.

Synaptogenesis

Once an axon has reached its target, the actual synapse must be formed, which includes the presynaptic membrane specialization, the synaptic vesicles containing neurotransmitters, the synaptic cleft, and the postsynaptic membrane specialization, comprising receptors for neurotransmitters (see Chaps. 3 and 4). Physiologic recordings have revealed the existence of miniature end-plate potentials in muscle cells even before any morphologic specializations appear either there or in the presynaptic elements. There ensues the gradual appearance of synaptic vesicles in the transforming, arrested growth cone, the thickening of the postsynaptic myocyte membrane, the formation of a basal lamina in the synaptic cleft, and the thickening of the presynaptic membrane.[25] At first, and even before the presynaptic element contacts the myocyte, acetylcholine receptors occur on the length of the myocyte membrane. Gradually, they cluster at synaptic sites as the latter differentiate. Junctional folds and cholinesterase also localize at these hot spots. The reorganization of the postsynaptic membrane is triggered by the presynaptic element, probably through chemical signaling and activity. The best known synapse in the mature state, the neuromuscular junction just described, is also the best known developmentally. How the formation of central synapses conforms to this model remains largely to be determined.

Choice of Neurotransmitters

For a long time, investigators believed that a given neuronal type expressed a single neurotransmitter in all its collateral and terminal branches (Dale's law).

With the advent of immunohistochemistry and its widespread application to the nervous system, the identification of more than one neurotransmitter at the same synaptic junction proved this assumption faulty. The use of a single neurotransmitter by a type of neuron, such as acetylcholine by motor neurons, now seems to be more the exception than the rule. Understanding how a single neurotransmitter could be expressed in a neuron—by simple genetic determination—was easier than explaining how multiple expression is controlled, a problem compounded by the finding that, in tissue culture, certain neurons could be made to switch neurotransmitters by manipulating the culture medium!

Although little is known even now about determination of neurotransmitters in the central nervous system, the elements influencing the "choice" of neurotransmitters by peripheral neurons during development are better understood.[31] Mature sympathetic ganglion neurons use norepinephrine as a transmitter. A small population of them, however, such as the neurons in the superior cervical ganglion that innervate sweat glands, use acetylcholine, the transmitter of parasympathetic neurons. Interestingly, in early development the neurons that are destined to innervate the sweat glands are noradrenergic, like all other neurons in the superior cervical ganglion, and *not* cholinergic. As they begin innervating their target, they cease synthesizing norepinephrine and gradually replace the norepinephrine with acetylcholine. A cholinergic differentiation factor released by the sweat glands induces such transformation, in addition to triggering the concomitant expression of certain neuropeptides. If a foreign target—for example, the parotid gland—replaces the normal one, no switch of neurotransmitters occurs, and the neurons continue expressing norepinephrine.

Other instances of the transient expression of neurotransmitters during development were mentioned with regard to path finding. Whatever its role, the phenomenon has now been described in varied systems. The specification of a neuroblast along a particular neuronal line may involve the concomitant acquisition of a given neurotransmitter as a "default" state. This transmitter would be retained unless the environment decides otherwise. Hence, the default transmitter could either be replaced by another one (or many), or other transmitters, such as neuropeptides, could be added to it.

Stabilization of Connections and Regressive Events

The different controls of development do not act solely before or while things happen. Even though the very complex connectivity is achieved with great accuracy, imprecisions and mistakes do occur and must be corrected. The numeric ratio of the elements connected must be finely adjusted. At the same time, the functioning of the connections must be validated as they are gradually used by the individual in behavioral functioning (i.e., all the types of functions mentioned in the introduction to this chapter). If they do not work at their best, they must be modified, eliminated, or replaced.

Rearrangement and Elimination

Many examples have been reported of the numeric adjustment of connections, probably resulting from competition or functional validation, although this relationship has not been ascertained in all cases. First, let us consider some illustrations of the reorganization and elimination of connections. Mention was made earlier of the great precision in the innervation of skeletal muscles by axons from motor neurons of the spinal cord. When studied in detail, however, the one-to-one adult ratio—that is, one axon innervating one (twitch) muscle fiber—is not obtained from the outset. A given axon terminal initially sprouts to several muscle fibers with which it establishes synaptic connections. It later retracts all sprouts and maintains connections only with a single muscle fiber. The size of the motor unit is obtained by synaptic elimination, not cell (motor neuron) elimination. Likewise, in the central nervous system, the adult ratio of one Purkinje cell in the cerebellum being innervated by one climbing fiber from the inferior olive results from synaptic elimination. Callosal connections are also more widespread during development than in the adult. Axons may sometimes grow longer than they should, without necessarily making synaptic connections, and later withdraw. In the adult, pyramidal tract axons distribute to a number of targets in the brainstem and spinal cord, sometimes by way of collaterals. During development, some of the axons destined to brainstem targets, such as the pontine nuclei, may extend more caudally, as far as

the medullary reticular formation, or even the spinal cord, and later withdraw their caudal extension.

The rearrangements of connections known to take place in the peripheral and central nervous system can be classified in three categories:[25] decrease of convergence onto a target; segregation of inputs across targets; and complete loss of projection to a target. Total cell death as a result of failure to survive (for cells that have passed the stage of normal cell death mentioned earlier) is not as common as the elimination of portions of cells; it is not the main way to achieve the fine tuning of connections. Elimination of elements, be they axon collaterals, synapses, or whole cells, is not a universal feature of neural development; it has not been observed in all the systems and regions investigated.

Competition and Functional Validation

While connections are being formed or rearranged, and even afterward, they must be validated to be retained, and functional validation is often exerted through **competition** for synaptic sites.[25] For the same target receiving afferents from multiple sources, the different types of inputs are in general segregated on the dendritic field. For example, red nucleus neurons receive two main types of afferents: axons from the cerebellar nuclei terminate preferentially on the soma and proximal dendrites, and those from the cerebral cortex on distal dendrites. If the cerebellar afferents are removed, cerebral axons distribute to the proximal dendritic field. In addition, if the lesion allows for regrowth of the cerebellar fibers, they displace at least part of the cerebral axons and reoccupy their original synaptic territory. Hence, cerebellar axons have "won the competition." Several other instances of competition have been documented after experimental manipulation; it is reasonable to assume that competition participates in establishing neuronal networks during normal development. Axon terminals may compete for a number of things, notably **trophic factors**. Activity in itself equally provides trophic support. Also, some axons may simply be more efficient than others at driving a target. The more efficient the activity, the better reinforcement a terminal gets. If the best-fit pattern of connections is not obtained from the beginning, it will be after some form of rearrangement.

The retinogeniculocortical projections are not established from the outset according to the pattern of alternate ocular dominance. The striped arrangement in the distribution of retinal axons into the dorsal lateral geniculate nucleus, or of geniculate axons within the visual cortex, results from binocular visual experience. (Remember the ocular dominance columns described in Chap. 11, on vision.) Of course, binocular experience does not begin until at least both eyes open. If one eye is occluded before gaining visual experience, stripes will not form, because the widespread distribution of afferents will be retained in the absence of competition from the inactive eye. If one eye is occluded after the establishment of the striped pattern, within certain temporal limits, afferents from the remaining side will invade the nonfunctional stripes, resulting in the nonstriped pattern of the visually naive animal. This case illustrates again the phenomenon of competition and functional validation. This illustration also has some significant clinical implications.

Some form of competition and functional validation at the synaptic level may well be involved in the processes of learning and memory, but it is not treated in this chapter. In a sense, development never really ends. This, as one gets older, is comforting.

Conclusions

It is hoped that this chapter has succeeded in giving you sufficient information and understanding of the development of the nervous system without making it too cumbersome. The most important information to remember is the general sequence of the main events of neural development, and the notion of compromise between the hard-wiring necessitated by a communication system made up of so many (and such complex) units, and the plasticity necessitated by the vocation of the nervous system—to communicate with the environment and, therefore, to adjust to it.

REFERENCES

1. Schoenwolf GC, Smith JL. Mechanisms of neurulation: traditional viewpoint and recent advances. _Development_ 1990;109:243–270.
2. Altman J, Bayer SA. The development of the rat spinal cord. _Adv Anat Embryol Cell Biol_ 1984;85.
3. Altman J, Bayer SA. Prenatal development of the cerebellar system in the rat: I. cytogenesis of the deep cerebellar nuclei and the cortex of the cerebellum. _J Comp Neurol_ 1978;179:23–48.
4. Altman J, Bayer SA, Prenatal development of the cerebellar system in the rat: II. cytogenesis and histogenesis of the inferior olive, pontine gray, and the precerebellar reticular nuclei. _J Comp Neurol_ 1978;179:49–76.
5. Altman J, Bayer SA. Development of the hippocampal region in the rat: I. neurogenesis examined with thymidine autoradiography. _J Comp Neurol_ 1978;190:87–114.
6. Altman J, Bayer SA. Development of the brainstem in the rat: I. thymidine-radiographic study of the time of origin of neurons of the lower medulla. _J Comp Neurol_ 1980;194:1–35.
7. Altman J, Bayer SA. Development of the brainstem in the rat: II. thymidine-radiographic study of the time of origin of neurons of the upper medulla, excluding the vestibular and auditory nuclei. _J Comp Neurol_ 1980; 194:37–56.
8. Altman J, Bayer SA. Development of the brainstem in the rat: III. thymidine-radiographic study of the time of origin of neurons of the vestibular and auditory nuclei of the upper medulla. _J Comp Neurol_ 1980;194:877–904.
9. Altman J, Bayer SA. Development of the brainstem in the rat: IV. thymidine-radiographic study of the time of origin of neurons in the pontine region. _J Comp Neurol_ 1980;194:905–929.
10. Altman J, Bayer SA. Development of the brainstem in the rat: V. thymidine-radiographic study of the time of origin of neurons in the midbrain tegmentum. _J Comp Neurol_ 1981;198:677–716.
11. Bayer SA. The development of the septal region in the rat: I. neurogenesis examined with H-thymidine autoradiography. _J Comp Neurol_ 1979;183:89–106.
12. Bayer SA. Quantitative H-thymidine radiographic analyses of neurogenesis in the rat amygdala. _J Comp Neurol_ 1980;194:845–875.
13. Bayer SA. H-Thymidine-radiographic studies of neurogenesis in the rat olfactory bulb. _Exp Brain Res_ 1983; 50:329–340.
14. Oppenheim RW. Cell death during development of the nervous system. _Annu Rev Neurosci_ 1991;14:453–501.
15. Williams RW, Herrup K. The control of neuron number. _Annu Rev Neurosci_ 1988;11:423–453.
16. Ramon y Cajal S. _Histologie du système nerveux de l'homme et des vertébrés._ Madrid: Consejo Superior de Investigaciones Cientificas (C.S.I.C.), 1911.
17. Rakic P. Principles of neural cell migration. _Experientia_ 1990;46:882–891.
18. Hatten ME. Riding the glial monorail: a common mechanism for glial-guided neuronal migration in dif-

ferent regions of the developing mammalian brain. *Trends Neurosci* 1990;13:179–184.

19. Rosen GD, Sherman GF, Galaburda AM. Birthdates of neurons in induced microgyria. *Brain Res* 1996;727: 71–78.

20. Black MM, Baas PW. The basis of polarity in neurons. *Trends Neurosci* 1989;12:211–214.

21. Chamak B, Prochiantz A. Influence of extracellular matrix proteins on the expression of neuronal polarity. *Development* 1989;106:483–491.

22. Ramon y Cajal SA. A quelle époque apparaissent les expansions des cellules nerveuses de la moëlle épinière du poulet? *Anat Anz* 1890;5:609–613.

23. Van Hoof COM, Oestreicher AB, De Graan PNE, Gispen WH. Role of the growth cone in neuronal differentiation. *Mol Neurobiol* 1989;3:101–133.

24. Dodd J, Jessell TM. Axon guidance and the patterning of neuronal projections in vertebrates. *Science* 1988; 242:692–699.

25. Purves D, Lichtman JW. *Principles of neural development.* Sunderland, MA: Sinauer Associates, 1985.

26. Maness LM, Kastin AJ, Weber JT, Banks WA, Beckman BS, Zadina JE. The neurotrophins and their receptors: structure, function, and neuropathology. *Neurosci Biobehav Rev* 1994;18:143–159.

27. Barde YA. Trophic factors and neuronal survival. *Neuron* 1989;2:1525–1534.

28. Kater SB, Mattson MP, Cohan C, Connor J. Calcium regulation of the neuronal growth cone. *Trends Neurosci* 1988;11:315–321.

29. Gordon-Weeks PR. GAP-43: what does it do in the growth cone? *Trends Neurosci* 1989;12:363–365.

30. Wong EV, Kenwrick S, Willems P, Lemmon L. Mutations in the cell adhesion molecule L1 cause mental retardation. *Trends Neurosci* 1995;18:168–172.

31. Landis SC. Target regulation of neurotransmitter phenotype. *Trends Neurosci* 1990;13:344–350.

Neural Mechanisms of Aging

CECILIA M. FOX, PhD
ROBERT N. ALDER, MS, OTR

Normal Aging in the Nervous System

• • •

Since the turn of the century, the average life expectancy for men and women has risen dramatically. In 1940, the average life expectancy for people of all races in the United States was approximately 61 years for men and 65 years for women. Currently, the life expectancies for men and women have risen to approximately 72 and 79 years, respectively.[1] This significant jump in life expectancy can be partially attributed to major changes in health care and medical technology. This positive trend continues, with projected life expectancies between 1987 and 2000 expected to increase 1.71 years for men and 1.51 years for women.[2]

As our population becomes older, problems associated with aging continue to increase. The term **aging** (or **senescence**) refers to a decrease in a person's probability of survival that is seen later in life.[3,4] Aging is commonly associated with impaired cognitive and physiologic performance, which makes people more susceptible to death. For example, the leading causes of death in almost all age groups are motor vehicle accidents and other accidents and adverse effects. In the age groups 45 to 64 and 65 years and over, however, the leading causes of death are heart disease and malignant neoplasms[5] (Table 20–1). In addition, some disorders, such as Alzheimer's disease, are specific to old age. Alzheimer's disease, characterized by a progressive loss of memory and intellectual abilities, virtually never appears in people younger than 45 years of age and is rare in the 45- to 64-year age group. In the 65 years and older age group, however, Alzheimer's disease is the ninth leading cause of death. Are these age-related disorders an inevitable result of longevity, or is it possible

TABLE 20–1

Death Rates for the 10 Leading Causes of Death: United States, 1995

Leading Causes of Mortality of All Races, Both Sexes, Ages 65 Years and Older	U.S. Death Rate per 100,000
1. Diseases of the heart	1,835.3
2. Malignant neoplasms	1,136.6
3. Cerebrovascular diseases	413.8
4. Chronic obstructive pulmonary disease and allied conditions	263.9
5. Pneumonia and influenza	221.6
6. Diabetes mellitus	132.6
7. Accidents and adverse effects	86.8
8. Alzheimer's disease	60.3
9. Nephritis, nephrotic syndrome, and nephrosis	60.2
10. Septicemia	50.4

Modified from Anderson RN, Kochanek KD, and Murphy SL. Report of final mortality statistics, 1995. Monthly vital statistics report. Vol. 45, No. 11, Supplement 2, Table 7. Hyattsville, MD: National Center for Health Statistics, 1997.

to age successfully? This chapter focuses on the changes to the nervous system that occur in normal aging as compared with two age-related disorders, Parkinson's and Alzheimer's diseases.

Normal Aging in the Nervous System

People experience some decline in functionality associated with aging of the nervous system. As people age, they experience difficulty sleeping and show an increase in wakefulness and arousal from sleep, as well as a decrease in their slow-wave sleep.[6] The acquisition of new information and the conversion of that information from working memory into long-term memory significantly declines with age.[7,8] Other studies have also shown age-related changes in neural conduction.[9,10] How do these changes manifest themselves in the central nervous system? As we will see, numerous alterations occur during normal aging at gross anatomic, cellular, and molecular levels that underlie these alterations in the nervous system.

Gross Anatomic Changes in the Nervous System Associated With Aging

A variety of postmortem and imaging studies have consistently shown an age-related decrease in total brain weight and volume.[8,11,12] This loss is not uniform; in certain regions of the brain, the volume loss appears to be more dramatic. In particular, the volumes of the frontal and temporal lobes decrease significantly with age.[8,12] Investigators have studied the atrophy seen in the hippocampal–amygdala complex of the temporal lobe because of its role in learning and memory[12–14] (Fig. 20–1). Age-related atrophy of the hippocampus has been positively correlated with both memory and cognitive impairments. As brain volume decreases with age, it is accompanied by enlargement of the ventricles.[8,12] This ventricular dilation has also been positively correlated with changes in memory and cognitive function.[8] Researchers are investigating what factors cause the regional decreases in brain volume and enlargement of the ventricles. Several lines of research suggest that the age-associated changes may be due to cell death, neuronal atrophy, or loss of white matter (Fig. 20–2).

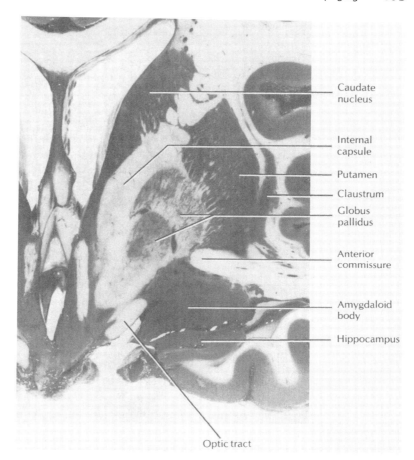

Caudate
nucleus

Internal
capsule

Putamen

Claustrum

Globus
pallidus

Anterior
commissure

Amygdaloid
body

Hippocampus

Optic tract

Figure 20–1. Coronal section through the amygdala and surrounding parts of the brain. This section was stained by a method that differentiates gray matter (dark) and white matter (light). (Reproduced with permission from Barr ML, Kiernan JA. *The human nervous system: An anatomical viewpoint.* 6th ed. Philadelphia: JB Lippincott, 1993.)

Cell Death and Age

Over the past four decades, an extensive body of research has evaluated the relationship between neuronal cell death and increasing age. Cell counting techniques and imaging studies have been used to estimate regional neuronal loss and gray matter shrinkage throughout the brain. The results of these studies have mostly supported the changes seen in brain volume; the areas of the brain showing the greatest amount of age-related neuronal loss and shrinkage are the frontal and temporal lobes and the amygdala–hippocampal complex[8,12,14–17] (Fig. 20–3). Until recently, almost all hippocampal cell density studies have indicated that a gradual loss of pyramidal neurons is associated with age. The important role of pyramidal neurons of the hippocampus in learning and memory is

well known; their loss would therefore impair such functions. Studies of this region have also shown significant increases in astrocyte and microglial proliferation associated with age. This finding indicates that these glial cells target degenerating neurons. Thus, these data support the concept of hippocampal cell loss. Cell loss has also been noted in the nucleus basalis and subcortically in the locus ceruleus and substantia nigra.[18,19,20] Interestingly, the nucleus basalis exhibits extensive neuronal loss in Alzheimer's disease and the locus ceruleus and substantia nigra specifically exhibit extensive neuronal loss in another age-related disorder, Parkinson's disease.

Some researchers have challenged the idea that neuronal cell death causes some age-related changes in the nervous system. Instead, they have suggested that previous techniques were imperfect.[21,22] The prep-

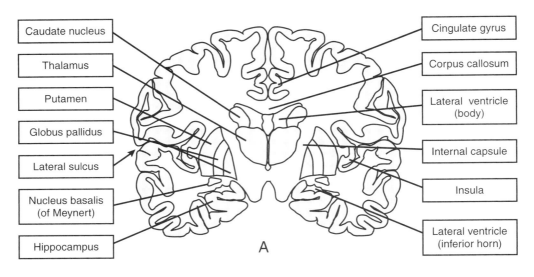

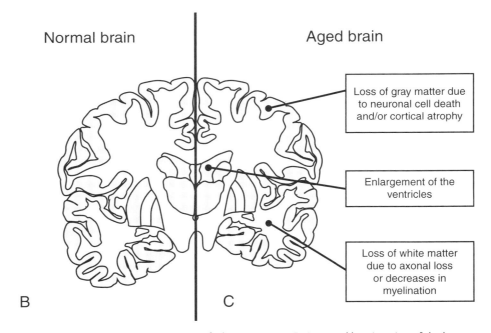

Figure 20–2. A: A normal coronal section of a human cortex. **B:** A normal hemisection of the human cortex compared with an aged human cortex. **C:** Researchers have observed several age-related gross anatomical changes, including a loss or atrophy of cortical neurons, a decrease in white matter (due to axonal or myelin loss) and an enlargement of the ventricles.

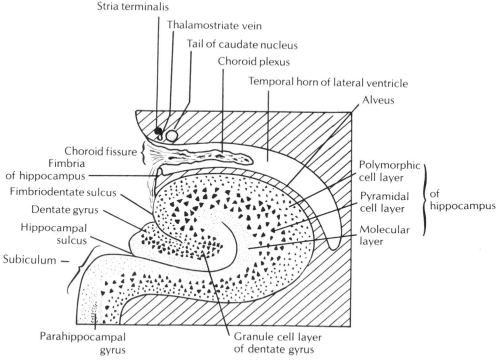

Figure 20–3. Coronal section through the hippocampal formation. Notice the pyramidal cell layer present throughout the hippocampus (medial surface at the left). (Reproduced with permission from Barr ML, Kiernan JA. *The human nervous system: An anatomical viewpoint.* 6th ed. Philadelphia: JB Lippincott, 1993.)

aration techniques for cell density analysis may cause shrinkage of nonaged tissue. Therefore, aged tissue may appear less dense even though it may contain the same number of cells. A new technique called optical fractionation allows an accurate calculation of the total number of neurons within a cortical region regardless of the density. Some critics of previous studies have also argued that the old screening techniques for pathologic brains were not sensitive enough.[21,22] Therefore, brains exhibiting neuronal cell death associated with a disease may have been included with the normal, aged brains. New screening techniques may ameliorate this problem. Researchers using these new techniques observed few signs of neuronal loss in the pyramidal regions, but did find significant losses in the hilus and subiculum of the hippocampus, and they found little or no loss of neurons throughout the rest of the cortex.[21,22] Neurons of the hilus and subiculum are not known to be major contributors to the processes of learning and

memory, and the effects of their loss on cognitive function are unknown. These studies suggest that we may not have the widespread neuronal loss once associated with aging. Instead, age-related changes in function may result from other factors.

Neuronal Atrophy and Age

Although some imaging studies that reported cortical atrophy suggested that their results corresponded with neuronal loss, this interpretation may not be entirely correct. The age-related decline in gray matter volume may actually be due to neuronal atrophy. One study observed a significant age-related decrease in large neurons in the frontal and temporal areas, with a corresponding increase in the number of small neurons.[16] This finding, which suggests that cortical neurons actually atrophy with age, is supported by the observation that the total number of neurons in the brain did not change. Therefore, as we age we may not necessarily lose the machinery for functioning, however its capacity to function at a normal level is altered. This change might be due to changes in membrane sensitivity and neurotransmitter function, or might even result from intracellular changes (i.e., DNA damage, accumulation of free radicals), all of which are addressed later in this chapter. If aging does not cause widespread neuronal loss, but rather causes neuronal atrophy, then perhaps drug therapies can be developed to combat the aging process in the nervous system.

Loss of White Matter and Age

Some imaging studies suggest that the shrinkage of brain volume associated with aging may be due not only to changes in gray matter volume; aging may also cause shrinkage in white matter because of axonal death or myelin degeneration.[11,23,24] Axonal death may result from the disuse of axonal collaterals or from neuronal death itself. Using imaging studies, one group of investigators found a greater loss in the volume of white matter than gray matter with age. This finding may indicate a loss of cortical neurons, because myelinated fibers are much larger in diameter than cell bodies.[24] Myelin loss might also play an important role in normal aging and explain the differences between white and gray matter volumes observed by some researchers. Degeneration of myelin could cause observable differences in neuronal conduction rates and difficulty processing in regions of the cerebral cortex where speed is crucial. Some evidence supports this idea. Studies of somatosensory and motor neural transmission demonstrate significant increases in the latency period with age and significant decreases in potential amplitudes.[9,10] Some preliminary studies using magnetic resonance imaging imaging techniques to analyze the degradation of myelin associated with normal aging have found age-related myelin degeneration throughout the cerebral hemispheres.

Cellular and Molecular Changes Associated With Aging

We have examined the current research regarding anatomic changes that occur during normal aging, but why do these changes occur? The decreases in function associated with aging may not be due

solely to widespread neuronal loss, but may also result from alterations at the cellular and molecular levels. A variety of age-related changes have been observed in the architecture of neurons as well as in their capacity for neural transmission.

Age-Related Changes in Neuronal Architecture and Neural Transmission

Normal aging in the nervous system is correlated with alterations in the architecture of neurons. Studies have shown significant degeneration of dendrites and dendritic spines in cortical pyramidal cells with advancing age.[25,26] In addition, increasing age and declining presynaptic terminal density are significantly related.[27,28] If a neuron decreases its dendritic arborization, it gradually decreases its rate of activation, which alters the state of neuronal plasticity. Synaptogenesis decreases, resulting in a decline in synaptic density. Over time, the lack of stimulation to a neuron results in cell atrophy or death. Therefore, these age-related alterations in neuronal architecture may underlie the neuronal loss or atrophy that occurs in cortical and subcortical structures.

A growing body of research indicates the occurrence of pathologic changes to neuronal architecture. These changes—the formation of senile or "neuritic" plaques (SPs) and neurofibrillary tangles (NFTs)—used to be associated only with Alzheimer's disease.[29] SPs are located outside the neuron and consist of spherical structures with a central core of beta-amyloid protein. Beta-amyloid protein ranges in length from 40 to 42 amino acids and aggregates into insoluble beta-pleated sheets.[30,31] These sheets form the core of the neuritic plaque. Some studies have indicated the presence of SPs throughout the neocortex of normal (control group) aged people, but other studies have suggested that the density of neuritic plaques does not increase with age and that the appearance of plaques may represent the onset of mild Alzheimer's disease.[32–35]

The research on NFTs and aging has yielded different results. NFTs, which are located inside the neuron, consist of bundles of filaments in cell bodies, axons, and dendrites. The primary element of the NFT is a paired helical filament composed of a microtubule-associated, hyperphosphorylated protein called tau.[29–31] In normal cells, tau is a critical protein of the cytoskeleton. The hyperphosphorylated form of tau prevents the association of the microtubules in the neuron and the consequent disruption of axonal transport as well as degeneration of the axon. The expression of NFTs is positively correlated with normal aging.[32–37] NFTs appear in the entorhinal cortex, in the pyramidal cells and the subiculum of the hippocampus, and in the inferior temporal cortex of a normally aging brain.[34,36] As you will see later, both SPs and NFTs are more prominent in the cortex of people with Alzheimer's disease.

Much evidence suggests that neurons alter their neural transmission with age, which directly affects the degree of neuronal activation. Research has shown age-related decreases in the number of receptors and the desensitization of the remaining receptors.[38–42] Studies have also shown decreases in the production, release, and metabolism of the neurotransmitters acetylcholine, dopamine, and norepinephrine, which are produced in the nucleus basalis, substantia nigra, and locus ceruleus, respectively.[43–49] As mentioned previously, these cortical and subcortical regions exhibit neuronal loss with advancing age. Also, significant reductions have been noted in the concentrations of second messengers and enzymes involved in signal transduction cascades.[50–52] All of these changes in neural transmission may therefore be important in the mechanisms that underlie the functional changes in the aging nervous system.

Hypotheses of the Cellular and Molecular Bases of Aging

Alterations in Gene Expression
In the past, DNA has been the target of many hypotheses explaining the theories behind brain aging. An accumulation of DNA strand breaks because of an increase in fragility of chromatin, as well as variations in DNA length, has been reported.[53] Several investigators have also observed a decrease in DNA synthesis for neuronal repair and an increase in intercellular variability in DNA content. Because the pattern of gene expression begins at the level of the DNA molecule, these changes can have deleterious effects on the process of transcription that, in turn, affect the process of translating this genetic information into protein.[53,54]

Total RNA synthesis in the brain decreases significantly with aging. Although all three types of RNA are affected, messenger RNA (mRNA) is more susceptible to the aging process than transfer RNA (tRNA) or ribosomal RNA (rRNA).[55] Because mRNA

is critical for the expression of genetic material into protein, several investigators have studied the age-related differences in mRNA expression.

Messenger RNA is characterized by the presence of numerous adenosine residues at the 3' end of the molecule. These multiple residues are known as the "poly-A tail." This poly-A segment allows for the identification and quantification of an mRNA molecule within the neuronal cell body as opposed to a tRNA or rRNA molecule.[54,56] Based on this principle, levels of mRNA as a function of age have been examined in rat brain tissue. The average life span of most laboratory rodents is between 2 and 3 years. Several studies have shown that as the animal approaches 2 years of age, levels of mRNA are significantly decreased in the neuronal cell body.[56] Other studies have shown that the translation of mRNA into protein is also decreased by at least 50% in the rat cortex and forebrain.[54,55]

A possible explanation for this decrease in brain mRNA levels is an alteration in the stability of the mRNA molecule. The control of gene expression is based on the stability of mRNA, which, in turn, is a critical factor for protein synthesis. Changes in poly-A tail length have been associated with decreased mRNA stability and translational efficiency in the aging heart, although the information about mRNA changes in brain tissue is limited.[56] Nonetheless, this finding is important and should be considered seriously.

Protein Synthesis and Degradation
As aging proceeds, protein turnover decreases, indicating a slowing of both protein synthesis and degradation. In the aging rodent brain, protein synthesis decreases by 17%.[53] Most research has focused on identifying specific proteins that are affected during the aging process. Among the affected proteins are enzymes designed to sequester **free radicals** (i.e., superoxide dismutase, glutathione peroxidase) and regulate calcium homeostasis (i.e., calbindin, calmodulin).[57,58] This decrease in protein synthesis has several possible explanations. A number of studies have reported defects in the aggregation of ribosomes and mRNA necessary for initiating protein synthesis. Furthermore, in neuronal cell cultures of the mouse, elongation of the peptide strand during protein synthesis is significantly impaired.[55]

In addition to the effects of aging on protein synthesis, decreases in protein degradation have been observed in the brain, liver, and kidney of aging rats.[55] Several investigators, however, have shown some variation in the rates of degradation. Therefore, all proteins may not be degraded in the same way. Intracellular protein degradation appears to be carried out by a number of pathways, ranging from a lysosome-dependent pathway to a calcium-dependent pathway. In addition, each pathway treats proteins differently depending on their amino acid sequence; folding and coiling patterns based on hydrogen bonding; and the relationship of multiple polypeptides within the protein.[55,56]

Free Radical Production

Increasing evidence has implicated oxidative stress in the pathogenesis of many neurodegenerative diseases, such as Parkinson's disease, Alzheimer's disease, Huntington's disease, and amyotrophic lateral sclerosis. The neuropathologic features of these diseases involve degeneration of specific neuronal populations that are functionally or neuroanatomically connected.[58] Each disorder is age related and progressive, although their etiologies are unknown in most cases.

One of the basic mechanisms proposed to explain neuronal cell loss in the aging brain is the production of toxic free radical species. A free radical is an oxygen molecule containing one or more unpaired electrons, such as the superoxide (O_2), hydroxyl (OH^-), and nitric oxide (NO^-) radicals. Most free radicals are highly unstable reactive species that remove an electron from nearby atoms to stabilize their own structure.[58–60] This process leads to the oxidation of neighboring molecules, thereby irreversibly damaging functional biologic units such as DNA, RNA, proteins, and lipids. The reaction of free radicals with lipids can initiate subsequent events leading to lipid peroxidation and breakdown of cellular membranes.[60]

There are multiple sources of oxygen free radicals in the neuron. Electrons escape from the electron transport chain located in the mitochondria to induce the formation of the superoxide and hydroxyl radicals.[60] The hydroxyl radical is the most prominent and reactive of the free radical species in the neuron. In contrast, the superoxide radical is less reactive and capable of limited direct oxidative damage. The integrity of the neuron can be effectively challenged, however, when superoxide interacts with nitric oxide, forming the highly reactive oxidizing peroxynitrite ($ONOO^-$).[58,60]

Both the superoxide and nitric oxide radicals can also be produced in response to increased levels of intracellular calcium.[60] First, calcium-activated phospholipase A_2 is stimulated to release arachidonic acid, which in turn breaks down to form the superoxide radical. Second, a calcium-activated protease converts xanthine dehydrogenase to xanthine oxidase. Xanthine oxidase subsequently catalyzes the oxidation of xanthine to produce uric acid and the superoxide radical. Third, calcium-activated nitric oxide synthetase results in the formation of nitric oxide from arginine. Thus, an increase in intracellular calcium has the potential to generate both the superoxide and nitric oxide radicals, which interact to promote neuronal degeneration[61] (Fig. 20–4).

The formation of free radicals can be enhanced in the presence of transition metals such as iron, copper, and manganese. These metals have a loosely bound electron in their outer shell that can accept or donate electrons, thereby promoting **redox reactions**.[58] Hydrogen peroxide is known to decompose spontaneously to form the hydroxyl radical. In the presence of iron (Fe^{++}), however, the rate of the reaction is greatly increased. The specificity of oxidative damage to DNA and proteins is thought to result from iron-binding properties on specific areas of these molecules. When the neuron is not experiencing oxidative stress, iron is usually bound to transferrin or ferritin, which maintains it in a nonreactive state.[58]

Under normal physiologic conditions, the neuron has the mechanisms needed to limit free radical production and oxidative stress. The mitochondria, where oxidative phosphorylation through the electron transport chain occurs, are equipped with endogenous free radical scavenging mechanisms.[59,60,62] Superoxide dismutase catalyzes the dismutation of superoxide to hydrogen peroxide. The hydrogen peroxide is then safely reduced to water by glutathione in a reaction catalyzed by glutathione peroxidase. Another free radical scavenger, alpha-tocopherol (vitamin E), protects against lipid peroxidation by donating an electron to satisfy the outer shell of reactive oxygen species. In addition, iron-binding proteins such as transferrin or ferritin can behave as antioxidants by maintaining iron and other transitional elements in an unreactive state.[62,63]

The aging brain may be particularly susceptible to the oxidative damage from free radical production for several reasons. First, the brain generates more free radicals per gram of tissue than any other organ

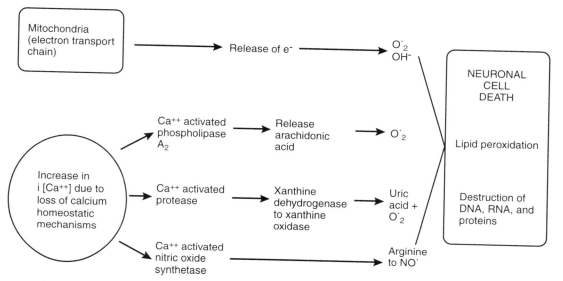

Figure 20–4. Diagram of the various pathways of free radical production within a neuron. i [Ca^{++}], intracellular calcium; O$_2^{\cdot}$, superoxide radical; OH$^-$, hydroxyl radical; NO$^{\cdot}$, nitric oxide radical; e$^-$, electron.

in the human body. Second, compared with other tissues, the brain is relatively deficient in antioxidants such as superoxide dismutase or glutathione peroxidase. Third, in focal areas in the brain, iron appears to accumulate at much higher concentrations than those found in the "iron-rich" liver. Fourth, the brain undergoes a higher rate of oxidative phosphorylation and uses a disproportionately large amount of the body's oxygen supply.[59,62] Therefore, based on this evidence, it seems reasonable that the brain is a good candidate for experiencing significant levels of oxidative stress.

Normally, free radical production and the antioxidant defense mechanisms are balanced. In the aging neuron, however, an imbalance between these two systems can lead to oxidative stress.[61,62] It is still unclear whether neuronal degeneration is a direct consequence of an overproduction of free radical oxygen species or whether there is a defect in the enzymatic processes in the neuron that is specifically designed to handle this stress. Later in this chapter, we discuss the free radical theory of neuronal degeneration and its role in the pathogenesis of certain illnesses such as Parkinson's disease and Alzheimer's disease.

Calcium Homeostasis

The calcium hypothesis of brain aging and neurodegenerative disorders is based on two principles. First, the cellular mechanisms responsible for maintaining normal cytosolic calcium levels play a key role in aging; second, sustained changes in calcium homeostasis could provide a common pathway for the pathologic changes observed in brain aging and neurodegenerative disorders.[64,65]

Calcium is a universal messenger for extracellular signals in a number of cell types. It regulates a variety of neuronal functions, such as neurotransmitter synthesis and release; neuronal excitability; and phosphorylation of proteins.[64–66] Under resting conditions, the level of intracellular calcium in a neuron is approximately 100 nmol/L, whereas the concentration outside the neuron is about 1 mmol/L. Neuronal activation induces a transient increase in intracellular calcium by its entry through voltage-gated calcium channels or ligand-gated calcium channels, or release from intracellular stores (e.g., mitochondria, smooth endoplasmic reticulum).[64] Once these events are completed, levels of intracellular calcium are immediately restored to normal by binding to calcium-binding proteins (i.e., calmodulin, calbindin), sequestration into the mitochondria or smooth endoplasmic reticulum, and expulsion from the cell by adenosine triphosphate-driven pumps specifically designed to remove calcium and the plasma membrane sodium–calcium exchanger [64,66,67] (Fig. 20–5).

The aging brain is characterized by slowly progressive alterations in the mechanisms related to calcium homeostasis. Several investigators have reported a significant increase in resting intracellular calcium levels in hippocampal, cortical, and substantia nigral neurons of aging rats compared with neonatal and adult animals.[30,65] Also, the amount of the calcium-binding protein, calbindin, has been shown to decline with age, therefore compromising the ability of the neuron to buffer against high intracellular calcium levels. Increases in calcium influx have also been observed due to age-related changes in the functioning of voltage-gated calcium channels.[66,67]

Several characteristics demonstrate the detrimental effects of disturbances in neuronal calcium homeostasis during aging as well as in the pathogenesis of neurodegenerative disorders. An excessive rise in intracellular calcium ultimately leads to lipolysis, proteolysis, changes in protein phosphorylation, loss of cytoskeletal integrity, and, finally, cell death.[30,64–67] These changes in intracellular calcium levels damage neurons in a time- and concentration-dependent manner. In pro-gressive neurodegenerative disorders such as Parkinson's disease and Alzheimer's disease, the neuronal damage may be due to small changes in calcium homeostasis that are maintained for long periods of time.

Calcium homeostasis regulation impairment and antioxidant protective mechanism impairment are two major causes of the neuronal degeneration observed during normal aging and in neurodegenerative disorders.[61] Although calcium may have a role in aging, it is still unclear whether the changes in calcium concentration are the result or cause of pathologic effects. By contrast, any change in the transport or storage of calcium, regardless of how minor, has significant consequences for aging.

Age-Related Diseases of the Nervous System

To understand aging in the central nervous system, you must understand that aging is a stage in development, albeit the end stage. During normal aging, time and use alter the functioning of the entire organism. As mentioned earlier, aging causes changes in mental ability, emotional and behavioral reactions, muscle activity, and motor coordination.[68]

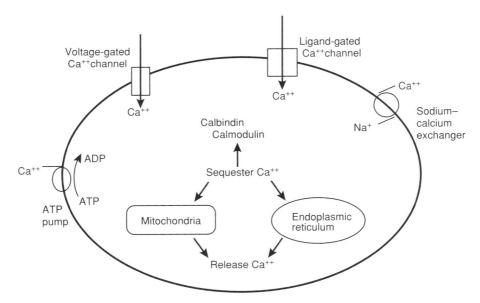

Figure 20–5. The release and sequestration of Ca++ in the neuron cell body. ADP, adenosine diphosphate; ATP, adenosine triphosphate.

As human life expectancy increases, investigators have become more interested in disease processes that alter cognitive and motor function as people age. The neuronal degeneration in diseases such as Parkinson's disease and Alzheimer's disease probably represents accelerated forms of the normal aging process. The following sections focus on the clinical features, pathologic processes, and current treatments of these two disorders.

Parkinson's Disease

Clinical Features

Parkinson's disease is a progressive neurologic disorder characterized by tremor at rest, muscular rigidity, flexed posture, slowness of voluntary movement, and impaired postural reflexes. Some "nonmotor" symptoms may also appear over time, including excessive sweating or other disturbances of the involuntary nervous system, and psychological problems such as depression or dementia.[68] Parkinson's disease develops in approximately 1% of the population older than 55 years of age. Within 10 years of onset, 60% of patients diagnosed with Parkinson's disease are either severely disabled or dead.[69,70]

Pathologic Process

Although the specific etiology of Parkinson's disease is unclear, the pathologic process is well known. As you learned in Chapter 14, the most prominent feature is a loss of dopaminergic neurons in the substantia nigra, which project from the medial forebrain bundle and internal capsule to the striatum.[70] This nigrostriatal pathway degenerates in Parkinson's disease. To some extent, this pathway also degenerates during the natural course of aging (Fig. 20–6). Symptoms of the disease become evident when 80% or more of dopaminergic neurons in the substantia nigra degenerate.[69,70] In addition to this neuronal loss, dopamine and its metabolites are depleted in both the substantia nigra and the striatum. Some evidence suggests a loss of cell bodies and depigmentation of the locus ceruleus in Parkinson's disease, although the role of this nucleus is poorly understood.

Possible Causes for Cell Death in Parkinson's Disease

Possible causes for the loss of dopamine neurons in Parkinson's disease include chronic toxicity and acceleration of the loss in dopaminergic neurons associated with normal aging. Several hypotheses are being studied to determine the causes of this disease: 1) the consequence of a loss in calcium homeostasis in dopamine neurons, 2) age-related changes in oxidative metabolism, and 3) changes in trophic support of specific growth factors that enhance the survival of dopamine neurons in culture and animal systems.[71]

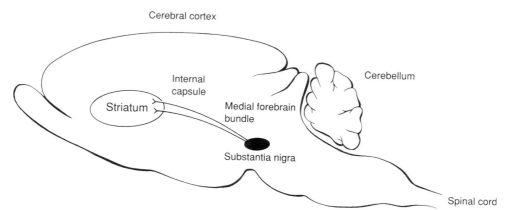

Figure 20–6. Diagram of the nigrostriatal pathway in the rodent. This pathway originates in the dopaminergic neurons of the substantia nigra and projects from the medial forebrain bundle and internal capsule to the striatum.

Several investigators have shown reductions in the expression and content of calcium-binding proteins essential for buffering internal calcium levels in postmortem brains of patients with Parkinson's disease. Calbindin-specific mRNA and protein levels are decreased in the substantia nigra, hippocampus, and raphe nucleus of patients with Parkinson's disease compared with age- and sex-matched control subjects.[69,71] This finding therefore suggests an impairment in calcium homeostasis.

Other evidence suggests that oxidative metabolism plays a major role in dopaminergic cell death in Parkinson's disease. Decreased levels of antioxidant enzymes such as superoxide dismutase and glutathione peroxidase and catalase have been detected at autopsy in the substantia nigra of patients with Parkinson's disease. Increases in lipid peroxidation have also been observed in these patients.[71] An accumulation of nonchelated iron and a decrease in ferritin content in the substantia nigra have been found during the later stages of the disease, suggesting impaired iron metabolism.[58,71]

Some evidence indicates that lack of trophic support from specific dopaminergic growth factors may play a role in cell death in the nigrostriatal pathway. Over the past decade, many studies have shown that the development, maintenance of function, and regeneration of neurons is influenced by proteins called "neurotrophic factors."[72–75] These neurotrophic factors stimulate mechanisms necessary for survival, neurite outgrowth, and functions related to transmitter production and release. Appel formulated a general hypothesis stating that the lack of neurotrophic factors may be responsible for the degeneration of selective neuronal populations as it occurs in Parkinson's disease or Alzheimer's disease.[76]

A number of neurotrophic factors exert their specific effects directly on dopamine neurons. Several investigators have shown that the removal of trophic support from dopamine neurons in culture leads to a rapid decrease in survival and neurite outgrowth. In light of this finding, it seems reasonable to postulate that the exogenous administration of trophic factors may have a protective or restorative property for dopamine neurons subjected to oxidative stress or calcium imbalance.[73–75]

Clinical Correlations

The marked degeneration of dopamine neurons and the dramatic reduction of dopamine and its metabolites in the nigrostriatal pathway provided a rational basis for the development of dopamine replacement therapy in Parkinson's disease. The most frequently used treatment involves the administration of a dopamine precursor known as levodopa (L-dopa). Dopamine itself cannot be used as a drug because it does not cross the blood–brain barrier, discussed in Chapter 5. L-dopa, however, is able to pass through this barrier and be converted into dopamine by substantia nigra neurons.[72] L-dopa treatment reduces the severity of the motor symptoms observed in Parkinson's disease and therefore improves the quality of life in most treated patients.[68]

Another current treatment is the use of dopamine receptor agonists, such as bromocriptine and pergolide. Agonists are compounds that mimic the action of the neurotransmitter itself by binding to its receptors. In most cases, however, these compounds are given as adjunct therapy to L-dopa, and may be helpful early or late in the disease.[72] Unfortunately, dopamine precursors and receptor agonists used in the therapeutics of Parkinson's disease gradually lose their effectiveness and have numerous side effects that include hallucinations, sleep disturbances, cardiac arrhythmias, vomiting, and choreic movements.[72,73,75] Therefore, identifying possible alternative therapies for alleviating or inhibiting the progression of this debilitating disease would be of significant benefit for these patients.

Current Research

Trophic Factors. The use of neurotrophic factors to protect or restore the phenotype and function of dopamine neurons damaged by disease processes or injured by trauma has been studied. A novel trophic factor identified in 1993, glial cell line–derived neurotrophic factor (GDNF), has been shown to be the most promising in protecting and restoring dopamine neurons in animal models of Parkinson's disease.[74,75] When administered in conjunction with L-dopa, GDNF decreases the dosage of L-dopa required as well as its side effects in hemiparkinsonian primates.[75] Furthermore, GDNF maintains the survival and phenotype of dopamine neurons and restores dopamine levels in the nigrostriatal pathway of parkinsonian rodents.[74] GDNF seems to have a promising future as a therapy for Parkinson's disease. It is currently in the early phases of clinical trials.

Surgical Treatment

Lesions of the Subthalamic–Globus Pallidus Pathway. The development of reliable and effective animal models and advances in anatomic and electrophysiologic techniques have improved our understanding of the functional organization of the basal ganglia and have led to new neurosurgical therapies. The nigrostriatal system's influence on motor function is primarily inhibitory.[72] Therefore, the loss of dopaminergic cells in the substantia nigra and the subsequent deficit in striatal dopamine induces an overactivity of the excitatory subthalamic–globus pallidus pathway[70,72] (Fig. 20–7). Based on this principle, there has been a resurgence of interest in the operative procedures aimed at decreasing the activity of the subthalamic–globus pallidus pathway. Lesions of this pathway, however, are somewhat variable. Although tremor and rigidity are decreased to some extent and lower doses of L-dopa are needed to obtain beneficial results, these areas of the brain

are more complex than originally thought.[70,72,73] More research must be done to understand the subtle variations within these brain regions as well as the long-term consequences of this type of surgical procedure.

Cell Transplantation. Another type of surgical intervention in the treatment of Parkinson's disease is the replacement of dopamine in the striatum. The first clinical trials using cell transplantation were carried out using grafts of chromaffin cells. Adrenal chromaffin cells are capable of synthesizing and releasing dopamine. Therefore, when transplanted into the striatum, these cells may compensate for the loss of dopamine observed in Parkinson's disease.[72,75] Although modest improvements have been reported,

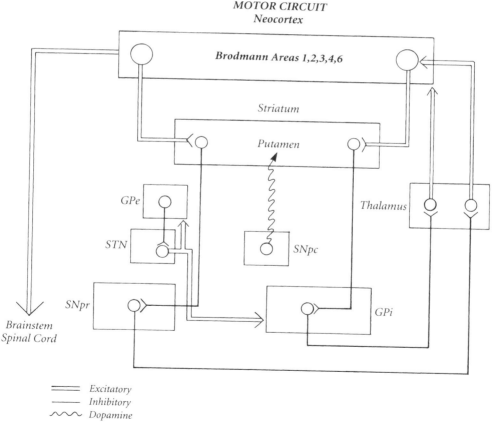

Figure 20–7. Diagram of the circuitry involved in motor control and function. Of intertest here are the inhibitory nigrostriatal and the excitatory subthalamic–globus pallidus pathways. GPe, globus pallidus externa; GPi, globus pallidus interna; SNpc, substantia nigra pars compacta; SNpr, substantia nigra pars reticulata; STN, subthalamic nucleus.

the viability of these grafts in patients remains problematic. Trophic factor support improves graft survival, but an optimal method for chronic administration of a trophic factor without initiating side effects has not yet been developed.

Intrastriatal transplantation of human embryonic mesencephalic cells has also been assessed. General improvement of motor function with no significant side effects has been observed, but several problems are associated with this procedure: 1) immunosuppression seems to be required to avoid graft rejection, 2) ethical issues with the use of this tissue have not been resolved, and 3) survival of this graft type has been poor unless chronic trophic factor support is administered.[61,70]

Gene Therapy. To compensate for the loss of striatal dopamine, research is focusing on the use of cell lines genetically engineered to synthesize and release dopamine. These cell lines have been produced by the insertion of a gene encoding tyrosine hydroxylase, the rate-limiting enzyme in dopamine synthesis. Recombinant viruses are also being used as vectors to deliver specific genes into the central nervous system. To convert striatal cells into L-dopa– producing cells, the human tyrosine hydroxylase cDNA is inserted into replication-defective forms of either herpes simplex virus or adenovirus.[61] To test the efficacy of these vectors, they have been delivered into the partially denervated striatum of parkinsonian rodents. Investigators have shown that tyrosine hydroxylase immunoreactivity is present in striatal neurons, with behavioral improvements evident for up to 1 year after treatment[61,72] (see Fig. 20–7).

This research, encompassing avenues such as trophic factor administration, surgical intervention, and gene therapy, may provide useful tools in the treatment of Parkinson's disease. Perhaps combinations of these techniques, in particular gene therapy and trophic factor-based protective therapy, will lead to improved reversal of clinical symptoms observed in this degenerative disorder within the near future.

Alzheimer's Disease

Clinical Features

Alzheimer's disease is a brain disorder of unknown etiology characterized by a progressive and irreversible loss of intellectual function. Approximately 4% of the population older than 65 years of age have Alzheimer's disease. The prevalence of this disorder increases with advancing age, especially after 75 years of age.[29,31]

In the early stages of the disease, memory impairment appears to be the only major cognitive deficit. Subtle personality changes begin to emerge as the person becomes more withdrawn and apathetic. By the middle stage, changes in appearance (due to poor self-care) and behavior generally become more noticeable, while the severity of intellect and personality disturbances becomes increasingly evident. In the late stages of the disease, patients show profound cognitive changes, including marked disorientation to time, place, and person. Depression or delusions have also been noticed in patients with Alzheimer's disease during this late phase.[31,35] The average course of the disease from onset to death is approximately 5 to 8 years.

Pathologic Process

Pathologically, Alzheimer's disease is characterized by SPs, NFTs, and neuronal loss in the hippocampus and cerebral cortex. Although some studies have indicated the presence of SPs during normal aging, other studies have suggested that diffuse SP formation may actually represent the onset of Alzheimer's disease.[35,77] The NFTs in the brains of patients with Alzheimer's disease are usually more dense in the hippocampus than NFTs seen in normal aging.[35] In addition, NFTs may also be found in the neocortex of patients with Alzheimer's disease and are rarely found in the neocortex of a normal aging brain. Although it is clear that beta-amyloid is present in abnormal levels in people with Alzheimer's disease, it is not clear if beta-amyloid is a neurotoxic protein that causes the destruction of neurons in Alzheimer's disease, or if it is a by product of neuronal damage caused by some other degenerative process.[77,78] Biochemical analyses of beta-amyloid and its toxic properties remain inconclusive. Several studies suggest that beta-amyloid is destructive to hippocampal neurons both in culture and in animal models. Neurochemical studies, however, fail to demonstrate a toxic effect of beta-amyloid on hippocampal neurons.[77]

Possible Causes for Cell Death in Alzheimer's Disease

The loss of hippocampal and cortical neurons in Alzheimer's disease has several possible causes. In fact, the three hypotheses of neuronal loss in Parkinson's disease, discussed earlier in this chapter, can also be applied to the pathogenesis of Alzheimer's disease: 1) the consequence of a loss in calcium homeostasis, 2) age-related changes in oxidative metabolism, and 3) changes in trophic support of specific growth factors that enhance the survival of hippocampal neurons in culture and animal systems.[76,77] In addition to these possibilities, a genetic component is probably involved in this disease process.

The loss of calcium homeostasis has been suggested as a cause of Alzheimer's disease as well as Parkinson's disease. Cultured rat and mouse hippocampal neurons show age-related increases in basal levels of intracellular calcium.[65,67] Furthermore, in postmortem brains of patients with Alzheimer's disease, calbindin and calmodulin protein levels are diminished.[66]

Considerable evidence suggests that the nitration of tyrosine residues in proteins, mediated by peroxynitrite, is involved in the neuronal degeneration of Alzheimer's disease. Peroxynitrite, a reaction product of nitric oxide and superoxide radicals, has been demonstrated in NFTs.[30,58] Protein nitration by peroxynitrite represents a major mechanism of oxidative modification in proteins. This modification renders nitrated proteins dysfunctional and rapidly kills hippocampal neurons in culture. In addition to the effects of peroxynitrate, some evidence of increased iron levels, alterations in protective enzymes, and lipid peroxidation associated with postmortem brains of patients with Alzheimer's disease suggests the theory of oxidative stress.[30,77,78]

Just as neurotrophic factors can enhance the survival and morphologic differentiation of dopamine neurons in culture, some trophic factors can enhance the survival of hippocampal neurons. The most potent trophic factor for these neurons is nerve growth factor.[73] It supports the survival of hippocampal neurons in culture as well as increases the outgrowth of neurite fibers. An extensive literature reports the protective properties of nerve growth factor on hippocampal neurons against axotomy-induced degeneration in rodents.[73,75]

Although most cases of Alzheimer's disease are sporadic, new research has identified a genetic component for the etiology of the disease. Families with early-onset, autosomal dominant Alzheimer's disease have genetic mutations at four separate chromosomal loci: chromosome 1, chromosome 14, chromosome 19, and chromosome 21.[29] These mutations have been linked to increases in production or alteration in the deposits of the beta-amyloid protein. Moreover, studies of humans with Alzheimer's disease or Down's syndrome and of transgenic mouse models all indicate that beta-amyloid accumulation in the cerebral cortex is an early and invariant event in the development of Alzheimer's disease.[29,30,77]

Clinical Correlations

Although treatments to prevent or delay the onset of Alzheimer's disease have yet to be developed, several therapeutic approaches to managing the symptoms of dementia are becoming more available in clinical practice. Cholinergic agents are the most promising and frequently used drugs in the treatment for Alzheimer's disease.[79] The rationale behind this method of treatment is based on the relationship between cognitive decline and a loss of cholinergic neurons (cells that produce the neurotransmitter, acetylcholine) in the cortex and hippocampus in patients with Alzheimer's disease. The two major classes of cholinergic agents are cholinergic agonists and cholinesterase inhibitors.[29,79] The agonists bind to two types of cholinergic receptors (muscarinic and nicotinic), thereby initiating a series of events in the neuron similar to those observed with the binding of acetylcholine.[79] Cholinesterase inhibitors, however, function by preventing the degradation of acetylcholine in the synapse and therefore lead to a greater amount of acetylcholine available at muscarinic and nicotinic receptors.[79] Both of these treatments probably result in improved cognitive function in patients with Alzheimer's disease; cholinesterase inhibitors may play an additional role in the regulation of the production and secretion of the beta-amyloid protein.

To combat the oxidative stress that occurs during Alzheimer's disease, chronic administration of selegiline, a selective monoamine oxidase inhibitor, may reduce the concentration of free radicals and other neurotoxins in the brain.[78] Both selegiline and another common antioxidant, vitamin E, are being studied in clinical trials.

Several other approaches are being studied in an effort to prevent the degeneration that takes place in Alzheimer's disease. One approach focuses on interfering with the formation of the insoluble beta-amyloid protein. Another method aims at preventing the formation of the hyperphosphorylated form of tau, whereas another approach is to enhance the function of cholinergic neurons of the hippocampus that are characteristically affected in this disease.[29,30,79] Also, to counteract the cholinergic atrophy, the use of nerve growth factor is being tested and attempts are being made to identify additional antioxidants and free radical scavenging enzymes that prevent toxic levels of oxidative stress.[73,78]

These new therapeutic approaches for the treatment of Alzheimer's disease focus on improving symptomatology and slowing the progression of the disease. Research in progress will support the eventual development of effective pharmacologic treatments to improve the quality of life of people suffering from the debilitating cognitive impairment characteristic of Alzheimer's disease.

Conclusion

Normal aging causes many changes in the nervous system that result in functional changes. These functional changes are exacerbated by disease processes. Rehabilitation professionals work with people who are disabled by the effects of aging, many of whom have age-related disorders as well, such as Parkinson's and Alzheimer's diseases. To develop the best possible treatments for elderly people, we must base those treatments on an understanding of the aging process in normal people and the mechanisms of age-related disorders.

REFERENCES

1. Singh GK, Kochanek KD, MacDorman MF. Advance report of final mortality statistics, 1994. *Monthly vital statistics report*. Vol. 45, No. 3, Supplement. Hyattsville, MD: National Center for Health Statistics, 1996:19.
2. Rockett IR, Pollard JH. Life table analysis of the United States' year 2000 mortality objectives. *Int J Epidemiol* 1995;24:547–551.
3. Rowe JW, Kahn RL. Human aging: usual and successful. *Science* 1987;237:143–149.
4. Partridge L, Barton NH. Optimality, mutation and the evolution of ageing. *Nature* 1993;362:305–311.
5. Anderson RN, Kockanek KD, Murphy SL. Report of final mortality statistics, 1995. *Monthly vital statistics report*. Vol. 45, No. 11, Supplement 2, Table 7. Hyattsville, MD: National Center for Health Statistics, 1997.
6. Prinz PN. Sleep and sleep disorders in older adults. *J Clin Neurophysiol* 1995;12:139–146.
7. Petersen RC, Smith G, Kokmen E, Ivnik RJ, Tangalos EG. Memory function in normal aging. *Neurology* 1992;42:396–401.
8. Sullivan EV, Marsh L, Mathalon DH, Lim KO, Pfefferbaum A. Age-related decline in MRI volumes of temporal lobe gray matter but not hippocampus. *Neurobiol Aging* 1995;16:591–606.
9. Mackenzie RA, Phillips LH II. Changes in peripheral and central nerve conduction with aging. *Clin Exp Neurol* 1981;18:109–116
10. Strenge H, Hedderich J. Age-dependent changes in central somatosensory conduction time. *Eur Neurol* 1982;21:270–276.
11. Double KL, Halliday GM, Kril JJ, et al. Topography of brain atrophy during normal aging and Alzheimer's disease. *Neurobiol Aging* 1996;17:513–521.
12. Coffey CE, Wilkinson WE, Parashos IA, et al. Quantitative cerebral anatomy of the aging human brain: a cross-sectional study using magnetic resonance imaging. *Neurology* 1992;42:527–536.
13. De Leon MJ, George AE, Golomb J, et al. Frequency of hippocampal formation atrophy in normal aging and Alzheimer's disease. *Neurobiol Aging* 1997;18:1–11.
14. Jack CR Jr, Petersen RC, Xu YC, et al. Medial temporal atrophy on MRI in normal aging and very mild Alzheimer's disease. *Neurology* 1997;49:786–794.
15. Lippa CF, Hamos JE, Pulaski-Salo D, DeGennaro LJ, Drachman DA. Alzheimer's disease and aging: effects on perforant pathway perikarya and synapses. *Neurobiol Aging* 1992;13:405–411.
16. Terry RD, DeTeresa R, Hansen LA. Neocortical cell counts in normal human adult aging. *Ann Neurol* 1987; 21:530–539.
17. DeKosky ST, Bass NH. Aging, senile dementia, and the intralaminar microchemistry of cerebral cortex. *Neurology* 1982;32:1227–1233.
18. Barr ML, Kiernan JA. *The human nervous system an anatomical viewpoint*. 6th ed. Philadelphia: JB Lippincott, 1993.
19. Tompkins MM, Basgall EJ, Zamrini E, Hill WD. Apoptotic-like changes in Lewy-body-associated disorders and normal aging in substantia nigral neurons. *Am J Pathol* 1997;150:119–131.
20. Lowes-Hummel P, Gertz HJ, Ferszt R, Cervos-Navarro J. The basal nucleus of Meynert revised: the nerve cell number decreases with age. *Archives of Gerontology and Geriatrics* 1989;8:21–27.
21. Wickelgren I. For the cortex, neuron loss may be less than thought. *Science* 1996;273:48–50.
22. West MJ, Coleman PD, Flood DG, Troncoso JC. Differences in the pattern of hippocampal neuronal loss in normal ageing and Alzheimer's disease. *Lancet* 1994; 344:769–772.
23. Scheltens P, Barkhof F, Leys D, Wolters EC, Ravid R, Kamphorst W. Histopathologic correlates of white matter changes on MRI in Alzheimer's disease and normal aging. *Neurology* 1995;45:883–888.
24. Meier-Ruge W, Ulrich J, Bruhlmann M, Meier E. Age-related white matter atrophy in the human brain. *Ann NY Acad Sci* 1992;673:260–269.

25. Feldman ML, Dowd C. Loss of dendritic spines in aging cerebral cortex. *Anat Embryol (Berl)* 1975;148: 279–301.
26. Jacobs B, Scheibel AB. A quantitative dendritic analysis of Wernicke's area in humans: I. lifespan changes. *J Comp Neurol* 1993;327:83–96.
27. Liu X, Erikson C, Brun A. Cortical synaptic changes and gliosis in normal aging, Alzheimer's disease and frontal lobe degeneration. *Dementia* 1996;7:128–134.
28. Masliah E, Mallory M, Hansen L, DeTeresa R, Terry RD. Quantitative synaptic alterations in the human neocortex during normal aging. *Neurology* 1993;43:192–197.
29. Peskind ER. Neurobiology of Alzheimer's disease. *J Clin Psychol* 1996;57(Suppl 14):5–8.
30. Mattson MP, Barger SW, Begley JG, Mark RJ. Calcium, free radicals and excitotoxic neuronal death in primary cell culture. *Methods Cell Biol* 1995;46:187–216.
31. Edelberg HK, Wei JY. The biology of Alzheimer's disease. *Mech Ageing Dev* 1996;91:95–114.
32. Miller FD, Hicks SP, D'Amato CJ, Landis JR. A descriptive study of neuritic plaques and neurofibrillary tangles in an autopsy population. *Am J Epidemiol* 1984;3: 331–341.
33. Yasha TC, Shankar L, Santosh V, Das S, Shankar SK. Histopathologic and immunohistochemical evaluation of ageing changes in normal human brain. *Indian J Med Res* 1997;105:141–150.
34. Morris JC, Storandt M, McKeel DW Jr, et al. Cerebral amyloid deposition and diffuse plaques in "normal" aging: evidence for presymptomatic and very mild Alzheimer's disease. *Neurology* 1996;46:707–719.
35. Finch CE, Cohen DM. Aging, metabolism and Alzheimer's disease: review and hypotheses. *Exp Neurol* 1997; 143:82–102.
36. Hof PR, Glannakopoulos P, Bouras C. The neuropathological changes associated with normal brain aging. *Histol Histopathol* 1996;11:1075–1088.
37. Dani SU, Pittella JE, Boehme A, Hori A, Schneider B. Progressive formation of neuritic plaques and neurofibrillary tangles is exponentially related to age and neuronal size: a morphometric study of three geographically distinct series of aging people. *Dement Geriatr Cogn Disord* 1997;8:217–227.
38. Antonini A, Leenders KL. Dopamine D2 receptors in normal human brain: effect of age measured by positron emission tomography (PET) and [11C]-raclopride. *Ann NY Acad Sci* 1993;695:81–85.
39. Hoyer S. Age-related changes in cerebral oxidative metabolism: implications for drug therapy. *Drugs Aging* 1995;6:210–218.
40. Decker MW. The effects of aging on hippocampal and cortical projections of the forebrain cholinergic system. *Brain Res* 1987;434:423–438.
41. Wong DF, Young D, Wilson PD, Meltzer CC, Gjedde A. Quantification of neuroreceptors in the living human brain: III. D2-like dopamine receptors: theory, validation, and changes during normal aging. *J Cereb Blood Flow Metab* 1997;17:316–330.
42. Nordberg A, Alafuzoff I, Winblad B. Nicotinic and muscarinic subtypes in the human brain: changes with aging and dementia. *J Neurosci Res* 1992;31:103–111.
43. Cohen BM, Renshaw PF, Stoll AL, Wurtman RJ, Yurgelun-Todd D, Babb SM. Decreased brain choline uptake in older adults: an in vivo proton magnetic resonance spectroscopy study. *JAMA* 1995;274:902–907.
44. Palmer AM, DeKosky ST. Monoamine neurons in aging and Alzheimer's disease. *Journal of Neural Transmission General Section* 1993;91:135–159.
45. Irwin I, DeLanney LE, McNeill T, et al. Aging and the nigrostriatal dopamine system: a non-human primate study. *Neurodegeneration* 1994;3:251–265.
46. Kabuto H, Yokoi I, Mori A, Murakami M, Sawada S. Neurochemical changes related to ageing in the senescence-accelerated mouse brain and the effect of chronic administration of nimodipine. *Mech Ageing Dev* 1995;80: 1–9.
47. Geula C, Mesulam MM. Cortical cholinergic fibers in aging and Alzheimer's disease: a morphometric study. *Neuroscience* 1989;33:469–481.
48. Shen J, Barnes CA. Age-related decrease in cholinergic synaptic transmission in three hippocampal subfields. *Neurobiol Aging* 1996;17:439–451.
49. Gottfries CG. Neurochemical aspects on aging and diseases with cognitive impairment. *J Neurosci Res* 1990; 27:541–547.
50. Meier-Ruge W, Iwangoff P, Reichmeier K, Sandoz P. Neurochemical findings in the aging brain. *Adv Biochem Psychopharmacol* 1980;23:323–338.
51. Sugawa M, Coper H, Schulze G, Yamashina I, Krause F, Dencher NA. Impaired plasticity of neurons in aging: biochemical, biophysical and behavioral studies. *Ann NY Acad Sci* 1996;786:274–282.
52. Halliwell B. Reactive oxygen species and the central nervous system. *J Neurochem* 1992;59:1609–1623.
53. Danner DB, Holbrook NJ. Alterations in gene expression with age. In: Schneider EL, Rowe JW, eds. *Handbook of the biology of aging*. 3rd ed. San Diego: Academic Press, 1990.
54. Lindell TJ, Duffy JJ, Byrnes B. Transcription in aging. *Mech Ageing Dev* 1986;19:63–71.
55. Reff ME. RNA and protein metabolism. In: Finch CE, Schneider EL, eds. *Handbook of the biology of aging*. 2nd ed. New York: Academic Press, 1985.
56. Colman PD, Kaplan BB, Osterburg HH, Finch CE. Brain poly(A) RNA during aging: stability of yield and sequence complexity in two rat strains. *J Neurochem* 1990;34:335–345.
57. Beal FM. Oxidative damage in neurodegenerative diseases. *The Neuroscientist* 1997;3:21–27.
58. Olanow CW, Arendash GW. Metals and free radicals in neurodegeneration. *Curr Opin Neurol* 1994;7:548–558.
59. Beal FM. Aging, energy and oxidative stress in neurodegenerative diseases. *Ann Neurol* 1995;38:357–366.

60. Halliwell B. Reactive oxygen species and the central nervous system. *J Neurochem* 1992;59:1609–1623.

61. De Erausquin GA, Costa E, Hanbauer I. Calcium homeostasis, free radical formation and trophic factor dependence mechanisms in Parkinson's disease. *Pharmacol Rev* 1994;46:467–482.

62. Yu BP, Yang R. Critical evaluation of the free radical theory of aging. *Ann NY Acad Sci* 1996;786:1–11.

63. Reiter RJ. Oxidative processes and antioxidant defense mechanisms in the aging brain. *FASEB J* 1995;9:526–533.

64. Gareri P, Mattace R, Nava F, De Sarro G. Role of calcium in brain aging. *Gen Pharmacol* 1995;26:1651–1657.

65. Khachaturian ZS. Calcium hypothesis of Alzheimer's disease and brain aging. *Ann NY Acad Sci* 1994;747: 1–11.

66. Muller WE, Hartmann H, Eckert A, Velbinger K, Forstl H. Free intracellular calcium in aging and Alzheimer's disease. *Ann NY Acad Sci* 1996;786:305–320.

67. Biessels G, Gispen WH. The calcium hypothesis of brain aging and neurodegenerative disorders: significance in diabetic neuropathy. *Life Sci* 1996;59:379–387.

68. Markham CH, Diamond SG. Clinical overview of Parkinson's disease. *Clin Neurosci* 1993;1:5–11.

69. Forno LS. Neuropathology of Parkinson's disease. *J Neuropathol Exp Neurol* 1996;55:259–272.

70. Youdim MBH, Riederer P. Understanding Parkinson's disease. *Sci Am* 1997;276:52–59.

71. Poirier J, Thiffault C. Are free radicals involved in the pathogenesis of idiopathic Parkinson's disease? *Eur Neurol* 1993;33(Suppl 1):38–43.

72. Ghika J. Treatment of Parkinson's disease: advances in the pharmacological therapy. *Eur Neurol* 1996;36:396–408.

73. Hefti F. Neurotrophic factor therapy for nervous system degenerative diseases. *J Neurobiol* 1996;25:1418–1435.

74. Kearns CM, Gash DM. GDNF protects nigral dopamine neurons against 6-hydroxydopamine in vivo. *Brain Res* 1995;672:104–111.

75. Gash DM, Zhang Z, Ovadia A, et al. Functional recovery in GDNF-treated parkinsonian monkeys. *Nature* 1996;380:252–255.

76. Appel SH. A unifying hypothesis for the cause of amyotrophic lateral sclerosis, parkinsonism, and Alzheimer's disease. *Ann Neurol* 1981;10:499–505.

77. Cotman CW, Su JH. Mechanisms of neuronal death in Alzheimer's disease. *Brain Pathol* 1996;6:493–506.

78. Good PF, Werner P, Hsu A, Olanow CW, Perl DP. Evidence for neuronal oxidative damage in Alzheimer's disease. *Am J Pathol* 1996;149:21–28.

79. Schneider LS. New therapeutic approaches to Alzheimer's disease. *J Clin Psychol* 1996;57(Suppl 14):30–36.

21

Recovery of Function After Brain Damage

JEAN M. HELD, EdD, PT
TIM PAY, PT

• • •

Our theoretic models of how the nervous system functions influence our treatment paradigms. Until recently, our fields have been heavily biased by the hierarchical model of motor control. In this model, the nervous system is seen as a rather rigid, inflexible structure, characterized by localization of function. Under this model, the consequences of damage to a particular area are expected to be quite severe because other areas would be unable to take over the function, and therefore true recovery would not occur.

Contemporary thinking favors a systems model of motor control, in which the nervous system, in conjunction with all other systems of the body, and in constant interaction with the environment, is much more flexible. In this model, the numerous reciprocal connections and redundant representations are seen to underlie a more distributed control of function, such that the center of command is determined instantaneously by the circumstances. In this model, the effect of brain damage is less catastrophic, and the system has greater potential for recovery of function.

Definitions

The term "recovery of function" is ambiguous. In the clinical literature, "good recovery" occurs when the person can resume normal life, even though there may still be minor impairments. In the research literature, an animal could be considered "recovered" if it is able to achieve a goal, or, using an even stricter definition, it would be "recovered" only if it achieves the goal in the same or similar ways as it did before the injury. These three definitions of recovery are distinct and different, thus making it difficult to discriminate between recovery and compensation, or between recovery and no recovery. "Compensation" means that the person has switched to different means of accomplishing the task. In other words, the goal is not accomplished in the same way, but by using alternate cues or tactics.

Almli and Finger have suggested that recovery be defined more precisely: the person must have an initial deficit from which he or she "recovers" as indicated by the ability to accomplish the goal in exactly the same way as before the injury.[1] The Almli and Finger definition allows for distinctions between recovery, compensation, and "sparing." Sparing is the absence of a functional deficit immediately after central nervous system (CNS) damage.

Theoretic Mechanisms Underlying Recovery

Numerous theoretic mechanisms have been proposed to explain recovery or sparing over the years. One concept is that unoccupied or unassigned regions of the brain can learn, or take over, the functions lost through damage to another area. The most convincing evidence for this notion comes from research on early brain damage. This work is discussed later in the chapter, when we consider age as a factor that influences the potential for sparing or recovery.

Another mechanism is based on the concept of redundancy: that is, functions are variously represented throughout the nervous system, so that when one area is damaged, several others still retain the capacity to control the function. This concept would logically explain sparing more so than recovery.

Other mechanisms are based on anatomic rearrangements and physiologic readjustments. Anatomic plasticity may be in the form of **regenerative** or **collateral sprouting**. Physiologic readjustments may include resolution of **diaschisis**, **denervation supersensitivity**, and increased effectiveness of **silent synapses**. These anatomic and physiologic phenomena are discussed in greater detail later in this chapter.

Recent research on mechanisms underlying stroke suggests that surrounding intact cortical tissue, or comparable cortical tissue in the contralateral cortex, may be responsible for the recovery seen.[2,3] In animal research, this reorganization of the adjacent cortex may take place within a few hours of the damage. Given this brief time period, the recovery is probably not due to formation of new synapses. Rather, it may be due to an "unmasking" of already existing neuronal connections that under normal conditions are inhibited.[2] Approximately 25% of corticospinal fibers remain uncrossed at the level of the pyramids, and perhaps 15% remain uncrossed throughout the spinal cord. These uncrossed pathways may also play a role in subserving recovery after unilateral cortical damage.[2]

Which of these mechanisms is operating may depend on two factors: the state of the system at the time of damage, and the nature of the insult. In the rest of this chapter, we examine the response of the system to CNS damage, and review the conditions that influence the potential for recovery of function after brain damage. Finally, we consider the implications of this information for practicing therapists.

Structural and Functional Responses to Damage

The brain can be damaged in many ways, including infection, tumor, or hemorrhage secondary to arteriosclerotic vessels. It can be caused by trauma at birth, the use of forceps, or by hypoxia, when the umbilical cord is wrapped around the neck. It can be caused by trauma later in life, in either closed head injuries, where the head impacts against a solid surface without the cranium being fractured or penetrated, or in an open head injury, in which the cranium is invaded. Symptoms can vary dramatically. For instance, a newborn infant sustaining insult at birth may not show any symptoms until several months later. A person whose spinal cord has been severed shows immediate loss of all sensation and muscle action below the level of the lesion. Someone who has had a cerebrovascular accident or closed head injury may or may not lose consciousness, and may show loss of sensation and muscle action, but usually demonstrates **spasticity**, muscular weakness, loss of dexterity, and sometimes involuntary muscular contractions within days to weeks of the insult. Improvement usually follows, although the degree of improvement varies from individual to individual.

Systemic Reaction to Damage

The Russian neurologist Alexander Luria has suggested that the symptoms we see after an insult to the CNS are due to two phenomena: actual cell death caused by the event, and secondary physiologic shut-down of other neurons near the area of damage, or associated with the area of damage.[4] Luria referred to these secondary effects as inhibition, and suggested that these could be reversed within a relatively short period of time.

This concept was best described by Constantin Von Monakow in 1914, when he suggested the term **diaschisis**, a functional standstill or abolition of electrical excitability transmitted to neuronal areas that are related to the damaged part of the system, and which could explain transient functional impairments after injury.[5] Diaschisis could be due to neural shock, edema, disruption of local blood flow, or partial denervation of postsynaptic neurons.

Luria et al., building on the concept of inhibition of related neural areas, suggested that one effect of therapy is **disinhibition** of intact neurons affected secondary to the insult.[4] Perhaps the proportion of symptoms after injury due to actual primary cell death versus secondary neuronal inhibition depends on the type of insult: sudden, localized damage would most likely result in both cell death and widespread inhibition; slowly developing lesions might produce cell death without diaschisis; and a **concussion** might have a higher percentage of physiologic dampening than actual cell death.

The work of Meyer and colleagues supports the notion that damage to the CNS can result in an inhibition, or reduced excitability, and even suggests that this effect can be more than transient.[6] They administered amphetamine (a stimulant) to cats whose entire neocortex had been removed 1 year previously, and who had shown a deficit in **placing responses** throughout the entire year. Within 20 minutes, the cats exhibited normal placing responses. When the stimulant wore off, the deficits returned. Meyer et al. suggested that the deficits after neocortical removals were due to the inability to retrieve "engrams" that were used to produce the function—in this case, the placing responses. In other words, engrams, or memory traces, were therefore not lost with damage, but access to them was.

LeVere[7] viewed the person's behavior after CNS insult as reflecting the function of the remaining, intact portions of the brain. The person uses whatever works best to accomplish the desired function, both on the neurophysiologic level and on the behavioral level. Consequently, systems that have been partially damaged or secondarily inhibited would probably not be the most effective. In other words, compensation would be attempted. LeVere suggested that if the compensation is successful in accomplishing the goal, the damaged part of the system will not be challenged to recover. If, however, compensation is unsuccessful, or if it is prevented by therapy, perhaps other mechanisms that might lead to recovery will be stimulated.

Neuronal Response to Injury

When damage to the CNS occurs in regions that are mature and are primarily composed of cell bodies, those cells will die. Those neurons cannot be replaced because the remaining intact cells in the area have withdrawn from the mitotic cycle and can no longer divide. Many types of insult to the CNS, however, occur in regions where the insult causes injury to axons rather than to cell bodies. Such injuries lead to complex, widespread effects.

When the axon is cut, the two ends close, swell and retract from each other. In the zone of trauma, as the axon and myelin sheath degenerate, **macrophages** absorb and destroy axonal debris. Glial cells, including fibrous astrocytes, proliferate and form a glial scar around the zone of trauma. Degeneration proceeds in both directions. Within 2 to 3 days, **retrograde** reaction occurs in the cell body, ranging from **chromatolysis** to cell death (Fig. 21–1A). The severity of the reaction depends on how close to the cell body the **axotomy** occurred and on whether connections are restored after regeneration. If the axotomy is beyond axon collaterals, the cell has a better chance of surviving (see Fig. 21–1A). In the distal part of the severed axon, degeneration begins within 1 day, and is referred to as wallerian degeneration (see Fig. 21–1B). Invading glial cells push the axon terminal away from the postsynaptic neuron.

Adjacent neurons may die as a result of biochemical effects stemming from the initial insult. With neuronal damage, cation pumps fail and cellular depolarization occurs, which results in an increased concentration of excitatory amino acid neurotransmitters in the synaptic cleft. The excitatory neuro-

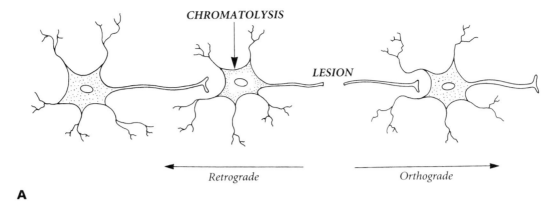

A

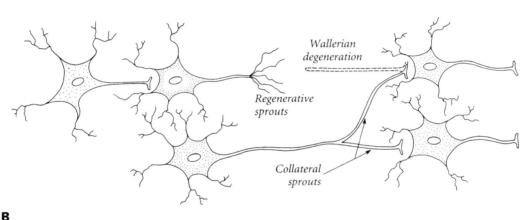

B

Figure 21–1. Neuronal response to damage. **A:** After a lesion of the axon, retrograde changes occur in the cell body, including chromatolysis or possible cell death. **B:** Later, orthograde degeneration of the axon occurs (wallerian degeneration), and collateral and regenerative sprouts grow.

transmitter glutamate has been shown to accumulate in extreme levels after CNS damage. Increased glutamate concentration results in overexcitation of postsynaptic neurons and increased intracellular calcium concentration, leading to further neurotransmitter release, thus creating an excitotoxic cascade. Excitotoxicity results in additional neuronal loss because of excessive release of excitatory amino acid neurotransmitters after an initial CNS injury. At the same time, damaged mitochondria and biochemical effects of the binding of oxygen with iron

released from protein-binding sites result in the production of free radicals, which probably contribute to further neuronal death.[8]

Transneuronal changes may also result from axotomy. Transneuronal degeneration may occur in both the **orthograde** and retrograde direction within 2 to 7 days of injury, and may account for more cell death than the primary injury. Other retrograde changes may include retraction of synapses. Orthograde changes may include the development of denervation supersensitivity, the unmasking of silent or inefficient synapses, and the replacement of lost synapses by terminals formed by collateral sprouts from nearby neurons (see Fig. 21–1B).

Denervation supersensitivity results from partial denervation of neurons. The postsynaptic neuron becomes more responsive to the neurotransmitters of the remaining **afference**. This phenomenon was described originally at the neuromuscular junction, and is more difficult to describe centrally. Denervation supersensitivity takes approximately 2 weeks to develop.

The increase in efficiency of so-called "silent synapses" may be related to denervation supersensitivity. The term refers to the fact that numerous synapses are so far from the axon hillock that their input normally does not cause sufficient depolarization to initiate an impulse. After the removal of more primary input because of damage and degeneration, however, these synapses become effective. Evidence for this phenomenon comes from research in the somatosensory system. When peripheral nerves are cut in adult animals, receptive fields in the spinal cord and cortex are shifted to represent other areas on the body surface.

Collateral sprouting from nearby undamaged neurons occurs within 4 to 5 days of injury. These collateral sprouts replace the vacant synaptic fields, increasing the residual inputs to the postsynaptic neuron and possibly preventing transneuronal degeneration. Although collateral sprouts do not replace the original circuitry, they do not occur randomly either. The new inputs occur only from systems most closely associated with the injured area.[9]

Denervation sensitivity, activation of silent synapses, and collateral sprouting may not always be beneficial. All three phenomena may contribute to spasticity, or abnormal reflexes or movement patterns, and collateral sprouts may create abnormal connections, or compete with regenerating sprouts.

Regenerative sprouts also begin to grow from the distal end of the cut axon, near the injury site, in approximately 4 to 5 days after injury. These sprouts must usually travel over longer distances than collateral sprouts, and under normal circumstances are usually unsuccessful in reconnecting to normal targets. At one time, the glial scarring at the zone of trauma was thought to form a physical barrier, preventing regenerative sprouts from growing through. The problem is now known to be much more complex. Astrocytes, as well as other cells in the injured area, do not provide a beneficial microenvironment for axonal growth. Either the reactive glia do not produce adequate neurotrophic substances, or surface-associated, neurite-promoting molecules, or they produce growth-inhibiting factors. Extensive research is examining ways to manipulate the microenvironment to allow and promote successful growth and reconnections of regenerative sprouts.

Factors Influencing the Potential for Sparing or Recovery

A number of factors influence the short- and long-term effects of brain damage. The nature of the damage itself is one very important consideration. The age and sex of the person also seem to influence the initial deficit or recovery. Experiences of the person, either before or after the injury, and either generalized or specific to the function affected, are known to influence outcome. In addition, various pharmacologic interventions have been used in attempts to enhance survival, promote growth, or increase excitability of the system. The most recent investigations have used fetal neural transplants to stimulate recovery.

The Nature of the Damage

The extent and placement of the lesion, the symmetricality of the lesion, and the rapidity with which the lesion is produced all affect the degree of deficit and recovery. The impact of the size of the lesion depends on the precise location. Depending on the cause of the damage, it may be diffuse, and spread relatively symmetrically throughout the brain, or it may be localized, and asymmetric. Some causes of brain damage are sudden, whereas others take time to develop. Various research paradigms have been used to simulate these conditions, to understand the effects of these factors better.

Size

The significance of size can be generalized by saying, "the smaller the lesion, the smaller the deficit." Size, however, is relative to the area of the brain involved. In other words, size really relates to whether an entire area, or only a portion of that area, is removed. Size also relates to how strictly localized the functions or subfunctions of the areas are (i.e., how tightly or loosely coupled they are).

Several studies illustrate the effect of lesion size on functional capacity in the motor system. Kennard summarized her experiments by saying that the size of the lesion affects the rate of recovery, such that recovery occurs more rapidly after a small lesion than after a large one.[10] She gave examples in which removal of the entire motor area produced a slower recovery in the hand and arm than if just the arm and hand areas were lesioned. Lesions of the motor and premotor area led to slower recovery than lesions of one or the other. Lesions extending beyond these motor areas (i.e., frontal cortex), however, did not increase the motor deficit.[10]

Glees and Cole reported the results of graduated-sized lesions of the motor cortex of thumb, fingers, and face, and showed more rapid recovery with smaller lesions.[11] Through stimulation of surrounding cortex after recovery, they also showed that the movements could now be elicited in areas not previously capable of producing those same movements.

The symmetric features of the lesions are also important factors in determining the initial impairment or the potential for recovery. Travis and Woolsey demonstrated greater sparing and more rapid recovery with small lesions of motor cortex.[12] In addition, they found that when the animals had large, bilaterally symmetric lesions, they regained locomotion more rapidly, and to a greater extent than those animals who had large, asymmetric lesions. Gentile et al. produced graduated lesions of the sensorimotor cortex in rats.[13] The smaller, bilaterally symmetric lesions failed to produce deficits in the locomotor tasks, whereas larger, symmetric lesions produced moderate deficits. The largest lesion, which was unilateral, produced the greatest deficit.

Rapidity of Onset

Clinicians generally accept the idea that slowly developing lesions in the CNS create less disruption of function than lesions of the same site and extent sustained suddenly. An example of this would be a slowly developing tumor, as illustrated in Figure 21–2. This photograph of a coronal section shows a benign meningioma located in the parietooccipital lobe on the right side, and occupying a large area of the right hemisphere. This patient was undiagnosed before his death from medical illnesses, and had few associated symptoms. He was hospitalized for medical reasons, and was said to demonstrate some mental instability. In retrospect, these symptoms may have been brought on by deficits in spatial perception, or left visual field impairments. Nonetheless, the lesion was probably present for at least 8 months, and possibly for years, without noticeable symptoms.

A research paradigm known as "the serial lesion experiment" has been developed to simulate the gradually expanding lesion. The serial lesion experiment entails the removal of nervous system tissue in sequential stages rather than all at once. The phenomena usually observed with serial lesion placement are 1) a partial sparing of function relative to initial deficits from the same damage imposed at one time (one-stage); and 2) a more rapid rate of recovery. Several factors seem to influence the serial lesion phenomenon. The first factor is the amount of tissue removed in each stage. The less tissue removed at one time, the less disruption to the system, and the greater the sparing or potential for recovery, despite possible complications of multiple surgeries and anesthetizations. This reduction in deficit, or improved recovery, occurs even though serially placed damage frequently exceeds the size of one-stage damage. The second factor is the interoperative interval, or the period of time between successive removals. There seems to be a minimum length of time between episodes of serially placed damage necessary to differentiate them from one-stage lesions. The third factor is the importance of interoperative experience in some situations. Under certain conditions, the general level of stimulation may be critical (e.g., light vs. darkness; sound vs. silence). Depending on the task used for analysis, interoperative training may be necessary to obtain serial lesion effects. Of course, the general care and maintenance of the animals between stages of damage is crucial. The fourth factor is the pattern of sequential placement of removals. As mentioned earlier, the outcome seems to differ if the lesions are symmetric with subsequent enlargement, or unilateral (asymmetric) with subsequent contralateral removal. Travis and Woolsey suggested that although asymmetric serial lesion patterns do demonstrate an advantage over one-stage removals, deficits are greater than in symmetric sequential removals.[12] The mode of reorganization may be different, depending on the symmetricality of the serial damage. In symmetric cortical lesions, the surrounding tissue, or subcortical tissue, may be reorganized, whereas with unilateral damage, the contralateral, homologous area of the cortex may be reorganized.

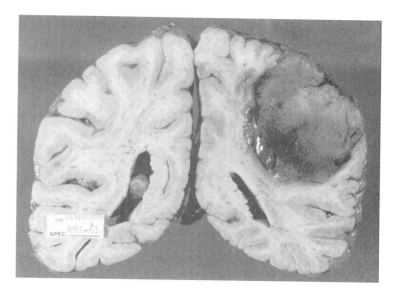

Figure 21-2. Slowly developing lesion. Coronal section demonstrates a benign meningioma that has compressed the right parietooccipital lobe. (Photograph courtesy of W. Pendlebury, University of Vermont, Burlington, Vermont.)

Various explanations have been offered for the serial lesion effect. Finger has suggested that sudden, large lesions create greater shock, or diaschisis, which would take longer to subside before reorganization can take place.[14] Also, slowly developing lesions might provide optimal conditions for sprouting or denervation supersensitivity, and, in fact, the minimal interoperative interval suggested in some studies corresponds with the time course of sprouting and denervation supersensitivity.[15] Finally, the gradual onset might make it possible for the person gradually to switch strategies for accomplishing the desired goal.

Age at the Time of Damage

At one time, early brain injury was thought to result in less deficit in function than the same injury occurring in adulthood. Research over the last 20 years, however, building and expanding on the work of Kennard, has demonstrated that this result is true only under limited circumstances, and that the effects of early brain damage are actually quite complex. To understand this complexity, consider the premise that Isaacson and Spear proposed for evaluating the consequences of brain damage at any age.[16] In contradistinction to the view of the loss of function due to the absence of the injured brain area, they suggested that the behavioral changes

seen after brain damage are due to the functioning of remaining intact parts of the brain. With this premise in mind, consider that with early brain damage the functions of the remaining, intact portions of the brain may be quite different from what they would be in adulthood or in old age. You should not be surprised, then, to learn that early lesions to certain areas produce the same functional deficits that result from damage in adulthood. In other cases, early damage causes no apparent deficit, but later on, deficits become evident. In rare circumstances, sparing of function seems to be permanent.

Some authors have related some of these findings to the functional maturation of the area of the brain damaged. Therefore, if the area was mature at the time of damage, regardless of the age of the subject, then the behavioral consequences would be the same. If, however, the damaged area was not mature when damaged, no initial deficit would be apparent. Several possibilities have been proposed: 1) another "unoccupied" or "unassigned" region could take on the function of the area damaged; 2) **anomalous** growth could develop in the undeveloped system eventually to control the function of the area damaged; or 3) when the damaged area would normally mature, behavioral deficits would become apparent. Isaacson and Spear pointed out that development after early brain damage is different from that in the normal animal because of the secondary changes produced in the remaining intact systems.[16] Consequently, it is hard to predict what the long-term effects of early damage may be, and they may be quite unexpected.

Kennard's work elegantly depicted the differences in initial deficit and recovery of motor function in infant versus adult monkeys. In a series of studies in monkeys and chimpanzees comparing unilateral, bilateral simultaneous, or bilateral serial lesions of areas 4, 4 and 6, frontal cortex, 4-6-3-2-1, and an entire hemisphere, she demonstrated in all cases that deficits in infant lesioned animals were much less than comparable adult operates. Unilateral lesions to areas 4 and 6 in infants produced almost unnoticeable deficits, with increasing loss corresponding to increased areas removed. Bilateral lesions in infants created greater deficits, although the animals could carry out most, if not all gross motor activities. Infants failed to exhibit paresis until the time when fine motor skills would have developed normally, and spasticity developed still later. In adults, paresis (or paralysis) developed immediately after damage and spasticity became evident within a matter of days at most.

Kennard interpreted her results as follows: in infancy, some cortical areas have not yet assumed specific functions, which allows for a greater functional reorganization than is possible in adults.[17] Although acknowledging that this potential for functional reorganization might be due to increased potential for morphologic restructuring, she did not believe that such functional reorganization had to entail structural anomalies. Hicks and D'Amato have demonstrated the development of anomalous ipsilateral corticospinal tracts after unilateral ablation of sensorimotor cortex in infant rats, providing evidence for structural remodeling.[18] The development of this tract was correlated with the sparing of a specific stride component of locomotion, which was altered in adult operates.

Smith et al. also demonstrated the infant lesion effect (i.e., unilateral cerebellar damage in adults produced greater and longer-lasting motor deficits than in infants).[19] Of the younger animals, the older groups (15- or 21-day-old) were less impaired and recovered more rapidly and to a greater degree than the youngest group (10-day-old). After recovery from cerebellar damage, secondary lesions were made in the motor cortex, which reinstated cerebellar symptoms. Under this condition, 10- and 15-day-old animals were most debilitated, whereas 21-day-old and

adult subjects were least affected. Smith et al. interpreted these results to suggest a greater potential for plasticity in neonates.[19] One might also infer an optimal time for plastic changes, and a differential mode of adaptation of the two youngest groups versus the 21-day-old and adult operates.

In addition to her research on monkeys and chimpanzees, Kennard reviewed cases of patients seen in a neurologic clinic.[17] She found some striking differences between children with prenatal or perinatal damage and children with postnatal injuries. In cases of early damage, almost no spasticity was present early in life, whereas it *was* present in those children with postnatal damage. Paresis was recognized later in development (4–12 months) in birth injury, whereas it appeared almost immediately after postnatal injury. In general, she noted a trend of increased deficits with development.

More recent studies have shown greater anatomic damage in both very young and older animals with less damage in those of an intermediate age. Yager et al. gave controlled ischemic brain damage to rats 1 to 24 weeks old.[20] The animals were sacrificed 7 days later. When their brains were examined for damage the authors found the most severe damage in the 1- and 3-week-old animals. Six- and 9-week-old rats had less injury compared with both older and younger animals. The authors concluded that brain damage as a result of ischemia is age dependent; however, the extent of damage does not progress linearly with increasing age.[20]

The notion that sparing, or recovery of function, after early brain damage is mediated by "unoccupied" areas of the brain taking over the function of the damaged areas has been established only in humans, and only with one function—speech. Milner and colleagues have demonstrated that speech functions are usually controlled by one hemisphere.[21] In right-handed people without brain injury, 96% have speech localized in the left hemisphere, whereas the remaining 4% show right hemisphere localization.[22] Speech is also localized in the left hemisphere of 70% of left-handers and ambidextrous persons, whereas 15% have right hemisphere localization and 15% have bilateral speech representation. In adult patients who have sustained left-hemisphere damage, however, these percentages shift, suggesting that the control of speech may shift from the usual left hemisphere to the right hemisphere under certain circumstances.[22] Milner has pointed out that speech *may be* spared if the injury occurs before a critical age (6 years), but at some cost.[21] Sparing of language functions after left hemisphere damage in young children is often accompanied by diminished capacity for spatial perception.

LeVere et al. found that age at the time of left hemisphere damage is only one of two critical conditions for the relocation of speech.[23] The second factor is the exact location of the injury. Apparently, a major involvement of either Broca's or Wernicke's speech area was required before speech would become lateralized in the right hemisphere, regardless of the actual size of the early lesion. In addition, only those speech functions controlled by the injured speech area were relocated to the other hemisphere.

Remember, the functions of particular regions of the brain may not be the same in infancy, adulthood, and old age. Therefore, damage in old age also may not produce the same deficits as that occurring in the mature organism. Stein and Firl gave aged rats bilateral frontal cortex lesions and compared them with age-matched controls, as well as to young lesioned and nonlesioned rats.[24] Both lesioned and nonlesioned aged rats learned the delayed spatial alternation task in about the same length of time, but were slower than the nonoperated young rats. The lesioned young rats, however, were severely impaired on the task. Stein and Firl suggested that the functions of the frontal lobes may be different at different points of the age span, and that early functions of the frontal lobes may be subserved by other parts of the brain later in life.[24]

To summarize, it is *not* the rule that early brain damage results in fewer deficits or greater recovery. Early brain damage may produce the same deficits as damage in adulthood, or an apparent initial sparing may be followed by greater deficits as the system (and the child) matures. The only instance of evidence for functional relocalization (speech) has a resultant cost: decreased normal function of the area to which speech has been relocated (visuospatial functional deficits). Finally, brain damage occurring late in the life span may also yield fewer or different deficits than that during midlife.

Differential Capacity for Recovery in Men and Women

A growing amount of evidence indicates morphologic and biochemical differences in the brains of men and women. During certain perinatal critical periods, exposure to sex hormones (estrogen, tes-

tosterone) influences the differentiation of certain aspects of brain function. Nance has shown that early exposure to androgens influences reproductive function regardless of the genetic sex of the animal.[25] He has also shown a similar effect of chronic exposure to androgens or estrogens during a critical period after septal lesions and suggested that the mechanisms of hormonal influence after lesions may be the same as those during normal development.

Roof et al. investigated the role of progesterone in limiting edema after brain damage by comparing brain edema in male, female, and pseudopregnant female rats 24 hours after experiencing controlled frontal cortex contusions[26]. Pseudopregnant female rats showed almost no edema, and male rats had significantly greater levels of edema when compared with either of the other groups. The authors hypothesized that the most notable difference among the three groups was the circulating levels of progesterone. A subsequent part of the study further tested this hypothesis by comparing posttraumatic cerebral edema in ovariectomized female rats 1) without hormone supplementation, 2) with estrogen implants, 3) with estrogen implants and progesterone injections, and 4) with progesterone injections alone. The results supported the presence of progesterone as the critical factor in limiting brain edema.[26]

Studies on the development of hemispheric specializations have demonstrated that men and women develop lateralizations of speech and visuospatial functions at different rates and to different degrees. Women are ultimately less highly lateralized in cortical functions than men. Also, some evidence suggests differences associated with gender in age-related changes in brain structure and metabolism.[27] Age-related decreases in total brain volume with age were greater in men than in women. This finding suggests that women may demonstrate greater sparing or recovery of function after brain damage.

Experience

Specific training, therapeutic intervention, and environmental exposures are experiential factors. In the cases of specific training and therapeutic intervention, the teacher or therapist encourages the client to perform certain activities that may enhance performance. Exposures to different environments may provide (or restrict) opportunities for generalized experiences.

Specific Training and Therapeutic Intervention

Numerous studies have demonstrated that representational maps in the somatosensory cortex in rats, cats, and monkeys may be altered by recent experiences of the animal. A growing body of evidence suggests that the same is true for the motor cortex—that is, experience of the animal leads to changes in the representations of movements.[28] Whether these changes in cortical representations provide some substrate for protection from deficits after brain injury is unclear.

Meager evidence in the literature supports the notion that specific training before brain injury leads to sparing of function after injury. Orbach and Fantz demonstrated that **overtraining** on various visual discrimination tests led to nearly total sparing of these skills after temporal neocortical damage in monkeys.[29] Similar findings were reported across modalities after brain injury in humans; those with previous experience with visual discrimination problems performed better on similar tactual problems than non–brain-injured control subjects without this prior experience.[30]

Conditioning also affects recovery. Preoperative conditioning of certain triggered responses, or voluntary acts, in monkeys later given pyramidal tract lesions led to an increase in the degree of recovery of responses that could not be elicited without such training, but monkeys demonstrated these responses only in the training situation and did not use them in spontaneous movements.[31] Goldberger suggested that the pathways mediating the conditioned responses may have been different from those mediating the unlearned movement. Therefore, the conditioned response would not have been affected by lesions to the areas subserving the unlearned movement.

Training after brain damage may also be important, if not critical, to recovery of function. In 1917, Ogden and Franz did one of the classic studies on the effect of postoperative training on therapy.[32] They destroyed motor cortex unilaterally, producing hemiplegia in monkeys. Postoperative training varied, as follows: 1) no treatment; 2) general massage to the involved limbs; 3) restraint of the noninvolved arm; and 4) a combination of restraint of the noninvolved arm, massage, and stimulation of the involved limbs to move using noxious stimuli at first, specific facilitation to more involved muscle groups, and forced active movement of the animal. The monkeys showed recovery in only the most rigorous and com-

prehensive condition (condition 4), but the recovery was complete within 3 weeks.[32] More recently, Black et al. removed the motor cortex forelimb area unilaterally and examined the effects of specific motor training in monkeys.[33] Training was given to the contralateral forelimb, the ipsilateral forelimb, or both forelimbs, initiated immediately or after 4 months, and lasting for 6 months. Training of the weak hand alone, or the weak and the normal hands together resulted in better recovery in the weak hand than did training in the normal hand alone. Training of both hands was no better than training the weak hand only. When training was delayed, final recovery was less complete than for those receiving immediate training.

Although still not well understood, many investigators have tested the hypothesis that the mechanism for recovery after brain damage is the reorganization of other parts of the nervous system to assume the function lost by the original lesion. Having established that training on specific motor tasks leads to expansion of motor representations in primary motor cortex of normal monkeys, Nudo and others studied changes in motor representations after focal cortical damage.[28,34] After lesions in the part of the primary motor cortex that represents the hand, animals had a decrease in the area of representation of the digits in the region immediately surrounding the lesion, and an increase in areas representing more proximal upper extremity segments. They found no evidence that movements originally represented in the lesioned region reappeared in the surrounding cortical tissue. In a follow-up study, monkeys received retraining of hand use, which prevented loss of representation of the hand in surrounding tissue. In some cases, the representation spread into areas that formerly represented more proximal portions of the upper limb.[34] This finding suggests that the reorganization depends on the specific training rather than general experience. In other studies, Schallert and colleagues have studied the effects of unilateral lesions to the forelimb areas of sensorimotor cortex in rats. They have found increased dendritic branching of pyramidal cells in the contralateral forelimb sensorimotor cortex if, and only if, the unimpaired forelimb is free to be used to compensate for the impaired limb.[35] Such growth of dendrites does not occur if the unimpaired limb is restrained. In addition, if the unimpaired limb is restrained immediately after the lesion to force the animal to use the impaired limb, the behavioral deficit is increased, with less ultimate recovery, accompanied by more neural injury. Thus, immediate forced use of the impaired limb appears to amplify the amount of secondary neuronal cell death that occurs after the brain lesion.

The findings of Schallert et al. may seem to contradict those of Nudo and associates. Taub, however, has suggested that there may be a critical period immediately after the injury that may coincide with the period of diaschisis, or neural shock, when forced use is detrimental.[36] He also suggested that when the animal attempts to use the impaired limb during this period of neural shock, it is usually unsuccessful. It therefore develops compensatory strategies that, if allowed to be used, lead to learned nonuse of the affected limb. This idea may be related to the findings of Schallert et al. that immediate forced use of the impaired limb after the lesion led to permanent behavioral deficit and greater neuronal cell death.[35] Nudo and colleagues, however, did not initiate rehabilitation training until 5 days after the lesion, which led to an expanded representation in the surrounding tissue as well as to behavioral recovery.[34] Perhaps this delay was long enough for the neural shock to decline, avoiding detrimental effects on the surrounding tissue. Then, use of the limb could cause the reorganization of the representational maps in undamaged areas. Taub and others have examined the strategy of forcing individuals with chronic stroke to use their impaired upper extremity by constraining the unimpaired limb, and have demonstrated functional improvements.[37] Therefore, therapeutic intervention too early may be detrimental, and may lead to prolonged functional deficits. After the period of neural shock, however, training or forced use of the impaired limb may lead to greater recovery.

Despite Taub and colleagues' interesting results, few clinical studies have addressed the effectiveness of therapy in the rehabilitation of neurologically impaired patients, and many of these studies have had negative results. A recent review of research on the efficacy of physical therapy in the management of cerebral palsy dating back to the 1940s suggested that some evidence supports the effectiveness of certain techniques under certain circumstances. In general, however, the available evidence does not support the notion of beneficial effects of physical therapy intervention on the motor problems of children with cerebral palsy.[38]

Several studies examining the effect of rehabilitation on outcome after stroke have demonstrated that functional performance improves over time. Unfor-

tunately, no control groups have been used to determine if rehabilitation was better than no therapy. Also, few studies have demonstrated any difference between different approaches to rehabilitation. The designs of many of the studies had numerous methodologic problems. Therefore, these results should not be accepted without further study. Unquestionably, sound clinical research is needed to evaluate the efficacy of therapy.

Environmental Exposures

The interest in studying the possible effects of environmental complexity on recovery of function is a direct outgrowth of evidence that differential environments affect anatomic and physiologic characteristics of the intact brain. Rosenzweig and Bennett varied the environments to which animals were exposed, and evaluated biochemical and morphologic differences between the brains of these animals after the exposure. Standard colony housing consists of a moderately sized cage housing four to six rats, and is sometimes described as "the social condition." Animals housed individually in small, rack-mounted or plastic laboratory cages are considered to be environmentally impoverished (IMP). The environment is considered enriched when several animals (6 to 12) are placed in a large cage with multiple levels, climbing apparatus, and "playthings" (Fig. 21–3). In animals with intact brains, exposure to the enriched environment was associated with increased cortical depth, increased brain weight, increased dendritic branching, and increased enzyme activity.[39]

Despite the apparently potent effect of enrichment on the physiology and anatomy of the CNS in normal animals, few studies have examined the effect of preoperative environmental exposures on recovery of function after brain damage. A differential effect of environment on exploratory behavior and fluid consumption was demonstrated among rats with septal lesions, but no environmental effect was shown on the learning of spatial alternation after septal lesions.[40] In exploratory behavior, animals reared in the enriched condition were more active than those in the standard colony and IMP groups. This finding is important because activity is usually decreased after septal lesions. Animals in the impoverished group consumed more fluid than those in the other two groups, although septal lesions usually lead to increased fluid consumption. Therefore, enrichment may have enhanced sparing of exploratory behavior,

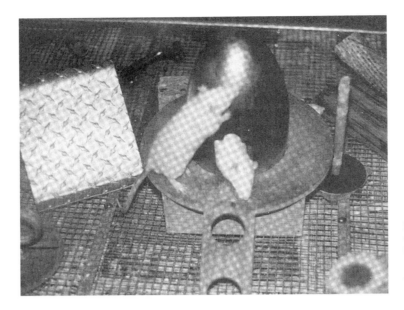

Figure 21-3. A view of the enriched environment used in the study by Held et al. Animals had enclosures, ramps, elevated platforms, a swing, climbing objects, wooden corks, and ping-pong balls to play with.

but impoverishment may have caused the deficits after septal lesions.

Smith and colleagues exposed rats to different environments before the removal of anterior or posterior cortex, and demonstrated that rats exposed to enrichment made fewer errors on the maze-learning problems than those that were impoverished. In fact enriched, lesioned animals performed better than impoverished animals without cortical damage.[41]

Held et al. evaluated the relative effects of preoperative or postoperative enrichment versus impoverishment on a constrained locomotor task with sensorimotor cortex lesions, and found that preoperative enrichment had a potent protective effect.[42] The animals that had been preoperatively enriched could run as rapidly as sham-operated control animals, and also demonstrated a normal pattern of hindlimb movement. In a follow-up study, Gentile et al. compared preoperative enrichment versus impoverishment to a third condition allowing exercise in a running wheel (WH), based on the hypothesis that the critical feature of an enriched environment is the opportunity for exercise to produce "fitness."[43] In this study, preoperative exposure to the enriched environment again led to sparing of constrained locomotion, whereas the IMP and WH animals were significantly impaired initially. The WH animals did recover

faster than the IMP animals. Therefore, enrichment yielded a protective effect, but exercise enhanced recovery. Unfortunately, it was not possible to discriminate between true restitution of function and compensation.

Postoperative effects of differential environmental exposures have been studied more extensively. Three studies explored the effects of environmental conditions to which rats were exposed after occipital cortex removals in neonates[44,45] or 30-day-old rats.[46] The enriched environmental exposure enhanced performance when begun immediately and lasting 60 days, or when begun 3 weeks later for 40 days,[45] and when the duration of exposure was reduced from 24 hours per day to 2 hours per day for 60 days.[46] Held et al. demonstrated that animals that had been enriched postoperatively (but not preoperatively) were initially less impaired on the locomotor task after sensorimotor cortex removals, and recovered more quickly than impoverished animals in terms of running times.[42] After their running times returned to preoperative levels, however, they still demonstrated an aberrant pattern of hindlimb movement.

Will et al. proposed three ways that enrichment might overcome the effects of lesions: 1) an increase in the number of synaptic connections may support the takeover of the functions lost; 2) it might protect against the loss of cortical cells in regions other than those lesioned; and 3) there might be a compensatory increase in RNA/DNA in hippocampus and ventral cortex.[46] Other processes that have been suggested to underlie enrichment effects are more rapid resolution of diaschisis; facilitation of effectiveness of silent synapses; facilitation of functional reorganization; and enhancement of the learning of multiple alternate strategies for problem solving.

From a clinical perspective, we might think of environment in relation to the setting in which the individual receives care during the recovery period. One study compared the outcomes of patients with stroke who were housed and treated on a stroke unit to patients in general wards.[47] Despite more physical therapy on the wards and comparable amounts of occupational therapy, the patients who received care on the stroke units recovered sooner, achieved higher scores on the Barthel Index (a functional skills assessment) at discharge, and had shorter hospital stays. Just as in the animal research on environmental enrichment, it is unclear what features of the stroke unit are responsible for the better outcomes. In another study, patients with stroke had better, more rapid recovery if they had high levels of social support.[48] Thus, environmental factors enhance recovery.

Pharmacologic Interventions

Some pharmacologic interventions may aid in recovery after brain damage. Such interventions may prevent glial scarring, stimulate excitability, and promote survival and growth. Although studies in the 1950s seemed to demonstrate a reduction in glial scarring after spinal cord transections in cats by using a pyrogenic substance, more recent attempts have failed to replicate these findings. For these reasons, drugs to prevent glial scarring are not discussed.

Research involving pharmacology in recovery from brain damage has grown dramatically since the mid-1980s. Ongoing studies are investigating the mechanisms behind a wide variety of endogenous substances that control neuronal and glial activity throughout the nervous system. Investigators are now looking into drugs to help in the prevention of neuronal death in a wide variety of conditions ranging from head trauma and epilepsy to stroke and Alzheimer's disease.

Facilitation, Inhibition, and Neurotransmitters

The stimulant, *d*-amphetamine, seems to facilitate some aspects of recovery. Meyer et al. reported the reinstatement of visual and tactile placing responses 1 year after decortication with the administration of *d*-amphetamine.[6] Further studies showed that *d*-amphetamine improved relearning of pattern discriminations after neocortex removals in rats and reinstated visual placing responses after visual cortex ablations. These effects were not maintained unless testing or retraining took place during the drug intoxication period.[49]

Feeney and Sutton found similar effects of *d*-amphetamine on recovery of constrained locomotion after sensorimotor cortex removals in rats and cats. Single doses of *d*-amphetamine 24 hours after surgery in rats or 10 days after surgery in cats produced immediate reinstatement of locomotion on a narrow beam. Again, experience during drug exposure was critical to the enhanced recovery.[49]

A single injection of haloperidol, a depressant, prevented recovery on the beam walking in rats for several weeks by blocking the effects of *d*-amphetamine. Haloperidol also reinstated deficits in placing responses in cats who had demonstrated recovery of placing approximately a year after cortical injury. Because haloperidol is a catecholamine blocker, *d*-amphetamine probably restores placing responses and locomotor capabilities through its agonistic action on catecholamines, particularly norepinephrine, which is a critical neurotransmitter.[49]

More recent investigations have compared the effects of injections of haloperidol, *d*-amphetamine, and saline on the performance of radial maze tasks in gerbils who have experienced global forebrain ischemia.[50] Results from this study supported the findings of previous studies. Gerbils treated with *d*-amphetamine demonstrated a reduction in the number of working memory errors more quickly than gerbils treated with saline. Conversely, the haloperidol-treated gerbils consistently made more errors than those in the *d*-amphetamine and saline groups.

The effects of *d*-amphetamine were also examined with hemiparetic stroke patients. Subjects were given one dose of *d*-amphetamine or a placebo, immediately followed by physical therapy. Patients who received *d*-amphetamine (a stimulant) performed better than the placebo group.[51] Unfortunately, haloperidol (a depressant) is often the drug used for the control of posttraumatic agitation in patients with head injury. For example, in clinical studies on the recovery of aphasia, subjects receiving various types of depressants (diazepam to control agitation and spasticity, or clonidine and methyldopa for hypertension) recover slower than those not on these medications.[49] Given these clinical studies, as well as the evidence from animal studies on the detrimental effects of catecholamine blockers on recovery of function after brain damage, depressants may be detrimental to recovery, and thus should be avoided unless absolutely necessary for medical reasons.

Some neurotransmitters have been examined to determine their effects on recovery after brain damage. Acetylcholine improves motor function after hemiplegia or brain trauma in rats, cats, monkeys, and humans, and improves cognitive functions in rats and humans with Alzheimer's disease. Dopamine and dopamine agonists enhance recovery after septal, basal ganglia and substantia nigra lesions. Gamma-aminobutyric acid, an inhibitory neurotransmitter, inhibits recovery after brain damage.[49] Further research is needed to examine other neurotransmitters regarding their influence on recovery.

Promotion of Survival and Growth

Since the mid-1980s, many studies have examined the specific cellular events that contribute to neuronal death after mechanical trauma, ischemia, hypoxia, hypoglycemia, and status epilepticus.[52] As investigators begin to understand the complex biochemical events that occur with almost any injury involving the brain, they are looking for ways to minimize the cellular death that occurs after the initial insult to the brain. Duhaime described components of a brain injury, which include *primary* and *delayed primary* injuries.[52] During the *primary* injury, irreversible neuronal death occurs at the immediate site of the lesion. *Delayed primary* injury is the term given to the additional loss of cells resulting from a cascade of biochemical events initiated at the time of the brain injury. This subsequent cell loss can be more detrimental to the patient than the effects of the initial injury or event. Therefore, many studies are aimed at learning more about the precise mechanisms involved in this biochemical cascade, so that methods of interrupting the process can be developed. Free radical scavengers, calcium channel blockers, and neurotransmitter modulators are among

a variety of compounds designed to interrupt the events leading to *delayed primary* injury.[53]

The role of amino acids as neurotransmitters has been examined extensively. Under pathologic conditions, such as stroke or traumatic brain injury, excitatory amino acids such as glutamate are released in excessive amounts. This release of excessive excitatory amino acids results in excitotoxicity, which ultimately leads to neuronal death.[52] After stroke, subsequent excitotoxic effects may proceed for hours or even days.[54]

As we have come to understand these processes better, research has focused on finding compounds that block excitotoxic events in the hope of limiting cell loss after brain injury. Research is investigating the effects of several neurotransmitter modulators in suppressing excitotoxicity.[49] Current experiments are looking at each of these drugs independently, but further studies may show that a combination of drugs results in better functional outcomes.[8] Many of the studies involving neuroprotective drug treatment for stroke have not yet progressed to the use of human subjects. The development of neuroprotective agents may lead to the ability to reduce the size of infarcts caused by stroke.[8]

Neuronotrophic factors are proteins that have one or more effects on neurons: promotion of the health and survival of nerve cells, stimulation and guidance of nerve fiber growth, or stimulation of the production of neurotransmitter-synthesizing enzymes. Nerve growth factor (NGF) was the first neuronotrophic factor discovered.[55] NGF has been found to affect cholinergic neurons in developing and adult brain. It is found endogenously in the CNS, and its concentrations increase in response to injury of the CNS of developing, mature, and aged rats.[56] Many other growth factors, as well as substances that specifically promote outgrowth of neuronal processes without other neuronotrophic activity, have been discovered and studied, as you learned in the chapter on support structures.

Nerve growth factor has been found to prevent cell death after axotomy caused by fimbria–fornix lesions.[49,57] It also facilitates behavioral recovery of learned habits after lesions of the caudate nucleus when administered at the time of bilateral damage.[58] Although initially impaired on a spatial reversal task, during the time they were tested, NGF-treated, lesioned animals recovered, whereas buffer-treated lesioned animals did not.

Deficiencies in **endogenous** neuronotrophic factors may account for certain types of degenerative nervous diseases.[59] Fischer et al. tested aged rats who had difficulties in identifying and remembering the location of a submerged platform in a swimming task, and rats who had no difficulties.[60] The impaired rats were divided into two groups, one receiving continuous infusion of NGF by an intraventricular cannula and one with the implanted cannula without infused substances. By 4 weeks after the beginning of NGF treatment, the treated group had reached performance levels of unimpaired rats, whereas the untreated, impaired rats showed little, if any, improvement. Thus, NGF has the ability to affect behavior in an animal model of aging with cognitive deficits when no lesions have been made. Varon et al. speculated that NGF treatment may be beneficial to patients with Alzheimer's disease or other age-related functional brain deficits.[59]

Several obstacles currently limit the beneficial effects of NGF in treating humans with Alzheimer's disease. Difficulty in delivering NGF to the target tissues remains a problem. NGF administered systematically does not cross the blood–brain barrier, necessitating some form of surgical administration. Researchers are now looking at other compounds that cross the blood–brain barrier and either stimulate production of NGF or enhance the effects of NGF.[61]

Gangliosides are substances that are endogenous to neuronal membranes and are highly concentrated in the CNS. Various authors have proposed that gangliosides promote sprouting, enhance the effects of NGF, reduce cerebral edema, and protect the Na^+/K^+ pump.[49] Behavioral effects of gangliosides after brain damage have also been reported. Karpiak demonstrated that treatment with gangliosides (after surgery, or before and after surgery) reduced the initial deficit and speeded recovery of a spatial alternation task after unilateral entorhinal cortex lesions.[62] The gangliosides also reduced surgical mortality. Sabel et al. reported that after ganglioside injections following bilateral caudate damage, rats demonstrated reduced deficits in spatial learning abilities.[63] Ganglioside treatments also have been shown to produce positive results in European clinical studies on diabetic and alcoholic **neuropathies**, polyneuropathies, and **dementias**. The actions by which gangliosides promote sprouting are poorly understood, limiting the clinical use of these substances.[64] Further

research is needed in this area before widespread use of gangliosides in humans is instituted.

Neural Transplantation

Research on fetal neural transplantation has been very productive. This paradigm involves the placement of neural tissue taken from aborted fetuses into the brains of host animals. Much of the work involving neural transplantation has been directed toward the treatment of Parkinson's disease because a good animal model of the disease is available and because this disorder primarily affects an isolated part of the brain and an isolated neurotransmitter.[65] Donor tissues have typically come from one of two sources: fetal neural tissue or tissue from the adrenal medulla of the host, used with the intention of implanting a living tissue that can synthesize dopamine. Fetal cell transplants have the supposed benefit of being more plastic, resulting in neural network reconstruction in the host brain.[66] Grafts from the adrenal medulla of the host (autografts), however, carry less risks of rejection by the host, and reduce the chance of infection. Ethical issues associated with the use of fetal tissues are also eliminated. Fetal neural transplants have been found to survive, become integrated in the host brain, and ameliorate behavioral deficits after brain injury in rats. The transplants may replace original circuitry, provide a source of neurotransmitters depleted by the damage, or provide neuronotrophic substances to enhance survival and growth of cells in the damaged host brain.

Parkinson's disease in rats has been the model used most extensively to examine the effects of fetal neural transplants. Studies in 1979 first demonstrated that transplants from fetal substantia nigra to dopamine-depleted striatum could survive, make connections with the host brain, and ameliorate motor symptoms caused by the damage.[67,68] Since then, a number of alterations of the paradigm have been tried. Blocks of fetal mesencephalon containing substantia nigra cells have been transplanted into cavities created through the cortex and corpus callosum, so that the transplants are next to the dorsal (Fig. 21–4A,C,E) or lateral surface of the striatum, or into the lateral ventricles, so that the transplants are next to the medial surface of the striatum (see Fig. 21–4A,C,F). These block transplants grew into the

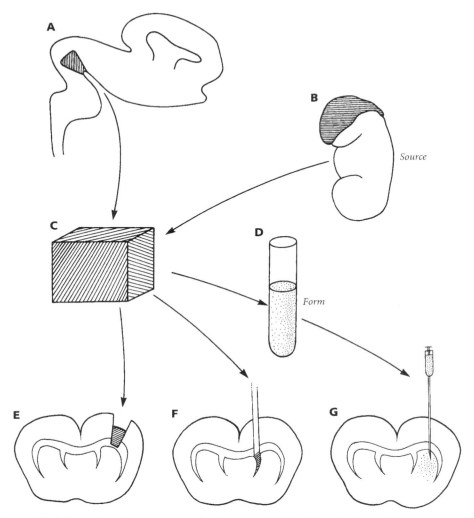

Figure 21–4. Transplantation procedures in the rat model of Parkinson's disease. Tissue was removed from the fetal mesencephalon *(A)* or the adrenal cortex *(B)*, in block form *(C)*, and either transplanted directly into cavities created in the cortex and corpus callosum next to the striatum *(E)* or into the lateral ventricle medial to the striatum *(F)*, or processed to produce a cell suspension *(D)* that is stereotaxically injected into the striatum *(G)*.

striatum and formed dense innervation within a few millimeters, and reduced the motor abnormalities by 50% to 100%.[69-71] Suspensions of fetal neurons were injected into the head of the caudate nucleus or into putamen (see Fig. 21–4A,C,D,G), innervated the striatum, and ameliorated behavioral deficits.[72] After adult chromaffin cells from the adrenal cortex were shown to transform into sympathetic neurons, adrenal cortex tissue was transplanted into the lat-

eral ventricles, or processed into **cell suspensions** and injected into the striatum of rats with induced Parkinson's syndrome (see Fig. 21–4B,C,F or B,C, D,G). This tissue survived and reduced behavioral deficits, although to a lesser degree than fetal substantia nigra tissue. These grafts did not form nerve processes; therefore, the chromaffin cells apparently produced dopamine which caused the behavior improvements.[71]

These techniques have now been used in humans with Parkinson's disease, with varying degrees of success. Transplants from the patient's own adrenal cortex, in the form of cell suspensions, as described previously, have produced modest and transient improvements in motor function.[73,74] Mexican neurosurgeons have developed an open surgical approach to placing pieces of adrenal cortex into a cavity in the head of the caudate nucleus.[75] They reported marked improvement in movement capabilities, accompanied by a reduction in rigidity. Reports of surgical complications and side effects, however, make this procedure less preferred.[71] Transplantation of human fetal substantia nigra tissue, in the form of cell suspensions, to people with Parkinson's disease has been done to a limited degree.[76] The results are promising; behavioral deficits have improved and performance has been maintained. Therefore, this approach is promising, although ethical concerns must still be resolved.

The use of neural transplantation in treating patients with Parkinson's disease remains experimental. A number of researchers are documenting a variety of outcomes, resulting from several different procedures. The actual number of patients having undergone this experimental surgical technique is unknown. Ahlskog reviewed outcomes up to 1993 and reported that no case had complete remission of symptoms. Even the patients who were markedly improved still had prominent signs of Parkinsonism.[65]

Several investigators have noted improved functional abilities in animal models of Parkinson's disease despite poor survival of grafted tissues.[65] Autopsy has revealed that in some animal models, even without survival of cerebral grafts, sprouting of endogenous dopaminergic tissues has occurred.[77,78] Investigators now believe that the benefits from these transplantations may not be related to the transplanted tissue's ability to produce dopamine. Instead, transplantation of these tissues may stimulate the host to begin sprouting tissues that produce dopamine.[65] Some of the tissues that have been used for transplantation are known to be sources of neurotrophic factors for dopaminergic neurons.[79] These neurotrophic factors may play critical roles in stimulating host tissues to begin to produce dopamine.[66]

One longitudinal study of subjects with advanced Parkinson's disease examined motor function and clinical recovery in 10 subjects 5 years after implantation of fetal ventral mesencephalic tissue.[80] All subjects demonstrated improvement 30 months after implantation and 7 of 10 subjects demonstrated improvement after 5 years. Despite their encouraging results, the authors caution that additional long-term studies are needed before such implantations can be considered as "a valid and therapeutic alternative" for patients with Parkinson's disease.[80]

Research into the transplantation of genetically engineered cell lines is in its infancy. Cells that would produce either dopamine or neurotrophic factors could potentially be engineered and implanted into the brains of patients with Parkinson's disease.[65] Although ethical concerns related to the use of fetal tissue would be eliminated, a variety of new ethical and logistical questions would be brought to light. Complications, including immune system rejection and the potential for tumor formation or transmission of viral infections, need further attention.

Transplants to other areas of the brain have also been successful in enhancing recovery after injury. Several laboratories have demonstrated short-term improvements in spatial alternation task performances after fetal frontal cortex transplants into damaged frontal cortex. Dunnett et al. demonstrated that on long-term follow-up, animals who had received fetal transplants performed worse than lesioned animals, suggesting that either the transplants caused a decrement in performance over time or prevented normal recovery processes.[81] Stein et al. also demonstrated improvement on a brightness discrimination task in animals who first received visual cortex lesions, followed by fetal frontal or occipital cortex transplants.[82] Surprisingly, the animals who received frontal cortex transplants into visual cortex performed better than those that received visual cortex transplants. The reason for this difference is unknown.

Many issues remain to be resolved in the area of fetal transplantation, including the optimal fetal age of the tissue to be transplanted, the questionable need for the transplant to be from the same region of brain to which it will be placed in the host brain, the optimal time after initial brain damage for transplantation, the risks of using fetal transplants, the precise procedures that are the most beneficial, and the effectiveness of transplantation used in the case of progressive degenerative diseases. It is also unknown whether it is the recreation of original circuitry that is critical to behavioral recovery, or the neurotransmitters or neurotrophic factors produced by the transplant.

As more is learned about transplantation, these techniques may be applied to other disorders. For example, studies are investigating the effects of fetal cell transplants on animal models of Huntington's disease. Current research may ultimately lead to neurosurgical treatment techniques for a variety of disorders ranging from Alzheimer's disease to spinal cord injury, traumatic brain injury, and stroke.

Clinical Correlations

Therapists who work with clients with CNS damage should understand the theories and scientific basis, or lack thereof, for the treatment approaches they use. The literature reviewed in this chapter supports the following concepts: 1) recovery is possible, 2) prognosis varies depending on many factors, and 3) therapists play important roles in enhancing recovery of function after brain damage.

Recovery Is Possible

The information presented in this chapter supports the notion that true recovery is possible under certain circumstances; because the definition of recovery has been loosely defined in both the clinical and research worlds, however, some of the findings probably represent compensation rather than true recovery. We must establish valid and reliable measurement tools that will not only help us to document improvements in our clients, but actually discriminate restitution of function from compensatory strategies. In the meantime, research findings suggest that if compensation is allowed, true recovery will not happen. Therefore, we must make wise decisions about when to intervene to prevent compensation, even if it means a slight delay in functional progress, because compensation is rarely as efficient and effective as normal functioning.

Prognosis Varies

The literature suggests that with lesions to certain regions of the brain, fewer deficits may result in neonates and in aged people than in mature adults. The long-term implications of those findings are complex. Deficits may develop later in the neonate, reflecting the loss of the damaged area or the limited capacity of other regions that have taken over the function of the area originally damaged. The aged patient may have already experienced age-related decrements in function, so that brain injury does not produce any greater deficit.

The research also suggests that deficits and potential for recovery may differ with the type of damage. Slowly developing lesions often produce fewer deficits than lesions that are produced all at once. Closed head injuries may produce different effects on the nervous system than cerebrovascular accidents, therefore causing different degrees and types of deficits, as well as potential for recovery. In fact, cerebrovascular accidents caused by thrombus may differ from those that are caused by hemorrhage.

Research on the effects of the environment suggests that the background, or premorbid experiences, of the patient may have important effects on the response to brain injury. In addition, the environment in which patients live and receive treatment after the damage will undoubtedly be critical. The typical acute care hospital (and many rehabilitation facilities) is essentially an impoverished environment in which we expect our clients to improve. Enriching the institutional environments should facilitate recovery.

The Role of Therapists

Clearly, as therapists we believe that our treatments are effective in enhancing recovery after brain damage, but we must examine what we do and how we do it. Research suggests that relatively early intervention is more effective than later intervention, and that the more intense the therapy, the better the outcome. With pressures being applied to cut health care costs, we must remember that the real desire is for cost effectiveness. Therefore, more intense therapy given early may be more effective, and therefore cost less than less intense therapy for longer periods with poorer results.

Does this intensity make a difference in the long-term cost to society? Do clients who receive less intense therapy require more services for the remainder of their lives than those who have the opportunity for intense, effective rehabilitation? Experimental results suggest that although the greatest amount of recovery occurs within a short period after the damage, recovery can continue for several years. Therefore, periodic reevaluations and selective intervention should not be ruled out in long-term cases.

The more specific the training, the better the functional outcome. In other words, to improve performance of specific motor skills, we should emphasize acquisition of that skill. From the motor learning and exercise physiology literature, we know that very little transfer of training occurs. For this reason we must question whether the emphasis on "normal movement patterns" in many of the traditional therapeutic approaches is really effective if these patterns are promoted outside of the context of specific, goal-directed tasks.

Finally, the literature suggests that therapy is critical in conjunction with drugs, transplantation, or other surgical interventions. Without therapy, these other interventions may not be effective at all.

As therapists who work with neurologically impaired populations, we have an obligation to carry out more clinical research studies to demonstrate clearly, carefully, and convincingly that therapy is effective. For the purpose of cost containment we must also determine which approaches are most effective under various conditions. Finally, we must coordinate our research with that of basic scientists to understand the mechanisms of action of our effective therapeutic approaches so that we may continually improve our techniques and develop new ones.

REFERENCES

1. Almli CR, Finger S. Toward a definition of recovery of function. In: Finger S, LeVere THE, Almli CR, Stein DG, eds. *Brain injury and recovery: theoretical and controversial issues*. New York: Plenum Press, 1988:1–14.
2. Lee RG, van Donkelaar P. Mechanisms underlying functional recovery following stroke. *Can J Neurol Sci* 1995; 22:257–263.
3. Silvestrini M, Troisi E, Matteis M, Cupini LM, Caltagirone C. Involvement of the healthy hemisphere in recovery from aphasia and motor deficit in patients with cortical ischemic infarction: a transcranial Doppler study. *Neurology* 1995;45:1815–1820.
4. Luria AR, Naydin VL, Tsvetkova LS, Vinarskays EN. Restoration of higher cortical function following local brain damage. In: Vinken RJ, Bruyn GW, eds. *Handbook of Clinical Neurology*. Vol. 3. Amsterdam: North Holland, 1969;3:368–433.
5. Von Monakow C. Diaschisis. In: Pribram KH, ed. *Brain and behavior: I. mood states and minds*. Baltimore: Penguin Publishers, 1969:27–36.
6. Meyer PM, Horel JA, Meyer DR. Effects of *d*-amphetamine upon placing responses in neodecorticate cats. *J Comp Physiol Psychol* 1963;56:402–404.
7. LeVere TE. Recovery of function after brain damage: a theory of the behavioral deficit. *Physiol Psychol* 1980;8: 297–308.
8. Koroshetz WJ, Moskowitz MA. Emerging treatments for stroke in humans. *Trends Pharmacol Sci* 1996;17:227–233.
9. Florence SL, Kaas JH. Large-scale reorganization at multiple levels of the somatosensory pathway follows therapeutic amputation of the hand in monkeys. *J Neurosci* 1995;15:8083–8095.
10. Kennard MA. Age and other factors in motor recovery from precentral lesions in monkeys. *Am J Physiol* 1936;115:138–146.
11. Glees P, Cole J. Recovery of skilled motor functions after small repeated lesions in motor cortex in macaque. *J Neurophysiol* 1950;13:137–148.
12. Travis AM, Woolsey CN. Motor performance of monkeys after bilateral partial and total cerebral decortications. *Am J Phys Med* 1956;35:273–310.
13. Gentile AM, Held JM, Muzii R. Recovery of locomotion following symmetrical and asymmetrical serial lesions in rats. *Soc Neurosci Abstr* 1980;6:650.
14. Finger S. Lesion momentum and behavior. In: Finger S, ed. *Recovery from brain damage: research and theory*. New York: Plenum Press, 1978:135–164.
15. Finger S, Walbran B, Stein DG. Brain damage and behavioral recovery: serial lesion phenomena. *Brain Res* 1973;63:1–18.
16. Isaacson RL, Spear LP. A new perspective for the interpretation of early brain damage. In: Finger S, Almli CR, eds. *Early brain damage: volume 2, neurobiology and behavior*. New York: Academic Press, 1984:73–98.
17. Kennard MA. Relation of age to motor impairment in man and in subhuman primates. *Archives of Neurology and Psychiatry* 1940;44:377–397.
18. Hicks SP, D'Amato CJ. Motor-sensory and visual behavior after hemispherectomy in newborn and mature rats. *Exp Neurol* 1970;29:416–438.
19. Smith RL, Parks T, Lynch G. A comparison of the role of the motor cortex in recovery from cerebellar damage in young and adult rats. *Behav Biol* 1974;12:177–198.
20. Yager JY, Shuaib A, Thornhill J. The effect of age on susceptibility to brain damage in a model of global hemispheric hypoxia-ischemia. *Dev Brain Res* 1996;93:143–154.
21. Milner B. Sparing of language function after early unilateral brain damage. *Neurosci Res Program Bull* 1974; 12:213–217.
22. Rasmussen T, Milner B. The role of early left-brain injury in determining lateralization of cerebral speech functions. *Ann NY Acad Sci* 1977;299:355–368.
23. LeVere ND, Gray-Silva S, LeVere TE. Infant brain injury: the benefit of relocation and the cost of crowding. In: Finger S, LeVere TE, Almli CR, Stein DG, eds. *Brain injury and recovery: theoretical and controversial issues*. New York: Plenum Press, 1988:133–150.

24. Stein DG, Firl A. Brain damage and reorganization of function in old age. *Exp Neurol* 1976;52:157–167.
25. Nance DM. Sex-steroid-induced alterations in the behavioral effects of brain damage. In: Finger S, Almli CR, eds. *Early brain damage: volume 2, neurobiology and behavior.* New York: Academic Press, 1984:313–325.
26. Roof R, Duvdevani R, Stein D. Gender influences outcome of brain injury: progesterone plays a protective role. *Brain Res* 1993;607:333–336.
27. Murphy DGM, DeCarli C, McIntosh AR, et al. Sex differences in human brain morphometry and metabolism: an in vivo quantitative magnetic resonance imaging and positron emission tomography study on the effect of aging. *Arch Gen Psychiatry* 1996;53:585–594.
28. Nudo RJ, Milliken GW, Jenkins WM, Merzenich MM. Use-dependent alterations of movement representations in primary motor cortex of adult squirrel monkeys. *J Neurosci* 1996;16:785–807.
29. Orbach J, Fantz RL. Differential effects of temporal neocortical resections on overtrained and non-overtrained visual habits in monkeys. *J Comp Physiol Psychol* 1958;51:126–129.
30. Weinstein S, Teuber HL. The role of preinjury education and intelligence level in intellectual loss after brain injury. *J Comp Physiol Psychol* 1957;50:535–539.
31. Goldberger ME. Recovery of movement after CNS lesions in monkeys. In: Stein DG, Rosen JJ, Butters N, eds. *Plasticity and recovery of function in the central nervous system.* New York: Academic Press, 1974:265–338.
32. Ogden R, Franz SI. On cerebral motor control: the recovery from experimentally produced hemiplegia. *Psychobiology* 1917;1:33–49.
33. Black P, Markowitz RS, Cianci SN. Recovery of motor function after lesions in motor cortex of monkey. *Ciba Found Symp* 1975;34:65–83.
34. Nudo RJ, Wise BM, SiFuentes F, Milliken GW. Neural substrates for the effects of rehabilitative training on motor recovery after ischemic infarct. *Science* 1996;272:1791–1794.
35. Schallert T, Kozlowski DA, Humm JL, Cocke RR. Use-dependent structural events in recovery of function. *Brain Plasticity, Adv Neurol* 1997;73:229–238.
36. Taub E. Constraint induced movement therapy: a new family of treatments for rehabilitation of movement after stroke. Presented at the Teachers College, Columbia University Conference on Movement Disorders Associated with Aging, April 5, 1997, New York.
37. Taub E, Miller NE, Novack TA, et al. Techniques to improve chronic motor deficit after stroke. *Arch Phys Med Rehabil* 1993;74:347–354.
38. Campbell SK, ed. Proceedings of the consensus conference on the efficacy of physical therapy in the management of cerebral palsy. *Pediatr Phys Ther* 1990; 2:121–176.
39. Rosenzweig MR, Bennett EL. Effects of differential environments on brain weights and enzyme activities in gerbils, rats, and mice. *Dev Psychobiol* 1969;2:87–95.
40. Donovick PJ, Burright RG, Swidler MA. Presurgical rearing environment alters exploration, fluid consumption, and learning of septal lesioned and control rats. *Physiol Behav* 1973;11:543–553.
41. Smith RL, Parks T, Lynch G. A comparison of the role of the motor cortex in recovery from cerebellar damage in young and adult rats. *Behav Biol* 1974;12:177–198.
42. Held JM, Gordon J, Gentile AM. Environmental influences on locomotor recovery following cortical lesions in rats. *Behav Neurosci* 1985;99:678–690.
43. Gentile AM, Beheshti Z, Held JM. Enrichment versus exercise effects on motor impairment following cortical removals in rats. *Behav Neural Biol* 1987;47:321–332.
44. Schwartz S. Effects of neonatal cortical lesions and early environmental factors on adult rat behavior. *J Comp Physiol Psychol* 1964;57:72–77.
45. Will BE, Rosenzweig MR, Bennett EL. Effects of differential environments on recovery from neonatal brain lesions, measured by problem-solving scores and brain dimensions. *Physiol Behav* 1976;16:603–611.
46. Will BE, Rosenzweig MR, Bennett EL, Hebert M, Morimoto H. Relatively brief environmental enrichment aids recovery of learning capacity and alters brain measures after postweaning brain lesions in rats. *J Comp Physiol Psychol* 1977;91:33–50.
47. Kalra L. The influence of stroke unit rehabilitation on functional recovery from stroke. *Stroke* 1994;25:821–825.
48. Glass TA, Matchar DB, Belyea M, Feussner JR. Impact of social support on outcome in first stroke. *Stroke* 1993;24:64–70.
49. Feeney DM, Sutton RL. Pharmacotherapy for recovery of function after brain injury. *Crit Rev Neurobiol* 1987;3:135–197.
50. Wishart TB, Ijaz S, Shuaib A. Differential effects of amphetamine and haloperidol on recovery after global forebrain ischemia. *Pharmacol Biochem Behav* 1994;47:963–968.
51. Crisostomo EA, Duncan PW, Propst MA, Dawson DB, Davis JN. Evidence that amphetamine with physical therapy promotes recovery of motor function in stroke patients. *Ann Neurol* 1988;23:94–97.
52. Duhaime AC. Exciting your neurons to death: can we prevent cell loss after brain injury? *Pediatr Neurosurg* 1994;21:117–123.
53. Siesjo BK. Pathophysiology and treatment of focal cerebral ischemia: part II. mechanisms of damage and treatment. *J Neurosurg* 1992;77:337–354.
54. Kirino T, Tamura A, Sano K. Delayed neuronal death in the rat hippocampus following transient forebrain ischemia. *Acta Neuropathol* 1984;64:139–147.

55. Levi-Montalcini R, Calissano,P. The nerve growth factor. *Sci Am* 1979;176:297–310.

56. Nieto-Sampedro M, Cotman CW. Growth factor induction and temporal order in central nervous system repair. In: Cotman CW, ed. *Synaptic plasticity*. New York: Guilford Press, 1985:407–455.

57. Kromer LF. Nerve growth factor treatment after brain injury prevents neuronal death. *Science* 1987;235:214–216.

58. Hart T, Chaimas N, Moore RY, Stein DG. Effects of nerve growth factor on behavioral recovery following caudate nucleus lesions in rats. *Brain Res Bull* 1978;3: 245–250.

59. Varon S, Hagg T, Manthorpe M. Neuronal growth factors. In: Seil FJ, ed. *Neural regeneration and transplantation*. New York: Alan R. Liss, 1989:101–121.

60. Fischer W, Wictorin K, Bjorklund A, Williams LR, Varon S, Gage FH. Amelioration of cholinergic neuron atrophy and spatial memory impairment in aged rats by nerve growth factor. *Nature* 1987;329:65–68.

61. Aisen P, Davis K. The search for disease-modifying treatment for Alzheimer's disease. *Neurology* 1997;48(Suppl 6):S35–S41.

62. Karpiak SE. Exogenous gangliosides enhance recovery from CNS injury. In: Ledeen RW, Yu RK, Rapport MM, Suzuki K, eds. *Ganglioside structure, function, and biomedical potential*. New York: Plenum Press, 1984:489–497.

63. Sabel BA, Slavin MD, Stein DG. GM1 ganglioside treatment facilitates behavioral recovery from bilateral brain damage. *Science* 1984;225:340–342.

64. Riggott M, Matthew W. Neurite outgrowth is enhanced by anti-idiotypic monoclonal antibodies to the ganglioside GM1. *Exp Neurol* 1997:145;278–287.

65. Ahlskog E. Cerebral transplantation for Parkinson's disease: current progress and future prospects. *Mayo Clin Proc* 1993;68:578–591.

66. Date I. Parkinson's disease, trophic factors, and adrenal medullary chromaffin cell grafting: basic and clinical studies. *Brain Res Bull* 1996;40:1–19.

67. Bjorklund A, Stenevi U. Reconstruction of the nigrostriatal dopamine pathway by intracerebral nigral transplants. *Brain Res* 1979;177:555–560.

68. Perlow M, Freed W, Hoffer B, Seiger A, Olson L, Wyatt R. Brain grafts reduce motor abnormalities produced by destruction of nigrostriatal dopamine system. *Science* 1979; 204:643–647.

69. Dunnett SB, Bjorklund A, Stenevi U. Dopamine-rich transplants in experimental parkinsonism. *Trends Neurosci* 1983;6:266–270.

70. Iversen SD, Dunnett SB. Functional compensation afforded by grafts of foetal neurones. *Prog Neuropsychopharmacol Biol Psychiatry* 1989;13:453–467.

71. Olson L. Grafts and growth factors in CNS: basic science with clinical promise. *Stereotact Funct Neurosurg* 1990;54 & 55:250–267.

72. Bjorklund A, Gage FH, Dunnett SB, Stenevi U. Regenerative capacity of central neurons as revealed by intracerebral grafting experiments. In: Bignami A, Bloom FE, Bolis CL, Adeloye A, eds. *Central nervous system plasticity and repair*. New York: Raven Press, 1985:57–62.

73. Backlund E-O, Granberg PO, Hamberger B, et al. Transplantation of adrenal medullary tissue to striatum in parkinsonism: first clinical trials. *J Neurosci* 1985;62: 169–173.

74. Lindvall O, Backlund E-O, Farde L, et al. Transplantation in Parkinson's disease: two cases of adrenal medullary grafts to putamen. *Ann Neurol* 1987;22:457–468.

75. Madrazo I, Drucker-Colin R, Diaz V, Martinez-Mata J, Torres C, Becerril JJ. Open microsurgical autograft of adrenal medulla to the right caudate nucleus in two patients with intractable Parkinson's disease. *N Engl J Med* 1986;316:831–834.

76. Lindvall O. Transplantation into the human brain: present status and future possibilities. *J Neurol Neurosurg Psychiatry* 1989;(Suppl):39–54.

77. Bohn MC, Cupit L, Marciano F, Gash DM. Adrenal medulla grafts enhance recovery of striatal dopaminergic fibers. *Science* 1987;237:913–916.

78. Hansen JT, Kordower JH, Fiandaca MS, et al. Adrenal medullary autografts into the basal ganglia of cebus monkeys: graft viability and fine structure. *Exp Neurol* 1988;102:65–75.

79. Unsicker K. The trophic cocktail made by adrenal chromaffin cells. *Exp Neurol* 1993;123:167–173.

80. Lopez-Lozano J, Bravo G, Brera B, et al. Long-term improvement in patients with severe Parkinson's disease after implantation of fetal ventral mesencephalic tissue in a cavity of the caudate nucleus: 5-year follow up in 10 patients. *J Neurosurg* 1997;86:931–942.

81. Dunnett SB, Ryan, CN, Levin PD, Reynolds M, Bunch ST. Functional consequences of embryonic neocortex transplanted to rats with prefrontal cortex lesions. *Behav Neurosci* 1987;101:489–503.

82. Stein DG, Labbe R, Attella MJ, Rakowsky HA. Fetal brain tissue transplants reduce visual deficits in adult rats with bilateral lesions of the occipital cortex. *Behav Neural Biol* 1985;44:266–277.

Glossary

•
•
•
•
•
•

3'5'-Cyclic adenosine monophosphate (cAMP; cyclic AMP): a second messenger in cells that is formed by activation of the enzyme adenylate cyclase. Adenylate cyclase splits adenosine triphosphate (ATP), releasing two phosphate molecules to form cAMP. cAMP, in turn, regulates the activity of protein kinase A (PKA).

5-HT: see *serotonin*.

Abducens nerve: cranial nerve VI, which innervates the lateral rectus muscle of the eye.

Abduction: yaw rotation of the eye away from the midline; the eye looks away from the nose.

Ablation: removal of a part of the brain, usually by cutting or aspiration.

Absolute refractory period: the interval after the discharge of an action potential during which the membrane cannot be stimulated to discharge another action potential regardless of the strength of the stimulus.

Accessory optic tract: projection from the optic tract to the dorsal cap of the inferior olivary nucleus.

Accommodation: adjustment of the lens of the eye to focus at various distances, especially associated with focusing for short distances.

Acetylcholine: neurotransmitter composed of an acetyl group and a choline group; a neurotransmitter released at cholinergic synapses. In the periphery, acetylcholine is the neurotransmitter for the somatic nervous system, all preganglionic neurons of the autonomic nervous system, postganglionic parasympathetic neurons, and sympathetic innervation to eccrine sweat glands.

Acetylcholine receptor sites: molecules located on the muscle membrane at the neuromuscular junction that recognize and bind with acetylcholine.

Acetylcholinesterase: an enzyme that catalyzes the hydrolysis of acetylcholine to choline and acetic acid.

Acoustic nerve: synonymous with *auditory nerve*.

Acoustic neuroma: a benign tumor of the Schwann cells of the vestibular nerve.

Action potential: the explosive change in membrane potential that results from a rapid and massive movement of ions across the membrane of excitable cells such as neurons, usually in response to a stimulus that causes a change in the ion conductance across the membrane.

Active tension: the tension produced in a muscle by cross-bridge activity (forms part of muscle length–force relation).

Activity-dependent neuromodulation (ADM): a form of associative neuronal plasticity in which contiguous activity in a facilitatory neuron and a postsynaptic cell produce pairing-specific changes in the properties of the postsynaptic cell. ADM is believed to contribute to associative learning in *Aplysia*.

Adaptation: in general, a decrease over time in sensory response to a maintained stimulus: 1) in the auditory system, the change in firing rate of a nerve caused by the depletion of neurotransmitter in the hair cell; 2) in the vestibular system, the change in the magnitude of the reflex response after repeated experience with a stimulus (i.e., a learned behavior). Note the differences in meaning when used in reference to different levels of analysis of the system.

Adduction: yaw rotation of the eye toward the midline; the eye looks toward the nose.

Adenosine triphosphate (ATP): a high-energy phosphate compound that is the energy storehouse of the body. ATP liberates energy for the synthesis of chemical compounds.

Adenylyl cyclase (AC): an enzyme that catalyzes the production of a second messenger, specifically 3'5'-cyclic adenosine monophosphate (cAMP).

Adequate stimulus: the necessary and sufficient input to a particular sensory system.

Adhesion: one of the mechanisms used by cells to migrate and extend their dendritic and axonal processes. A nerve cell can adhere to another nerve cell or to a glial cell as well as to the extracellular matrix.

Adrenaline: a neurotransmitter, one of the catecholamines.

Adrenergic: associated with catecholamine neurotransmission or catecholamine receptors.

Adrenergic neurons: nerve cells that release epinephrine as a neurotransmitter at a synapse.

Aerobic metabolism: metabolic process occurring in the presence of free oxygen.

Affective defense behavior: a form of aggressive behavior that is elicited by stimulation of the medial hypothalamus or dorsal aspect of the midbrain periaqueductal gray of the cat. It is characterized by marked autonomic signs such as increased heart rate and blood pressure, pupillary dilation, piloerection, hissing and growling, arching of the back, unsheathing of the claws, and striking at a moving object in its visual field.

Afference: input.

Afferent: going from the periphery toward the central nervous system.

Afferent element: the component of a system that carries information toward a central point; the afferent element of a synapse carries an action potential toward the synapse.

Afferent nerve: a nerve that carries sensory information from the periphery toward the central nervous system. Synonymous with *sensory nerve*.

Ageusia: loss of taste sensation.

Aging: synonymous with *senescence*.

Agonist: an agent that binds to a target organ receptor and produces an excitatory or inhibitory response. Agonists can be endogenous neurotransmitters or drugs.

Akinesia: poverty or absence of movement.

Akinetopsia: inability to perceive objects in motion. Perception of stationary objects is unimpaired.

Alar plate: the part of the developing neural tube concerned mainly with the reception of sensory afferents, delimited from the basal plate by the sulcus limitans in the wall of the neurocele. In the adult, it corresponds to the dorsal horn of the spinal cord and the part of the brainstem lateral to the sulcus limitans in the floor of the ventricle.

Alkaloids: ring compounds of plant origin that contain nitrogen and combine with acids to form bitter salts.

Alpha$_1$-adrenergic receptor: an adrenergic target organ receptor that is normally stimulated by sympathetic neural release of norepinephrine. This receptor mediates primarily excitatory effects except in the gastrointestinal tract, where inhibition occurs.

Alpha$_2$-adrenergic receptor: an adrenergic receptor found predominantly on presynaptic nerve terminals. It inhibits release of norepinephrine from these nerve terminals.

Amacrine cells: neurons without axons, the cell bodies of which are located in the inner nuclear layer of the retina. They synapse with ganglion cells and bipolar cells.

AMPA receptor: a type of glutamate receptor that is activated by the glutamate agonist against alpha-amino-3-hydroxy-5-methyl-4-isoxazolepropionate (AMPA).

Ampullae: the specialized receptor areas in the semicircular canals of the vestibular labyrinth. At the ampulla, the canal is wider to accommodate the crista ampullaris.

Amygdala: one of the basal ganglia; the large, almond-shaped ganglion in the anterior medial portion of the temporal lobe, which is involved in mediation of emotions.

Anabolism: creation of energy stores.

Anaerobic metabolism: metabolic process occurring in the absence of free oxygen.

Anastomose: to communicate by joining together; many blood vessels in the brain anastomose, increasing the innervating blood supply of a region.

Anatomical position: the standard reference position of the human (i.e., standing erect, facing forward, palms outward).

Anencephaly: a developmental defect; incomplete development of the brain results from the failure of the anterior neuropore to close. Anencephalic infants are usually lacking a forebrain and may also lack the entire cerebrum and diencephalon.

Anesthesia: the numbing effect of a substance that blocks sensory input to the nervous system, commonly used to block pain.

Anhidrosis: absence or loss of sweating.

Anomalous: markedly different from normal.

Anosmia: loss of smell sensation.

Antagonist: a substance that binds to a receptor and produces no response, thereby blocking or -interrupting the actions of agonist agents on the receptor.

Anterior: toward the front.

Anterior canal: synonymous with *superior vertical canal*. The most anterior of the semicircular canals of the vestibular labyrinth. It detects pitch rotation of the head.

Anterior commissure: a bundle of nerve fibers interconnecting the two sides of the cerebrum, including projections from the olfactory bulb and amygdala on each side. It passes through the head of the caudate nucleus.

Anterograde axoplasmic transport: the ratchet-like mechanism used to transport substances from the neuron soma to the periphery of its processes.

Aphasia: a disturbance in language expression or comprehension, usually as a result of brain damage.

Aplysia: a marine mollusk used in neuroscience to investigate learning and memory at the level of nerve cells.

Apnea: transient suspension of respiration.

Apraxia: loss of ability to carry out purposeful movements in the absence of paralysis or sensory loss.

Aqueous humor: the clear, watery fluid that fills the anterior and posterior chambers of the eye. It provides metabolic support to the cornea and lens of the eye.

Arachnoid: the highly vascularized middle layer of the meninges.

Arachnoid villi: protruding tissue processes of the arachnoid that are involved in cerebrospinal fluid reabsorption.

Astrocyte: star-shaped neuroglial cell of ectodermal origin that surrounds neurons in the central nervous system.

Ataxia: impairment or irregularity of muscle action, resulting in an inability to coordinate movements; may be associated with hypotonia, dyssynergy, and unusual postures.

Atherosclerosis: a degenerative arterial disease that can lead to reduced blood flow in blocked vessels.

Auditory: referring to hearing or the ear.

Auditory brainstem response (ABR): the recording of brain activity in response to tones or click stimuli presented to a person through earphones. The recorded brain activity represents the synchronous firing of auditory nuclei along the auditory pathway to the inferior colliculus.

Auditory labyrinth: obsolete name for the *cochlea*.

Auditory nerve: cranial nerve VIII, a double nerve, which includes the cochlear nerve, innervating the cochlea, and the vestibular nerve, innervating the vestibular labyrinth.

Autogenic facilitation: reflex activation of a muscle through activation of its own sensory receptors.

Autogenic inhibition: reflex inhibition of a muscle through activation of its own sensory receptors.

Autonomic dysreflexia: condition found in patients with high spinal cord lesions above T6–T7 where a potentially profound, reflexive increased sympathetic outflow occurs because of activation of sympathetic afferent nerves. Also called *sympathetic hyperreflexia*.

Autonomic nervous system: the component of the peripheral nervous system that controls smooth muscle, glands, and cardiac muscle. The autonomic nervous system comprises two major divisions, the sympathetic and the parasympathetic nervous systems. Also called the visceral, vegetative, and involuntary nervous system.

Autophosphorylation: a process in which kinase attaches phosphate molecules to itself, thereby regulating its own activity. This process can be used to turn the kinase off or on, thus increasing or decreasing the duration of inactivity or activity, respectively.

Autoradiography: a neuroanatomic technique used to trace a fiber pathway in the nervous system by using compounds labeled with minute amounts of radioactive substances that are incorporated into neurons.

Axon: one of the neuronal processes, responsible for propagating electrical messages from the neuron soma toward the periphery. Most neurons have only one axon each.

Axon hillock: that portion of the neuron soma that tapers into the initial segment of an axon.

Axoplasm: cytoplasm contained inside the boundary of the unit membrane of an axon.

Axotomy: the severing of an axon.

Babinski's sign: an indicator of central nervous system damage. It includes extension of the great toe and abduction of the toes in response to stroking of the sole of the foot.

Bacterial meningitis: a disease state characterized by inflammation of the meninges often due to a bacterial infection.

Bandpass filter: a device that selectively attenuates frequencies above and below a band of frequencies selected to "pass through" the filter.

Baroreceptors: sensory receptors found primarily in the aortic arch and carotid sinus regions. These sensory receptors respond to stretch of blood vessels due to changes in blood pressure, and thus send sensory or afferent information regarding the level of blood pressure to the central nervous system.

Basal ganglia: the deep subcortical nuclei of the cerebrum.

Basal lamina: a layer of extracellular matrix that surrounds most blood vessels.

Basal plate: the part of the developing neural tube comprising mainly the motor regions. In the adult, it corresponds to the ventral horn of the spinal cord and the part of the brainstem medial to the sulcus limitans in the floor of the ventricle.

Basilar artery: a major brain artery that is formed by the vertebral arteries at the brainstem; it anastomoses with the internal carotid arteries to form the circle of Willis.

Basilar membrane: a membrane that forms the floor of the cochlear duct or scala media of the cochlea. The organ of Corti, containing the sensory transducers of the cochlea, rests on top of the basilar membrane.

Bed nucleus of the stria terminalis: the nucleus of the stria terminalis, located in the dorsomedial part of the forebrain adjacent to the head of the caudate nucleus and the septal area. It receives an important input from the amygdala and projects its axons to well known visceral nuclei of the forebrain and midbrain, such as the medial hypothalamus and midbrain periaqueductal gray, and the subiculum of the hippocampal formation.

Behavioral neurology: a branch of neurology that specializes in analyzing higher cortical function (complex behaviors such as language, emotion, attention and memory).

Bell-Magendie's Law: the assumption that in the spinal cord, dorsal roots are sensory and the ventral roots are motor.

Beta$_1$-adrenergic receptor: a target organ receptor for the sympathetic nervous system that is found on the heart and mediates increases in heart rate and cardiac contractility.

Beta$_2$-adrenergic receptor: a target organ receptor for the sympathetic nervous system mediating dilation and inhibitory effects such as vascular dilation, bronchial dilation, and inhibition of the gastrointestinal tract.

Binocular cells: cortical neurons that respond to the specific contributions by both eyes simultaneously.

Bipolar cells: neurons that have their cell bodies in the inner nuclear layer of the retina. They connect rods and cones with ganglion cells.

Bipolar neuron: a nerve cell that possesses only one axon and one dendrite.

Blood–brain barrier: a structural and physiologic attribute of brain blood vessels that functions to restrict the movement of nonlipid substances in and out of the central nervous system environment.

Brachial plexus: peripheral nerve network innervating the upper extremity.

Brachium of the superior colliculus: a central visual pathway connecting the lateral geniculate nucleus and optic tract to the superior colliculus.

Bradycardia: a reduction in heart rate.

Bradykinesia: slowness of movement.

Brain: the part of the central nervous system inside the skull.

Brainstem: the most caudal part of the brain, the lower end of which joins the spinal cord through the foramen magnum. It controls reflexes and essential processes such as respiration.

Broca's area: the inferior frontal gyrus in the left hemisphere. This region plays a crucial role in the generation of fluent utterances, perhaps by allowing sentences and phrases to be assembled in working memory.

Brodmann's areas: a numbering system for cortical regions that is based on cytoarchitectonic differences in different cortical layers. Brodmann described the results of his analysis on only one hemisphere in one postmortem brain, but the system has proved remarkably useful to comparative neuroanatomists, psychologists, neurologists, and physiologists as a means of locating functionally significant boundaries between regions. Many area boundaries are found in the depths of sulci.

Brown-Séquard syndrome: the neurologic deficits resulting from a hemisection of the spinal cord: paralysis and loss of dorsal column function on the same side of the body and deficits of pain and temperature sensation on the other.

Calcarine sulcus: the groove on the medial aspect of the occipital lobe running from anterior to the parietooccipital fissure to the occipital pole. It is the anatomic termination of the visual pathway.

Calcium (Ca^{++}): one of the elements essential for life. It is important in development and learning. Neurons have channels specific to calcium ions.

Caloric testing: the use of warm or cool water or air injected into the external ear canal to cause an artificial vestibular stimulus. Used to diagnose disorders of the peripheral part of the vestibular system.

Cardiac output: the blood volume pumped by the heart. Normally expressed in liters or milliliters per minute.

Catabolism: any destructive process by which complex materials or molecules are converted by living cells into more simple compounds or molecules.

Catecholamine: a group of compounds composed of a catechol group and an aliphatic amine group, which produce effects similar to those observed with stimulation of the sympathetic nervous system. Examples are norepinephrine (noradrenaline), epinephrine (adrenaline), and dopamine.

Cauda equina: literally, "horse's tail." It is the collection of nerve roots at the base of the spinal cord.

Caudal: literally, "toward the tail"; antonym of rostral.

Caudate nucleus: one of the basal ganglia (i.e., part of the striatum), a large nucleus deep in the center of the cerebrum surrounding the lateral ventricles.

Cell suspensions: solutions containing cells that have been abstracted from blocks of tissue.

Central canal: the space that runs through the center of the spinal cord, throughout its length. In the brainstem it widens into the fourth ventricle. It contains cerebrospinal fluid.

Central command: the signal from the motor cortex relayed down to the spinal cord and brainstem for the execution of a movement.

Central delay: refers to that portion of reaction time that accounts for signal transmission within the brain and spinal cord.

Central fissure: the space between the two cerebral hemispheres, which is virtually a very deep sulcus.

Central nervous system (CNS): those parts of the nervous system inside the spinal column and skull, including the spinal cord and brain.

Central pattern generators: neural circuits capable of generating coordinated activity patterns in the absence of sensory input.

Central process: an axon or dendrite that extends from the soma of a neuron into the substance of the central nervous system.

Central sulcus: a large sulcus that divides the frontal lobe from the occipital lobe, also known as the *fissure of Rolando.*

Centrifugal: directed from a more central to a more peripheral location in the nervous system.

Cephalic: toward the head.

Cephalic flexure: the bend in the developing nervous system of the embryo. It forms at approximately the level of what will become the midbrain.

Cerebellum: the hindbrain, a semicircular structure at the base of the cerebrum with a deeply folded cortex and several deep nuclei, connected with the rest of the brain by three peduncles. The cytology of its cortex is remarkably uniform throughout, and is well documented. Its functions are less well understood, but seem to involve regulation and fine tuning of motor commands.

Cerebral cortex: the outer layers of gray matter of the cerebrum of the brain associated with higher functions.

Cerebral hemispheres: the large, hemispheric-shaped structures at the most rostral end of the neuraxis, the outside of which are wrinkled in appearance because of folds (gyri) of cerebral cortex.

Cerebrospinal fluid (CSF): protein-free fluid that comprises the second circulatory system of the central nervous system. It circulates in the brain ventricles and around the brain and spinal cord.

Cerebrovascular accident: a general term applied to brain damage as a result of ischemia or hemorrhage; a stroke (from the expression "stroke of God").

Cerebrovasculature: blood vessel network that supplies blood to the brain.

Cerebrum: the large structure rostral to the brainstem, and overlying the thalamus. It has two halves, the cerebral hemispheres, each containing a cortex, white matter, and deep nuclei known as the basal ganglia.

Cervical: refers to the most rostral seven vertebrae or eight spinal nerves or cord segments. They are in the neck.

Cervical flexure: the ventral bend in the developing nervous system of the embryo that forms at approximately the level of the differentiation between the brain and the spinal cord.

Characteristic delay: the time required after presentation of an auditory stimulus for a particular neuron to fire in response to that sound.

Characteristic frequency (cf): that frequency to which an auditory hair cell or nerve fibers responds best—that is, the frequency to which it has the lowest threshold. Also known as the "best frequency" (bf).

Chemotropism: the attraction, at a distance, of the growing axon by its target by means of a gradient of diffusible chemicals.

Cholinergic: associated with acetylcholine neurotransmission, including nerves that contain acetylcholine, synaptic release of acetylcholine, and target organ receptors for acetylcholine.

Cholinergic neurons: nerve cells that release acetylcholine as a neurotransmitter at a synapse.

Cholinesterase: an enzyme that destroys and inactivates acetylcholine.

Chorda tympani nerve: branch of facial nerve (cranial nerve VII) containing sensory fibers innervating the front two thirds of the tongue.

Choroid: the part of the vascular tunic of the retina posterior to the ciliary body, between the retina and the sclera. It provides metabolical support to the retina.

Choroid plexus: ependymal cells in the ventricles of the brain that produce cerebrospinal fluid.

Chromatolysis: disintegration of Nissl bodies of a neuron as a result of injury, fatigue, or exhaustion.

Cilia: hairlike organelles that line the cell surface of certain cells, which in most forms beat in unison (singular form, *cilium*).

Ciliary body: the part of the vascular tunic of the eye between the iris and choroid. It is internal to the sclera and external to the posterior chamber.

Ciliary muscle: the intrinsic smooth muscle of the ciliary body of the eye innervated by the ciliary nerves of cranial nerve III. Its primary function is to facilitate accommodation.

Circle of Willis: the arterial circle on the ventral surface of the brain, formed by the anastomosis of internal carotid and basilar artery branches.

Circumvallate papillae: circular elevations on the top surface of the back part of the tongue, containing taste buds in the encircling trenches.

Clarke's column: synonymous with *nucleus dorsalis*.

Clarke's nucleus: a column of cells located in the medial part of the dorsal horn, usually extending from the eighth cervical segment to the third or fourth lumbar segment; it gives rise to the posterior spinocerebellar tract.

Clasp-knife: a term used to describe muscle spasticity as increasing resistance against increasing passive stretch followed by a sudden collapse of resistance.

Classical conditioning: a type of associative learning in which presentation of a reinforcing (uncon-ditional) stimulus is contingent on the presentation of a preceding (conditional) stimulus. Also known as Pavlovian conditioning in honor of the Russian scientist who first described and studied this example of learning.

Clonus: oscillation of a limb segment due to the alternating pattern of stretch reflex and inverse stretch reflex of a spastic muscle.

Closed class: small words such as to, and, with, and so forth. They are called "closed class" because there are only approximately 30 of these words in English and no more can apparently be generated, in contrast to nouns, adjectives, and verbs, which are continually added to the language.

Coactivated: simultaneously activated.

Coccygeal: related to the most caudal one to three vertebrae or spinal nerves.

Cochlea: the coiled, snail-like, bony portion of the inner ear containing three scalae or compartments, the scala media or the cochlear duct, scala vestibuli, and scala tympani. It has five coils in humans. An obsolete name is the *auditory labyrinth*.

Cochlear duct: the fluid-filled space bounded on one side by the basilar membrane and the other by Reissner's membrane. It contains endolymph, which is high in potassium (K^+) ions. It houses the organ of Corti, on which rest the sensory transducers. Also called the *scala media*.

Cochlear microphonic: an electrical potential that is recorded usually from the round window of the cochlea in response to sound. It is called "microphonic" because it mimics the incoming sound. It is generated by the outer hair cells.

Cochlear nerve: that part of the eighth cranial nerve innervating the cochlea.

Cochlear nucleus: the neural structure in the medulla that receives direct synaptic input from the cochlear nerve. It is divided into an anterior, posterior, and dorsal portion according to the pattern of cochlear nerve innervation.

Cochlear partition: see *scala media*.

Cogwheel rigidity: a term used to qualify muscle spasticity; the ratchet-like resistance to passive stretch, seen in patients with Parkinson's syndrome.

Common chemical sense: in the context of the oral and nasal cavities, it is the sense of irritation caused by chemical stimulation of the free nerve endings buried deep in nasal and oral mucous membranes.

Compensation: 1) recovery of impaired behavior after central nervous system damage; 2) more precisely, switching to a new way to perform a task after a central nervous system lesion.

Competition: nerve cells "compete" with each other for space, for targets, for afferents, for growth factors, and so on. The winner remains and the loser may die out or at least lose processes and synapses.

Complex cells: cortical neurons in areas V2 and V3 that respond maximally to unidirectional movement of a stimulus with the correct orientation.

Computed tomography (CT): cross-sectional imaging technique using a rotating x-ray beam; detectors send information to a computer, which reconstructs a two-dimensional image based on the relative absorption of x-rays passing through body tissues.

Concentric contraction: the active shortening of a muscle due to sliding of the actin filaments.

Concussion: loss of consciousness, transient or prolonged, due to a blow to the head.

Conduction velocity: the speed of propagation of an action potential along a neuron process.

Cone: a type of photoreceptor.

Conjugate: movement of both eyes in the same direction.

Conjunctiva: a mucous membrane running from the eyelid margins to the corneal limbus. It forms the anterior layer of the eyeball (bulbar conjunctiva) and the posterior layer of the eyelids (palpebral conjunctiva).

Connexons: protein channels that form gap junctions between two electrically coupled neurons.

Contact guidance: one mechanism used by growing axons to reach their targets, relying on contacts of membrane molecules with the substrates on which the axons grow.

Contact inhibition: the growth of an axon can be inhibited by physical contact with certain substrates, such as cartilage, or by chemical contact.

Contractility: the ability of a muscle to generate force in response to stimulation. Cardiac contractility refers to the property of the heart to contract more vigorously or forcefully.

Contralateral: located on the other side.

Convergence: simultaneous adduction of both eyes so that the lines of sight point toward each other.

Convergence: the termination of more than one neural input onto a single neuron.

Cornea: the transparent anterior portion of the fibrous tunic of the eye. It serves as the first refracting medium of the eye.

Corollary discharge: an internal loop relaying descending motor signals back to the higher centers.

Coronal: referring to the top of the head.

Coronal section: a slice separating the front from the back.

Corpus callosum: the thick band of fibers connecting the two cerebral hemispheres.

Cortex: part of a structure that surrounds or partially surrounds an inner core. In the brain, cortex regions usually consist of several layers.

Cortical column: visual cortex cells organized into columns running superficial to deep containing cells of a single receptive field axis of orientation.

Corticomesencephalic tract: voluntary fibers that arise in the frontal eye field, decussate in the pons, and innervate the motor nuclei of cranial nerves III, IV, and VI.

Corticosteroids: any of the steroids of the adrenal cortex.

Cranial nerves (CN): the 12 peripheral nerves originating from the brain rather than the spinal cord. They include sensory and motor innervation to the head and neck. They are numbered rostral to caudal, with roman numerals: I, olfactory; II, optic; III, oculomotor; IV, trochlear; V, trigeminal; VI, abducens; VII, facial; VIII, vestibulocochlear or acoustic; IX, glossopharyngeal; X, vagus; XI, spinal accessory; and XII, hypoglossal. Most people remember these nerves in order by using a mnemonic sentence.

Craniosacral division: another term for the parasympathetic nervous system, especially with regard to the origin of parasympathetic preganglionic cell bodies from the cranial region (cranial nerves III, VII, IX, and X) and the sacral spinal cord (S2–S4).

Cribriform plate: thin, perforated, horizontal part of the ethmoid bone of the skull.

Crista: the hillock containing hair cells inside the ampulla of one of the semicircular canals of the vestibular labyrinth.

Crista ampullaris: the cilia-covered hillock (*crista*) and related structures in the *ampulla* of the semicircular canal of the vestibular labyrinth. The cilia, at the apical ends of the *hair cells*, are covered by the *cupula*. The entire set of structures makes up the receptor area of the canal.

Cross-bridges: the extensions of the myosin filament.

Crossed extensor reflexes: reflex extension of the opposite limb that occurs during a flexor withdrawal response.

Cuneate fascicle: ascending fibers at high levels of the spinal cord in the lateral dorsal columns carrying input from the ipsilateral upper thoracic and cervical segments. Synonymous with *fasciculus cuneatus*.

Cupula: the inverted gelatinous cup covering the hair cells in the crista ampullaris.

Cytoarchitectonic: pertaining to the cell morphology and packing density that characterizes different cortical regions. Sensory cortex tends to have more small (granular) cells and motor cortex tends to have more large pyramids.

Cytoarchitectonic area: an area of cortex defined by the structure of its neurons.

Cytoarchitecture: the arrangement and structure of cells and their constituent parts within a structure; this includes laminar organization, packing density, fiber direction, and the like.

Cytokines: chemical substances secreted by certain cells that usually have a localized effect on tissue.

Decerebrate: experimental animal in which cerebral function is eliminated by transecting the brainstem at the level of the midbrain.

Decerebrate rigidity: hypertonus of the physiologic extensors after decerebration.

Declarative memory: also known as explicit memory, encompasses the memory for facts and concepts (semantic memory), as well as the memory for events (episodic or autobiographic memory).

Decorticate: experimental animal in which cerebral function is eliminated by transection of the forebrain from the remainder of the central nervous system.

Decussate: to cross the midline.

Deep cerebellar nuclei: the nuclei inside the cerebellum, to and from which the cortical areas project.

Defecation: elimination of fecal material from the bowels.

Defensive withdrawal reflex: habituation: a decrement in a behavioral response during repeated presentations of the eliciting stimulus. Habituation is an example of nonassociative learning and can induce both short- and long-term memories.

Degeneration: deterioration.

Deiter's nucleus: synonymous with *lateral vestibular nucleus*.

Dementia: organic loss of intellectual function.

Dendrite: one of the neuronal processes responsi-ble for propagating electrical messages from the periphery toward the neuron, commonly more than one per neuron.

Dendroplasm: cytoplasm contained inside the boundary of the unit membrane of a dendrite.

Denervate: to remove the nervous system innervation to a tissue.

Denervation supersensitivity: the increase in the responsiveness to neurotransmitter of the cell membrane of the postsynaptic neuron that occurs after presynaptic terminals are removed.

Depolarization: making a membrane potential less negative, the shift of a membrane potential in the positive direction, shifting a membrane potential toward threshold.

Dermatome: an area of skin supplied with primary afferents that travel through a single dorsal root.

Diabetic autonomic neuropathy: dysfunction of the autonomic neural control of visceral organs resulting from diabetes-induced damage of peripheral autonomic nerves.

Diaschisis: loss of function and electrical activity due to cerebral lesions in areas remote from the lesion but neuronally connected to it.

Dichotic listening: an experimental procedure developed by Doreen Kimura in an attempt noninvasively to identify the hemisphere governing language. Words and nonwords are played into the two ears simultaneously through headphones. There is a statistical bias for improved word recognition in the right ear because of more secure access to the language processing mechanisms in the left hemisphere.

Diencephalon: a subdivision of the brain when it is at the five-vesicle stage in the embryo. It becomes the hypothalamus, thalamus, and epithalamus. When referring to the mature brain, this term refers to the entire group of those structures, which are located rostral to the midbrain and covered by the cerebral hemispheres.

Dilator muscle: a radial band of smooth muscles intrinsic to the eye, innervated by sympathetic autonomic fibers traveling with cranial nerve V. The muscles enlarge the pupil in dim illumination.

Diplopia: double vision.

Disconjugate: movement of both eyes in opposite directions.

Disdiadokokinesia: loss of ability to perform rapid alternating movements, such as repeatedly turning the palms face up and face down.

Disinhibit: to reverse the inhibition; to excite.

Disinhibited: removal of inhibitory input to a population of neurons, resulting in return to their tonic activity levels.

Divergence: 1) the output of one neuron affecting two or more neurons; 2) simultaneous abduction of both eyes so that the lines of sight move away from rather than toward each other.

Dorsal: toward the back, top, or upper surface; antonym of *ventral*.

Dorsal acoustic stria: the pathway sending processed auditory signals to the lateral lemniscus and the inferior colliculus from fusiform cells in the cochlear nucleus.

Dorsal column–medial lemniscal system: sensory pathway of fibers ascending in the dorsal funiculus of the spinal cord and in the medial lemniscus in the brainstem, carrying proprioceptive information.

Dorsal column nuclei: brainstem nuclei of the fibers ascending the spinal cord in the dorsal columns.

Dorsal columns: ascending bundles of fibers in the posterior aspect of the spinal cord, carrying input from joint receptors and low-threshold mechanoreceptors.

Dorsal horn: dorsal portion of the spinal cord gray matter, posterior to the central gray; concerned mainly with sensory functions, it derives from the embryonic alar plate.

Dorsal root: a bundle of nerve fibers immediately outside the spinal cord, carrying mostly efferent but also some afferent fibers, on the dorsal side of the cord.

Dorsal root ganglia: synonymous with *spinal ganglion*. A group of sensory nerve cell bodies located outside of the spinal cord, on its posterior aspect. The nerve processes are found in the dorsal root.

Dorsal spinocerebellar tract: ascending tract from the spinal cord carrying proprioceptive input to the cerebellum.

Dorsolateral tract of Lissauer: white matter occupying the region between the dorsal edge of the dorsal horn and the external dorsolateral surface of the spinal cord where the dorsal roots attach.

Double-labeling: an anatomic tracing technique in which two different stains or radioactive compounds are used to trace the projections of neurons.

Dual innervation: refers to organs receiving innervation from both the sympathetic and parasympathetic nervous systems.

Dura mater: the inelastic, outermost layer of the meninges.

Dynamic index: the measure of dynamic sensitivity of a muscle spindle afferent.

Dynamic sensitivity: the sensitivity of a muscle spindle afferent to rate of change in muscle length.

Dysgeusia: abnormal, unpleasant, persistent taste sensation.

Dyslexia: a developmental reading disorder that occurs in the absence of impaired cognition or motivation, or of a neurologic disorder. It runs in families and is more common in boys. Current research suggests that most dyslexics have difficulty imaging and manipulating the sounds of words (phonologic awareness). They make mistakes reading nonsense words, for example. Kindergartners who cannot rhyme are at risk for dyslexia. Many dyslexics excel at sports, architecture, computers, and science. Few become writers.

Dysmetria: inability to control the appropriate range of muscle actions, such that the distances of targets are misjudged by the motor system; in hypometria, the voluntary movement undershoots and misses the goal, and in hypermetria the voluntary movement overshoots and misses the goal.

Dysosmia: abnormal, unpleasant, persistent odor sensation.

Dyssynergy: impairment of motor coordination of different body parts, often associated with intention tremors and disturbance of muscle tone.

Early receptor potential: first response of a retinal rod or cone cell to stimulation. It is purely biochemical, not electrophysiologic.

Eccrine sweat glands: glands of the body involved in temperature regulation through sweat secretion. Sweating promotes heat loss through evaporation of sweat (i.e., body water) from the skin.

Edge enhancement: the phenomenon of perceptual amplification of surface borders.

Effector organ: the organ or tissue that produces an effect as a result of stimulation of a nerve or hormone. *Effector organ* is essentially the same term as *target organ*.

Efferent: conveyed away from a structure; efferent signals are outgoing signals.

Efferent element: the component of a system that carries information away from a central point; the efferent element of a synapse carries an action potential away from the synapse.

Efferent nerve: nerves that carry information from the central nervous system. Efferent nerves are also called *motor nerves*.

Emergent property: functions or behavior of a system that are not apparent from the structure, but arise out of the combined functions of groups of cells or groups of structures.

Emesis: vomiting; the forced expulsion of stomach contents through the mouth.

Encapsulated Paciniform endings: receptors found in the fibrous periosteum.

End-plate potential: the action potential generated in the muscle fiber at the neuromuscular junction in response to the release of acetylcholine.

Endogenous: produced in or caused by factors in the organism.

Endolymph: the viscous fluid inside the cochlea and the labyrinth.

Enteric nervous system: the nerve plexuses in the wall of the gastrointestinal tract that function to control the motor and secretory activities of the gastrointestinal tract. Influences of the sympathetic and parasympathetic nervous systems on the digestive system probably act through effects on the enteric nervous system.

Entorhinal cortex: the area in the temporal lobe surrounding the hippocampus, which it strongly influences.

Ependyma: one-cell–thick epithelial lining of the central canal of the spinal cord or ventricles of the brain. Ependymal cells are usually cylindrical in shape and have cilia that beat in the canal or ventricles.

Epinephrine: a hormone secreted by the adrenal medulla; a potent activator of sympathetic receptors. Synonymous with *adrenaline*.

Epithalamus: the dorsal diencephalon.

Epithelium: layer of cells on the surface of a tissue.

Erection: in the male, the condition during which the penis is made rigid when erectile tissue is filled with blood.

Excitation–contraction coupling: the process by which the electrical activity of the muscle membrane is converted into a mechanical contraction.

Excitatory postsynaptic potential (EPSP): a change in the ion conductance of the postsynaptic membrane that results in a tendency to depolarize the postsynaptic membrane.

Excitotoxicity: a pathologic condition resulting from the release of toxic amounts of excitatory neurotransmitters after brain injury.

Exit nuclei: the two nuclei through which most output leaves the basal ganglia. They comprise the internal segment of the globus pallidus and the pars reticulata of the substantia nigra.

External auditory meatus: the ear canal that leads from the external ear to the eardrum, or tympanic membrane.

External ear: the parts of the auditory system lateral to the tympanic membrane, also known as the outer ear.

External germinal layer (EGL): a germinal zone formed late in development on top of the developing cerebellum, the cells of which give rise to the cerebellar granule cells.

External limiting membrane: layer 3, the innermost limit of the retina.

Exteroceptive: stimuli received from the immediate external environment; the receptors of this information would be those in the external body surfaces, such as skin and mucous membranes.

Extorsion: roll rotation of the eye such that the superior pole of the eye rotates toward the temple and inferior pole of the eye rotates toward the nose.

Extracellular matrix (ECM): molecules of the extracellular space that can serve as substrate for growing neurites that possess membrane receptors for them.

Extrafusal: striated muscle fiber that is not part of the muscle spindle.

Extraneuronal reuptake: nonneuronal reuptake mechanism that assists in terminating the action of synaptically released norepinephrine through uptake of norepinephrine into nonneural tissues. Also known as uptake-2.

Extraocular: referring to the structures outside of the globe of the eye, such as the extraocular muscles, which move the globe in the orbit.

Facial nerve: cranial nerve VII. It innervates muscles and glands of the face.

Facilitatory neurons (FN): neurons that release modulatory transmitters, which in turn alter the properties of the postsynaptic cell by activating a complex array of second messenger and protein kinase systems. For example, a facilitatory neuron synapses with a sensory neuron that mediates the monosynaptic withdrawal reflex in *Aplysia*. The transmitter that is released by this facilitatory neuron (i.e., 5-HT) activates at least three second messenger and kinase systems in the sensory neurons, which work in concert to modulate the biophysical properties of the sensory neuron and to enhance (i.e., facilitate) the release of neurotransmitter from the sensory neuron.

Fasciculation: the formation of a nerve fascicle by the growth of axons on the surface of earlier established or pioneer axons as a result of homophilic chemical binding.

Fasciculus cuneatus: synonymous with *cuneate fascicle*; lateral portion of the spinal cord dorsal column, composed of ascending fibers that terminate in the nucleus cuneatus.

Fasciculus gracilis: synonymous with *gracile fascicle*; medial portion of the spinal cord dorsal column, composed of ascending fibers that terminate in the nucleus cuneatus.

Fast fatigue-resistant muscle fiber: the muscle fiber type that is fast contracting, has high aerobic and anaerobic capacity, and does not fatigue easily.

Fast muscle fiber: the muscle fiber type that is fast contracting, has high glycolytic capacity (anaerobic), and fatigues easily.

Fast pain (initial or first pain): A delta (Aδ) primary afferent fiber stimulation that results in pain that has a sharp, pricking quality; can be localized on the body and diminishes quickly.

Feedback: information provided after an event or process has occurred, about the outcome of that event. This information can be used later to modify or change the process or event at the next occurrence.

Feedforward control: anticipates the relation between the system and the environment and accordingly influences the output of the controller.

Fibrin: an insoluble protein in blood found in clots when blood coagulates.

Field defect: see *scotoma*.

Filopodia: long, thin extensions of the growth cone that do not adhere much to the growth substrate but rather "sense" the environmental clues that direct growth.

Filum terminale: the caudal end of the pia mater.

Final common pathway: the last point at which information is collected before being sent to the motor efferents for control of movement. In the axial motor system, the spinal motor neurons are the last point in the central nervous system for controlling muscle activity. In the oculomotor system, the final common pathway is the medial longitudinal fasciculus.

First-order neuron: all sensory stimuli from the periphery have their first-order neuron cell bodies (primary afferent neurons) in the dorsal root ganglia, and enter the spinal cord by the dorsal roots of spinal nerves.

Fissure: a deep sulcus.

Fissure of Rolando: synonym for *central sulcus*.

Flexor reflex afferents: cutaneous afferents that, when stimulated, evoke a flexor withdrawal response.

Flexor withdrawal reflex: reflex activation of limb flexors in response to noxious stimulation of the distal limb.

Fluency: an attribute that suggests effortless, rapid, and flexible generation of motor sequences.

Foliate papillae: folds on the sides of the back part of the tongue containing taste buds.

Foramen magnum: the hole in the skull through which the spinal cord connects with the brain.

Forebrain: most rostral (anterior) part of the brain, including the thalamus and cerebrum.

Fovea: a small depression in the retina of the eye, approximately 1.5 mm in diameter, located in the macula lutea and composed primarily of cone cells. This area is important for color vision and is an area specialized for higher visual acuity than the periphery of the retina.

Foveola: the center of the fovea. It contains the cone cells most adapted for high visual acuity; each cone is connected to a single ganglion cell.

Free radicals: molecules or molecular fragments with an unpaired electron in the outer orbital. They are highly reactive, unstable species capable of extracting an electron from neighboring molecules, leading to oxidative damage.

Frequency: number of oscillations per second, expressed in cycles per second or herz (Hz).

Frontal lobe: the most anterior section of the cortex.

Frontal operculum: portion of frontal lobe, a flap deep within the lateral fissure of cerebrum.

Functional lateralization: the concept that the two hemispheres have different priorities in regulating behavior and processing afferent stimuli. The right hemisphere appears to process stimuli more globally, whereas the left hemisphere is more analytic and better at extracting perceptual detail. The mechanisms by which these specializations are implemented are not understood.

Functional magnetic resonance imaging (fMRI): a new technique to visualize brain function. When neurons fire, the surrounding astrocytes signal the vasculature to increase blood flow. More oxygen is supplied than needed and the excess drains off in capillaries, changing the magnetic properties of the tissue. This change can be detected with special magnetic resonance imaging procedures as a change in brightness in the region containing more oxygen. It is thus an indirect way of visualizing regional differences in brain activation in different cognitive and motor tasks. Because no radiation or injection is necessary, it is safe to use in children, patients, and research subjects.

Functional synergism: the condition where the sympathetic and parasympathetic nervous systems act together to promote a single response in an organ. Functional synergism normally is found through inhibition of outflow of one system and increased outflow from the other system; for example, a decrease in heart rate is mediated by a decrease in sympathetic outflow and an increase in parasympathetic outflow.

Fungiform papillae: round bumps on the top surface of the front part of the tongue, containing taste buds.

Galvanotropism: the direction of neuritic growth by electrical fields.

Ganglion: a mass of neural tissue, primarily cell bodies.

Ganglion cell: an aggregation of nerve cell bodies located outside the central nervous system.

Ganglion cell layer: layer 8 of the retina.

Gangliosides: a class of galactose-containing glycolipids found in the central nervous system.

GAP 43: growth-associated protein present in axonal growth cones that may be involved in the regulation of calcium, itself implicated in the integration of the various signals that influence neuritic growth and guidance.

Gap junction: a nonsynaptic connection between two neurons, mediated by pores that allow the movement of molecules between the cells, for electrical rather than chemical transmission of signals from one neuron to the other.

Gastrula: the embryo when it is composed of three layers of cells. The nervous system starts to form at this stage.

Germinal zone: the portion of the neural tube around the neurocele comprising actively dividing cells at the origin of the nerve cells and glial cells of the central nervous system. Once a cell becomes postmitotic, it leaves the germinal zone. At the end of the proliferative period, the germinal

zone is reduced to one cell layer and transforms into the ependymal epithelium.

Glia: the nonneural cells that support, protect, and nourish neurons of the central nervous system. Synonymous with *neuroglia*.

Glioblasts: cells on the glial lineage that are not yet differentiated morphologically.

Globe: the eyeball.

Globus pallidus: one of the basal ganglia; forms the lentiform nucleus with the putamen, part of the striatum.

Glomerulus: small, rounded mass in the brain containing tangles of neuronal processes forming synapses with one another, but no nerve cell bodies.

Glossary: a list of specialized words and their definitions, often at the back of a book. From the Middle English *glosarie*, derived from the Latin *glossarium*, from *glossa*, meaning "foreign word." (*The American Heritage Dictionary of the English Language*, 3rd ed. Boston: Houghton Mifflin, 1992.)

Glossopharyngeal nerve: cranial nerve IX, innervating the posterior one third of the tongue for taste. It also carries nerves involved in respiration and blood pressure.

Glutamate: an amino acid; L-glutamate is the primary excitatory transmitter in the spinal cord and brain. L-Glutamate interacts with three classes of receptors: ionotropic receptors (two types) and metabotropic receptors.

Glutamate receptor: a receptor that specifically responds to glutamate. Glutamate receptors can be divided into several broad categories: those that directly gate ion channels (ionotropic receptors) and those that indirectly gate ions through second messengers (metabotropic receptors). Ionotropic receptors are divided into two major subtypes, NMDA and non-NMDA. These ionotropic subtypes are classified based on the agonist that activates them and the antagonists that inhibit them.

Golgi endings: proprioceptive receptors found in the joint ligaments.

Golgi tendon organ: an encapsulated mechanoreceptor that is the force-measuring organ of the muscle. Named for an Italian scientist, Nobel-prize winning neuroanatomist Camillo Golgi.

Gracile fascicle: ascending fibers at high levels of the spinal cord in the medial dorsal columns carrying input from the ipsilateral sacral, lumbar, and lower thoracic segments. Synonymous with *fasciculus gracilis.*

Gray matter: nonmyelinated brain matter, which appears gray in ordinary light. Often refers to nuclei, but can include unmyelinated processes.

Growth cone: a distal enlargement of a neuronal process by which most of the growth occurs. The growth cone is said to "sense" the substrate to direct the growth appropriately.

Growth factors: proteins synthesized by most tissues that are involved in the developmental processes of proliferation, differentiation, and survival. Their effects vary depending on cell type. See *nerve growth factor.*

Gustducin: member of G protein family involved in taste transduction that is located exclusively in taste receptor cells.

Gyrus: a wrinkle on the surface of the cerebral cortex (plural, *gyri*).

Habituation: a decrement in a behavioral response during repeated presentations of the eliciting stimulus. Habituation is an example of nonassociative learning and can induce both short- and long-term memories.

Hair cell: a specialized epithelial cell that contains cilia and is involved in transduction. The cochlea and the vestibular labyrinths each have two types of hair cells. In the cochlea, inner hair cells are the true sensory transducers, and outer hair cells modulate the activity of inner hair cells. In the labyrinths, the functional distinctions between type I and type II hair cells are less well understood.

Hair follicle: a long keratinous filament located in the skin and sensitive to mechanical pressures.

Helicotrema: the opening at the apex of the cochlea, through which the scala tympani and vestibuli communicate.

Hemianopsia: blindness in one half of the visual field of one or both eyes.

Heterophoria: latent tendency toward heterotropia that is prevented by binocular fusion. Also called phoria.

Heterotropia: eye misalignment so that one fovea is not directed to the same point in space as the other. Also called *strabismus*, squint, or tropia.

Hippocampus: a structure in the temporal lobe, involved in memory and spatial orientation. It is phylogenetically ancient, and is sometimes called the archicortex.

Homeostasis: the regulation of specific physiologic and chemical processes in the body to maintain a consistent internal environment.

Homonymous: refers to symmetric halves of the visual fields (e.g., the nasal half of one field and the temporal half of the other).

Homunculus: literally means "little man," but refers here to body representation in brain structures; it can refer to the body parts represented by receptive fields on the surface of the sensory cortex, by movement control sites on the motor cortex, or other regions of the brain.

Horizontal canal: synonymous with *lateral canal.* One of the semicircular canals of the vestibular labyrinth. With the head pitched down 25 degrees, it detects yaw rotation of the head.

Horizontal cells: neurons with their cell bodies in the inner nuclear layer of the retina. The dendrite receives information from up to several photoreceptors and the axon transmits it to up to several distant photoreceptors, all of which are in the outer plexiform layer.

Horner's syndrome: syndrome resulting from loss of sympathetic innervation to the head and face due to damage of sympathetic nerves or cells bodies in the spinal cord. Characterized by loss of sweating in the head, miosis, ptosis, and vasodilation of the skin of the face.

Hydrocephalus: accumulation of cerebrospinal fluid in the brain as a result of impeded fluid circulation or absorption.

Hydrophilic: having an affinity for or capable of dissolving in water.

Hydrophobic: tending not to combine with or incapable of dissolving in water.

Hypercomplex cell: visual cortical cells in areas V2 and V3 that have elaborate response properties, such as responses to bidirectional movements.

Hypermetria: a condition in which impairment of motor control results in voluntary movements that overshoot their target.

Hyperpolarization: making a membrane potential more negative than the resting membrane potential.

Hyperreflexia: a state of abnormally high reflex responsiveness.

Hypersomnia: a state of slow-wave electroencephalographic activity, low respiration, and relaxation.

Hypertension: high blood pressure.

Hypogeusia: partial loss of taste sensation.

Hypoglossal nerve: cranial nerve XII. It innervates most muscles of the tongue.

Hypokinesia: abnormal decrease in motor activity and mobility.

Hypophysis: also known as the pituitary gland; has important endocrine functions.

Hyporeflexia: a state of abnormally low reflex responsiveness.

Hyposmia: partial loss of olfactory sensation.

Hypothalamus: portion of the brain located ventral to the thalamus, to which the pituitary is connected by a stalk. Through the pituitary it controls the endocrine functions of the body. It also influences autonomic functions.

Immunocytochemistry: a tool for determining pathways that use specific biochemical compounds and for identification of putative neurotransmitters. The technique involves the use of antibodies to specific neurotransmitters or specific enzymes. When these antibodies are placed in the synaptic cleft, they are taken up at the nerve terminal along with the neurotransmitters to which they bind.

Impedance: similar to resistance, but it varies depending on the frequency.

Implicit memory: see *nondeclarative memory*.

Incus: the middle bone of the three ossicles.

Induction (neural): the action of the notochord on the overlying ectoderm that results in the transformation of the latter, leading to neurulation. Neural induction is chemically mediated and acts over a concentration gradient.

Infarction: death of neural tissue due to ischemia.

Inferior: toward the bottom of the body; antonym of *superior*.

Inferior canal: synonymous with *posterior canal*. One of the vertical semicircular canals of the vestibular labyrinth. It detects pitch rotation of the head.

Inferior colliculus: the auditory relay and reflex center of the midbrain. It receives synaptic input from all lower auditory structures and sends axons to the medial geniculate body.

Inferior oblique muscle: a striated, extrinsic muscle of the eye that originates at the anterior, medial portion of the orbital floor and inserts on the posterior, temporal portion of the eyeball. It is innervated by cranial nerve III and elevates, abducts, and extorts the eye.

Inferior olivary nucleus: also known as the inferior olive. The large group of nuclei in the ventro-lateral medulla, heavily involved with vision. In cross-section, the nucleus looks wrinkled.

Inferior rectus muscle: a striated, extrinsic muscle of the eyeball that originates at the annulus of Zinn and inserts inferiorly near the limbus cornea of the eyeball. It is innervated by cranial nerve III and depresses, abducts, and extorts the eye.

Information processing: the internal process of evaluating and acting on input or information from the environment, combined and recombined with other knowledge either concurrently obtained or stored; the act of thinking.

Inhibitory postsynaptic potential (IPSP): a change in the ion conductance of the postsynaptic membrane that results in a tendency to hyperpolarize the postsynaptic membrane.

Inner nuclear layer: layer 6 of the retina, between the inner and outer synaptic layers. It contains amacrine, bipolar, and horizontal cell bodies.

Inner plexiform layer: layer 7 of the retina, between the inner nuclear and ganglion cell layers, where neurons from these two layers and amacrine cells synapse.

Insula: a part of the cerebral cortex that is hidden in the Sylvian fissure.

Intermediate acoustic stria: the pathway through which neurons of the posteroventral cochlear send their axons to the superior olivary complex and nuclei of the lateral lemniscus.

Intermediate zone: portion of the neural tube around the germinal zone formed by the incoming postmitotic and postmigratory nerve cells.

Internal arcuate fibers: decussating fibers from the dorsal column nuclei.

Internal capsule: the sheet of fibers that separates the caudate nucleus from the putamen and thalamus, connecting the cerebral cortex with more caudal centers.

Internal carotid artery: a branch of the carotid artery that supplies blood to all levels of the brain and anastomoses with the basilar artery to form the circle of Willis.

Internal limiting membrane: layer 10 of the retina, between the nerve fiber layer and the vitreous, made of collagen fibers and Müller cells, forming the inner limit of the retina.

Interneuron: a neuron that is contained in one region of the nervous system and that links other neurons.

Intorsion: roll rotation of the eye such that the superior pole of the eye rotates toward the nose and the inferior pole of the eye rotates toward the temple.

Intrafusal: striated muscle fiber of the muscle spindle.

Intralaminar nuclei of the thalamus: pain and temperature information is projected along the spinothalamic tract and spinoreticular tract to this thalamic structure, which in turn distributes the information to widespread areas of the cerebral cortex.

Intrinsic: a structure that lies completely within a delineated region (e.g., an axon intrinsic to the motor cortex is one that arises from and remains within the motor cortex).

Inverse myotatic reflex: see *tendon organ reflex*.

Inverse stretch reflex: see *tendon organ reflex*.

Involuntary nervous system: a synonym for the autonomic nervous system denoting that autonomic control is normally not at the conscious level.

Ipsilateral: located on the same side.

Iris: the most anterior part of the vascular tunic. It is composed of a pigmented, circular membrane perforated to form the pupil. It is the colored part of the visible eye.

Ischemia: a pathologic condition of reduced or absent blood supply.

Ischemic: affected or damaged by a lack of blood because of obstruction or constriction of a blood vessel.

Isometric contraction: muscle contraction without an appreciable decrease in the length of the whole muscle.

Jendrassik's maneuver: the technique by which the excitability of a motor neuron pool is enhanced by activating a remote muscle.

Joint receptor: a mechanoreceptor that responds to deep pressure and to other stimuli such as stress or change in position, located near joints.

Kinematic: refers to physical aspects of motion.

Kinesthesia: the sense of movement and limb position.

Kinocilium: largest of the cilia on vestibular hair cells. It indicates the orientation vector of the hair cell bundle.

L-type Ca^{++} currents: ionic membrane currents that underlie neuronal excitability. They are classified based on the type of ion that can pass through the pore (e.g., Na^{+}, K^{+}, Ca^{++}), their voltage- and time-dependent properties, and the pharmacologic agents that interact with the channel. L-type Ca^{++} currents are a class of Ca^{++} found in many neurons and are characterized by a low threshold of activation, slow inactivation, and sensitivity to dihydropyridine (i.e., nifedipine).

Lamellipodia: thin, veil-like extensions of the growth cone that do not adhere much to the growth substrate but rather "sense" the environmental clues that direct growth.

Lamina I to lamina VI of the spinal cord: The gray matter in the spinal cord is divided into 10 layers, or laminae, on a cytoarchitectural basis. Laminae I to VI constitute the dorsal horn.

Lateral: toward the side, antonym of *medial*.

Lateral canal: synonymous with *horizontal canal*.

Lateral geniculate nucleus: a subcortical primary visual nucleus located lateral to the pulvinar of each thalamus. It receives input from the optic tract and sends secondary neurons to visual cortex. It is pierced by fibers projecting to the superior colliculus.

Lateral horn: portion of the spinal cord in between the dorsal and ventral horns containing the visceral motor neurons at thoracic and sacral levels.

Lateral lemniscus: the tract in which axons project from the superior olivary complex to the inferior colliculus.

Lateral motor column: longitudinal organization of the ventral horn motor neurons that innervate the upper and lower limbs, thus found at the levels of the brachial and lumbosacral enlargements.

Lateral rectus muscle: striated, extrinsic muscle of the eye that originates at the annulus of Zinn and inserts temporally near the limbus cornea of the eyeball. It is innervated by cranial nerve VI and abducts the eye.

Leading process: motile extension of a migrating neuroblast that senses the guiding cues. It extends toward the pial surface when the cell migrates radially.

Levator palpebrae superioris muscle: striated muscle that inserts into the upper eyelid. It is innervated by the oculomotor nerve (cranial nerve III) and elevates the eyelid.

Limbic system: refers to the structures of the so-called limbic lobe, comprising the amygdala (also part of the basal ganglia), hippocampus and fornix, parahippocampal gyrus, olfactory gyri, cingulate gyrus, parts of the thalamus, parts of the hypothalamus, and parts of the periaqueductal gray. This complex set of cortical and subcortical pathways is probably involved in emotions, learning, and memory.

Limbus: the border between the cornea and the sclera. It is highly vascularized and metabolically supports the cornea.

Lipid peroxidation: a process in which free radicals attack adjacent fatty acid side chains or membrane proteins, resulting in the breakdown of the cell membrane.

Lipophilic: having an affinity for lipids (i.e., fats).

Lissencephalic: smooth, lacking gyri or sulci.

Lobe: a section of cortex.

Local circuit neurons: a chain of neurons that make a complete pathway with in the same level or region of the CNS.

Long-term depression (LTD): a long-lasting depression in synaptic effectiveness that follows some types of electrical stimulation. Several broad types of LTD may be distinguished. Heterosynaptic LTD can occur at synapses that are inactive during high-frequency stimulation of a converging synaptic input. Homosynaptic LTD can occur at synapses that are activated at low frequencies. Associative or pairing-specific LTD can be induced by conjunctive activity of converging synaptic inputs or by conjunctive activity of presynaptic and postsynaptic cells.

Long-term potentiation (LTP): an enduring synaptic enhancement that follows brief, high-frequency electrical stimulation. Like LTD, two types of LTP may be distinguished. Homosynaptic LTP can occur at synapses that are activated at low frequencies. Heterosynaptic or associative LTP can be induced by conjunctive activity of two converging synaptic inputs or by conjunctive activity of presynaptic and postsynaptic cells.

Lower motor neurons: spinal motor neurons and the motor nuclei of the cranial nerves located in the brainstem that directly innervate muscles.

Lumbar: refers to the five vertebrae, spinal nerves, or cord segments of the low back between the thoracic and sacral areas.

Lumbosacral plexus: the network of nerves innervating the lower extremities, usually said to originate from L2 to S3.

Macrophage: any of the large, mononuclear cells derived from monocytes that occur in the walls of blood vessels and in loose connective tissue, and that ingest microorganisms or other cells and foreign particles.

Macula (plural, maculae): 1) In the saccule and utricle of the vestibular labyrinth, the sensory surface covered with hair cells, overlaid by the otolithic membrane. 2) In the eye, an oval area of the retina 3 to 5 mm in diameter containing the fovea in its center and providing the best visual acuity under normal conditions; also known as the macula lutea.

Macula lutea: see *macula.*

Macular sparing: retention of macular function in the presence of adjacent visual field losses.

Magnetic resonance imaging (MRI): cross-sectional imaging technique using the magnetic spin of molecules in a strong magnetic field to detect a spatial image based on mathematically transformed signals.

Malleus: the lateral-most bone of the three ossicles.

Mamillary bodies: nuclei in the posterior hypothalamus, part of the limbic system.

Mantle: synonymous with *intermediate zone*, particularly in cortical regions.

Marginal zone: the portion of the neural tube around the intermediate zone, formed by the incoming axons of the differentiating nerve cells in the intermediate zone.

Matrix metalloproteinases: family of enzymes that cleave and degrade extracellular matrix proteins.

Mechanoelectrical transduction: the process of changing the signal input from acceleration, the adequate stimulus, from mechanical bending of stereocilia to electrochemical transmission coded by the nervous system.

Mechanoreceptors: receptors that are excited by mechanical pressures or distortions, as those responding to sound, touch, and muscular contractions.

Medial: toward the middle, antonym of *lateral.*

Medial geniculate nucleus: the thalamic auditory relay center that receives input from the inferior colliculus and sends axons to the auditory cortex.

Medial lemniscus: a tract arising from axons of the nuclei cuneatus and gracilis, which crosses to the opposite side of the medulla and ends in the ventral posterior part of the thalamus.

Medial longitudinal fasciculus: large-fiber tract extending from the midbrain to the cervical spinal cord. It carries mostly vestibular and oculomotor signals.

Medial motor column: longitudinal organization of the ventral horn motor neurons that innervate the neck and trunk muscles, thus found at all levels of spinal cord.

Medial rectus muscle: a striated, extrinsic muscle of the eyeball that originates at the annulus of Zinn and inserts nasally near the limbus cornea of the eyeball. It is innervated by cranial nerve III and adducts the eye.

Medulla oblongata: the most caudal section of the brain, often simply called the medulla.

Meissner corpuscle: a medium-sized, rapidly adapting, encapsulated tactile receptor sensitive to pressure, located near the skin surface and found most commonly in the glabrous skin of the palms and soles.

Melanocytes: the cells containing dark pigment that determine the color of the iris.

Meninges: the membranes that surround and protect the central nervous system.

Merkel's disc: a small, slowly adapting, tactile receptor composed of several modified epithelial cells, located near the skin surface.

Mesencephalon: the middle subdivision of the embryonic brain when at the three-vesicle stage. It does not subdivide and is thus found at the five-vesicle stage; synonymous with *midbrain*.

Metencephalon: a subdivision of the brain when at the five-vesicle stage. It will become the pons and cerebellum.

Microneurography: study of conduction in individual nerve fibers or bundles of fibers using a recording microelectrode.

Microvilli: microscopic projections from the surface of a cell.

Micturition: urination.

Midbrain: a section of the brain located at the rostral end of the brainstem, above the pons.

Middle ear: the air-filled space between the eardrum or tympanic membrane and the cochlea. It contains the three ossicles, which form a bony chain attached to the eardrum at one end (malleus) and the oval window at the other end (stapes), with the incus in the middle.

Middle ear transfer function: the frequency response of the middle ear is produced by the mechanical properties of the middle ear and results in attenuation of sounds above 3 kHz.

Miosis: constriction of the pupil or reduction in pupillary diameter.

Mitral cell: a type of neuron in the olfactory bulb that has a cell body that resembles a bishop's miter (hat).

Mixed nerve: a nerve that has both sensory and motor axons.

Modality: a specific sensory entity, such as the perception of light touch or temperature; this also refers to nonsomatosensory perception such as taste, smell, and so forth.

Mononuclear phagocyte system: cells that engulf and digest relatively large particles such as tissue debris and dead cells as part of the body's defense system against foreign organisms and injury; includes macrophages, monocytes, and microglia.

Monosynaptic: involving a single synapse.

Motor control: the control and coordination of posture and movement.

Motor eye fields: the posterior portion of the middle frontal gyrus of each frontal lobe that controls voluntary, contradirectional, conjugate eye movements. It is also known as Brodmann's area 8.

Motor neuron excitability: the motor neuron's capability to respond to an input.

Motor neuron pool: a group of spinal motor neurons that innervate a single muscle.

Motor program: an algorithm of neuronal activities that encodes the movement strategy for execution of a desired motor behavior.

Motor unit: a spinal motor neuron, its axon, and all of the muscle fibers it innervates.

Mucosa: mucous membrane; a layer of tissue that secretes mucus.

Müller cells: neuroglial cells that extend through all nine layers of sensory retina. They provide mechanical and metabolic support to the retinal neurons.

Multiple sclerosis: disorder characterized by demyelination of nerve fibers.

Multipolar neuron: nerve cell with numerous processes, commonly one axon and many dendrites.

Muscarinic receptor: a type of cholinergic receptor primarily activated by stimulation of the parasympathetic nervous system or by sympathetic stimulation to sweat glands.

Muscle fibers: the cells of skeletal or cardiac muscle tissue.

Muscle spindles: mechanoreceptors, found in skeletal muscle in between muscle fibers, that respond to changes in muscle length.

Muscle tone: the resistance to passive movement or change of muscle length.

Mutism: inability to speak.

Myasthenia gravis: an autoimmune disease characterized by a decrease in acetylcholine receptor sites in the postjunctional muscle membrane.

Mydriasis: dilation or opening of the pupil.

Myelencephalon: a subdivision of the brain when at the five-vesicle stage. It will become the medulla oblongata.

Myelin: a nonneuronal lipid sheath that is formed around many nerve axons by oligodendrocyte and Schwann cells, which helps to increase conduction velocity.

Myofibril: a muscle fibril composed of numerous myofilaments.

Myogenic diseases: impaired muscular performance due to disorders of muscle tissue.

Myoglobin: the oxygen-transporting protein pigment of muscle.

Myotatic reflex: see *stretch reflex*.

N-type Ca++ currents: Ca++ currents are classified on the basis of their voltage- and time-dependent properties and the pharmacologic agents that interact with the channel. N-type Ca++ currents are a class of Ca++ currents found in many neurons and are characterized by a high threshold of activation, fast inactivation, and an insensitivity to dihydropyridine.

Negative feedback: a corrective mechanism that causes the controller to respond by opposing a deviation from the desired output.

Nerve: 1) a neuron, or 2) a bundle of fibers from several neurons.

Nerve fiber layer: layer 9 of the retina, between the ganglion cell layer and the internal limiting membrane, containing axons of the ganglion cells.

Nerve growth factor (NGF): a trophic growth factor important for the development of nerve cells and processes. Discovered by a remarkable woman, the Jewish Italian neuroscientist, Rita Levi-Montalcini.

Neural crest: portions of the neural plate and folds adjacent to the general ectoderm that, during neurulation, separate from the latter without being incorporated into the neural tube, and form a crescent-shaped structure between the neural tube and the dorsal ectoderm. It marks the origin of peripheral nervous system.

Neural folds: the lateral margins of the neural plate that elevate to create a gutter, and eventually fuse on the midline to form the neural tube.

Neural groove: the midline depression created by the elevation of the neural folds during neurulation.

Neural plate: the thickening of the dorsal ectoderm of the gastrula caused by elongation of the cells as a result of induction from the notochord.

Neural tube: the tubular epithelium formed by closure of the invaginated neural plate, at the origin of the central nervous system.

Neuraxis: the central nervous system, but sometimes refers just to the brainstem and spinal cord.

Neurectoderm: the dorsal part of the embryonic ectoderm that has been specified to become nervous tissue by the inductive action of the underlying notochord.

Neurite: an undifferentiated neuronal process, more often the growing axon.

Neuroblasts: newly postmitotic cells on the nerve cell lineage that are not yet differentiated morphologically.

Neurocele: the lumen of the newly closed neural tube; the forerunner of the central canal of the spinal cord and the ventricles of the brain, lined by the ependyma.

Neuroepithelium: usually refers to the epithelium of the neural plate and the newly closed neural tube—that is, before it becomes highly stratified and differentiated into zones.

Neurogenic diseases: impaired motor performance due to lesions of the nervous system.

Neuroglia: nonneuronal cells of the central nervous system, including astrocytes, oligodendrocytes, microglia, and ependymal cells. Sometimes known as *glia* or glial cells.

Neuromuscular junction: the synapse between a spinal motor nerve and the muscle fiber that it innervates.

Neuron: a nerve cell, including the soma, dendrites, and axons. The neuron is the basic functional unit of the nervous system.

Neuronal reuptake: mechanism for terminating the effects of synaptically released norepinephrine through transport of norepinephrine back into nerve terminals. Also known as uptake-1.

Neuronotrophic: having one or more effects on neurons: promotion of the health and survival of nerve cells; stimulation and guidance of nerve fiber growth; stimulation of the production of neurotransmitter-synthesizing enzymes.

Neuropathy: any functional disturbances or pathologic changes in the peripheral nervous system.

Neuropil: network of axons, dendrites, and synapses.

Neuroplasm: cytoplasm of a neuron.

Neuropores: the openings of the neurocele at both ends of neural tube into the amniotic cavity, which close later than the rest of the neural tube.

Neurotransmitter: a substance of complex molecular structure, released from the presynaptic nerve terminal at a chemical synapse for the purpose of propagating an electrical message across the synapse, and which interacts with target organ receptors to produce an excitatory or inhibitory response; effects are relatively long lasting.

Neurotrophic: providing nourishment to neurons.

Neurotrophic factors: proteins primarily detected in the nervous system that influence the regulation of neuronal differentiation and survival, axon sprouting, and synaptic rearrangement.

Neurotrophism: the process of cell maintenance by innervation.

Nicotinic ganglionic receptor: subtype of nicotinic receptor found on postganglionic cell bodies of both the sympathetic and parasympathetic nervous systems.

Nicotinic receptors: receptors that are activated by low doses of nicotine and blocked by high doses of nicotine. The nicotinic receptor is one type of receptor activated by the neurotransmitter acetylcholine. There are two types of nicotinic receptors, nicotinic ganglionic receptors and nicotinic receptors at the neuromuscular junction in skeletal muscle.

Nissl substance: the neuronal organelle that consists of rough endoplasmic reticulum and ribosomes.

NMDA receptors: a type of glutamate receptor that is activated by the glutamate agonist N-methyl-D-aspartate. The NMDA receptor has two unusual characteristics. First, the ion channel of the receptor has a binding site for Mg^{++}, which blocks the flow of ions through the pore. The Mg^{++} block of the channel can be relieved by depolarization of the postsynaptic cell. Second, the ion channel of the receptor is nonspecific and allows Na^+, K^+, and Ca^{++} to pass through the pore. NMDA receptors have been found to be important in several forms of associative neuronal plasticity, including long-term potentiation (LTP), as well as during the development of the nervous system.

Nociceptor: a sensory receptor that responds to noxious stimuli and can signal pain.

Nodes of Ranvier: small areas of bare axon membrane between segments of myelin.

Nodulus: the most caudal part of the central section of the cerebellum. Part of the vestibulocerebellum and functionally and structurally similar to the ventral uvula.

Nondeclarative memory: also known as *implicit memory*, operates at an unconscious level. Nondeclarative memory encompasses the memory for skills and habits, priming, examples of associative learning such as classical conditioning, operant conditioning, and types of nonassociative learning such as sensitization and habituation. Memories are formed during nonepisodic learning of complex information in an incidental manner, without conscious awareness.

Noradrenergic neurons: nerve cells that release norepinephrine as a neurotransmitter at a synapse.

Norepinephrine: neurotransmitter released by postganglionic neurons of the sympathetic nervous system. Norepinephrine also represents 20% of the catecholamine secretion from the adrenal medulla.

Notochord: rodlike structure serving transiently as vertebral skeleton in the early embryo and which is the inductor of neurulation.

Nuclear bag fibers: one type of intrafusal muscle fiber.

Nuclear chain fibers: another type of intrafusal muscle fiber.

Nucleus: mass of neuron cell bodies, and sometimes interneurons, in the central nervous system.

Nucleus cuneatus: a nucleus in the medulla oblongata in which the fibers of the fasciculus cuneatus synapse; its axons travel to the thalamus by way of the medial lemniscus.

Nucleus dorsalis: a column of large cells on the medial side of the dorsal horn of the spinal cord from C8 to L3 that receives ascending primary afferents carrying proprioceptive information from the lower extremities. Second-order neurons give rise to the dorsal spinocerebellar tract.

Nucleus gracilis: nucleus in the medulla oblongata, in which the fibers of the fasciculus gracilis synapse; its axons travel to the thalamus by way of the medial lemniscus.

Nucleus Z: nucleus in the medulla that receives proprioceptive input and sends it to the thalamus.

Nystagmus: an eye movement pattern of alternating rapid and slow phases in one direction and resetting quick phases in the opposite direction.

Occipital lobe: portion of the cerebral hemispheres that contains the primary visual areas, visual associative areas, and areas involved in oculomotor control. It is the most posterior lobe of the cerebrum, located posterior to the parietal lobes.

Occipital pole: the most dorsal aspect of the occipital lobe, which is furthest from its equator.

Oculomotor nerve: cranial nerve III; it innervates most of the extraocular muscles.

Olfactory bulb: the ovoid structure at the anterior end of the olfactory lobe that sends sensory impulses to the olfactory nerve (cranial nerve I).

Olfactory cortex: the portion of the cerebral cortex closely related to the sense of smell; paleocortex.

Olfactory mucosa: the receptor surface in the nose.

Olfactory nerve: (CNI) the afferent fibers projecting from the olfactory mucosa in the nose to the olfactory bulb.

Olfactory tract: the group of axonal processes connecting the olfactory bulb to the olfactory cortex.

Olfactory tubercle: a region of the basal forebrain caudal to the olfactory tracts, which receives olfactory input.

Oligodendrocyte: one member of the category of glial cells; produces myelin for neurons in the central nervous system.

Olivocochlear bundle: the pathway that connects the superior olivary complex with the cochlear hair cells to modulate the action of the cochlea.

Operant conditioning: a type of associative learning in which the reinforcing stimulus is contingent on the behavior rather than on a conditioning stimulus produced by a researcher. The animal learns the consequences of its own behavior and alters its behavior as a result of training.

Opsin: transmembrane protein constituent of rhodopsin found in rod photoreceptors.

Optic chiasm: structure formed by the junction and partial decussation of the optic nerves just above the pituitary body. The nasal fibers of each optic nerve decussate and enter the contralateral optic tract.

Optic nerve: cranial nerve II; the cranial nerve that innervates the retina of the eye. It is embryologically and histologically derived from the forebrain and carries visual information.

Optic radiations: fibers that arise in the lateral geniculate body and project in a fanlike pattern to the primary visual cortex.

Optic tract: the continuation of the optic nerve from the optic chiasm to the brain.

Optic vesicles: invagination of the lateral walls of the diencephalic vesicle at the origin of the nervous component of the retina of the eye.

Optokinetic nystagmus: conjugate eye movements in the direction of a visual stimulus, elicited by low-frequency movement of the entire visual field to stabilize gaze.

Orbicularis oculi muscle: sheet of striated muscle in the eyelid forming concentric rings around the palpebral aperture. It is innervated by the facial nerve, cranial nerve VII, and functions as a sphincter, closing the eyelid.

Orbit: the cavity in the skull that contains the eyeball, orbital fat, fascia (connective tissue sheaths), the levator muscle of the upper lid, the lacrimal gland, extraocular muscles, and the nerves and circulatory supply (blood vessels) for the orbital contents and some of the face.

Orbitofrontal cortex: a part of the frontal lobe that is involved with executive functions, particularly emotional behavior.

Organ of Corti: the structure composed of supporting and hair cells that rests in the scala media on top of the basilar membrane.

Orthograde: occurring in a forward direction.

Oscillopsia: apparent movement of stationary objects in the visual field due to vestibular or oculomotor disorder.

Ossicles: the three tiny bones of the middle ear. They transmit airborne sounds to the inner ear.

Otoconia: the tiny calcium carbonate crystals imbedded in the otoconial membranes that act as inertial masses in the otoliths of the vestibular labyrinth.

Otolithic membrane: the protein matrix that holds the otoconia in place in the otoliths. During linear acceleration, deflection of underlying otolithic hair cells is caused by sliding of the membrane.

Otoliths: the two saclike membranous structures in the vestibular labyrinth that respond to linear acceleration, gravity, and tilt.

Outer nuclear layer: layer 4 of the retina, between the external limiting membrane and outer synaptic layer. It contains photoreceptor cell bodies.

Outer plexiform layer: layer 5 of the retina, between the internal and outer nuclear layers where these two layers and horizontal cells synapse.

Oval window: the membranous entrance to the cochlea from the middle ear, in which the stapes footplate is embedded.

Overtraining: training that has extended far beyond the time when the learner has become skilled at the task.

Pacinian corpuscle: a large, rapidly adapting, encapsulated tactile receptor sensitive composed of layers of connective tissue, located deep in the skin; it responds to pressure and vibration.

Pain thresholds: the point at which a stimulus is first perceived as painful.

Pain tolerance: the amount of pain a person can bear, which differs between individuals.

Paleocortex: cerebral cortex that has less than six layers. It is phylogenetically older than neocortex, most of which has six layers.

Palpebrae: the eyelids.

Parabrachial nucleus: nucleus in the pons located next to the brachium conjunctivum (superior cerebellar peduncle).

Parallel processing: the simultaneous transmission of bits of information.

Parasagittal: refers to a sagittal section taken away from the midline of the head.

Parasympathetic nervous system: a division of the autonomic nervous system most active during resting conditions, which acts to promote conservation and restoration of energy stores. The parasympathetic nervous system is also called the craniosacral division of the autonomic nervous system.

Parasympatholytic: an agent or an effect that blocks the effects of the parasympathetic nervous system.

Parasynaptic neurotransmission: communication between neurons when the postsynaptic receptor is some distance away from the presynaptic element.

Paresis: partial paralysis.

Parietal: a lobe of the cerebral cortex, located between the frontal and occipital lobes, rostral to the temporal lobe.

Parietooccipital sulcus: the sulcus that forms the border between the parietal and occipital lobes.

Parosmia: abnormal persistent, usually unpleasant odor sensation or phantom odor sensation.

Parvocellular: small-celled.

Passive tension: the resistance that the noncontractile elements of a muscle offer when a muscle is stretched (forms part of muscle length–force relation).

Path finding: the process of directed growth of axons in response to guiding clues.

Pedicle: the narrow foot of the cone photoreceptor cell.

Peduncle: a large bundle of tracts.

Peptidergic neurons: nerve cells that release a peptide, a short chain of amino acids, as a neurotransmitter at a synapse.

Periaqueductal gray matter: an area in the midbrain surrounding the cerebral aqueduct, which seems to be involved in pain inhibition and affective defense behavior.

Pericyte: a cell type found in blood vessel walls of the nervous system that appears to have phagocytic traits.

Periglomerular cell: type of neuron in the olfactory bulb near the glomeruli.

Perilymph: the fluid in the bony labyrinth and cochlea that surrounds and cushions the membranous vestibular and auditory labyrinths.

Peripheral nervous system: that part of the nervous system outside of the brain and spinal cord, not encased in protective bony enclosures.

Peripheral process: an axon or dendrite that extends from the soma of a neuron away from the substance of the central nervous system.

Peripheral resistance: the hindrance or impediment to blood flowing through a blood vessel, primarily used in reference to arterial blood flow.

Perseveration: the persistence of a response after the cessation of the stimulus; it refers here to persistence of a movement beyond the effectiveness of the movement.

Phantom limb: illusory sensory and motor sensations arising from a limb or limb segment that has been amputated or no longer has functional nerves.

Phase locking: the tendency of auditory neurons to fire during a particular phase or time of the auditory stimulus.

Pheochromocytoma: tumor of the adrenal medulla resulting in excessive secretion of the catecholamines norepinephrine and epinephrine.

Phonemic awareness: an understanding that syllables can be broken down into separate abstract units that can be recombined to form different sounds and words. A metalinguistic process, a conceptual understanding of language form.

Phospholipase C (PLC): an enzyme that cleaves membrane lipid chains producing two second messengers: inositol (IP3) and diacylglycerol (DAG). IP3 acts to release Ca^{++} from intracellular stores and DAG is necessary for activation of protein kinase (PKC).

Photoreceptor layer: layer 2 of the retina, containing the rods and cones.

Photoreceptors: sensory receptor of the eye, activated by light stimuli.

Pia mater: the thin, innermost layer of the meninges that follows the gyri and sulci surfaces of the brain and spinal cord.

Pineal body: a gland near the diencephalon, probably involved in the body's response to light, innervated by the autonomic nervous system.

Pinna: the cartilaginous external ear structure surrounding the concha, which serves to "catch" sound waves; often used to support eyeglasses, sometimes decorated by earrings.

Pioneer axons: the first axons of a fascicle to grow.

Piriform cortex: a pear-shaped cortical region that is situated on the medial part of the temporal lobe, immediately below the amygdala. It receives major olfactory input.

Pitch: 1) The psychophysical correlate of frequency: how high or low a sound sounds. 2) From anatomical position, up/down rotation of the head about an axis that goes through the ears.

Placing responses: when an animal's limb is moved toward an elevated support surface, it reflexively lifts the limb and puts it on the surface. There are two types: visual and tactile placing.

Plaque: an area of demyelination, characteristic of multiple sclerosis.

Plasmalemma: the unit membrane that envelopes a cell.

Plexiform: referring to a region of brain containing a network of neuronal processes.

Pons: a section of the brainstem immediately rostral to the pontine cistern, rostral between the midbrain and medulla.

Positional cues: in neuroembryology, cell surface molecules distributed according to a gradient within two fields, source and targets, that allow the formation of precise topographic connections between them.

Positron emission tomography (PET): scanning technique that combines computed tomography with radioisotope imaging, and that requires injection of a radioactive tracer. Depending on the chemical to which the radioactive tracer is attached, receptors or blood flow changes can be visualized. No structural information is provided, and because the signal/noise ratio is relatively low, the data from several subjects are usually averaged.

Postcentral gyrus: gyrus of the cerebral cortex, on the lateral surface, just behind the central sulcus.

Posterior: toward the back.

Posterior canal: synonymous with *inferior semicircular canal*.

Posterior commissure: a small bundle of fibers posterior to the thalamus.

Posterior fossa: the space in the skull in which the medulla, pons, and cerebellum are located.

Postganglionic neuron: the second neuron of the autonomic nervous system that innervates the target organs or tissues. The cell bodies of postganglionic neurons are located in the autonomic ganglia, and postganglionic neurons are unmyelinated.

Postmitotic: no longer dividing.

Poststimulus time (PST) histogram: a histogram of the response to a stimulus (firing rate) plotted as a function of time after the stimulus onset. The histogram is collected over many repetitions of the stimulus.

Postsynaptic density: the ground substance and filaments in the postsynaptic element that serve to anchor intercellular filaments that span between the presynaptic and postsynaptic elements.

Postsynaptic element: the component of a synapse that receives the transmission of an action potential.

Postsynaptic potential (PSP): a graded change in the membrane potential of a postsynaptic cell that results from currents flowing through ionotropic receptors that are activated by the binding of molecules of neurotransmitter released by presynaptic cells. Postsynaptic potentials either depolarize the postsynaptic cell (i.e., excitatory PSP) or hyperpolarize the postsynaptic cell (inhibitory PSP).

Postural hypotension: the fall in blood pressure associated with dizziness or light-headedness upon standing. Also called orthostatic hypotension.

Presynaptic element: the component of a synapse that transmits an action potential.

Precentral gyrus: the gyrus rostral to the central sulcus.

Predatory aggression: a directed attack by a predator toward a natural prey object.

Predatory attack behavior: a form of aggression elicited by stimulation of the lateral hypothalamus or ventral periaqueductal gray in the cat, characterized by the initial stalking and subsequent biting of the back of the neck of a prey object.

Preganglionic neuron: the first neuron of the autonomic nervous system that innervates postganglionic cell bodies in the autonomic ganglia. Preganglionic neurons are myelinated, release acetylcholine, and their cell bodies are located in the central nervous system.

Prejunctional terminal: an enlargement of the spinal motor nerve at the neuromuscular junction.

Presynaptic inhibition: inhibition of neurotransmitter release due to the depolarization of the nerve terminal by a second neural input.

Pretectum: area immediately caudal to the superior colliculus, concerned with eye movements.

Primary afferent fiber: a nerve fiber that transmits signals from sensory receptors and has its cell body in a dorsal root ganglion.

Primary somatosensory cortex (S-I): located in the postcentral gyrus, it comprises Brodmann's areas 3a, 3b, 1, and 2; the neurons in this region respond to somatosensory stimuli.

Priming: an example of nondeclarative memory in which recognition of words or visual cues is facilitated by prior exposure to the words or visual cues.

Projection neuron: neuron with a single long axon that connects to other nervous system areas.

Proprioception: sensation of movement or static limb position, mediated by muscle spindles, tendon organs, and joint receptors. Sometimes synonymous with *kinesthesia*.

Propriospinal fibers: dorsal column fibers carrying proprioceptive input that terminate in the spinal cord.

Prosencephalon: the rostral-most subdivision of the embryonic brain when at the three-vesicle stage. It subdivides into the diencephalon and the telencephalon.

Protein kinase: a group of enzymes that catalyze the phosphorylation of other proteins by using adenosine triphosphate. This changes the function of the proteins. Examples include protein kinase A (PKA) and protein kinase C (PKC).

Pseudounipolar neuron: a nerve cell that processes an apparent single process that functions as both an axon and a dendrite.

Psychogenic tearing: weeping or crying.

Ptosis: drooping of the eyelid, normally due to loss of neural innervation.

Pupil: aperture in the iris through which the image forming light enters the eye.

Pursuit: conjugate eye movements used to follow a moving target.

Putamen: one of the basal ganglia; with the globus pallidus, it forms the lentiform nucleus; with the caudate nucleus, it forms the striatum.

Pyramids: the raised areas on the ventral surface of the medulla containing descending fibers from the pyramidal tracts.

Pyriform cortex: the cortical region that is situated immediately below the amygdala. It receives significant olfactory inputs and is intimately linked with functions of the amygdala.

Quadrantanopia: loss of vision in a quarter sector of the visual field of one eye.

Quadrantanopsia: see *quadrantanopia*.

Quantum: the smallest amount of light energy needed for a photoreceptor to respond. It is equal to the product of the frequency of the light and Planck's constant (6.624×10^{-27} erg), a very small unit of energy.

Radial glial cell: a transient category of glial cells spanning the thickness of the developing neural tube and serving as substrate for the postmitotic neuroblasts to migrate from the germinal zone to the intermediate zone. After migration, it either degenerates or transforms into an astrocyte.

Radial migration: migration of postmitotic nerve cells from their germinal zone of origin to the intermediate zone, following a radial course in relation to the neurocele and pial surface. It is generally mediated by the radial glial cells.

Ramon y Cajal, Santiago: the great Spanish neuroanatomist largely responsible for developing the science of the structure of the nervous system. He shared the Nobel prize with Camillo Golgi.

Ramus: Latin word for "branch." Used to refer to branches of cortical sulci.

Rapidly adapting: characterized by rapid responsiveness to mechanical stimulation and rapid accommodation to sustained deformation of the skin.

Rate coding: the speed or frequency of motor nerve excitation causing an increase in muscle force.

Reaction time: the time interval between the application of a stimulus and the response it evokes.

Reactive gliosis: a reactive state in which stimulated glial cells migrate to a central nervous system injury site and form a glial scar during the repair process.

Receptive field: the area of a receptive sheet, such as the skin or retina, within which the activity of a neuron can be influenced.

Receptive field axis of orientation: the axis of orientation of a stimulus that maximally influences a cell.

Receptor: protein commonly found in plasma membranes specialized to identify and bind with specific substances. The neurotransmitter binds with the macromolecule in a precise orientation to produce a response in an effector organ.

Receptor potential: the change in the electrical potential of the receptor organ in a sensory system. In the auditory system, it is synonymous with *cochlear microphonic*.

Reciprocal excitation: refers to the spinal circuitry resulting in an excitation of the motor neurons of the antagonist muscle due to activation of the agonist muscle's tendon organ.

Reciprocal inhibition: the spinal circuitry resulting in decreased excitability of the motor neurons of the antagonist muscle due to stretch of the agonist muscle.

Recovery of function: after a central nervous system lesion, 1) the ability to perform at a level defined before the lesion; 2) more precisely, achieving a goal or performing in the same way as before the lesion.

Recruitment: refers to the activation of motor units.

Redox reactions: the tendency of a redox couple (a mixture of oxidized and reduced species) to donate electrons.

Referred pain: deep, dull, poorly localized pain arising from the viscera is perceived by higher centers as coming from superficial regions of the body because of convergence of visceral and somatic inputs onto these same neurons.

Reflex-reversal: a dramatic change in reflex action as a function of posture or action (e.g., locomotion).

Reissner's membrane: the membrane that bounds the scala media or cochlear duct on one side.

Relative refractory period: the interval after the discharge of an action potential during which the membrane can be stimulated to discharge another action potential only by a normally suprathreshold stimulus.

Release phenomenon: the overt effect caused by the cessation of normal activity. Often this activity is inhibition, and part of a balanced system.

Repolarization: moving a membrane potential toward the resting membrane potential from a hyperpolarized state.

Resonating: having a large-amplitude vibration in a mechanical system in response to a sinusoidal stimulation at the natural vibration frequency of the system.

Response area: the range of frequencies and intensities to which the neuron can respond with an action potential; synonymous with *tuning curve*.

Rest length: the muscle length at which active tension is maximum.

Restiform body: synonymous with *inferior cerebellar peduncle*.

Reticular activating system: the brainstem formation involved with states of wakefulness.

Retina: the receptor surface of the eye.

Retinal pigment epithelium: layer 1, the outermost layer of the retina. A nonneural structure, it provides metabolic and optical support to the inner layers of the retina.

Retrograde: occurring in a backward direction.

Retrograde axoplasmic transport: the ratchet-like mechanism used to transport substances from the axon terminal to the soma.

Rhombencephalon: the caudal-most subdivision of the embryonic brain when at the three-vesicle stage. It subdivides into the myelencephalon and the metencephalon.

Rhombic lip: the most lateral portion of the germinal zone of the metencephalic vesicle, which remains proliferative over an extended period of time and from which derive the cerebellum and several brainstem structures, such as the precerebellar nuclei.

Rigidity: a state of abnormal muscle tone characterized by resistance to passive movement that is unaffected by movement velocity and does not involve an exaggerated tendon jerk.

Rod: a type of photoreceptor.

Roll: from anatomic position, the tilting motion of the head as it rotates about an axis from the front to the back of the head, to bring the left ear toward or away from the left shoulder.

Romberg's sign: an indicator of disease manifested by loss of balance while standing with the feet together and the eyes closed.

Rostral: toward the top of the head, the antonym of *caudal.*

Ruffini endings: slowly adapting, encapsulated tactile receptors sensitive to continuous pressure and skin stretch, located at an intermediate depth in the skin.

Saccade: conjugate, rapid eye movement used to scan a stationary visual field, to catch up when the eye lags a moving target, or to reset the position of the eye in the head during nystagmus.

Saccule: one of the two otoliths of the vestibular labyrinth. It responds primarily to vertical linear acceleration.

Sacral: refers to the five vertebrae, spinal nerves, or cord segments just rostral to the coccygeal area.

Sagittal: refers to an anteroposterior section, separating left from right sides.

Saltatory conduction: propagation of an action potential along a myelinated neuron moving from one node of Ranvier to the next.

Sarcolemma: the excitable plasma membrane covering every striated muscle fiber.

Sarcomere: the contractile unit of a myofibril.

Sarcoplasm: the cytoplasm of a striated muscle fiber.

Sarcoplasmic reticulum: a membranous system in the muscle fiber that acts as a storage site for calcium ions.

Scala media: the middle, endolymph-filled compartment of the cochlea, bounded by the basilar membrane and Reissner's membrane. Also known as the *cochlear partition.*

Scala tympani: the lower compartment of the cochlear spiral, which communicates with the middle ear by the round window.

Scala vestibuli: the upper compartment of the cochlear spiral, which communicates with the middle ear by the oval window.

Scarpa's ganglion: the ganglion of the vestibular nerve.

Schwann cells: glial cells of the peripheral nervous system.

Sclera: the white, opaque, fibrous, outer tunic of the eye. It covers the entire eye except for the small, anterior segment that is covered by the clear cornea.

Scotoma: an isolated area of decreased or absent visual sensitivity in the visual field, surrounded by a more sensitive area.

Second-order sensory axon: conveys sensory information to higher centers of the central nervous system.

Second-order sensory neuron: sensory neurons in the central nervous system on which primary sensory neurons make their first synapse.

Secondary somatosensory cortex (S-II): lies at the lateral edge of the primary somatosensory (S-I) and motor cortices; receives input from S-I and ascending pathways regarding general sensory modalities.

Section: a slice of the brain or spinal cord.

Segmental: a cross-sectional component of the brainstem or spinal cord containing neural inputs and outputs.

Semicircular canals: the three curved bony spaces in the vestibular labyrinth of the inner ear of the temporal bone, or the membranous tubes contained in the bony canals. They are oriented approximately at right angles to each other, so that rotation of the head through any plane in space stimulates at least one of them.

Senescence: a decrease in an individual's probability of survival later in life.

Sense of effort: centrally mediated sensations of the force or effort used to perform a movement.

Sense of force: synonymous with *tension.*

Sensitization: the enhancement of an elicited behavior after a strong or noxious stimulus. Sensitization is an example of nonassociative learning and can induce both short- and long-term memories.

Septal area: part of the limbic system that lies in the dorsomedial position at the level of the rostral forebrain. Its axons project to the hypothalamus and play an important role in regulation of functions associated with the hypothalamus.

Serial processing: the consecutive transmission of bits of information.

Serotonin (5-hydroxytryptamine, 5-HT): a low–molecular-weight molecule that is used as a neurotransmitter by several different types of neurons. Serotonin is a member of a class of neurotransmitters, the biogenic amines (i.e., dopamine, norepinephrine, epinephrine, serotonin, and histamine). Biogenic amines, such as 5-HT, often function as modulatory transmitters, that is, they activate second messenger and protein kinase systems that regulate the properties of the postsynaptic cells. The projections of cells that use biogenic amines as transmitters are widely distributed throughout the central nervous system and regulate complex cognitive functions such as attention, learning, and memory.

Shortening contraction: see *concentric contraction*.

Silent synapses: connections between neurons that, under normal circumstances, cannot produce sufficient depolarization of the cell membrane to initiate an action potential in the postsynaptic neuron.

Simple cells: cortical cells of area V1 that have a proper receptive field axis of orientation with on/off areas. They respond to a stimulus of specific size and orientation but not to movement.

Size principle: refers to the principle governing the orderly recruitment of motor neurons by the size of the neuronal cell body, from the smallest to the largest.

Sliding filament model: the model that describes the sliding of actin filaments over the myosin filaments by cross-bridge formation during muscle contraction.

Slowly adapting: characterized by relatively sustained responsiveness to sustained deformation of the skin.

Slow muscle fibers: refers to the muscle fiber type that is slowly contracting, has high oxidative capacity (aerobic), and does not fatigue easily.

Slow pain (delayed or second pain): C primary afferent fiber stimulation that results in diffuse, persisting pain that has an aching, throbbing, burning quality; poorly localized on the body.

Sodium/potassium pump: an energy-dependent mechanism in the plasma membrane that moves sodium and potassium ions across the membrane. Ions are moved in a ratio of three sodium ions out of the cell to two potassium ions into the cell.

Solitary tract nucleus: also called nucleus tractus solitarius; nucleus in the medulla that receives information from cranial nerves VII, IX, and X, including the sensory fibers for taste. When viewed in coronal sections, it gives the impression of sitting off by itself.

Soma: the central region or body of a cell, the central region or body of a neuron.

Somatic motor system: the division of the peripheral nervous system innervating skeletal muscle.

Somatic senses: the senses with receptors located in the skin or muscle structures, including light touch, deep pressure, vibration, temperature, and kinesthesia.

Somatosensory: pertaining to sensory input form the body, including pain, temperature, touch, vibration, and proprioception.

Somatosensory cortex: the portion of the anterior parietal cortex that processes sensory information about touch, proprioception, and some special senses.

Somatotopic organization: inputs from the sensory receptors in the periphery are conveyed to the central nervous system in a manner that reflects their actual positional relationships; these positional relationships are conserved in areas of the central nervous system.

Sparing of function: the absence of a functional deficit immediately after central nervous system damage.

Spasticity: increased resistance to passive motion of a limb that is proportional to velocity of the motion, and is accompanied by increased deep tendon reflexes; characterized by the clasp-knife phenomenon.

Spatial summation: the integration of multiple postsynaptic potentials that arrive at a neuron simultaneously but in different locations.

Special senses: the senses with receptors located in specific structures on the head, including smell, taste, the chemical sense, vision, hearing, and the sense of head movement.

Specific language disorder: a developmental disorder in acquiring expressive and comprehensive language abilities. It runs in families and is more common in boys. Cognitive decline and reading disability usually result. Synonymous with developmental aphasia and learning disability.

Spherules: the end bulbs of the rod photoreceptor.

Sphincter muscle: a muscle that surrounds an opening, such as the pupil, and acts to reduce the size.

Spina bifida: developmental defect that consists of the incomplete development of the caudal spinal cord resulting from the failure of the posterior neuropore to close.

Spinal accessory nerve: cranial nerve XI. It innervates the sternocleidomastoid muscle and the upper part of the trapezius muscle.

Spinal cord: the part of the central nervous system outside of the skull, encased in the vertebrae.

Spinal nerves: peripheral nerves of the spinal cord, carrying afferent and efferent fibers.

Spinal shock: transient hypoactivity of the spinal cord immediately after spinal cord injury.

Spinal trigeminal (spinal V) nucleus: second-order neurons for sensory impulses from the face conveyed by the trigeminal nerve; these trigeminal neurons project this information to the ventral posteromedial (VPM) nucleus of the thalamus.

Spinoreticular pathway: a major ascending pathway of pain and temperature information that ascends as part of the contralateral anterolateral pathway; some fibers form uncrossed projections.

Spinotectal tract: a tract carrying mixed signals from the spinal cord and the medulla to the superior colliculus.

Spinothalamic pathway: an ascending somatosensory pathway, traveling from spinal cord to the thalamus by way of the lateral spinothalamic columns, that mediates information about pain, temperature, and some touch.

Sprout: 1) v. To begin to grow. 2) n. New growth. Generally divided into two types: regenerative sprouting, new growth at the severed end of the axon; and collateral sprouting, new growth of a side branch from a nearby intact axon.

Stapedius: the muscle attached to the stapes that contracts in response to loud sounds and dampens the movement of the ossicles.

Stapes: the medial-most bone of the three ossicles, shaped like a stirrup. The footplate of the stapes covers the oval window.

Static sensitivity: the sensitivity of a muscle spindle afferent to static muscle length.

Stereotropism: the path-finding strategy of neurites by mechanical guidance.

Stereocilia: the cilia located at the apical ends of the hair cells in the vestibular and auditory labyrinths.

Strabismus: inability to direct the foveal line of sight of both eyes at the same time to an object of regard; commonly called a squint, or crossed eyes.

Stretch reflex: the reflex contraction of a muscle in response to a sudden, rapid increase in its length.

Stria vascularis: the blood supply to the cochlea located in its lateral wall.

Striate cortex: cerebral cortex in area 17, the primary *visual cortex*, characterized by its striped appearance.

Striatum: part of the basal ganglia, usually includes the caudate nucleus and the putamen. Synonymous with neostriatum.

Striola: the vector of orientation in each otolithic macula.

Stroke: from the expression "stroke of God," a lay term for a cerebrovascular accident.

Subacute combined degeneration: degeneration of the dorsal and lateral columns of the spinal cord with preservation of the gray matter, often due to a vitamin B_{12} deficiency. This disorder is most often seen in pernicious anemia.

Subarachnoid space: region between the arachnoid and pia mater, filled with cerebrospinal fluid.

Subliminal excitation: excitation with no overt effect, which brings the neuron, or population of neurons, closer to threshold.

Substantia gelatinosa: lamina II of the dorsal horn; receives input from nociceptive C fibers.

Substantia nigra: darkly pigmented structure in the brainstem, considered to be one of the basal ganglia-related structures.

Subthalamic nucleus: a nucleus in the diencephalon, near the thalamus, that receives input from the basal ganglia.

Sulcus: the valley between two gyri (plural, *sulci*).

Sulcus limitans: small dimple on the lateral wall of the neurocele of the developing spinal cord and brainstem demarcating the dorsal, sensory alar plate from the ventral, motor basal plate.

Summation of contractions: the contractile response of the whole muscle or motor units to repeated excitatory impulses.

Superior: toward the top; antonym of *inferior*.

Superior canal: synonymous with *anterior canal*.

Superior colliculus: the rostral eminence of the dorsal midbrain located near the pineal gland. It is the integrative and relay center for visuospatial information to the skeletal muscles.

Superior oblique muscle: striated, extrinsic muscle of the eyeball that anatomically originates near the annulus of Zinn but functionally at the trochlea on the anterior, superior, medial aspect of the orbit. It inserts superiorly and posterotemporally on the eyeball. Innervated by cranial nerve IV, it depresses, abducts, and intorts the eye.

Superior olivary complex: a group of three nuclei in the pons to which neurons of the ventral cochlear nucleus project. The major nuclei are the medial and lateral nuclei (MSO and LSO) and medial nucleus of the trapezoid body (MNTB). It seems to be important for localizing sound in space.

Superior rectus muscle: a striated, extrinsic muscle of the eyeball that originates at the annulus of Zinn and inserts superiorly near the corneal limbus of the eyeball. Innervated by cranial nerve III, it elevates, adducts, and intorts the eye. It also assists in raising the upper eyelid.

Supersensitivity: in pharmacology, the increase in responsiveness of a tissue or organ that occurs as a result of functional denervation.

Suture: the junction between immovable bones.

Sylvian fissure: deep sulcus that divides the frontal lobe from the temporal lobe.

Sympathetic hyperreflexia: synonymous with *autonomic dysreflexia*.

Sympathetic nervous system: the thoracolumbar division of the autonomic nervous system. The sympathetic nervous system helps the body deal with stressful conditions.

Synapse: the point of functional connection or association between the various elements of a neuron. *Axoaxonic synapse:* the functional connection between the axon of one neuron and the axon of another neuron. *Axodendritic synapse:* the functional connection between the axon of one neuron and the dendrite of another neuron. *Axosomatic synapse:* the functional connection between the axon of one neuron and the soma of another neuron. Often in a synapse, the presynaptic element is the termination of an axon and the postsynaptic element a dendrite (possibly a spine) or the soma.

Synaptic cleft: the microscopic space that separates the elements of a synapse.

Synaptic vesicles: small spherical structures in synaptic terminals in which neurotransmitter substances are stored until released.

Synaptogenesis: the formation of synapses, the connections between axon terminals and their targets: muscle cells (neuromuscular junction), or nerve cells.

Synergistic: acting together to enhance the effect of another force; synergistic muscles act together at one or more joints to produce voluntary movement.

Syringomyelia: formation of a cyst in the spinal cord; as the cyst expands, it causes a progressive, asymmetric lesion of the cord.

T tubules: see *transverse tubules*.

Tabetic syndrome: synonymous with *tabes dorsalis*; a slowly progressive degeneration of the spinal cord dorsal columns that occurs 15 to 20 years after an initial infection of syphilis.

Tachycardia: an abnormal increase in heart rate.

Tangential migration: migration of postmitotic nerve cells from their germinal zone of origin to the intermediate zone after an oblique course in relation to the neurocele and pial surface. It usually uses the surface of other nerve cells for substrate (rather than radial glia) and is often secondary to radial migration.

Target organ: the organ or tissue that produces an effect due to stimulation by a hormone, the nervous system. The term is essentially equivalent to *effector organ*.

Tectorial membrane: the gelatinous structure covering the organ of Corti, with grooves into which the tips of the cilia of outer hair cells fit. It facilitates bending of the hair cells on stimulation.

Tectospinal tract: a tract carrying visual signals from the superior colliculus to the rostral spinal cord.

Tectothalamic tract: a tract carrying signals from the superior colliculus to the pulvinar of the thalamus.

Telencephalon: a subdivision of the brain when at the five-vesicle stage. It will become the basal forebrain and cerebral hemispheres.

Temporal: 1) the most lateral lobe of the cerebral cortex; 2) related to time.

Temporal summation: the integration of multiple postsynaptic potentials that arrive at the same location on a neuron but at different times.

Tendon organ reflex: reflex inhibition of a muscle due to stimulation of its tendon organ.

Tension: peripherally mediated sensation of the force or effort used to perform a movement.

Terminal bouton: the enlarged end of an axon or dendrite.

Tetanus: prolonged contractile response of the whole muscle or motor unit to rapidly repeated excitatory impulses.

Thalamic pain syndrome: severe, persistent pain resulting from lesions in multiple regions of the thalamus.

Thalamus: large, egg-shaped structure located at the rostral end of the brainstem, containing nuclei that are major relay centers for ascending pathways to the cerebral cortex.

Thermoreceptor: a sensory receptor that responds to a change in temperature.

Thoracic: refers to the 12 vertebrae, spinal nerves, or cord segments related to the trunk, between the cervical and lumbar areas.

Threshold: the membrane potential that triggers the change in ion conductance that leads to the firing of an action potential.

Tip links: the fine filaments that connect the tips of the stereocilia in the hair cell bundle of the hair cell. Deflecting the hair bundle causes the tip links to be unloaded, opening ion channels in the stereocilia.

Tone: the background or resting amount of neural activity to an organ or tissue.

Topography: orderly organization of fibers in a bundle, or neurons in a nucleus, or whole projection systems reflecting the functional and anatomic organization of the periphery, such as the skin (somatotopy) or the visual field (visuotopy).

Trailing process: extension of the migrating neuroblast that is on the opposite side of the nucleus in relation to the leading process. In cortical regions, the leading process of some cells is the one that becomes the axon.

Transcutaneous electrical nerve stimulation (TENS): a treatment for pain reduction in which external electrical current is repetitively applied to areas associated with painful sensations to alter neuronal electrical properties in these areas and thus produce analgesia.

Transducer: a mechanism that changes one form of energy into another form.

Transducin: special G protein family member that is found in photoreceptor cells.

Transduction: the process of changing one signal into another. For example, in the auditory system, it is the process by which channels in the inner hair cells are opened to allow release of neurotransmitter into the synaptic cleft between the hair cell and auditory nerve fiber.

Transient ischemic attack (TIA): temporary episode of ischemia characterized by blurred vision, lightheadedness, slurred speech, numbness, and paralysis. A series of TIAs may precede a cerebrovascular accident.

Transneuronal: occurring across synapses such that more than one neuron is involved.

Transverse tubules: series of folds of the sarcolemma that run through the muscle cell; also known as T tubules.

Traumatic brain injury (TBI): any injury to the head that causes damage to the brain.

Trigeminal complex: group of four nuclei that carry sensory and motor information from and to the face, located chiefly in the pons and medulla oblongata.

Trigeminal ganglion: a collection of cell bodies with a peripheral process transducing sensory information from the head and face and a central process conveying the information to the midbrain.

Trigeminal nerve: cranial nerve V. It inserts into the pons and has three divisions, ophthalmic, maxillary, and mandibular, consisting of motor fibers to muscles of mastication and sensory fibers from the face and head.

Trigeminal pathway: carries somatosensory information from the head and face to various nuclei in the thalamus; also known as trigeminoreticulothalamic tract or trigeminothalamic tract.

Trochlea: a cartilaginous, ringlike structure of the frontal bone through which the tendon of the superior oblique muscle passes. It serves as the functional origin of the superior oblique for all force dynamics.

Trochlear nerve: cranial nerve IV. It innervates the superior oblique muscle.

Trophic factors: diffusible chemical agents that sustain a neuron's life. The best known is nerve growth factor.

Tuning curve: all of the frequencies to which a hair cell in the cochlea or an auditory nerve fiber respond; also known as *response area*.

Twitch: the contractile response of the whole muscle or motor unit to single excitatory impulse.

Two-point discrimination: point of separation at which two closely spaced stimuli are perceived as separate and distinct rather than as one stimulus.

Two-tone suppression: the phenomenon in the auditory system in which hearing one tone can reduce the response to another tone of similar but not identical frequency. It results from the nonlinear mechanics of the basilar membrane.

Tympanic membrane: the membrane separating the external auditory meatus from the middle ear. The malleus attaches to it at one end; also known as the eardrum.

Unilaterally: occurring on or affecting one side.

Utricle: one of the otoliths of the vestibular labyrinth, it responds primarily to horizontal acceleration.

Uvula: a posterior part of the cerebellum. The ventral uvula is considered part of the vestibulocerebellum and is similar to the nodulus.

Vagus nerve: cranial nerve X, the major cranial nerve of the autonomic nervous system, which also carries some fibers for taste.

Varicosity: dilated regions of adrenergic neuronal axons containing large numbers of synaptic vesicles, and the site of the neuron from which norepinephrine is released.

Vegetative nervous system: an alternative term for the autonomic nervous system that describes the involuntary or unconscious control of the visceral organs.

Velocity storage integrator: a mechanism in the central vestibular pathways that collects, stores, and gradually releases information about head velocity; it may be involved in vestibular contributions to spatial orientation.

Ventral: toward the belly side, synonym of *anterior*; antonym of *dorsal*.

Ventral acoustic stria: one pathway leaving the cochlear nucleus through which axons of bushy and multipolar cells travel to other parts of the brainstem.

Ventral amygdalofugal pathway: a second major pathway of the amygdala, which projects from more lateral regions of the amygdala to the hypothalamus and midbrain periaqueductal gray.

Ventral commissure: a region ventral to the central canal in which axons transmitting pain and postural information cross the spinal cord.

Ventral horn: ventral portion of the spinal cord concerned mainly with motor functions and which derives from the embryonic basal plate.

Ventral posterior lateral (VPL) nucleus: the thalamic nucleus to which proprioceptive fibers from the limbs and trunk project as they ascend to somatosensory cortex.

Ventral posterior medial (VPM) nucleus: the part of the ventral posterior nucleus of the thalamus that receives somatosensory input from the face, including afferents from the tongue.

Ventral roots: the bundle of primarily efferent fibers emerging from the spinal cord at a particular spinal level.

Ventricles: spaces inside the brain filled with cerebrospinal fluid.

Ventroposteriomedial thalamus: medial portion of the posterior ventral nucleus of the thalamus; it receives input from the trigeminal tract and sends its axons to somatosensory cortex.

Vergence: disjunctive rotational eye movement such that a point of reference on the two globes moves in opposite directions. For example, convergence moves the right eye leftward and the left eye rightward.

Vertigo: the illusion of self-motion.

Vestibular labyrinth: the bony or membranous set of spaces and structures in the inner ear in the temporal bone. It detects rotatory and linear head acceleration.

Vestibular nuclei: the nuclei in the rostral medulla that receive input from the vestibular labyrinth.

Vestibule: the space in the inner ear that contains the otoliths.

Vestibulo-ocular reflex (VOR): the conjugate, compensatory eye movement stimulated by head movement to stabilize gaze in space.

Vestibulocerebellum: the parts of the cerebellum that respond to vestibular input and communicate with the vestibular system.

Vestibulocochlear nerve: synonymous with *auditory nerve*.

Vestibulospinal tracts: pathways that descend into the spinal cord from the vestibular nuclei and are the basis for the vestibular system's influence on postural control.

Visceral nervous system: an alternative term for the autonomic nervous system, referring to autonomic control of the visceral organs such as the heart, lungs, and gastrointestinal tract.

Visceral: referring to the internal organs (viscera) such as the heart, lungs, and gastrointestinal tract.

Visual cortex: the cortex of the occipital lobe, composed of Brodmann's areas 17, 18, and 19. It is the primary cortical receptive area for visual information. It is also thought to be involved in reflex fixation, smooth pursuit, accommodation, convergence, and pupil size.

Visual field: the extent of physical space represented on the retina of an eye in a given position. On average it is 65 degrees up, 75 degrees down, 60 degrees in, and 95 degrees out when the eye is in the null position, straight ahead in the orbit. The 60 degrees in may vary for those of us with more distinguished noses.

Vitreous humor: the transparent, gelatinous fluid (humor) that fills the vitreous chamber of the eye, the space between the lens, ciliary body, and the retina. It supports the eye mechanically and optically.

Vocabulary burst: Most normal children start the acquisition of language slowly and repeat the same words and two-word combinations frequently. In the first part of the same year, the acquisition curve starts to accelerate rapidly and many new words are acquired every day. The neural mechanisms underlying this rapid increase are not understood, but it is one of the many linguistic phenomena that clearly separate human from ape.

Wada test: a test that can identify the "eloquent" hemisphere (i.e., the hemisphere housing language function). It is used as a surgical planning guide for epilepsy patients. Injection of a briefly acting barbiturate into the vascular supply of the "dominant" (language supporting) hemisphere halts speech output.

Wallerian degeneration: degeneration of an axon distal to the site of lesion.

Wernicke's area: the posterior half of the superior temporal gyrus and middle temporal gyrus in the left hemisphere. The region is thought to contain specialized information processing mechanisms for phonologic, semantic, and syntactic analysis. When this region is damaged, verbal output remains fluent but becomes filled with errors and sometimes is incomprehensible.

White matter: parts of the central nervous system that appear white in ordinary light because they are covered with myelin, usually fiber tracts.

Working memory: a temporary storage process that allows information to be brought in from the long-term store and manipulated to regulate behavior. It can be constantly updated. Imaging and lesion experiments suggest that working memory for different modalities is located in different parts of the frontal lobe.

Yaw: from anatomic position, rotation of the head back and forth (e.g., from left to right).

Zonula adherens: the tight, nonpermeable junction between cells that acts as a biochemical barrier.

Index

- - - - - - - - -

O

Occipital lobe, 16
  in visual system, 178, 179–180f, 179–184, 183f
Occipital petalia, in language, 363
Occipital pole, 179, 182
Octopus cells, in auditory system, 142, 144f
Oculomotor abnormalities, 191–192
Oculomotor control, 158–162, 160f
Oculomotor nerve, 24t
  in autonomic nervous system, 281, 290
Odor, 201–202, 203
OKN (optokinetic nystagmus), 187, 189–190
Old age. *See* Aging
Olfactory bulb, 201, 201f, 203–204, 203f
Olfactory nerve, 24t, 202
Olfactory receptor mucosa, 200f, 200–201, 201f
Olfactory system, 200–205f, 200–204
Olfactory tracts, 204, 205f
Olfactory tubercle, 204
Oligodendrocytes, 30f, 72–74, 73f
  development of, 388
Olivocerebellar projection, 265
Olivocochlear bundle, 140
Open-loop control, of movement, 211–213, 212f
Operant conditioning, 322, 324
Optical fractionation, 405
Optic chiasm, 176
Optic nerve, 24t, 176
  damage to, 173, 192
Optic radiations, 178–179
Optic tract, 176
  accessory, 178
Optokinetic nystagmus (OKN), 187, 189–190
Orbicularis oculi muscle, 171
Orbit, 170
Orbitofrontal cortex, in gustation, 200
Organizational principles, 3–8
Organ of Corti, 136, 137f, 138f
Oropharyngeal cavity, 197f
Orthograde changes, after brain damage, 422–423
Oscillopsia, 166
Ossicles, 131, 132f, 135, 135f
Otoconia, 154, 155
Otolith(s), 149–154, 150–152f, 155
Otolithic membrane, 151–154
Outer ear, 131, 132f, 134–135
Outer nuclear layer, of retina, 175
Outer plexiform layer, of retina, 175
Oval window, 132f, 133, 135, 135f, 138f
Overtraining, and brain damage, 428
Oxygen free radical production, with aging, 407, 408–409, 409f

P

Pacinian corpuscles
  in discriminative touch, 95, 97
  in proprioception, 119
Pain
  delayed, 79
  fast, 79
  first, 79
  gate control theory of, 81–82, 82f
  initial, 79
  phantom limb, 90–91
  receptors for, 78
  referred, 83
  second, 79
  slow, 79
  transcutaneous electrical nerve stimulation for, 82–83
Pain modulation, descending pathways in, 88–90, 89f
Pain perception, 77–91
  anterolateral system pathways in, 83–86, 84f, 86f, 87f
  cerebral cortex in, 88
  clinical correlations of, 90
  laminae of dorsal horn of spinal cord in, 80f, 80–81
  primary afferent neurons in, 78–81, 79f, 80f
  spinoreticular tract in, 84f, 86–87
  spinothalamic tract in, 83–86, 84f
  in thalamic pain syndrome, 88
  trigeminal pathways in, 87
Pain thresholds, 90
Pain tolerance, 90
Paleocerebellum, 262
Paleocortex, in olfactory system, 204
Paleostriatum, 255
Pallidum, 255
Palpebrae, 170–171
Palpebral aperture, 170
Papillae, 196
Parabrachial nucleus, in gustatory system, 199
Parallel fibers (PF), in long-term depression, 339, 340f, 341f
Parallel processing, 6
  in motor system, 273
Paralysis, 226
Paramedian reticular nucleus, 235–236
Parasagittal section, 12
Parasympathetic nervous system (PNS)
  anatomy of, 278f, 279f, 279–281, 280t
  physiology of, 287–292, 289–290t
Parasympatholytic agent, 287
Parasynaptic neurotransmission, 46
Paraventricular nucleus, of hypothalamus, in stress, 317–318, 318f
Paresis, 226
Parietal lobe, 16
Parietooccipital sulcus, 16
Parkinson's disease, 411f, 411–414, 413f
  basal ganglia in, 261
  neural transplantation for, 433–436, 434f
  neurotransmitters in, 60
Parosmia, 204
Paroxysmal hypertension, 301
Pars opercularis, in language, 353
Pars orbitalis, in language, 353
Pars triangularis, in language, 353, 356f, 364
Passive tension, 218, 219f
Passive touch, 98–99
Patch-matrix organization, of striatum, 259, 260f
Path finding, 393–395, 394f
Pavlovian conditioning, 322, 323–324
Pedicles, of cones, 175
Peduncles, 20, 22
Penis, erection of, 296–298, 297f

Peptidergic neurons, 32
Peptides, as neurotransmitters, 50, 52f, 53, 60
Periaqueductal gray matter, midbrain, in aggression, 305, 308f, 309, 309f
Pericytes, in blood-brain barrier, 69, 69f
Periglomerular cells, of olfactory system, 202, 203, 203f
Perilymph, 136, 137, 137f, 151
Peripheral motor system
  clinical correlations of, 225–226
  contractile unit of, 214–217, 215f, 216f
  excitation of muscle fibers of, 217–218
  functional unit of, 220–221
  mechanical properties of, 218–220, 219f
  in motor control, 214–226
  sensory organs of, 222–225, 223f
Peripheral nerve(s), in discriminative touch, 94–100, 95f, 96t, 99f, 100f
Peripheral nerve injury, 225–226
Peripheral nervous system (PNS)
  cell migration and proliferation in, 378–379
  defined, 11
Peripheral process, 32
Peripheral receptors, in discriminative touch, 94–100, 95f, 96t, 99f, 100f
Peripheral resistance, 290
Peroxynitrite, in Alzheimer's disease, 415
Perseveration, 254
PET (positron emission tomography), 352
PF (parallel fibers), in long-term depression, 339, 340f, 341f
Phantom limbs, 90–91, 126–127
Phase locking, 138, 141
Pheochromocytoma, 300
Phonemic awareness, 364
Phospholipase C, in learning, 327
Photoreceptors, 173–175
Phylogenetic layers, 7
Pia mater, 67
"Pie-in-the-sky" defect, 192
Pineal body, 21
Pinna, 131, 132f, 134
Pioneer axons, 390
Piriform cortex, in olfactory system, 204
Pitch, 132
Pitch rotation, 150
Pituitary gland, 21
Pivot words, 360
PKA (protein kinase A), in learning, 329
PKC (protein kinase C), in learning, 329
Placing responses, 421
Planum temporale, in language, 354–356, 361–364
Plaques
  in multiple sclerosis, 47
  senile, 406, 414
Plasmalemma, 29–31
  electrochemical properties of, 33–35
Plasticity, of motor cortex, 254–255
Plexiform layer, of olfactory system, 203, 203f
PM (premotor) area, 245, 246f, 247, 249f, 253
  lesions of, 254
PNS (parasympathetic nervous system)
  anatomy of, 278f, 279f, 279–281, 280t
  physiology of, 287–292, 289–290t